Praise for
Laughing Your Way to
Passing the Pediatric Boards™

"While I chose not to go to medical school, I got 'close' — I survived majoring in Biology at Yale and graduated with honors despite all the pre-meds in my major! After all the time and money you've spent on your education, you owe it to yourself to pass your boards the first time and this book can help but only if you read it! Dr. Stu Silverstein knows the value of being prepared and he's darn funny."

—Eric Tyson, Syndicated Columnist; Best-Selling author of **Personal Finance for Dummies** and **Investing for Dummies** (IDG Books)

"After failing 3 times, I realized I had not seen the salient points they were asking. Your book more than anything else helped pass the exam by scoring in the 500 range."
— S.J., now certified.

"The book arrived about 10 days before the exam and after reading the first few pages, I realized, "Hey, this guy really has his finger on the pulse of the boards."
— R.J.

"Just took the Boards last October and know I nailed several questions just for having read the book (three times). My only regret is that I didn't have it last year."
— E.B.

"Your Pediatric Board Review book made all the difference. It is well organized, with short chapters trimmed of all fat!! But the most important element of this book is its test taking strategies. Every chapter reminds you how to focus on what is important!!"
— A.R.

Laughing Your Way to Passing the Pediatric Boards, 5th Edition!®

The Seriously Funny Study Guide™

"Taking the boredom out of Board Review"®

By Stu Silverstein, M.D., FAAP

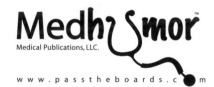

MedHumor Medical Publications, LLC.

www.passtheboards.com

MedHumor Medical Publications, Stamford, Connecticut

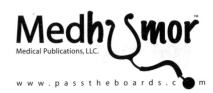

Published by:
Medhumor Medical Publications, LLC
1127 High Ridge Road, Suite 332
Stamford, CT 06905 U.S.A.

ISBN: 978-1-60743-533-4

Printed in the United States of America

This book is designed to provide information and guidance in regard to the subject matter covered. It is to be used as a study guide for physicians preparing for the General Pediatric Certifying Exam administered by the American Board of Pediatrics. It is not meant to be a clinical manual. The reader is advised to consult textbooks and other reference manuals in making clinical decisions. It is not the purpose of this book to reprint all the information that is otherwise available, but rather to assist the Board Candidate in organizing the material to facilitate study and recall on the exam. The reader is encouraged to read other sources of material, in particular picture atlases that are available.

Although every precaution has been taken in the preparation of this book, the publisher, author, and members of the editorial board assume no responsibility for errors, omissions or typographical mistakes. Nor is any liability assumed for damages resulting from the direct and indirect use of the information contained herein. The book contains information that is up-to-date only up to the printing date. Due to the very nature of the medical profession, there will be points out-of-date as soon as the book rolls off the press. The purpose of this book is to educate and entertain.

**If you do not wish to be bound by the above,
you may return this book to the publisher for a full refund.**

Publisher: MedHumor Medical Publications, LLC
                        Stamford, CT.

President: Stuart Silverstein, MD, FAAP

                        Medical Director
                        Firefly After Hours Pediatrics, LLC
                        Stamford, CT

                        Assistant Clinical Professor Emergency Medicine
                        New York Medical College

Vice-President: Brian Cahn

Senior Editor: Daisha Seyfer, MD, FAAP

Assistant Editor: Lourdes Geise, MD, FAAP
                        Windrose Health Network, Indianapolis, IN.

Layout Designer: Antoinette D'Amore, A.D. Design
                        addesign@videotron.ca

Cover Designer: Rachel Mindrup
                        www.rmindrup.com

Illustrations: James A. Phalen, MD, FAAP
                        © Medhumor Medical Publications, LLC

Comic Strip Cartoon: Conceived / Stu Silverstein, MD, FAAP
                        © Medhumor Medical Publications, LLC

About the Author

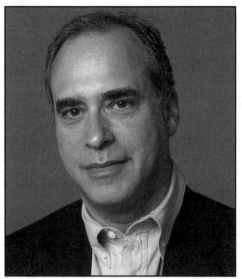

Dr. Stu Silverstein is the founder and CEO of Medhumor Medical Publications, LLC which began with the publication of the critically acclaimed *Laughing Your Way to Passing the Pediatric Boards®* back in the spring of 2000. Word spread quickly that finally there was a book out there that turned a traditionally daunting process into one that was actually fun and enjoyable. This groundbreaking study guide truly "Took the Boredom out of Board review"® with reports from our readers that they were able to reduce their study and review time in half. Those who were taking the exam for the 2nd time not only passed but increased their scores dramatically. We are now beginning our 2nd decade of helping pediatricians prepare for their boards through fun and innovation.

Our pediatric titles have also been critically acclaimed. Medhumor Publications, LLC has since expanded our catalogue, which now includes USMLE Step 3, Neonatology and the Neurology titles.

The concept of the *Laughing your way to Passing the Boards®* and Medhumor Medical Publications, LLC were conceived by Dr. Silverstein. He brought his years of experience in the field of Standup Comedy and Comedy writing after he realized the critical need for a study guide that spoke the language of colleagues rather than the language of dusty textbooks. His work as a Standup Comedian and Medical Humorist has frequently been featured in several newspapers, radio programs and TV shows, including the New York Times, WCBS newsradio in NY City, as well as World News Tonight with the late Peter Jennings.

Dr. Silverstein has also served as a contributing editor for the <u>Resident and Staff Physician</u> annual board review issue and has authored numerous articles on medical humor. He has served on the faculty of the Osler Institute Board Review course, UCLA Pediatric Board Review course and several local board review courses. He is the co-author of "What about Me? Growing up with a Developmentally Disabled Sibling" written with Dr. Bryna Siegel, professor of Child Psychiatry, the University of California San Francisco. Dr. Silverstein is in demand as a lecturer for residency programs on successful preparation for the pediatric board exam.

In addition to writing, lecturing, and expanding the scope of Medhumor Medical Publications, LLC., Dr. Silverstein is the Clinical Director for Firefly After Hours Pediatrics, a subacute emergency practice. Dr. Silverstein is an Assistant Clinical Professor of Emergency Medicine at the New York Medical College in Valhalla, New York.

The 5th Edition

In putting together the 5th edition of *Laughing Your Way to Passing the Pediatric Boards*® we updated and added material based on the content specifications published by the American Academy of Pediatrics as well as the AAP Red Book and sources noted in our bibliography.

We are always humbled and honored to hear from so many board candidates who give us credit for passing this difficult exam. This is even more fulfilling when this praise comes from those taking the exam for the 2nd time.

We hope that this, our 5th edition will continue to serve those for whom passing the pediatric board exam is the next ticket to be punched.

—Stuart Silverstein, MD, FAAP
Stamford, CT

This book is once again dedicated
to my wife Guita and
my children, Isra, Daniel, and Ariel
whose very existence gives life meaning
and keeps things in perspective.

Every day they remind me
that it is never too late
to have a happy childhood.

Acknowledgments

I would like to acknowledge Daisha Seyfer, MD, FAAP who initially contacted us as one of our readers noting improvement which we could make in our next edition. It wasn't long before we realized that her keen eye for detail and wide fund of knowledge made her an ideal technical and copy editor for this 5th edition. We know that much of the improvement in this edition can be attributed to her due diligence while working under a tight deadline without hesitation. We look forward to having her on our team as we expand our publication list. We would like to also thank Lourdes Geise, MD, FAAP for her assistance with the final proof reading. We also look forward to her continued involvement with our projects in the future. We also wish to thank Malcolm Kushner for editing the original manuscript and for being there for us from the beginning.

The layout and design of our books are the result of the talented, diligent eye and creativity of our layout designer, Antoinette D'Amore. Without Antoinette's assistance, the book you are holding would be a bunch of random uneven paragraphs with no adherence to standard paging and layout.

Brian has been the glue that holds our company together. As Vice President, Brian has been instrumental as our project manager, operations director, and marketing coordinator. Since coming on board last fall, Brian has brought Medhumor to the next level.

Judy Falbel, our business manager and accountant, has been instrumental in keeping our financial books balanced so we can focus on publishing and producing board review books.

I would like to acknowledge my parents Richard and Beverly Silverstein of Boynton Beach, Florida for their encouragement early on and for instilling in me the importance of diligence and staying the course despite adversity.

I would like to thank my family, in particular my children, for understanding when I had to be invested in the project. This includes my precious son, Daniel, who has grown to be a young man. Daniel was a mere 3 year old when we put together the first edition and is now a handsome bright young man of of thirteen who also provides us with tech support when needed and assists Brian with our e-marketing efforts. Among other things Daniel, is a talented pianist, but most of all a kind boy who also cares deeply about the environment. My daughter, Isra, has gone from a young girl to a self sufficient adult and copy editor for our companion texts since we started the series. Isra has also moved on to become a Masters Candidate, School of Middle East and North African Studies, University of Arizona. A special shout out to my baby son, Ariel who at 8, is no longer a baby, and is a student of science as well as an aspiring hockey and guitar player.

Most of all, I would like to thank my wife, Dr. Guita Sazan for always believing in me and encouraging me to use my talents. I am thankful for her staying the course while going through the toughest and the best of times without letting me get too low or high on myself.

I wish to acknowledge my friends and colleagues from back in my medical school days, especially Dr. Dan Mierlak with whom I have traveled the unconventional road with for more than 20 years now ever since we first sat next to each other in medical school. Also, I extend my thanks to Dr. Jim Celentano for inspiring me and playing a key role in my working in the field of pediatric emergency medicine.

To my friend Darren Kessler who is as close to me as a brother and proving that doctors and lawyers can indeed be close friends. I would like to thank Darren for always encouraging me and reminding me of the big picture when I doubted myself the most. Your ever-present encouragement has been a driving force in more ways than you realize.

I would be remiss if I didn't acknowledge Eric Tyson, who has coincidentally moved closer from San Francisco to Connecticut which reflects in many ways our growing friendship as well. Eric's encouragement and sharp business insight were the pillars of this project when it was simply a notion discussed over a sandwich. He reminds me by word and example that going with one's instincts and following through on talent brings success, happiness, and help to society in the long run in spite of any short-term challenges.

Finally, I would like to acknowledge the support, counseling, and/or friendship I have received from Glen Karow, Dr. Sid Nachman and my colleagues at the pediatric emergency room at Our Lady of Mercy Medical Center.

I apologize to anyone not listed; it is difficult to remember everyone when facing a deadline to go to press!

Table of Contents

Section A: Successful Techniques for Preparing for the Exam 1

Chapter 1: A User's Guide to Laughing Your Way to Passing the Pediatric Boards 3

Creating a Bell from the Few, The Proud, The Murines 3

Organizing and Scheduling Your Study 5

How to Use This Book 5

Guideposts Along the Way 5

Chapter 2: What, Me Worry? Proven Strategies for Reducing Test Anxiety 9

Anxious Over Being Anxious 9

The Day Before the Exam 11

The Day of The Exam 11

Arriving at the Room 12

Summary 14

Chapter 3: Time in a Bottle: Proven Strategies for Efficient Studying (for Those with a Life) 15

Sprint vs. Marathon Running 16

Setting Up Mini Deadlines : Artificial Intensity 16

The 80/20 Rule: 18

Chapter 4: Games Boards Play: Seeing the Answers in the Questions and Other Successful Test Taking Techniques 19

Arriving at the Exam 20

Easy to Forget the Basics, But Don't 21

Finish Line 24

Clinical Case Scenarios/ Vignettes 27

8 Simple Steps for Each Question (How to Approach a Lion... Very Carefully) 28

Final Word 30

Section B: Pearls and Perils: Specific Core Facts and Details........31

Chapter 5: Biostatistics (& Other Number Games) and Ethical-Legal Issues...33

Studying Studies...38

Ethical Considerations...39

Ethics of Genetic Studies and Screening.................................41

Failure to seek Medical Care and Abuse/Neglect Parameters 41

√ Chapter 6: Growth and Development.................................43

Physiologic Growth...43

Intelligence and Learning 48

Intelligence Screening..52

Normal Developmental Milestones......................................53

Developmental Milestone Mnemonics 57

√ Chapter 7: Nutrition...65

Fat Soluble Vitamins...65

Water Soluble Vitamins...66

Vitamin Deficiencies and Toxicities...66

Nutritional Needs 73

Nutritional Deficiencies..78

Nutritional Needs of the Premature 80

Nutrition and Weight...86

√ Chapter 8: Preventive Pediatrics 95

Lead Exposure...95

Vaccines 96

Getting through the Screen Door 114

Ounce of Prevention: When is Prophylactic Treatment Necessary? 122

Injury and Illness Prevention 123

Preparing Families for International Adoption 127

Cigarette Cessation in Adolescents 127

First Aid Considerations 128

✓ **Chapter 9: Poisons and Environmental Toxins**..**129**

   Procedures and Acute Management..**129**

   Toxidromes...**132**

      PCP...137

      The Masquerade Party of Toxicology: Managing Unknown and Multiple Agents...........146

   Bioterrorism..**149**

✓ **Chapter 10: Born Yesterday: Fetus and Newborn**.................................**151**

      Apnea...151

      Assessing Comatose and Lethargic Infants Without Becoming Lethargic.........153

      Antenatal Screening..154

      Respiratory Distress Syndrome (RDS)....................................155

      Sepsis...158

   Birth Trauma...**161**

   Facts and Definitions to Watch Out For.....................................**164**

   Lytes and Bytes, Sweets and Treats..**170**

      Metabolic Issues of the Newborn..174

✓ **Chapter 11: Fluids and Lytes, and Everything Nice**..............................**187**

   Acid Base Metabolism..**187**

      Fall into the Gap...190

      Renal Tubular Acidosis...191

   Sold on Sodium...**194**

   Potassium..**201**

      Degree of Dehydration...209

   Fluids and Lytes in Specific Clinical Conditions........................**212**

✓ **Chapter 12: Genetics: Everyone Into the (Gene) Pool**..........................**217**

   Chromosomes and Genetics...**217**

   Teratogens...**233**

   Malformations..**235**

   Celebrity Dysmorphology...**239**

✓ **Chapter 13: Allergy and Immunology**..**245**

      Prevention...245

Specific Allergic Conditions 246

Allergic Reactions **252**

Immunodeficiencies **254**

Testing the Immune System..262

Peritonitis 271

Chapter 14: You Give Me Fever: Infectious Diseases **265**

Bacterial Infections **265**

Opportunistic Infections 273

Hemolytic Uremic Syndrome 294

Antibiotic Antics...297

Viral Infections..**302**

Influenza...316

Parasitic Infections **318**

Fungal Infections...**322**

Modes of Transmission **326**

Chapter 15: Inborn Errors of Metabolism...**329**

Approaching Inborn Errors of Metabolism **329**

Metabolic Disorders presenting with Acidosis 330

Defects in Fatty Acid Metabolism...332

Urea Cycle Defects **333**

Hypoglycemia in Infants **333**

Disorders of Carbohydrate Metabolism..333

Inborn Errors of Metabolism that Defy Categorization **337**

Amino Acid Metabolic Disorders **339**

Mucopolysaccharidoses 342

Purine and Pyrimidine Disorders...343

Glycogen Storage Diseases **344**

Lipoprotein Disorders **345**

Lysosomal Disorders **347**

Lipid Storage Diseases (Sphingolipidoses)...**347**

Vitamin Therapy that Works **350**

✓ **Chapter 16: Is That an Orchidometer in Your Pocket?:**
Endocrinology...**353**

Sexual Differentiation **353**

Congenital Adrenal Hyperplasia (CAH)...358

Cushing Syndrome..362

Short Stature..362

Tall Stature...367

Thyroid Disorders..**368**

Diabetes Mellitus **372**

Metabolic Syndrome...376

Calcium Metabolism...376

✓ **Chapter 17: GI: What to Know!** **387**

GI **387**

Acute Abdominal Pain...387

Recurrent or Chronic Abdominal Pain...390

Diarrhea **394**

Vomiting **403**

Going From Top to Bottom..**412**

Constipation 423

GI Bleeding..424

A Liver Runs Through It/Liver Diseases 426

Pancreas..428

Bad Gall Bladder..429

The Alphabet Soup of Hepatitis..431

✓ **Chapter 18: Catching Your Breath: Pulmonary** **435**

Asthma 435

Calling All Coughs (Chronic)...445

Hypercarbia vs. Hypoxia 449

Newborn Pulmonary Disorders...449

Managing Tuberculosis...458

Managing Chest Wall Trauma...460

ARDS..461

Drowning 461

Hemoptysis 462

Pneumonia **463**

Chapter 19: Don't Go Breaking My Heart: Cardiology.........................**467**

Congestive Heart Failure **467**

Congenital Heart Disease **468**

I say Murmur, you say Mummur **483**

EKG Findings and the Disorders that Love Them................................**486**

Chapter 20: Heme Onc...**493**

Oncology **493**

Oncologic Emergencies 503

Side Effects of Chemotherapeutic Agents..504

Disorders of Red Cells **506**

Abnormal White Cells 523

Platelet Abnormalities 529

Chapter 21: Renal **537**

Microscopic Hematuria..**537**

Proteinuria **542**

Renal Dysplasia **544**

Collecting System Pathology...**546**

Infections (UTI)...**548**

Nephrotic Syndrome **550**

Specific Nephropathies/Nephritides..**551**

Hypertension **558**

Dysuria..561

Urinary Frequency and Incontinence...562

Neonatal Renal Numbers 563

Nephrotoxic Medications..564

Chapter 22: Genital-Urinary **565**

GU Conditions / Infants **565**

Vaginal Conditions...**567**

Male Conditions **570**

Dermatological GU Disorders **576**

Abdominal Pain **579**

√ **Chapter 23: The Neuro Bureau: Neurology** **583**

Encephalitis 583

What a Headache 584

California, Oregon and Other Altered States of Consciousness 587

Ataxia Attackia 589

Strange Movements (in D Minor) 591

Tips on Tics 594

Space Occupying CNS Lesions and Other Anatomical Problems 596

Muscle Weakness and Hypotonia **599**

Spinal Neurology 606

Hail Seizure **609**

Adrenoleukodystrophy 619

Cerebral Palsy **619**

Cerebrovascular Accident **621**

Neurodiagnostic Testing 622

Vertigo 622

√ **Chapter 24: Musculoskeletal** **623**

Defining Orthopedics 623

Sprains, strains, and pains 624

Specific Orthopedic Conditions 624

√ **Chapter 25: Skin Deep: Dermatology** **649**

Puffing up: Neonatal Pustular Lesions **649**

Dry Scaly Skin **652**

Infectious Rashes **659**

Staphylococcal Scalded Skin Syndrome (and other Skin Disorders that can "Burn" you) 659

Pests of Life (Scabies, Lice and Other Creatures) 663

Acne Vulgaris 668

Alopecia Hairpecia 673

Pigmented Lesions 675

Neurocutaneous Syndromes 676

Sun, Skin, and Melanoma 681

Erythema Confusiosum 681

Chapter 26: Rheumatology: Rheum With a View **683**

Specific Conditions 683

Synovial Fluid 709

Chapter 27: The Eyes Have It **711**

The Rhythm of Nystagmus 711

Pseudostrabismus and True Strabismus 711

Specific Conditions 712

Don't Shoot if you see the Red in their Eyes 716

Papilledema, Papillitis and Picking Out the Differences 717

Keep Your Eyes on the Retina 717

Chapter 28: See No Evil, Hear No Evil, Speak No Evil: ENT **721**

Ears 721

Know Your Nose/Rhinos 731

Throat..735

What About the Mouth?...740

Stridor Cider and Epiglottitis..742

Craning Your NECK 750

Chapter 29: Adolescent Medicine and Gynecology **755**

Adolescent Physiologic Development 755

Tools of the Trade 761

Gynecology..762

Adolescent Behavioral Health 767

Sexually Transmitted Diseases..770

Abdominal Pain: Special considerations in Adolescents 773

Chapter 30: Sports Injuries...**777**

Specific Injuries in the Athlete..778

Conclusions on Concussions...783

The Juice on Steroid Use..787

Sports, Fluids, and Electrolytes..788

The Growth of Growth Hormone 789

Wrestling with Weight Control in Athletes 789

Normal and Abnormal Cardiac Findings in the Athlete...790

The Diabetic Athlete 791

Chapter 31: Substance Abuse **793**

How Are High School Students Getting High?..793

Confidentiality..794

Anticipatory Guidance 795

Specific Drugs of Abuse...795

Chapter 32: Psychosocial Issues..**807**

Toddler and Preschool...**807**

Family and Environmental Issues **810**

Conversion Disorder 812

Psychosomatic Illness 813

Somatizations of Stress 814

Organizing the Non-Organic 814

Recurrent Pain 815

Impact of TV and other Media **815**

Sleep Disorders **816**

Chronic Illness and the Family **817**

Extracurricular Activities and School Performance..818

Enabling Cain and Abel (Sibling Rivalry) 818

Sexual Orientation...818

International Adoption 819

Pediatricians' Role with Children in Foster Care...820

Chapter 33: Critical Care **821**

Impending System Failure **821**

Conditions Requiring Life Support **824**

The ABC's of CPR 830

✓ Chapter 34: ER **831**
Codes Facts **831**
Specific ER Situations 832
Risk Factors for Abuse and Neglect 843
Fractures 846
Electric Burns 851
Thermal Burns 851
Lacerations 852
Biological Chemical Weapons 855

✓ Chapter 35: Pharmacology **857**
Alternative Drugs and Herb interactions **857**
You Watch What you Eat 858
Dare not take Dairy 859
Drug Eat Drug World 859
How to be Cognizant of Conscious Sedation 863

✓ Chapter 36: Behavior and Mental Health **865**
Behavioral Concerns **865**
Adolescent Parents 870
Mental Health Concerns **870**
Distinguishing a Tic from a Toc 874

Bibliography **877**

Index **881**

Section A: Successful Techniques for Preparing for the Exam

Chapter 1

A User's Guide to Laughing Your Way to Passing the Pediatric Boards®

So you've completed high school.[1] That was a proud moment and you have the crème colored tassel dangling from your rearview mirror to prove it. Then came *college* and you graduated Summa Cum (Very) Laude and got your Phi Beta Kappa Key, which opened the door to additional student debt. Then it was off to *med school* and you got the Golden MD degree.[2]

Then you "matched" and were given the opportunity to be paged and hounded every 3rd or 4th night into a sleep-deprived stupor and depression while making less per hour than the guy with the strange deodorant fixing the elevators.

All along the way you had to get your "admission ticket" punched by passing a gauntlet of Standardized Exams.[3] In doing so, you've proven that you are good at taking standardized exams. Let's face it; if you have made it to this point, you are at the tip of the pyramid. You've graduated from the *23rd grade.*[4]

Therefore, anyone who is reading this has reached the top of the food chain.[5] Just when you thought it was safe, you have to go through one more hoop, grab one more brass ring, one more audition before you're off to Hollywood, one more item on the managed care credentialing application: *change Board Eligible to Board Certified.*

Creating a Bell from the Few, The Proud, The Murines

No big deal for the Standardized Test Veteran? You would think so, but think again. The makers of the test create a bell curve out of a group that is already jammed into the nose cone at the far right of the general population curve. Here, we are the experimental mice, the murines. This is no small task, and there will be a host of tough questions to separate the greatest test takers from the great, the mice from the murines.

The Foreign Medical Grad

If you are from another country, I don't even want to think about from what grade you are graduating. Chances are you have had to come here and start from scratch, which meant becoming an Intern taking orders from someone half your age and half your experience and completing another residency, even though you were Professor Emeritus of Neonatology back in your country of origin. In addition, you had to pass all those standardized exams in a foreign language.

---

[1] With honors.   [2] Or the lesser known but equally as Golden DO degree.

[3] Which you did or you would not be reading this.   [4] Don't bother adding it up, I am correct.

[5] Unless you are the significant other of a Board Candidate, in which case I can assure you that there is nothing interesting here, so just put this down and watch the re-runs of American Idol.

You can get information from the Board directly:

The American Board of Pediatrics
111 Silver Cedar Court
Chapel Hill, NC 27514

Voice: 919-929-0461
Fax: 919-929-9255
www.apb.org

So How Many Pass?

Approximately 20% of first time test takers fail. However, around 40% of total test takers fail. The latter includes those who have failed previously. These are only estimates. For more information, log onto the ABP website and search for "Pass rate."

Raw Scores, Scores, and Who's Keeping Score?

The number of questions you get correct is called the "raw score." The average score of the reference group[6] is determined to be 500 with a standard deviation of 100. *So who cares about this?* You want to know how many questions you need to get correct in order to pass the exam. Again, this information is not released, but the rumor mill has proposed two rumors:

- some say in the mid 80's
- others say 68 is passing

The truth is that 65% will not get you a passing grade. While I am sure there is variation from year to year, **I would shoot to get 85% correct; this will likely result in a passing grade.**

Why is Passing the Pediatric Boards Sometimes Such a Challenge?

This is why it could be a challenge to pass and why so many intelligent, good clinicians do fail. It is also the reason why people take it more than once, and go to the same review courses, and take the exam in the same rooms and avoid eye contact with those in the same position.[7] You know who you are, so go ahead and make eye contact and say hello.

When I was taking the Boards I would hear so many colleagues tell me things like:

- ❑ "I didn't study, I just looked over Nelson the night before."
- ❑ "I took it cold."
- ❑ "I memorized Harriet Lane and looked through Rudolph."
- ❑ "I slept with Rudolph, Nelson AND Harriet Lane." [8]
- ❑ Rudolph slept with John McCain

I really don't think you can pass the exam without studying, or by reading a massive column of words like Rudolph or Nelson or baby Nelson for that matter. These are reference books that can help in clinical decisions, but they will not provide you with the tools needed to pass the Boards. This book and the suggestions made here will help you pass the exam.

---

[6] The gang taking it for the first time.

[7] As if nobody realizes you are there with them every year.

[8] Doing so while crossing state lines is a federal crime punishable with 3 extra years of residency with not less than 2 of those years spent in the dog labs.

The only people I know who can walk into the exam after 3 years of Residency and no additional preparation or study are those who live, breathe and eat Pediatrics.[9] These are folks who spend their leisure hours reading journal articles, often in lieu of sex. In very extreme cases these folks may be reading journal articles while having sex. These folks have not made eye contact with anyone since their last visit to an optometrist.[10]

Organizing and Scheduling Your Study

This exam is special. It requires a system for organizing the material so that you can have it at your fingertips when you take the exam. For many folks, anxiety is also a problem so you also need a *system to control anxiety*.[11]

Organizing the Material So That You Remember It Cold

In addition to helping you develop a strategy for organizing your study and controlling your anxiety, this book will show you how to organize and memorize the material with techniques and mnemonics that work. We have included a sample study schedule to help you get started.

We will include:

1. Key words and phrases in the question that point to the correct answers.
2. Proven memorization techniques and systems that maximize retention and recognition.
3. Tips for the exam day.
4. Methods that maximize your ability to recognize the graphics and illustrations.

How to Use This Book

You can go through this book cover to cover, or choose your own order. We suggest you read section A, and then go through the chapters of section B in the order you prefer.

Guideposts Along the Way

As you read the book, you will notice pictures in the margin that emphasize important points. These "Guideposts" will indicate a particular category of information.

---

9 You know who they are.

10 THESE are the folks with whom you should not be making eye contact; it is similar to staring into the sun.

11 We cover this in another chapter, and we don't mean pharmacology.

Clinical Case Studies

DEFINITION	*Definition*	This points to a "definition."[12]
PERIL WARNING	*Perils*	This alerts you to possible big mistakes and traps that can be laid down for you on the exam.
MNEMONIC	*Mnemonic Device*	This indicates a mnemonic that will help you memorize difficult but important information.
HOT TIP	*Hot Tip*	"This draws attention to a "Board Pearl," to help you on potential trouble areas in the exam.
MYTH	*Myth*	This signifies a popularly held myth that isn't true. This is a classic trap laid by Board Examiners.[13]
BUZZ WORDS	*Buzz Words*	This describes buzzwords or key phrases that are typical for a given disorder. By learning this, you will often be able to recognize the answer in the wording of the question itself.
EITHER OR CHOICES	*Down to two choices*	This points out minute differences between similar disorders, which are critical to answering many questions correctly.
TAKE HOME MESSAGE	*Take Home Message*	Important take home points to remember.
TREATMENT	*Treatment*	This points to specific treatments for a given diagnosis or disorder.

---

[12] Knowing the definition will save you from being tricked. For example, LGA is greater than the 90th %ile. Should they describe a child in the 88th percentile this would NOT be LGA.

[13] For example: Sugar causes ADHD.

On the exam you may be presented with specific case scenarios. In these instances, just knowing the material is not enough. Understanding how you can be diverted away from the correct answer and even falling prey because you know too much can often be the difference between passing and failing the exam.

We call your attention to these case studies with the following icons:

CASE STUDY	*Case Study*	Here we will present you with a case study or summarize how they might present a given vignette.
THE DIVERSION	*The Diversion*	As is common in most examinations, the test writers try to dissuade you from the correct answer by tripping you up if you are unsure of the subject matter. Here we explain how you might be diverted from the correct answer. The diversion can come in many forms: · **Understatement:** The understatement minimizes information that is key to answering correctly: "Other than ibuprofen the patient is not taking any medications." · **Abnormal physical findings in a forest of normal findings:** A list of normal findings with the word *hepatomegaly* mixed in, making it easy to overlook. · **Emphasis on diversionary factors:** An example would be implying purpura of the lower extremity is child abuse by noting the child is being raised by a single mother in the first sentence, rather than emphasizing findings consistent with actual diagnosis, Henoch Schönlein Purpura. We also use this guidepost throughout the text to call attention to specific diversions that may be used on the exam.
ANSWER REVEALED	*Answer Revealed*	Here we reveal the correct answer and show you how the correct answer can be deduced by carefully teasing out the important information and filtering out the diversionary material.

Chapter 2

What, Me Worry?
Proven Strategies for
Reducing Test Anxiety

Anxious Over Being Anxious

We are frequently approached by readers who feel that they know the material well, have used some memory techniques, retain the material in long-term memory, and yet still fail the exam. Often this is a result of test taking anxiety. This is truly a pity!

It is a pity because anxiety is a physiological reaction, nothing more. And its effects can be reversed. Our anxiety response has more to do with a perceived threat than how well we are or aren't prepared.

- **Motivational speaker Zig Ziegler defines** "FEAR" as "*False Evidence Appearing Real*," and this could apply to anyone taking the Boards.

- One can also define FEAR as "*Fluids Electrolytes And Residency.*"

Extreme Anxiety is as Useless as a Stethoscope Around a Psychiatrist's Neck

When I performed standup comedy in clubs, I got to know many comedians and saw them in action backstage. We all needed some anxiety to get us going, to give us that "edge" on stage (discussed in more detail below). Some would get very anxious; others wouldn't get anxious at all. What I noticed most was that the level of anxiety was independent of talent and prep time they had put into their routine.[1] I would see very talented comics be nauseated, and some with virtually no talent—folks who would make Larry King seem animated by comparison—walk out confident that they were funny. The same applies to those taking the Board Exam.

---

[1] This is very similar to parental anxiety in the practice of pediatrics. One can rarely use a parent's anxiety as a gauge for the severity of a child's disease. Some parents are frantic over an ear infection while others are unfazed over a child with signs of meningitis.

Do not mistake your anxiety as an indication of your ability to pass:

You need to counter the physical response of stress and anxiety. No matter what your level of preparedness, excess anxiety will only work against you. You need only a little anxiety to get your blood going.

Everyone who takes the Pediatric Board exam experiences anxiety. *Some of you experience anxiety about not experiencing anxiety,* and that can make anyone anxious—even those claiming that they experience no anxiety. Even writing about all this is making me anxious!

Stress and Necessary Anxiety

Let's face it; some anxiety is good and even necessary. Without anxiety, you wouldn't have any motivation to turn off reruns of *Lost* and study hypoparathyroidism. Too much anxiety, however, and you feel like John Edwards taking a paternity test.

Anxiety Level

Watching the season recap on Chess Channel 2.	Discovering that your photos taken at the congressional gym have been sent out on Twitter and Facebook and are on *Meet the Press*.

HOT TIP

Take systematic steps to reduce anxiety. Consider meditative tapes, progressive relaxation, aromatherapy, books on CD by Thich Nhat Hanh and the Dalai Lama; or just watch Larry King interviewing (or counting out loud the names of all his ex-wives).

Let's Get Physical

Remember, anxiety is a physiological response and "taking it easy" is often not enough to prepare you to focus solely on the task at hand. Steps to reduce the physiological response are equally important.

Here are a few proven techniques for reducing the physiological effects of stress.

If You Think You Will Fail or If You Think You Will Pass, You are Right

What do all of these quotes have in common?

Henry Ford once said,

> *"If you think you will succeed you are correct. If you think you will fail you are also correct."*

Your Mother once said,

> *"You're not going out to play until you finish your homework!"*

My friend the ophthalmologist's mother once said:

> *"Stop fooling around with those darts, you're not going to be happy until you take someone's eye out"*

What they have in common is this: They were all correct.

You need to stop negative self-talk in its tracks and your self-talk must be about passing. The first step is to envision yourself passing. You cannot begin taking the steps to pass unless you do this first!

If you send this message to your subconscious, it will find the means to pass the exam!

The Day Before the Exam

Do Not...do NOT...and in case you missed it the first two times, DO NOT study the day before the exam. I would even say do not (DO NOT) study 2 days before the exam. Your brain needs to recuperate and the material needs to marinate. Your brain will be working overtime on the day of the exam and it needs some R and R. It is very similar to weightlifting, and all weightlifters know you cannot lift every day.

The Day of The Exam

The day of the exam, you want to wake up and do whatever it is that gets you pumped up and energized. For some it means music, for some it means no sound at all and, *in extreme cases, a hyperbaric sensory deprivation tank.* Do whatever it takes, even if it is naked jumping jacks in front of a tinted mirror. The one thing you should NOT do is study some more.

There is really nothing you will learn in the hour before the exam that will be the difference between passing and failing. What **could be** the difference is a stressed out fatigued brain vs. a rested one. *The material has to marinate, so don't stir-fry.*

Dressed to Kill and What's Eating You And What are You Eating?

The word out there among test taking gurus is to avoid taking caffeine before the exam. Well, **if you drink coffee every day, this is not the day to quit.** Some additional nutritional tips can come in handy:

- Sugar and other forms of junk are not a good idea.
- Enjoy a well-balanced breakfast with fruits.
- Have a few peeled fruits available (*peeled so your chomping doesn't disturb your neighbor trying to take a call on his cell phone without interruption*).
- A multivitamin in the morning and then again at noon would be a good idea as long as you take it with food.

 Feel free to take some extra Vitamin B12 and Folic Acid. Both are good for the nerves and get flushed out the kidneys during times of stress and high caffeine intake.

Warning, do not take vitamins or supplements on an empty stomach!

Stretch and do whatever it takes to relax. Make sure you have a sweater in case the proctor has untreated hyperthyroidism and is as clammy as Donald Trump's comb-over.

On the other hand, you want to have something very light in case the person is as anxious as you are and has the heat turned up to the temperature on the planet Mercury during Oktoberfest.

Arriving at the Room

Folks will be pacing.

Folks will be chomping on gum.

Folks will be distorted beyond recognition trying to pretend to be calm and relaxed.

Folks will be ballroom dancing without moving their feet or leaving their seats.

Silly Zitelli

In the back of the room, you will notice 6 people reading the Zitelli Picture Atlas. They haven't read the book you are now holding. It is a waste of time "looking over" the pictures at this point.

Do you really think that one last look at the kid with Prader Willi Syndrome chomping on a fistful of Planters® peanuts will be the difference between passing and failing?

C'mon, you would be doing them a favor if you just walked up to them, pulled it away, and invited them to get with the program and get a life.

Lady with the Blue Hair, Blue Hair, Blue Hair...On!

In the front of the room there will be 2 proctors. One is a Board Certified Pediatrician glad that it is YOU taking the exam, and the other is the same lady with the Blue Hair from elementary school (or sometimes she IS the pediatrician). She's there to give you the same 20-minute lecture on using a #2 pencil and to warn about the nuclear meltdown that will occur should you use a #1 or #5 pencil.

Still Doing # 2

As of October 2011, the pediatric board-certifying exam is still using technology that was first developed during the Eisenhower administration. Hopefully at some point somebody at the ABP will realize that computers are all the rage and will actually put the Scantron® with its number 2 pencil and fill-in grid into the Smithsonian Institute in Washington, DC. As of today, the word on the street is that the Scantron® will be heading to the dustbin of history as of the 2012 exam. Again, the best place to check on this would be the American Board of Pediatrics website.

You will get a 1 hour tirade and instruction drill on how to write in your name and fill in the corresponding dots. You will actually complete this 5 minutes before they start reading the instructions. Let's face it, if you haven't mastered the concept of filling in dots with a number 2 pencil by now, you might as well leave at that point.

When they say, "read the question," they are not merely stating the obvious. This means pay close attention what they are asking. Key words in the last sentence of the question are very important. Words like "least" "most," "first," "etiology," "diagnosis," and "treatment" are important to note before moving on to the listed choices.

Summary

- No matter how prepared or unprepared you are, extreme anxiety will not help you.
- A bit of adrenaline coupled with a calm clear attitude will help you tap into the techniques and material you studied.
- We outlined some ways to reduce anxiety.
- Go ahead and take advantage of outside resources; you are entitled to do so.

If you are taking the exam for the second or nth time, and you did not take steps to reduce anxiety in the past, this can be one of the things you do "differently" to increase your chances of passing this time.

Chapter 3

Time in a Bottle:
Proven Strategies for Efficient Studying
(for Those with a Life)

You cannot possibly go into this test without preparation. If you are taking this exam for the 2nd, 3rd, *...nth* time, then past methods, by definition, will not work.

If you actually have a job, family, friends and hobbies, then over the next few months there will certainly be things that you would prefer to do besides memorizing the atomic structure of Botox®. If you don't have a job, family, friends, hobbies, then consider yourself lucky (for once).

Better Late Than Never

If you are reading this and actually are a few weeks away from the exam, and are a good memorizer, then some of the memorization techniques are still better than memorizing and cramming without any method at all.

Spread out the Spreadsheet

Baseball philosopher *Casey Stengel* once said, *"If you don't know where you're going, you might end up somewhere else."* Keep this in mind when preparing for the Boards. You need a plan. You've got to know where you're going.

For those of us who were fortunate enough to go to medical school while we were in extended adolescence (single with no responsibilities), life consisted of 2 things:

- leisure activities
- studying.

If you add family and actually earning a living, where does studying come in? Study time only fits in with a well-organized plan. *Peace of mind that you are getting the job done and not ignoring those you love only comes from a well organized plan. It is worth the effort.*

Sprint vs. Marathon Running

Was this you in College?

- ❑ "I pulled an all nighter and passed. Whooooo !!!!!"
- ❑ "We Passed...Quadruple Mocca Latte Espresso and me."
- ❑ "I work better under 1,000 PSI pressure."
- ❑ "Did we give up when the Germans bombed Pearl Harbor?" – John Belushi in *Animal House*.

While these methods worked well in college and maybe even in med school, they will not work for this exam unless you were among the select few who studied during residency in lieu of eating.

If you procrastinate, you will find yourself at the 11th hour with too little time to adequately prepare. This is a **Marathon** you are preparing for, not a sprint. You must take steady *small* steps to prepare for the big event.

Setting Up Mini Deadlines : Artificial Intensity

Somebody once said:

> " *If it wasn't for the last minute nothing would ever get done"*

Some of us need the "adrenaline rush" to get going and motivated, yet leaving studying to the last month is not going to work. On the other hand, without deadlines most of us won't be productive and other more pleasant activities will take over.

The solution is a compromise called ***"mini-deadlines."*** Mini-deadlines means breaking the Boards into smaller subcategories, making the project less formidable. If you set strict deadlines for completing each category, you get the benefit of working "under the gun."

First, break the Boards into the subspecialties outlined in this book.

Next- Break these into smaller subcategories.

Divide your study week so that you put in at least 2 hours a night, 3 nights a week.

Schedule this as you would schedule any appointment and you will stick to the plan.

Next, schedule the topics you will study and review in each of these "appointment slots". This will ensure that you are not short at the end of the program.

Allow some blank spots in between and for the last few weeks in case you underestimate the amount of time a given topic actually takes. In fact, *add 20% to the time you think it will take to cover a subcategory.*

Identify what material you do not like to study or is less "crammable." These are the subjects with which you should start. You have more energy early on and if you leave the topics that are of more personal interest to you for later, your interest will be maintained longer. Subjects like Fluids and Lytes, which really cannot be memorized and require you to think through and learn the physiology, should be done first. It is difficult to go over this material when you are anxious and pressed for time. And this is an important part of the exam.

Take Me Out to the Ball Game

By viewing your study time as set appointments with deadlines, you're more likely to stick to your study schedule, especially when fun alternatives present themselves—things like free tickets to a ball game. If you have a deadline to complete "thyroid disorders" this week and treat it like "an appointment," you'll probably pass on the tickets. However, if you have to complete "endocrine" sometime this month, you might figure, "What the heck. I'll catch up next week." We strongly encourage you to utilize a variety of electronic scheduling devices/tools, including things like "Remember the Milk®" and "Google® Calendar."

The actual schedule needs to be organized by you. You may be tempted to say that setting up a study schedule is a waste of precious time. You're wrong! In fact, you can't afford NOT to take the time.

This system gives you the advantages of advanced organized study along with the rush and thrill of cramming at the last minute. After all, if you "have to" get through Cardiology, it will be difficult to study when the "*going gets boring.*"

Gas Expands to Fill the Void

If you take a small amount of gas and put it into a large container, it will fill the entire space (kind of like those political talk shows on Sunday morning). We tend to do the same thing with our time. If we have a lot of time, or we *perceive* that we have a lot of time (for example, 3 months to get ready for the boards), then less stressful activities will look more enticing. You'll say things like "Gee, I haven't updated my Facebook® status in the past 3 minutes." That is why this proven method works. You won't be sidetracked from a 2-hour *appointment* to "study thyroid disease."

As a result of this organized study, you will actually have *more time to do the things you enjoy,* **with half the guilt.** Heck, if you are one of the fortunate souls whose main source of joy and pleasure is studying calcium metabolism, you are in even better shape. Setting and completing goals feels good. By having your goal defined, it will be easier to actually sit down and study, which is the most difficult step in any given study session.

The 80/20 Rule:

In the *5th edition of " Laughing your way to Passing the Pediatric Boards®* " we have focused on the material outlined in the most recent content specifications of the American Academy of Pediatrics and confirmed by recent board takers.

You may have heard that the exam emphasizes a different area each year. The truth is that there is a core set of material that they have to test, and 80% of the material will come from these topics with 20% at most coming from new or updated material.

The 80/20 rule can apply to board preparation as follows:

· 80% of the exam will derive from the core material

· Spending 80% of your time on this material will improve your score 20%

· Make your study time 20% more efficient and you will retain 80% more material.

Think of the the 80/20 rule as you begin preparing for the exam.

Knowing the core material cold will put you in a great position to pass. Fluids and Lytes, Immunology, and Endocrinology are heavy areas of concentration. Don't fret about the 20% esoteric material; focus on the 80% core and the rest will take care of itself.

Zebras may not be common in clinical practice, but they are very common "on the Boards"! However, there are only some zebras you need to know and these zebras are well represented in the core material we cover. Leave the Albino Zebras to those clustered around the 99th %ile. In fact, these are the folks we want to avoid making eye contact with.

Chapter 4

Games Boards Play: Seeing the Answers in the Questions and Other Successful Test Taking Techniques

Some Things Change and Some Things Don't

The good news is that the General Pediatrics Certifying Examination has been switched from a two-day examination to a one-day examination. At least when you leave at the end of the day, you can actually relax without having to wake up the next day to the nightmare of taking the exam for another 8 hours.

The bad news is, the exam is still paper/pencil based Scantron® format (at least until 2012, as far as we have heard). You will have to continue to wait if you wish to see the day when the exam enters 20th Century technology (let alone 21st Century technology).

So what will that day be like?

· There will be a morning session and an afternoon session
· Each session will be 3.5 hours long[1]
· There will <u>not</u> be a separate book for "graphics"[2]
· There will <u>not</u> be a separate book for "clinical scenarios"[3]
· These items will be integrated within the morning and afternoon booklets
· The total number of questions will be 330-350

So will you find out if you passed sooner?

The answer is No! You will still need to be tortured for approximately 3 months before finding out if you passed or failed the exam.

---

[1] This is 30 minutes longer than the sessions for the two-day examination, but still worth getting it all done in one day.
[2] What used to be referred to as Book C of mind-boggling pictures and drawings.
[3] What used to referred to as Book D or the last straw.

Will the cost of the examination be the same?

Best to check with the American Board of Pediatrics website for the latest fees, although at last check the fees have not gone down as a result of this being a 1 day rather than a 2 day exam.

Arriving at the Exam

So now, the moment has arrived: you prepared according to schedule, you have taken steps to reduce anxiety, and you have attended and memorized the credo of several 12-step groups. Now it is time to arrive and take the exam.

As you enter the room, you wade past the 6 candidates with thin paste-on mustaches reading through Zitelli. You ignore the pagers that are going off. You encounter the lady with the blue hair who tells you the history of the #2 pencil. You sit down to begin the process. You fill in the circles with a #3 pencil, get reprimanded and handed a #2 pencil. You marvel at the fact that the American Board of Pediatrics is using the same exam technology as doctors who took the boards in 1952. You also wonder if there ever was such a thing as a # 1 or a #3 pencil. Your mind drifts back to the exam room.

Circling the Wagon with a Pen

In previous editions of our book, we suggested using a highlighter in the question booklet. Highlighters, however, are no longer allowed in the exam room. Apparently, they were leaving yellow marks in the exam booklets.

Instead of a highlighter, you can use another number 2 pencil to make important margin notes or circle important information in the question so it stands out.

You should circle

- Pertinent negatives and positives
- Physical Findings
- Abnormal Labs
- Key words at the end of the question (that tell you what they are specifically asking)

Clinical vs. Test Taking Skills

It's the Boards' World—We Just Live In It: The Boards vs. Clinical Practice

Passing the Boards requires a different set of skills than being a good clinician. You can be a great clinician and fail the boards if you do not prepare correctly or if you have poor test taking skills (despite getting to this point in your life). On the other hand, you can be a master test taker, pass the Boards, and be a mediocre clinician. I'm sure you've never encountered anyone like this. Yeah right!

Organized planning and study will get you 1/3 of the way to passing the exam. Good solid focused test taking strategies is another 3rd.
Of course, the remaining 1/3 piece of the puzzle is having the information at your fingertips, and we cover this in Section 3.

Easy to Forget the Basics, But Don't

The basics in all this are often forgotten. Unfortunately, this can result in careless errors negating all your hard work and focus.

Read the Question

When we get to a standardized exam we are told to "read the question." This is such a cliché that most of us glaze over when we hear it, since who *isn't* going to read the question? However, it is critical advice when you realize that reading the question means focusing on what they are really asking. Once again, this is often found in the last sentence.

Circling key words like "except," "most," "the cause," and "most likely" best accomplish this. By paying close attention to this, you will avoid careless errors.

Tripping on the Slippery – Except for Rocks

We are trained to look for the correct answers. When the question contains words like "except," "not," or "least," take more time with the question. Most questions have you look for the "correct" choices, and your mind is trained that way and is going to look for "correct" choices automatically. If you are tired or it is late in the exam, *it is easy to get sloppy and choose one of the "correct" choices when the question is* **asking you to pick the incorrect choice**. Take the extra time to be careful when going through this type of question. Cross out the "correct" choices as you read through the choices.

Know Thy Foe

Be familiar with the format of the questions. This can usually be found online at www.abp.org.

Know Your Own Way

Some folks like to read the question first; others like to read the choices first. Personally, I like to read the questions first and circle the words I think are important and then read the answers. The other way, I find myself tricked by the traps and decoys they leave in the answer. Others swear by reading the answers first.

 Best to try both methods while taking practice questions and see which works better for you.

Invest in Rest

We've said this before, but it bears mentioning again: do not study the day before and, if possible, do not study 2 days before the exam. This will pay off. If you have organized your study and treated it like the marathon it is, then anything you study during the last day will be counterproductive. Your brain needs to recharge and the information has to "marinate." Think of it as a muscle—you would not want to lift weights just before an athletic competition, and the same applies here.

THE FOUR FACES OF ABP: QUESTION FORMATS

FIVE ITEM MULTIPLE-CHOICE: This is pretty straightforward. **"Multiple Guess,"** as my medical school roommate called it. Here you pick the "Best" answer from among five choices. There is an answer and four distractions called "choices." Your job is to not be thrown off by the distracters that are carefully placed there by professional test writers and their collaborators. One approach is to cross out the answers you know are not correct, in order to avoid distraction. This will increase the chances of "guessing" the correct one if you are not sure. Other techniques are:

❏ Cover the choices and read the entire question first.
❏ Come up with your own answer before looking at the choices.
❏ Compare each choice with what you thought it should be.
❏ Follow your gut reaction even if you don't know why.

Even if the correct answer jumps up at you, take the extra minute to read over the other choices. You might be surprised to find a "better" and therefore "BEST" answer.

If you find yourself between two answers that seem correct, look for the word or phrase that might make it "second best." Recheck the last sentence of the question to make sure you have read the question correctly.

If you are truly in the dark, choices which contain terms like "Always" and "Never" are usually not the correct answer. They need to get in a lot of information to have it be correct, and as a result the longest answer is often the correct one. Try this with your practice questions and see if it works. It often will.

CLINICAL VIGNETTES FOLLOWED BY 3 QUESTIONS: Here they provide you with a volume of facts and data that would make your most manic patient glaze over from boredom. They then ask three questions in a row. They won't just expect you to know the diagnosis.

Often they want you to:

- ❏ Question 1: Come up with a Diagnostic Test
- ❏ Question 2: Figure out something with the Disorder or the Inheritance Pattern
- ❏ Question 3: Determine treatment and management

By using solid memory techniques like the ones in this book, you will have the details locked in and linked to each other. Answering 3 questions in a row will be as easy as answering one.

Here's where circling the important points really comes in handy, by making pertinent pieces of information stand out and come together.

Multiple Guessing

Remember, there is no penalty for wrong answers. There will be questions to which you just have no clue. Statistically, you will get 20 -25% correct if you pick the same choice each time you are making a "wild guess." My favorite is B or C. You decide which is your favorite, but be consistent, and choose the same letter each time you are making a wild guess.

One Peg Down

Remember to make sure that the questions on the answer sheet match the ones you are reading, and that you did not skip a line on the Answer sheet. If you verify this every 10 questions, it will not take up a lot of time AND if you catch an error it will be easy to correct.

Look Over the Bored Materials

Once again, check the ABP website for updates on the question format.

Timing is Everything

You are given 3-1/2 hours to complete each book. It is best to divide the test into 15-minute blocks. First look over the entire test and get the lay of the land, and then decide where you should be at every 15-minute block. You can even set up a silent timer on your watch to keep on track.

For example, you could pace yourself so that at

> 9:15 – you are at Question 13
>
> 9:30 – you are at Question 25
>
> 12:30 – you take the last bite of your meatball sandwich, and then you remember that you're a vegetarian.
>
> 12:45 – You realize that iatrogenic is a Greek, not a Latin word and you say to yourself, "Who Cares!"

PERIL WARNING If you have a difficult time with the first three questions, don't panic. Take a deep breath and put a mark next to them, and do the next questions. You will find those questions that you know cold. Slam-dunk a few of those to get your confidence back.

HOT TIP Not only will you get your confidence back (which will allow you to go back to those initial difficult questions in a better mental state), but you may also find the key to the answer in questions found later in the exam. Yes, this does happen.

Match the Book and Answer Sheet

It is very easy to place the answer in the wrong number on the computer-scoring sheet, and then you are off all the way down. It is also easy to put two answers down for a given question. Be forewarned: this results in it being scored as incorrect automatically. Every 10 questions or so, double-check. It is well worth it, since it is much easier to go back 10 questions than an entire page. You knew that!

Finish Line

You don't have to (or want to) be the first person to leave the exam. The folks who leave first have either given up, are the ones who read up on pyloric stenosis in lieu of sex, or are simply arrogant. Having said that, there is also no reason to stay and torture yourself if you finish early. Leave, but wait until a few have gone before you so they can be the ones people stare at.

Before you leave, do a quick review of the questions you weren't sure of. Make sure you did not mark any of the answers by the wrong number.

Change the answers only if you are sure you chose the wrong answer. Your instincts are usually correct when taking an educated guess. You can test this in the practice questions you take.

Feel free to leave early and use the time to rest, but do rest. Do NOT look up the answers and torment yourself. Don't chit chat with fellow exam takers torturing yourselves by going over what answers you chose for specific questions. Your brain will serve you better if you rest it during the lunch break.

Gotten Down to the Core

There are a few key principles that one needs to know. These are the facts, clinical principles and specific pieces of information that the Boards expect you to know.

There are also some general rules, e.g., "the least invasive test" is often the answer, "the child is normal; do nothing" is often the answer, etc. Going in with these rules will often score big points on the test.

If the words include *"grandmother has told parents"* the answer will, more likely than not, be "reassurance."

Phrases and Mazes: Answers Found in Questions

Often the key to the answer can be found embedded in the question. This is because there are only so many ways to *classically* describe a disorder. Therefore, becoming familiar with these hot phrases and buzzwords will allow you to pick up on the answers immediately. (How many ways can you describe a child with Henoch Schönlein Purpura or Rocky Mountain Spotted Fever?) The specific buzzwords are noted in Section B.

Compass Points to Passing

The following principles can serve as a compass to help through the fog of anxiety or difficulty that you may encounter while taking the exam.

1. No Cutting Edge Here

If there is some raging controversy going on, it will not be tested on the exam. If there is, it is probably an experimental question for those who get their jollies from writing test questions. Recent developments will not appear on the test either.

2. Zebras and Geezers

Often, if there is a bizarre polysyllabic disorder that you read about in the *Accta Taurus Excretia*[4], it may very well be the correct answer.

3. That's "Mr. Vitamin A" To You

You will have to know the formal names for all vitamins and viruses. You will not see Vitamin A listed anywhere in the answer. Instead you will see Retinol. What, you wanted them to make it easy for you?

4. Bus Full of Hemophiliacs

You will have to be familiar with the complications of common disorders and typical treatments of common diseases. This is more important than knowing about uncommon disorders.

5. Know Where You Come From

Just because you have never seen a case of Measles, Mumps, Rubella and, apparently now for those younger than me (gulp!), *Haemophilus influenza*, it doesn't mean they are not going to appear on the Boards. These, plus nutritional deficiencies, are all common occurrences on the Boards.

6. The Generalist is Always Right (Almost)

Calling in a consultant or a surgeon is often the wrong answer on the Boards. Choose this only if you are sure it is the correct answer. The one exception is the Ophthalmologist, which is usually the correct answer. Likewise, again, the less invasive the test, the more likely it is going to be the correct answer.

7. Waiting to Develop

Often they have a mother come to the office complaining about a child's lack of development, compared to the child down the street. Again, the correct answer is often to "reassure the mother" unless there are real developmental delays described.

---

[4] Latin for Journal of BS.

8. Déjà Vu All Over Again

You will be sitting there taking the test. You will put down an answer to question 18 that you are not quite sure of, and suddenly there you are on question 128, and the answer to 18 is right there in the wording of question 128. You are not imagining things; this often happens. I am not sure if this is deliberate or coincidence, but it does happen. Unwrap it when it does: it is a gift. Of course, you might suddenly hear someone shout out DAMMIT. That is because you just found the answer to question 17, from Book 1 in the morning, and you are now at the end of Book 2 in the afternoon..

Clinical Case Scenarios/ Vignettes

This is a potentially intimidating part of the exam, but it need not be if you follow a few strategies to "tame" the "jungle of information" they throw at you.

Steps to Simplify the Question

1. The disorders here are presented in their "classic" presentation. Follow the bouncing

   buzzwords that are sprinkled throughout our text 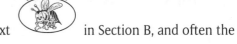 in Section B, and often the diagnosis will jump out at you.

2. The labs and physical findings are all there for a reason. They are there to rule in or rule out something.

3. Sometimes they have you read a lengthy diatribe. You're so proud that you have recognized the buzz words and identified the diagnosis, and then in the last sentence they tell you the diagnosis you just came up with and the following three questions are just "related" to the diagnosis. So why did they have you read the question? I don't know. But here is a solution:

If you see a lengthy clinical scenario taking up a half a page, read the last sentence to see if the diagnosis is sitting there. If so, read the question just in case, but you will be able to read it much faster already knowing what the diagnosis is.

Again, some folks suggest that you read the choices first. I don't usually recommend this since it may cause you to be tricked by the "distracters" they place there for you. Remember: often they are asking something you know cold, but it is foggy with a smokescreen of misinformation, numbers and data. Once you note the important points and put them into "words" in the margin, the answer will be obvious and all your hard studying will work for you. We go over the importance of "putting numbers into words" later in this chapter.

PERIL **WARNING** If you get distracted and deceived, you will be led down the primrose path to the wrong diagnosis. The traps will be laid in the subsequent (usually 3) questions that follow the vignette. You will then order the wrong diagnostic test and come up with the wrong treatment. This is where knowing the key descriptive word or phrase is critical.

HOT TIP Often considering the complications vs. the benefits will make the correct choice more apparent. If you have studied the limited number of case scenarios in each specialty, the correct answer will become a reflex that only involves your spinal cord; you will even be able to check your cerebral cortex at the coat check.

8 Simple Steps for Each Question (How to Approach a Lion... Very Carefully)

1. Line up the Facts: Use a Flashlight

Remember, one of the best ways to approach a dangerous and tricky situation is with a flashlight, and on the boards that means using a pencil to circle important points so they stand out. This will enable you to add up the clinical facts with minimal distraction.

This serves two purposes. One, you are **making important pieces of information stand out**. This allows you to go back and read just that which facilitates formulating a diagnosis. Two, there are pieces of information that **seem irrelevant** but are very relevant. We will call these the "**Windows,**" since they are often the windows to the answer. Most of the points in the question are there for a reason; don't discount them unless you are certain that they are there as a deliberate distraction.

This extra step may seem time consuming at first, but if you do this on practice questions[5] it will be second nature on the exam, and in the end it will help you better focus on the questions, making them a fun puzzle to solve, and will save you time and energy.

2. Analysis Leads to Paralysis

Often the question is simpler than you think. Over-reading and looking for tricks is how you can turn a slam-dunk into a missed lay-up. Too many of these can turn the tide to a failing grade. This is how fellows in endocrinology, for example, can often end up with this section being their lowest score.

---

[5] Although those taking the Compuprep® exam will find it is hard to highlight a computer screen.

3. Read the Whole Thing

On the other hand, even if you are sure of your answer, read the whole question to make sure you are not missing a better choice.

4. When Faced with 2 Choices

Often you will be down to 2 choices. You will have to choose one as being more correct. They might ask, "What is the first thing you should do in clinical practice?" In clinical practice it seems like you would be doing them all first but on the Boards, you must make a choice. This is the gray zone, which is where the real thinking goes in. At this point, pay attention to the following:

- ❏ Is one choice more invasive?
- ❏ Is there any harm in choosing one treatment over the other and will it affect outcome if you try it first?
- ❏ Consider what would absolutely be done first in clinical practice.

5. The Devil is in the Details

Pay attention to certain details like gender. Often this will give you a clue. For example, if the patient is a female, it is unlikely to be an X-linked disorder. If they describe the patient as coming from a certain ethnic group, they are not being politically incorrect; they are trying to point you to the diagnosis. Likewise, pay attention to the age of the patient. A 3-year-old with upper airway stridor is more likely to have croup than a teenager returning from a weekend out in the woods.

HOT TIP

If they describe a patient who is visiting or immigrating from a third world country[6], the answer will often be a chronic condition that is not diagnosed (e.g., sickle cell disease) or a disease that is rare in the US due to immunization. This disease may be common in other parts of the world, because of perceived or real inconsistent immunization practices outside the US. The same would apply for parents who they note are "against immunizations."

6. Put Numbers into Words

When you study the clinical descriptions, you are memorizing terms like "microcytic anemia," "febrile" "tachycardia," "tachypneic," "neutropenia," and "cyanotic mouth breathing drone."[7]

The main point is that you are memorizing the descriptions and not the numbers and the data. This is why it is important to actually write down in words what they are describing. Write it down in the margins.

---

6 "Developing Nation" for those with a Politically Correct scorecard.

7 Oh sorry, the last one is a description of my college roommate who failed pre-med and is now in charge of claims at one of the HMO's for which I am a "provider."

For example, if you note that the platelet count is low, *write down thrombocytopenia in the margin.* If the respiratory rate is high, write down "tachypnea." In doing so, the picture they are drawing will come into focus.

HOT TIP

Write in the margins - if they're going to charge more than a thousand dollars to take this exam, you might as well get your money's worth.

7. Cross It Out

Cross out all the wrong choices as you encounter them. In the matching section, even though they tell you that any choice can be used more than once, they rarely are used more than once. So you are better off crossing out the ones you use and eliminating the distraction. Certainly, if you are sure that a choice should be used twice, by all means go ahead.

8. Hit the Road: Move On

Don't be afraid to move on if you have no idea what the answer is. Put an asterisk there so you can return to it if the answer shows up in a later question or if you have time. Some books suggest not filling it in and coming back. I don't agree. Best to fill it in, just in case you run out of time. You will have a chance of getting it and once again, you increase your odds if you choose the same answer each time you are making a wild guess.

Another reason to not spend a lot of time on these bizarre questions: they may be experimental questions for the sheer enjoyment of the professional test writer or they may be thrown out due to a technicality. It would be a pity if you spent a lot of time on something like this.

Final Word

Remember, with a large number of candidates scattered around the middle of the curve, most folks who fail are within 10- 15 questions of passing. Following these test-taking techniques can often be an important deciding factor in answering these pivotal 10-15 questions correctly and thus the difference between passing and failing.

Section B:
Pearls and Perils:
Specific Core Facts and Details

Humorously Coded for Easy Memorization and Long Term Memory

Chapter 5

Biostatistics (& Other Number Games) and Ethical-Legal Issues

Even though you will probably never be a bench scientist or personally engage in clinical trials, you will be required to know the basics of biostatistics and answer some questions on biostatistics on the exam. The good news is there are only a few core formulas and topics you need to be familiar with in order to score some easy points. So let's roll the dice and play the numbers game.

You will be called upon to distinguish between sensitivity and specificity. In all likelihood, this will take place at a time in the exam when you yourself have been completely numbed and desensitized, to the point that you can't even distinguish light from dark. However, keeping a few basics in mind will help keep all this straight so you can get these predictable questions answered correctly.

Sensitivity

The sensitivity of a test is the probability that the test will produce a <u>True Positive</u> (TP) result when used on a population with the disease. We will explain sensitivity and specificity in three ways:

  1) Equation form
  2) 2x2 table form
  3) Narrative

It is calculated by taking the True Positives (TP) and dividing by the total number with the disease[1] [True Positives (TP) + False Negatives (FN)], thus:

$$\frac{TP}{TP+FN}$$

In a test with high sensitivity, *positive test results may or may not be reliable* (this depends on the specificity and the number of false positives). But *negative* results can **RULE OUT** disease, since there are very few false negatives. Therefore, a test that is seNsitive could be a good screeN. If it is negative, it is probably truly negative and you can cease and desist.

---

[1] The total number with the disease would include those with true positive test results and those with the disease who test negative (false negatives).

Tests that have a high seNsitivity have a sNOUT. A **N**egative result rules disease **OUT**. If you don't want to miss the diagnosis, choose a test with high sensitivity. Depending on the specificity, you may have a lot of false positives, but at least you'll be catching the true positives as well.

Specificity

The specificity of a test is *the probability that a test will produce a true negative* (TN) result when used on a population without disease [True Negatives (TN) + False Positives (FP)].[2]

$$\frac{TN}{TN+FP}$$

Therefore, in a test with high specificity, there are very few false positives; so *positive test results would be reliable.* Likewise, the test would have very *few false negatives* when testing the general population. Therefore, rather than being a good screen, it would be a good test to *confirm* the presence of a disease.

High s**P**ecificity is good for confirming **P**ositive disease.

Physicians may prefer high specificity if it is very important not to create false positives (i.e., if being positive has consequences). Highly s**P**ecific tests s**P**IN. If they are **P**ositive, you can rule **IN** disease.

Positive Predictive Value

The positive predictive value of a test is the probability that someone who has the disease tests positive. This is usually much more important to clinicians than sensitivity or specificity (or it should be).

This is a much simpler calculation; it is the True Positives divided by all positive test results [Total Positives plus False Positives].

$$\frac{TP}{TP+FP}$$

Positive predictive value is most useful when the prevalence is high. As prevalence increases, PPV increases. As prevalence falls, PPV falls.

---

[2] False positives would be those who do not actually have the disease but tested positive anyway, and the true negatives don't have the disease and tested negatively as expected.

Negative Predictive Value

The negative predictive value of a test is the probability that someone who does not have a disease will have a negative test result.

The opposite caveat that applies to a positive predictive calculation applies to a negative predictive value. That is to say, they are highest when the prevalence is low. As prevalence increases, NPV falls. As prevalence falls, NPV increases.

The calculation is, of course, predictable by now. It would be the True Negatives divided by [True Negatives plus False Negatives].

$$\frac{TN}{TN+FN}$$

	Disease	No Disease	Positive Predictive Value	Negative Predictive Value
Test Positive	True Positive (TP)	False Positive (FP)	TP/TP+FP	
Test Negative	False Negative (FN)	True Negative (TN)		TN/FN+TN
Sensitivity	TP/TP+FN			
Specificity		TN/FP+TN		

Null Hypothesis

Are we proving the null hypothesis or rejecting the null hypothesis when research confirms our results? Are you left with a giant null in your head when you think about this? Good — so are we, which is why we are here to help.

Null must have been a cynic. The null hypothesis basically claims that the results that were obtained are due to chance factors and not the variables being studied. Rejection of the null hypothesis and "statistically significant" are generally synonymous.

In other words, the null hypothesis represents the cynic claiming that the research is not significant and is only a result of chance.

Therefore, the ideal goal of research is to be able to prove that the results are not due to chance, and *reject the null hypothesis.*

P Value

The P value represents the chance that the null hypothesis was rejected in error. The P value is one of the most misunderstood values, especially by clinical physicians. The P value is the probability of getting results as or more extreme by chance alone (i.e., if the null hypothesis is true). Therefore, a P value <0.01 means there is a less than 1% chance that the null hypothesis was rejected in error and that the results are due to chance alone.

For purposes of the exam:

· P<0.05 is significant enough to reject the null hypothesis.
· P<0.01 is highly significant enough to reject the null hypothesis.

Therefore, if you have a choice between 0.05 and 0.01, the latter will be correct.

This is a good place to mention Type I and Type II errors.

A Type I error is what we think of as a big OOPS – that we thought something was significant (or different, or better) when it really wasn't. That is, we rejected the null hypothesis in error. You can see that the probability of a Type I error is the same as the P value!

A Type II error is just the opposite of a Type I – with your study results, you found that you could not reject the null hypothesis – but in reality, there is a difference between your groups and the null hypothesis is not true. You just couldn't figure that out based on what you had to study.

Obviously, in most cases of clinical medicine, a Type I error is worse than a Type II error. (Remember primum non nocere).[3]

Chi Square

No, the Chi square has nothing to do with Chai or Russian tea.

---

[3] Latin phrase which means "First, do no harm."

The Chi Square is used to determine whether the differences between an observed result and the expected result can be attributed to the parameter studied, or are a result of chance. The Chi square is a statistical tool to test the Null Hypothesis.

CASE STUDY

Invariably, you will be presented with 4 part table with values. From this, you will be expected to determine the sensitivity and specificity. This will be worth several points on the exam. You might as well study how to approach this now, so it will be on automatic pilot on exam day.

	Positive Test	Negative Test
Patient actually doesn't have the disease	Test falsely labels a healthy person with a disease (FALSE POSITIVE)	Test correctly identifies somebody who is healthy (TRUE NEGATIVE)
Patient does have the disease	Test correctly identifies somebody who has the disease (TRUE POSITIVE)	Test falsely claims somebody is healthy when they have the disease (FALSE NEGATIVE)

THE DIVERSION

Watch Out: Don't get confused when being asked to determine sensitivities and specificities. Don't let your eyes glaze over this information, and don't get thrown off by either calculating incorrectly or just putting down any number to move on. If you simply take a deep breath, these are actually easy questions to answer.

ANSWER REVEALED

You already know that **specificity identifies true negatives**.

True negative goes on top and is divided by the total population who actually do not have the disease. The population who do not have disease are True negatives plus False positives.

You know that sensitivity tests true positive. Sensitivity is TP divided by those who actually have the disease. The population who actually has the disease is true positive plus false negatives.

Therefore, this only involves the bottom row: TP divided by (TP plus FN).

Studying Studies

In a **cohort study**, you start with those with risk factors and those without to determine who gets disease (either prospectively or retrospectively). You can also have a single cohort with a commonality (e.g., risk factor, like similar blood pressure) and follow over time to find out frequency or incidence of some outcome.

In a **case-control study**, you start with those with disease and those without and then check for risk factors. Remember, the risk factor must come before the outcome!

Cross Sectional Study

In a cross sectional study, specific information is obtained from a cross section of a given population or sample.

Prospective study

In a prospective study, members of a given risk group are followed over time and assessed for outcomes.

Eany Meany Miney Mode

Just in case your mind freezes on the exam, it is worth noting some of the basics of *mean, median, and mode*

• **Mean** – To obtain a mean, you add up the sample values and divide by the size of the sample

• **Median** – The median value is one in which half of the data is smaller and half is larger. To obtain the median, you simply line up the values in order and pick the middle value

• **Mode** – The mode is the most frequently occurring number

---

Retrospective study

Old information (medical records, for example) of a group with a given disorder or outcome are reviewed to determine risk factors.

Retrospective Cohort Study

The retrospective study, as the name implies, looks backwards, comparing those with a risk factor and those without and checking for disease (or other outcome). It doesn't mean that the risk factor is there now and you are looking backwards for disease. It just means that the risks and disease (or other outcome) occurred in the past (risk before outcome!)

Prospective Cohort Study

Again, as the name implies, the prospective study moves forward, studying those with a risk factor and those without and assessing development of disease (or another outcome) over time.

Meta-analysis

Meta-analysis is simply the analysis of data from several studies, comparing the results to draw conclusions.[4]

Ethical considerations

Invariably, you will be asked some questions that are ethical dilemmas. These typically have to do with divulging information between teenagers and their parents. Ethical issues regarding HIV also pop up.

Rights of Children regarding treatment

The wishes of children should be honored, except regarding life-threatening situations. For example, if parents give informed consent for a child to participate in a research study, but the child does not want to, the child's wishes should be honored. All decisions are made on the basis of the needs of the child. Physicians are expected to provide information on risks/benefits and make recommendations accordingly.

Parental wishes can be overridden only when they conflict with the interests of the child. Parents cannot force a physician to make choices that the physician believes will be harmful to the child.

In terms of palliative care issues, there is no difference ethically between withdrawing a treatment and not starting it in the first place.

Emancipated Minors

Emancipated minors can make independent decisions regarding their treatment.

A teen with a child of their own should be considered an emancipated minor even if this is not explicitly stated in the history. Even though they do not have a child of their own, if a teenager is living independently with a source of income, they should be considered to be an emancipated minor.

---

4 Or it can be discussing the New York Mets' rapid decline and subsequent elimination from the playoffs prior to the start of the season for the next 200 years.

HOT TIP A teenager brought in by his parents for drug testing cannot be tested without the teenager's permission, even if he is not an emancipated minor.

Court Orders

If parents, and presumably the child/teenager, wish to refuse important treatment, then you need to obtain a court order. You cannot just plow through and implement the treatment against their wishes.

PERIL WARNING Life-threatening situations do not require parental consent (and, subsequently, do not require court order).

PERIL WARNING **In order to be considered an emancipated minor, the patient must be at least 16. If they are younger than 16, they are still not considered to be emancipated minors, regardless of other factors.**

Treatment over Religious Objections

You may be questioned regarding treating a patient over parental religious objections. The standards set forth by the AAP adhere to the principle that children are deserving of treatment which is likely to prevent harm and suffering. This overrides religious objections by the parents.

If presented with a situation like this on the exam, the first step is to try to work with the parents to remove their objections. If this is unsuccessful, then a court order may be sought.

In the face of life and death situations that cannot await a court order, the correct answer would be that the physician should treat over parental objections.

DNR

At this point in the chapter, you yourself may feel like you should be placed on DNR status. Regardless, here are some important points to know should this topic appear on the exam.

DNR orders may be implemented at the request of the parents, when the risks and downside of resuscitation outweigh any expected benefits. Even when DNR is ordered, you as the physician can still implement palliative measures, short of resuscitation and prolonged intensive care. DNR orders can be reconsidered, rescinded, and/or modified.

The goal of palliative care is management and alleviation of pain and suffering.

If you are asked what you are to do when you as the physician cannot comply with the parents' wishes, the correct answer will be to transfer the care to another physician and/or bring in consultants to assist you.

Ethics of Genetic Studies and Screening

Newborn screening must show benefit to the child. It cannot be done for the benefit of genetic counseling alone. In reality, it usually serves both purposes. However, if you were questioned on the exam regarding a situation where the testing was only for the purpose of determining carrier state, and not directly beneficial to the child, it cannot be done.

Likewise, adolescents should not be routinely screened to see if they are carriers of known inherited disorders. Adolescents can decide if they want this information or not when they become adults.

Similarly, regarding testing for "late-onset diseases," you need to know that the ethical standard is to wait until the child is old enough to decide (given the psychological implications of knowing you have a disease that will manifest later in life).

Failure to seek Medical Care and Abuse/Neglect Parameters

If a parent fails to seek medical care when a child is clearly seriously ill, it is considered to be child neglect.

If parents are not compliant with immunizations due to specific concerns or objections, it is not considered to be neglect, although you are expected to encourage compliance.

Chapter 6

Growth and Development

Physiologic Growth

Normal Growth

The following are some important facts and numbers to keep in mind when distinguishing between normal growth and abnormal growth — which is an area fertile for getting tripped up on the exam through deception.

Weight

The average newborn loses up to 10% of birthweight and regains it by the 3rd week.

- Birthweight doubles by 5 months
- Birthweight triples by 1 year
- Men's weight triples during their first year of marriage, especially if they become fathers for the first time that year

Infants may not regain their birthweight until 3 weeks of age. Therefore, if you are presented with an infant younger than 3 weeks who has not regained the birthweight, the correct answer will be to reassure and re-evaluate in one week.

Length

The average height (50th percentile) is easy to remember, since it is 50 cm

- Birth length/height goes up 50% by age 1
- Birth length/height is doubled by age 4
- Birth length/height is tripled by age 13

Head Circumference

Normal Head Circumference

You will be expected to know the average head circumference of a full term newborn and the normal growth following birth:

· Normal head circumference at birth for a full term newborn is **35cm**
· Normal growth: ~1 cm/month for the first 6 months
~ 1/2 cm/month from 6 months to 12 months

Big Heads

Here we are not talking about Donald Trump's swollen ego. We are talking about **macrocephaly** and **hydrocephaly** and how to distinguish between them. Let's start with definitions:

Macrocephaly

Macrocephaly is a head circumference at the **98th percentile for age.** It is by definition "normal."

Often these normal children **won't be born with large heads but will "head up" to their position by the 6th month. This would be an easy way to trick you into picking a major workup as the correct answer when no workup is necessary.**

If they describe an infant with an increasing head circumference but make a point to mention normal development, the first thing you should do is measure the parents' heads.[1] Parents with big heads usually have kids with big heads; this is macrocephaly.

---

[1] Tell them you would like to buy them a Stetson cowboy hat for National Texas Appreciation Day.

Hydrocephaly

Hydrocephaly, on the other hand, will have signs indicating that there is more going on. The *large head may be present at birth.*

"Irritability" or "lethargy and loss of appetite" and other neurological findings would tell you that you are dealing with hydrocephaly.

Macrocephaly vs. Hydrocephaly

· **Macrocephaly** is associated with normal development, which means there are no signs of increased intracranial pressure and, most importantly, there are often parents with large heads.

· **Hydrocephaly,** on the other hand, would be associated with *irritability, vomiting, bulging fontanelle and impaired upward gaze.*

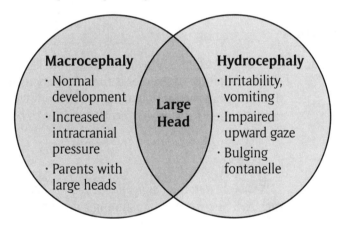

A **"large" anterior fontanelle** is a very general finding, and does not distinguish hydrocephaly from macrocephaly.

A **bulging fontanelle**, however, is associated with hydrocephaly. Read the question and watch the wording.

Neither condition is associated with papilledema since they are both chronic, not acute conditions.

Small heads

Acquired microcephaly

Microcephaly is a head circumference that is more than 3 standard deviations below the mean for age and gender. *Acquired* microcephaly would occur after a history of *normal head circumference at birth.*

If you are presented with an infant whose head circumference decreases, while the weight and height remain normal, there needs to be a cause.

Failure to Thrive

Non-organic causes

Most cases of FTT are due to *nonorganic factors.* Sophisticated tests and labs are *not the first steps to be taken.* Evaluation of the diet is the first step. If this has already been done, then a look at the mother/child interaction (with a focus on feeding technique) is the next step. **Often this needs to be done on an inpatient basis.**

Watch for signs in the history that would suggest a change, such as a new caretaker assuming care of an infant. In this case, *improper mixing of formula* might be the reason behind the failure to thrive.

Organic Causes

Organic causes include

· Chronic renal failure

· Thyroid problems and other metabolic disorders

· Disorders leading to inadequate absorption

· Disorders leading to inadequate utilization

In these cases, however, there would have to be something in the presenting history to suggest these as the causative factors.

Short, long and Dysmorphic

You will need to determine the likely cause of a measurement discrepancy as follows:

Inadequate Caloric Intake – Weight will drop initially, followed by decreased length

Endocrine disorders – Presents with short stature with normal weight

Chromosomal abnormalities – Microcephaly and dysmorphic features

---

You may be presented with a child whose height and weight are normal for age; however, the *growth rate may be abnormal, warranting a workup.* Children growing less than 5 cm/year should be evaluated for growth hormone deficiency or hypothyroidism.

You are presented with a 4 year old child who was at the 50th percentile for both height and weight at birth. She is now at the 25th percentile for weight, but her height is below the 5th percentile. There is no family history of short stature. Physical exam is otherwise non-contributory. What is the cause of the short stature?

You will be given lots of diversionary choices such as *poor nutrition, constitutional growth delay, or neglect.*

This time, the choice you might ignore (because it would be the obvious choice to even those who have no medical training) would be right. In this case, the masses would have picked **growth hormone deficiency** correctly and you, the well-trained pediatrician that you are, would have picked the wrong answer.

Constitutional growth delay would be ruled out by their telling you the parents have no significant history. The weight is at a reasonable 25th percentile, so inadequate nutrition is not a factor. If she went from the 50th percentile for height down to less than the 5th percentile, then she has not tripled her height or grown 5 cm/year. As noted above, this would most likely be due to growth hormone deficiency. Hypothyroidism could also be correct if it were one of the choices.

Intelligence and Learning

Intellectual Disability

You are expected to know how to go about identifying the possible etiology of intellectual disability. This prevents unnecessary testing and allows for appropriate management.

This includes

History –focusing on specific behavioral patterns consistent with known diagnoses.

Family history – look for history of stillborn infants, miscarriages, or consanguinity.

Physical exam – looking for dysmorphism or unusual features.

Genetic testing – there are genetic causes of intellectual disability.

Imaging studies – would be limited to those with features that warrant them, i.e. microcephaly. MRI is the imaging study of choice.

 In the absence of seizures, EEG is not indicated.

Metabolic screening should be considered if indications are given in the history.

 Routine metabolic screening is not indicated in the absence of physical findings or history that support the testing.

Mild intellectual disability[2] is the most common form.[3] It is often identified soon after enrollment in school. Ultimately, those with mild intellectual disability may receive vocational training and may live independently.

Genetics is the most common cause of intellectual disability; however, other causes to consider are **perinatal infections** or prenatal exposure to **teratogen**s.

 Intellectual disability must include limitations in **intellectual functioning** as well as **adaptive behavior/skills,** *originating before age 18.*

 This must be considered within the context of the community and cultural and linguistic factors.

---

[2] Also known as mental retardation.

[3] Up to 85%.

Degrees of Intellectual Disability

Intellectual disability is categorized as outlined in the table below:

Degree of Intellectual Disability	IQ
Mild	50-69
Moderate	35-49
Severe	20-34
Profound	Below 20

Language development in young children is often a better gauge of cognitive function than gross motor development.

· Severe intellectual disability is usually picked up at a younger age

· Mild intellectual disability is usually picked up at a later age, often at the time of entry into school

Visual impairment may result in delay of motor development

Autism

A diagnosis of autism is based on the clinical behavioral presentation, with no single definitive diagnostic test.

Characteristics include:

· Serious impairment of social skills
· Delayed language development
· Repetitive behaviors/restricted interests
· Presentation prior to 36 months

Autism is one of the **autistic spectrum disorders**, **along with pervasive developmental disorder-NOS** and **Asperger syndrome**. Asperger syndrome is characterized by impaired social interactions and rigid or repetitive behaviors, but does not have a component of language impairment.

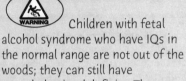

3 Potential Causes of Intellectual Disability

It could help to know that the 3 most common known causes of intellectual disability are:

1) Fetal alcohol syndrome
2) Fragile X syndrome
3) Down syndrome

Fetal alcohol syndrome is the most common preventable cause of intellectual disability.

Children with fetal alcohol syndrome who have IQs in the normal range are not out of the woods; they can still have neurobehavioral deficits. They are at increased risk for psychiatric disorders as well.

Children with Down syndrome are at increased risk for ADHD and oppositional-defiant disorder.

Family history is crucial; if you are presented with a question where they note a family tree full of "uncles with learning problems," they may be presenting an x-linked disorder such as Fragile X.

Remember that even an infant w significant hearing loss may demonstrate normal 'language' development until 6-9 months, right up to where babbling does not progress to definite 'mama' and 'dada'."

Consonant Counseling

If you are presented with a child younger than 6 years who is having difficulty pronouncing certain consonants, reassurance is all that is needed.

Se*ual Orientation

Sexual orientation is determined by mid-adolescence.

There is growing evidence for the biological/genetic/hormonal basis for sexual orientation. One thing to remember for the Boards is that there is no evidence for parental influence or various adverse life events "causing homosexuality."

An important component of autism, and one that distinguishes it from other causes of language delay is the **lack of eye contact and lack of social engagement**. It would be important to know about the child's **interactions with other family members**.

Delayed and atypical language, along with odd interests and activities, may distinguish autism and autistic spectrum disorders from intellectual disability. Good social interaction for the most part rules out autism.

With **Asperger syndrome,** there is no language delay. In **Rett syndrome,** development may be normal until age 1, after which it regresses. *Acquired microcephaly* will often be included in the history of Rett syndrome.

A **hearing test** is important in any child undergoing evaluation for autism, in order to make sure that the cause of the language delay component cannot be attributed to hearing loss.

Language and Hearing

Hearing is an important part of normal development

Newborn hearing loss may not be picked up by routine screening. Newborn hearing screens are done using OAE, ABR, or both. Screening may also be done in two steps, where an abnormal OAE triggers the ordering of an ABR to confirm results. Congenital hearing loss impacts language milestones of infancy, including cooing and babbling.

Clinical observation to assess hearing in an infant is not reliable.

50% of congenital deafness is due to genetic causes.

A wait and see approach will not likely be the correct answer if you are presented with an 18 month old with language delay.

This is especially the case if they note that despite the absence of hearing loss, language development is delayed.

If you are presented with a patient with delayed language development and normal hearing, a referral to a developmental specialist will be the correct answer.

Learning Disabilities (LD)

HOT TIP

Read the family history carefully and look for signs of a genetic predisposition or signs of specific disorders such as Fragile X syndrome.

Pay close attention to any mention of other family members with speech or language difficulties.

PERIL WARNING

A child can have a **learning disability** with normal or even superior **intelligence**.

Having a learning disability means there is a specific difficulty in one of the following areas:

· *Listening*
· *Speaking*
· *Reading*
· *Writing*
· *Reasoning*
· *Math skills*

PERIL WARNING

If you are presented with a child **younger than 7** who reverses letters such as "**b**" and "**d,**" do not be quick to make a diagnosis of dyslexia or another learning disability. This can be a **normal finding** up to age 7.

PERIL WARNING

Social problems may be a manifestation of a learning disability, but they are not considered learning disorders in and of themselves. A learning disability can often be compensated for in the early grades. They are then **picked up in the later grades** when things get tougher and more challenging. The key point you are expected to know is that the earlier a learning disorder is discovered, the easier it is to implement methods that give the child an increased chance to overcome or compensate for the disability.

Grandmothers

If the following phrase appears anywhere in the question — "the child's grandmother feels that (fill in the blank) and he isn't doing (fill in the blank again)" – the answer will likely be to **reassure the mother**.

LD Red Flags

Some of the specific red flags you may be presented with include delay in speech and language development, as well as:

• Inability to recognize letters and numbers by the end of kindergarten

• Speech delay in a preschooler

• Inability to read simple words by the end of the first grade.

On grade retention: There can be a significant negative social impact when children are held back and made to repeat a grade. However, moving children who are failing on to subsequent grades does not address their academic problems.

Medications and Medical Conditions

Read the history carefully for medical conditions, keeping in mind that anticonvulsants and antihistamines can alter school performance.

Watch for signs of depression as an underlying cause of poor school performance. On the other hand, poor school performance may lead to depression. You might have to distinguish the chicken from the egg.

Children with learning disabilities are at increased risk for behavioral and mood disorders in general.

Learning disabilities are not outgrown. Engagement in extracurricular activities may be important for the self esteem of a child with a learning disability. In addition, special tools that help a child overcome a specific learning disability are to be encouraged and used; this may include private tutoring, resource room help, etc. Early intervention is the key; delay in recognizing learning disabilities may result in repeated academic failures, which often negatively impacts a child's school motivation.

Unless there is a profound inability to read the letters on a page, the most commonly-encountered ophthalmological disorders generally do not impact reading ability. Gimmicks like tinted eyeglasses and eye gymnastics will be incorrect choices to improve reading ability (no matter how cool the described exercises are).

If you are presented with a child who is having difficulty in classes such as history or social studies, they may describing a child with difficulty reading or with short term memory problems.

Intelligence Screening

Performance and Verbal IQ Differential

Discrepancy between performance IQ (which measures visual-spatial interpretation) and verbal IQ (language-based learning) may mean that a child is **at risk for a learning disability.**

Achievement Test

Achievement tests distinguish between overall (potential) and achievement (actual) intellectual performance.

 Intelligence testing can be influenced by many factors (which may be included with the history you are presented with), including:

Genetics, cultural or language bias, emotional and/or psychosocial factors, as well as ability to focus and pay attention.

Sub test profile scores are more important than overall test scores on IQ tests such as the Wechsler Intelligence Scale for Children (WISC-IV), since the subtest scores allow for more detailed information on the child's difficulties.

If you are presented with a patient with below normal scores on an achievement test despite a normal IQ, they are probably pointing you toward a specific learning disability.

The predictive validity of IQ testing increases with age.

Normal Developmental Milestones

For many of us, remembering the details of the normal developmental milestones are about as exciting as memorizing the speed dial numbers on your cell phone. Unfortunately, you will be expected to identify a child's age by their developmental milestones. Knowing this cold will be worth several points on the exam, perhaps the few points that stand between you and a passing grade. The following are the key milestones to commit to memory.

I have found the most effective way to do this is to raise a child. However, at this point unless you are a PGY-1 preparing for the boards in advance, there probably isn't enough time to conceive and raise a few kids before the exam.

It is important to remember these milestones both using *months* and *years*. As you can see, much of the first year is spent growing and developing motor skills, while fine motor, language and social skills (one hopes) are the focus thereafter.

Age	Motor	Cognitive/ Behavioral	*Expressive/ Receptive* Language	Social
Full Term Infant	· Moro reflex	· Becomes alert with the sound of a bell or voice		· Fixates on face / object and briefly follows
2 months	· Follows objects past mid-line · Lifts head and shoulders off bed in prone position		· Cooing	
4 months	· Head lag disappears by 5 months · Moro disappears by 3-6 months · Bears weight on forearms while prone · Rolls from prone to supine · Bears weight while held standing		· Laughs out loud and squeals	· Imitates social interaction
6 months	· Ability to transfer object from one hand to the other · Reaches for objects · Sits with support · Rolls over in both directions	· *Turns* directly to *sound and voice*	· Babbles consonant sounds · Imitates speech	
9 months	· Bangs two blocks together · Sits without support	· *Turns* when *name* is called · *Plays peek a boo*	· Mama and Dada (non-specific)	· Stranger anxiety · Recognizes common objects and people
12 Months (1 year)	· Takes a few steps · Pincer grasp · Drinks from a cup held by another person · Pulls to stand and cruises	· Assists with dressing	· Speaks 1 additional word besides Mama and Dada · Mama and Dada specific	· Follows a single step command with gesture - Points for requests

Age	Motor	Cognitive/ Behavioral	*Expressive/ Receptive Language*	Social
15 month old	· Gives and takes a ball · Drinks from a cup · Scribbles with a crayon · Puts cube into a cup · Walks independently · Stoops to floor and recovers to standing position		· Speaks 3-6 additional words besides Mama and Dada · Points to one body part · Follow single step command without gesture (In this case a gesture is not needed, the child understands without gesturing.)	
18 months	· Self feeding with a spoon · Stacks 2 cube tower · Throws ball · Walks upstairs while holding hand	· Imitates household chores like sweeping vacuuming etc.	· 10-20 word vocabulary	- Points to show interest
16-19 months	· Builds a tower of 4 blocks · Releases a raisin into a bottle · Spontaneous Scribbling (18 months)			
24 months	· Builds a tower of 6 cubes · Washes and dries hands · Removes clothing · Kicks a ball · Jumps with 2 feet		· Greater than 50 word vocabulary · Starts using pronouns such as I, me, and you · Speech is 50% intelligible to a stranger	· Pretend play

Age	Motor	Cognitive/ Behavioral	*Expressive/ Receptive Language*	Social
36 months (3 years)	· Copies a circle · Puts on a T-shirt / shorts · Stacks a tower of 8 cubes · Stands on one foot for 1-2 seconds · Pedals tricycle · Climbs stairs *alternating feet*	· Imitates a vertical line drawn with a crayon · Knows the name of a friend · Understands basic adjectives, tired, hungry etc.	· Speaks with 5-8 word sentences · 75% of what is said is intelligible · Starts using what and who	- Imaginary play - Concepts of good and bad predominate
4 year old	· Walks up and down stairs · Draws a simple drawing of a person · Walks up and down steps · Balances on 1 foot for 4 seconds	· Dresses and brushes teeth without help · Names 4 colors	· Asks questions, Where? Why? How? What? · 100% intelligible to a stranger	· Pretend play more advanced
5 year old	· Draws a person with 6 body parts · Prepares a bowl for food · Skips alternating feet	· Plays board games · Counts 5 blocks · Names all the primary colors	· Defines words	- Can cooperate with chores - Complex roles and stories in play
6 year old	· Ties shoelaces · Rides a bicycle	· Writes name · Knows right from left	· Counts ten objects	

Ripe for Confusion

 The following areas are ripe for confusion:

· Throwing a ball: an 18-month-old can throw a ball. However, they cannot usually throw overhand until 2 years of age (24 months).

Making up for Lost Time/ Developmental Milestones of Preemies

· A premature baby who is chronologically now at full term (e.g. 38 weeks) would be expected to have the milestones of a full term baby: i.e., A 30 week-old preemie at 8 weeks of age would have the developmental milestones of a FT baby, not of a 2-month-old.

· You no longer have to factor in the prematurity after age 2 years.

Developmental Milestone Mnemonics

The following are some mnemonics that should help keep the sometimes confusing milestones straight.

2 Months Old

They can follow an object through a **180-degree arc**, which is really **2 sides**; **2 months = 2 sides**.

A 2-month-old can lift his or her head and chest while prone (picture it as a number 2 rolling up), **coo** (**rhymes with 2**), and can follow their mother around the room (with their **2** eyes, of course).

4 Months Old

A 4-month-old scratches and grabs clothes, and will clutch at and hold onto a rattle. They can also place objects deliberately in their mouths.

Picture a number 4 as a rattle.

6 Months Old

A 6-month-old can sit up.

Picture a number 6 sitting with the bottom of the number as its butt. They can transfer a cube from one hand to another (picture a 6 transforming into a 9 from hand to hand), and they can crawl on their bellies.

You can also change the word "six" to "sit" as in: **"sit month olds can sit."**

1 year (12 months)

A **one**-year-old can walk with **one** hand held, wave bye-bye, and say mama and dada. They have a fine pincer grasp by age one and can build with 2 blocks. They can cruise while holding on with one hand, and walk with support.

 Age 1 = can **one**-hand walk; waves good-bye with **one** hand

18 Months Old

Gross Motor: An 18-month-old walks fast, falls occasionally, walks upstairs with hand held, and climbs into and sits in a chair.

Fine Motor: An 18-month-old **turns book pages 3 at a time**[4] and builds a tower with 3 blocks. They will feed themselves, but it is quite messy.

 Picture two #3's coming together to form an 8 to remember that this occurs at 18 months.

Language: 18-month-olds can speak around 10 words, and identify *only one part of their bodies*.

All very similar to the average 18-*year*-old.

2 years (24 months)

Fine Motor: A 2-year-old builds a 6-cube tower

---

[4] Don't you wish you could too, and still retain it all?

3 Years Old

A **3**-year-old can walk up stairs **alternating** *feet,* ride a tricycle (**3** wheels), and hop **3** times.

4 Years Old

4-year-olds can identify opposites.

Drawing skills will be included in any question in a preschool aged child. Well, this one is easy. A **4**-year-old can draw **4** body parts.

Rule of 4's

- · Count to 4
- · Recite a 4-word sentence
- · Identify 4 primary colors
- · Draw a 4-part person
- · Build a gate out of blocks (picture a #4 as a gate)
- · A stranger will understand 4/4 of what they are saying[5]

5 Years Old

Fine Motor: He can tie a knot, correctly grab a pencil, and print letters. (These are all skills required in school, making it easy to remember.) At 5 they can draw a square.

Gross motor: A 5-year-old walks backward.

This is often the age they start school, so picture a child trying to avoid school by walking backwards.

---

[5] Which is everything, for those who have difficulty with fractions.

Age	What they can draw
3	(circle)
4	(cross) [6]
5	(square)
6	(triangle)
7	(diamond)

Now, you draw the shapes here and see the progression in complexity:

_____

_____

_____

_____

_____

_____

[6] This is easy to remember since the cross can be imagined to be a 4 and associated with age 4.

Troubling signs

The following table provides some **age-related abnormal findings**. If you are presented with these age-related deficiencies, then monitoring or intervention may be required.

Age	Deficiency requiring intervention
2 months	Lack of visual attention/fixation
4 months	Lack of visual tracking Lack of steady head control
6 months	Failure to turn to sound or voice
9 months	Inability to sit Lack of babbling
18 months	Inability to walk independently
24 months	Failure to use single words
36 months	Failure to speak in at least three words sentences

> ## Age by cubes
>
> You will need to know the number of cubes or blocks a child can pile up at any given age. Follow the bouncing block.
>
> 2-3 cubes by 18 months
>
> 4-6 cubes by 24 months
>
> 8 cubes by 36 months

Language Skills

The following will make it quite easy to keep language development straight. It might even allow you to get the question right without even knowing the other parameters.

They often ask how much of what a child says is intelligible at different ages. The following chart should help:

Age	% of what they say is intelligible
Age 2	2/4 = 50% intelligible
Age 3	3/4 = 75% intelligible
Age 4	4/4 = 100% intelligible
Pediatric Intern	1/3 intelligible
PGY 2	2/3 intelligible
PGY 3	3/3 (100%) intelligible
Chief Resident	I better try to sound intelligible
Chairman	What's intelligible?
Professor Emeritus	2/4 = 50% intelligible

Stuttering

Stuttering can **be normal up to age 3 or 4**. It often disappears once vocabulary rapidly increases. Therefore, this is one of those cases where "normal and reassurance" is often the correct answer.

Persistence **beyond preschool age** will require a workup. Other indications for a workup would be: if stuttering persists for more than 6-8 weeks, if there is marked parental concern, or if there are associated symptoms such as facial tics. In such cases, a referral would be indicated.

Language Deficits

A bilingual home, a second child with sibs, and parents speaking for the child do not explain language delays. While this is debatable, you cannot debate dots and circles on the Boards. Serious language delay cannot be explained by these circumstances.

A hearing evaluation is the first thing to do with any language delay, and is often the answer on the Boards, especially if they mention a history of TORCH infections, hyperbilirubinemia, or meningitis.

Chronic hearing loss, including hearing loss due to chronic otitis media, not only impacts language development, it can also impact emotional development, as well as the ability to read. Hearing loss that begins after 5 has less of an impact than hearing loss that occurs before then.

Although it may seem counterintuitive, the most important intervention for language development in an infant with a congenital hearing loss is family involvement, including non-verbal communication. Family use of both verbal and nonverbal communication has been shown to have the most positive impact on language acquisition in children with hearing loss.

This is considered to be more important than specific formal interventions.

Developmental Screens

The "Denver Developmental School Readiness Screen," and anything with the word "screen," including screen "door", are just that – screens. They do not rule out anything; instead they identify which children may require further testing and workup.

Early Intervention

Infants and young children identified early with developmental delays will benefit from early intervention, the goal of which is to provide services to aid in developmental progress (such as speech therapy, occupational therapy, or physical therapy).

The Individuals with Disabilities Education Act (IDEA) outlines guidelines for the education of children in the United States who have developmental delays or other problems that may interfere with learning.

Part C of IDEA covers early intervention services for children under age 3 years. The goal of this program is to allow children to reach their developmental potential and improve cognitive outcome in some cases. Programs must be family-based and culturally relevant to the family.

Fading Fads and Assessing CAMs

Parents of children with developmental concerns, behavioral problems, or autism may sometimes turn to complementary and alternative medicine to help their child. Here are some things to keep in mind:

The Feingold diet has not been shown to be beneficial in managing ADHD or learning disabilities.

Likewise, sugar restriction has not been shown to be beneficial in managing or treating ADHD or other behavioral disorders.

However, sugar or candy should not be used as a reward for good behavior.

Megavitamin therapy has actually been shown to increase disruptive behavior, and certainly has no role in managing learning disabilities or behavioral problems.

For purposes of the boards, complementary or alternative medicine solutions for autism and other developmental disorders have not been proven to be effective. This includes *sensory integration therapy, eye exercises, chelation therapy, or hyperbaric oxygen chambers.*

Chapter 7

Nutrition

Fat Soluble Vitamins

Not Fat

The only vitamins that are **not** fat-soluble are vitamins B and C. Fat-soluble vitamins are the ones that come in the gelatin tablet with the oil in the center.

 The fat soluble vitamins can be remembered with the acronym FAKED (Fat-soluble - AKED).

Vitamins on a First Name Basis	
Vitamin	**Formal Name**
Vitamin A	Retinol
Vitamin D	Has many forms and variations which are way too boring to bog down this nice table. It gets to sit in its own "Teak Table on the deck" on the side.
Vitamin E	Tocopherol Just remember it as "Toke-of-**E**thanol" to remember it as vitamin E.
Vitamin K	Phylloquinone To help remember that the formal name of vitamin K is phylloquinone, remember the term "**File-O-Kanines:**" Picture a file cabinet full of dogs that are shaped like the letter "K." This will jog your memory that **phylloquinone is vitamin K**, if this is what they call it.

Water Soluble Vitamins

 The water-soluble vitamins include the B vitamins (all of them) and vitamin C.

Vitamins on a First Name Basis	
Vitamin	**Formal Name**
Vitamin B_1	Thiamine
Vitamin B_2	Riboflavin
Vitamin B_3	Niacin
Vitamin B_5	Pantothenic Acid MNEMONIC — Change to Pentothenic acid
Vitamin B_6	Pyridoxine MNEMONIC — Pyrido6ine
Vitamin B_9	Folate MNEMONIC — If a fool comes late it is benign (B_9)
Vitamin B_{12}	Cyanocobalamin
Biotin	Biotin (only has a formal name but is considered to be a B vitamin).
Vitamin C	Ascorbic Acid

Vitamin Deficiencies and Toxicities

Being familiar with the clinical presentations of all vitamin toxicities and deficiencies is worth spending time on, because it will certainly be worth several points on the exam. They will likely describe patients with classic symptoms. They will most likely be identified by their **formal names**, which you must link somehow to the vitamin letter. Fortunately, you've come to the right place because we have already done this for you.

Vitamin	Deficiency	Toxicity
Vitamin A (Retinol)	**Worldwide, vitamin A deficiency is the most common cause of blindness in young children.** With the formal name retinol so similar to "retina," it is easy to link this to blindness. Vitamin A deficiency can also lead to dryness of the eyes (AKA **xerophthalmia**), **nyctalopia** (a fancy word for night blindness, but the word you are likely to see on the exam), and complete blindness.	Vitamin A intoxication can result in intracranial hypertension (i.e. **pseudotumor cerebri).** MNEMONIC Picture a giant **A** causing intracranial pressure.
Vitamin B$_1$ (Thiamine)	B1 deficiency results in "**Beri Beri.**" This consists of mental confusion, peripheral paralysis, muscle weakness, tachycardia, and cardiomegaly. MNEMONIC Change it to "**Thigh-Man**" and picture two **giant #1's** in place of thighs to remember it is B$_1$ deficiency. **Too little thiamine** and the "**thighs become weak;**" Thigh-Man falls down, becomes **confused**, and his **heart races**.	There is no documented toxicity, except when it is **given IV in too large a dose**. I would not expect to see it on the exam.
Vitamin B$_2$ (Riboflavin)	B2 deficiency results in **anemia**, **angular stomatitis**, and **seborrheic dermatitis**. MNEMONIC Change it to "**Rib-O-Flavor:**" Ribs so good that they are eaten and only **2 (B$_2$)** are left (from the original 12). If you have only **2** ribs that is **SAD** = **S**tomatitis (remember it is angular for the picture section) **A**nemia **D**ermatitis (seborrheic) HOT TIP **Phototherapy** gobbles up riboflavin, so **preemies** on prolonged phototherapy are at risk for riboflavin deficiency. Thus phototherapy is ordered in 12-hour intervals. MNEMONIC Picture a premature baby with 2 letter B's to protect their eyes, to remember that phototherapy is associated with Vitamin B$_2$ deficiency risk.	Riboflavin toxicity is not typically tested.

Vitamin	Deficiency	Toxicity
Vitamin B$_3$ (Niacin)	Pellagra consists of 3 D's: **D**ermatitis, **D**iarrhea, and **D**ementia. Remember it as the *3D's of B$_3$*. *MNEMONIC* Remember the "Nice Scene." Picture a nice scene on a frozen lake. You are skating on the lake and have a cheery outlook because you think you will be free (=B3). You accidentally take "Pellagra" instead of Viagra® and now have Dementia, Diarrhea, and Dermatitis (from falling so many times). Skating with dementia leads to Vertigo with your tongue hanging out, resulting in glossitis – another finding in B$_3$ deficiency.	Toxicity can result in **vasodilation.**
Vitamin B$_6$ (Pyridoxine)	Swelling of the tongue, rash. Neuropathy when a patient is also given INH for TB.	**Neuropathy.**
Vitamin B$_9$ (Folate)	Large tongue and macrocytic anemia.	**Irritability.** *PERIL WARNING* When given for macrocytic anemia due to folate deficiency, it masks the B12 deficiency.
Vitamin B$_{12}$ (Cyanoco-balamin)	Macrocytic anemia. Bowel disease leading to pernicious anemia (due to poor absorption secondary to decreased intrinsic factor).	Expensive electric urine, but harmless.
Vitamin C (Ascorbic Acid)	Besides bleeding gums and scurvy (remember the stories of Columbus), they might also describe **leg tenderness and poor wound healing**.	Vitamin C is well tolerated even in large doses. However, it is escorted out the door through the kidneys, so **excessive mega doses can cause oxalate and cysteine nephro-calcinosis** (also known as kidney stones). *HOT TIP* It is one of the agents that can **trigger a hemolytic crisis** in a patient with **glucose-6-phosphate dehydrogenase deficiency**.

Vitamin	Deficiency	Toxicity
Vitamin E (Tocopherol)	Vitamin E deficiency consists of **hemolytic anemia in preemies** and neurological effects in older children. However, it would have to be a severely prolonged deficiency. MNEMONIC **Picture the E as a fork puncturing the red cells**, and the association with **ethanol** (see first page of this chapter) should remind you of the potential for **neurological damage.** **Vitamin E deficiency is characterized by neuropathies and muscle weakness**	Vitamin E toxicity is controversial and they should not ask, but if they do, liver toxicity is the answer.
Vitamin K (Mr. Phylloquinone to you)	Vitamin K deficiency results in **hemorrhagic disease of the newborn**, because vitamin K **does not cross the placenta well** and the **newborn can't produce it well because gut flora hasn't been established.** Therefore, vitamin K dependent factors are only 30% of normal in the first 2-3 days of life. HOT TIP **Breast fed babies are particularly vulnerable** because breast milk does not contain much vitamin K. PERIL WARNING They could describe a child, who is born at home, and **did not receive vitamin K at birth** and is being exclusively breast-fed and is bleeding. Your answer will be to **give vitamin K[1] followed by fresh frozen plasma[2]** if there is active bleeding. TAKE HOME MESSAGE They could ask right out, "What are the **vitamin K dependent factors**?" They are **2, 7, 9, and 10.**	Vitamin K toxicity is not often an issue and is never really tested on the exam.

---

[1] For production of vitamin K dependent factors, which are 2, 7, 9, & 10.

[2] For clotting factors right now.

CASE STUDY You are presented with a toddler who is noted to be quite yellow.

THE DIVERSION Buried in the question is the fact that this is a child who has eaten many foods rich in beta carotene,[3] such as carrots, sweet potatoes, and apricots. The child looks or is described as being yellow.

The sclerae and oral mucosa are not yellow. This is the key to answering the question correctly.

ANSWER REVEALED The child is not jaundiced or icteric, and therefore no further evaluation is necessary. Changing the diet might also be the correct answer to the question.

However, the decoy answer, "get a serum bili," is not correct.

PERIL WARNING **Isotretinoin**, used to treat acne in teens, is an analog of vitamin A; however, it is a **significant teratogen,** and is contraindicated in pregnant teens, so beware when this is part of the question. Pregnancy needs to be ruled out before isotretinoin is used.

Managing Vitamin D Toxicity

This results in the mobilization of calcium and phosphorus from bones and deposition into soft tissue. It is treated with **hydration**, correction of **Na and K depletion, and Lasix®**.

Vitamin D

Vitamin D Excess

Vitamin D excess results in disturbances in calcium metabolism, specifically **hypercalcemia** and **hyperphosphatemia**. In addition, it will produce non-specific signs such as **nausea, vomiting, and weakness.**

The more specific findings include **polyuria**, **polydipsia**, **elevated BUN**, **nephrolithiasis**, and **perhaps renal failure**. It can also be fatal.

MNEMONIC Symptoms of polydipsia, polyuria, and poor growth are **similar to diabetes**. **D**iabetes and vitamin **D** both have "**D**." In addition, vitamin D toxicity and diabetes can both result in kidney failure.

---

[3] Beta carotene is converted to vitamin A (retinol) by the body, and is therefore a precursor to vitamin A.

The Faces and Phases of Vitamin D

Just when you thought it was going to be easy, in walks vitamin D, along with all its aliases and accomplices. D has different numbers and each has its own name.

Vitamin	Formal Name	Mnemonic
Vitamin D_2	Ergocalciferol	It has 2 C's in the name; therefore, D_2.
Vitamin D_3	Cholecalciferol	It has 3 C's in the name; therefore, D_3.
25-hydroxy vitamin D	Calcidiol, which is hydroxylated in the liver[4]	There is only one liver; therefore, only one number.
1,25 hydroxy-calciferol[5]	This is the same as activated calcitriol, which is hydroxylated in the kidney	There are 2 kidneys, therefore, 2 hydroxy groups.

D is the only vitamin known to be converted to a hormone form. There is no dietary requirement when the child is sufficiently exposed to UV sunlight.

Vitamin D Deficiency

Rickets occurs with vitamin D deficiency before the bone epiphyses have closed. It can be diagnosed with **a lower 25 OH-vitamin D level and an elevated PTH level**. Radiological findings include wide wrists and metaphyseal flaring of the long bones.

The serum calcium and phosphorus levels may be normal in the face of rickets, so don't be tricked. However, *serum alkaline phosphatase levels will likely be elevated.*

Liver Disease and Rickets

When rickets occurs with chronic liver disease, it is not due to the lack of hydroxylation. **It is usually a result of reduced availability of bile salts in the gut and subsequent decreased absorption of vitamin D.**

The Ticket to Rickets

Here is what they will describe and what you will see:

Head/ Craniotabes: Delayed suture and fontanel closure, skull thickening, "frontal bossing," and bad tooth enamel.

Extremities: Widened physes of wrists and ankles, femoral/tibial bowing.

Chest: "Pigeon chest," rachitic rosary (the costochondral joints are enlarged). They will likely show this in the picture section.

Rickets can occur with liver disease.

 To remember that Rachitic Rosary is associated with Rickets, change it to "RICKETIC Rosary."

---

[4] 25-hydroxy vitamin D (25 (OH) D3).

[5] 1,25 dihydroxy vitamin D (1,25 (OH)2 D3 or 1,25 (OH)2 D as it is referred to in the illustration of Vitamin D and Calcium Metabolism.

Vitamin D Metabolism

Calcium Metabolism

Skin Door   Diet Door

Vitamin D2

Liver

25(OH)-D

Kidney

1,25(OH)2-D

Intestine   Bone   Kidney

Adequate Vit D = 🙂   Low Vit D = rickets

Dietary Ca, P

GI Tract   Vit D   Kidney

Ca, P

P

ECF

Ca, P

Bone

Dietary Ca, P

PTH

GI Tract   Kidney

Ca   P

Urine

ECF

Ca,P

Bone

PTH

Mineral Deficiency

Zinc: Acrodermatitis enteropathica

Copper: Menkes Kinky Hair syndrome

HOT TIP

Picture kinky hairs as hands grabbing pennies, to remind you that it is due to copper deficiency.

HOT TIP

A common finding in both vitamin B12 (**cyanocobalamin**) deficiency and vitamin B9 (**folate**) deficiency is **macrocytic anemia.**

Nutritional Needs

Caloric Needs

Caloric Requirements should be easy to remember. It is similar to calculating fluids:

- ❏ 100 kcal/kg (1st 10 kg)
- ❏ 50 kcal/kg (next 10 kg)
- ❏ 20 kcal/kg (any more kgs.)
- ❏ 1500 kcal for the first 20 kg, then 20 kcal/kg for each additional kg

Caloric intake for children is based on body surface area

The optimal caloric intake is based on a child's body surface area. This of course varies from child to child.

PERIL WARNING   The RDA (recommended daily allowance) is only a starting point for estimating the caloric requirements in children.

> ### Relationship between dietary protein and renal solute load in infants
>
> The infant's kidney cannot handle the same osmotic load of an adult during times of stress, even if:
>
> • an infant is receiving adequate nutrition
>
> • there are no increased insensible water losses
>
> • there is no evidence of renal failure
>
> They can still lose weight due to renal fluid loss as a result of increased solute load.

CASE STUDY   A 3 year old child whose caloric intake is consistent with the RDA is at the 5th percentile for weight.

THE DIVERSION   The question specifically notes that the child is taking the recommended daily caloric intake, with all other clinical criteria within normal limits. What steps can be taken to have the patient gain weight appropriately?

ANSWER REVEALED   The correct answer will be to increase the child's caloric intake. This is because this particular child's caloric requirements exceed the RDA. You need to know that the RDA is a ballpark figure for the general population, which may not apply to any particular patient.

Fat Storage in the Premature

Preemies have lower levels of fat storage and may have difficulty maintaining appropriate body temperature. Because of this, they expend more energy in heat production that term babies. Premature infants also require more energy for organogenesis and to develop fat stores.

All of this increases nutritional and energy requirements in comparison to term babies.

Nutrition Fruition/Nutritional Needs in the Newborn Period

Nutrition is a fairly large part of the exam. They love to ask detailed questions on the differences between formula and breast milk, formula and whole milk, whole milk and 5% fruit juice, fruit juice and scotch, blended scotch and single malt scotch – well, I got carried away there, but you get the picture.

Remember that both term and preterm infants require 100-120 kcal/kg/day. Of course, a preterm infant's requirement is closer to 120 and a large term infant's requirement is closer to 100.

However, if you were faced with a choice that states, "both term and preterm infants require 100-120 kcal/kg/day to grow," it would be correct.

Protein Requirements

Premature infants require *3.5 g/kg per day* in order to achieve growth and weight gain close to that expected in utero.

Full Term infants, on the other hand, grow well with protein intakes of approximately ***2.0 to 2.5 g/kg per day*** for the first 6 months.

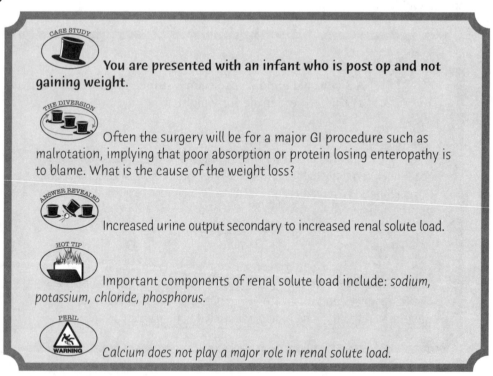

CASE STUDY You are presented with an infant who is post op and not gaining weight.

THE DIVERSION Often the surgery will be for a major GI procedure such as malrotation, implying that poor absorption or protein losing enteropathy is to blame. What is the cause of the weight loss?

ANSWER REVEALED Increased urine output secondary to increased renal solute load.

HOT TIP Important components of renal solute load include: *sodium, potassium, chloride, phosphorus.*

PERIL WARNING *Calcium does not play a major role in renal solute load.*

Fatty Acids

No cow's milk under 12 months. Nothing but whole milk should be given from age 1 until at least age 2. Children who are overweight should be on low fat milk after age 12 months. If they ask you to pick out an essential fatty acid, then **linoleic acid** will be the answer.

Formula for Success

Fluoride

Commercially available formula does not have adequate fluoride. This must be obtained from outside sources, such as drinking water.

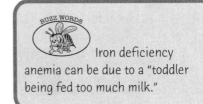

BUZZ WORDS

Iron deficiency anemia can be due to a "toddler being fed too much milk."

Ironing out the Need for Iron

You will be expected to iron out fact from fiction regarding iron fortified formula. The recommended concentration of iron in iron fortified formula is 12mg/L.

PERIL WARNING   Iron supplementation is not routinely required at birth since full term babies have adequate iron stores. It would, however, be required for those at high risk (e.g., LBW, preterm) in supplement form before 6 months of age, even in breast fed babies. All babies, including breast fed infants, should receive supplementation in their food (e.g., iron-fortified cereals), starting around 4-6 months of age.

CASE STUDY   You are doing a routine sports physical on a 16-year-old female. She has a hemoglobin of 11 and an SMR of 5. She proudly notes that she is a strict vegetarian.

What other physical findings would you expect to note in this patient?

THE DIVERSION   You will be tempted with choices such as tachycardia, marked pallor, weakness, and perhaps oral lesions. You will be tempted to pick these choices because they note that she is a vegetarian.

ANSWER REVEALED   The correct answer will be that no other physical findings should be expected. Vegetarians in general tend to have low iron stores. However, in this specific case, her hemoglobin is only consistent with mild iron deficiency anemia, and no other physical findings would be expected.

There is an association between obese children and adolescents and iron deficiency anemia.

 Low iron formula 1.5mg/L is not to be used. It will always be the incorrect choice.

 Iron fortified formula does not cause constipation. This is a trap often laid on the boards so beware.

CASE STUDY

An infant around 5-6 months of age who is on iron fortified formula (12mg/L) presents with constipation. How would you manage this problem?

THE DIVERSION

The question casually mentions that the infant is on iron fortified formula, 12mg/L. Here they are capitalizing on the myth that iron fortified formula causes constipation. One of the choices is to switch to "reduced iron fortified formula 1.5 mg/L."

ANSWER REVEALED

Do not change to low iron formula - this is incorrect.

• *Do not dilute the formula, this has nutritional consequences*
• *Do not change to whole milk*
• *Adding cereal will make the constipation worse*
• *The correct answer **will be to add fruit juice, to increase the osmotic load**.*

Formula Intolerance

Keeping Allergies Straight

Remember, with bona fide milk allergy there is a significant cross reactivity with soy-based formula. Therefore, elemental formula will be the correct answer.

DEFINITION

Formula intolerance also goes under the alias of "adverse reaction to formula," and therefore allergy is just one form of formula intolerance.

EITHER OR CHOICES

You are expected to know the differences between milk protein allergy (IgE-mediated), milk intolerance (non IgE-mediated), and lactose intolerance.

Both milk protein allergy and milk intolerance can cause rash, vomiting, and irritability (see GI Section).

Milk Protein Allergy is due to an IgE-mediated response, and presents with rash, vomiting, and irritability.

Lactose intolerance can cause irritability, but not vomiting or rash.

Lactose intolerance can be due to secondary lactase deficiency. This can occur following a GI infection, such as rotavirus.

This may be presented as an infant with bloating and worsening diarrhea after formula is reintroduced into the diet following an episode of viral gastroenteritis.

Most children who have GI infections do not develop secondary lactase deficiency. However, you need to be aware that this can occur.

Holding off on lactose-containing formula in a very young infant would be appropriate until diarrhea resolves. However, holding off on breastfeeding would not be the correct answer, even if lactase deficiency is hinted at in the question.

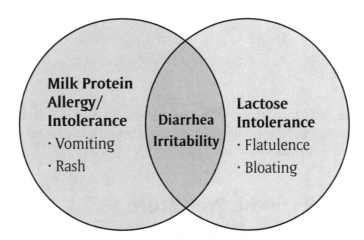

FPIES (Severe Milk Protein Intolerance)

FPIES is actually "food protein-induced enterocolitis syndrome," which is way too convoluted to include in the title heading. This is a **non IgE-mediated** severe cow milk protein (or other protein) intolerance.

FPIES typically presents in the first 3 months with either heme positive stools or hematochezia along with a normal abdominal exam.

Even though this is primarily due to cow milk intolerance, it can affect breast fed infants as well, because cow milk protein ingested by the mother can get into the breast milk.

Switching to soy formula will not be the correct answer since the symptoms frequently continue on soy formula. Therefore, the correct answer would be to switch to a **protein hydrolysate formula, or to completely eliminate the implicated protein from the mother's diet.**

Nutritional Deficiencies

Essential Fatty Acids

This will be described as "scaly dermatitis," with alopecia and thrombocytopenia.

Treatment would be with IV lipids, with a focus on linoleic acid.

Since this can easily be confused with other rashes, consider this: it is a fatty acid deficiency. Think of a thin fish with scales coming off (scaly rash) that turn into platelets (low platelet count) and, of course, the fish is then bald (alopecia).

Osteopenia/Rickets in the Premature

This is mainly due to poor phosphorus and calcium intake. Calcium and phosphorus are poorly absorbed in the gut of preemies, so large amounts must be given to compensate for this. This can lead to rickets in premature infants.

Vitamin E Deficiency

Vitamin E deficiency is often manifested as "hemolytic anemia," "peripheral edema," and "thrombocytosis."

Consider the triple E of vitamin E deficiency: **E**dema, **E**rythrocyte explosion (hemolytic anemia), and **E**levated platelet count.

Zinc Deficiency

This too is fair game on the Boards: "dry skin," "poor wound healing," and "perioral rashes" are your buzzwords.

Picture a dry mouth that does not heal well and turns into a Sink (Zinc).

Breast milk contains a protein which facilitates zinc absorption, so if you are presented with an infant with the above findings who was recently weaned from breast-milk, zinc deficiency is the most likely cause.

CASE STUDY

A 7 month old girl who was weaned from breast-milk one month ago now presents with facial dermatitis, including a similar rash on the hands and feet. In addition, the baby has been less energetic, with diarrhea and thin hair. The most likely cause of this is:

THE DIVERSION

The question suggests that this is due to milk allergy or milk intolerance.

ANSWER REVEALED

The correct answer is zinc deficiency. The key is to not fall for the diversionary implication of milk allergy. The pattern described, especially the thin hair coupled with the fact that the child was recently weaned from breast milk, is consistent with zinc deficiency.

Formula Facts

Which formula contains lactose? Lactose is found in:
- Human milk.
- Cow based formula.
- Evaporated cow milk.

Infants fed "non traditional" formula will suffer from nutritional deficiencies, especially on the boards, so watch for this description in the history.

Protein hydrolysate formula is indicated in infants with:
- Allergy to intact milk protein
- Allergy to soy protein

Nutritional Needs of the Premature

Preemies with RDS

If the mother of a preemie wants to breast-feed, the correct management is to have the mother pump so the milk is available for the infant. Breast-feeding can then begin when the baby is ready.

Vitamin D

The vitamin D requirements are higher in premature infants.

Vitamin E

Preterm infants taking formula high in polyunsaturated fatty acids must have vitamin E supplementation to avoid hemolysis.

Vitamin E deficiency can also have neurological consequences, including decreased deep tendon reflexes.

Too Young to Absorb Fat

Premature infants have a **decreased amount of bile acids,** which makes it **difficult for them to absorb long chain triglycerides** and **fat-soluble vitamins**.

Fat Facts

Difference in preterm and full term ability to digest fat:

Fat is absorbed less efficiently in premature babies; they can lose up to 20% of ingested fat through the stool. Medium chain triglycerides are absorbed better, since they do not require bile salts.

Preemie Formula – **50%** of **total fat** is from **medium chain triglycerides**.

Mature Breast Milk – **12%** of the **total fat** content is **medium chain triglycerides**.

 Breast milk does not contain or need a high amount of medium chain triglycerides because of its high absorptive abilities. Breast milk contains sufficient linoleic and linolenic acid, which are both essential (long chain) fatty acids.

Medium chain triglycerides enhance lipid absorption in formulas, but they are not sufficient to provide the essential fatty acids.

Phosphorus and Calcium

Inadequate phosphorus (often secondary to prolonged parenteral nutrition) in the very low birthweight preterm infant may result in demineralization of bone.

This may occur after 1 month of TPN. Typical lab findings would include normal serum calcium and phosphorus. However, **alkaline phosphatase** will be elevated.

Inadequate calcium can also lead to bone demineralization.

If excessive phosphorus is provided to a very low birthweight infant, it can lead to hypocalcemia, tetany, and seizures.

Milk: the Facts, the Breast, the Fiction

Breast Milk

Breast milk is good for virtually every reason. The AAP suggests exclusive breast-feeding until at least 6 months, and continued use of breast milk up to 12 months. The milk at the end of a breastfeeding session (hind milk) is higher in calories.

 Supplement with water? The answer they want is "No!"

Squeezing and Freezing

When pumping breast milk, the rule to remember is that it can be frozen for quite a while, but after it is thawed it needs to be used within 48 hours. And do not use the microwave.

There is no longer any need to sterilize formula bottles and water (provided well water is not being used),[6] no matter how much the grandmother in the question insists.

Cold tap water, rather than hot tap water, should be used to protect from lead contaminating the water.

Colostrum vs. Mature Milk

There are a variety of differences between colostrum and "mature" breast milk that could come up on the exam. Try to remember the following mind numbing facts for the exam!

Arachidonic Acid (AA) and **Docosahexaenoic acid (DHA)** – decrease in mature milk. This is true for mothers of premature babies as well. This is important for neurological development.

Zinc – Same as with AA, and is needed in premature infants especially to prevent skin lesions, poor wound healing, and decreased immune function.

Ergo-cholecalciferol – low levels in colostrum, which increases the risk for rickets.

The **H**ind milk is **H**igher in fat. (Hind milk is the milk at the end of the feeding).

The colostrum over the first few days postpartum is higher in protein, especially because of the high levels of immune globulins, including secretory IgA. This provides initial protection against infection. It is **yellow in color**, primarily because it is **high in carotene**. Colostrum provides a dose of enzymes that stimulate gut maturation and facilitates digestion, especially of fats. It also stimulates the gut to pass meconium (hence the frequent diaper changes).

	Colostrum	Mature Milk
Protein	More (2.3 g/dL)	Less (1.2 g/dL)
Fat	Low (1.7 g/dL)	High (4 g/dL)
Lactose	A bit less (6 g/dL)	A bit more (7g/dL)
Energy Content	Less (49 kcal/dL)	More (69 kcal/dL)
Minerals	Constant throughout lactation	Constant throughout lactation

---

[6] This assumes that "treated" municipal water is being used — not well water, which may not be treated enough.

Breast Milk vs. Cow's Milk

Breast milk contains more lactose and is, therefore, sweeter.[7]

Cow's milk contains a significantly **higher** amount of **phosphorus** than human milk. The infant kidney cannot get rid of it fast enough, and since phosphorus and calcium hate each other, when one goes up the other goes down. The result is **hypocalcemia**. Remember that hypocalcemia can occur if they describe an infant on cow's milk prior to one year of age.

"Hypo - cow – lcemia."

Breast is Best, but Know the Facts

It is safe to assume that breast milk is advantageous for everything. However, here are a few exceptions to watch out for.

When Breast Isn't Best

There are times when breast-feeding is contraindicated, and this is very much fair game.

Metronidazole - It is important to note that Flagyl® (metronidazole) is the most effective treatment of *Trichomonas vaginalis*; however, it is contraindicated with breast-feeding. Therefore, mothers taking this drug must stop breast-feeding during treatment.

Diazepam – is sufficiently concentrated and absorbed by a breast-feeding infant to cause him/her to be shlogged. Therefore, it is contraindicated. Any medication with sedative effects can make its way into breast milk.

Breast fed infants are at risk for vitamin D deficiency.

Breast milk contains **little vitamin K and can contribute to hemorrhagic disease of the newborn,** especially if they have not received IM vitamin K at birth.

Technetium -99: the half life is only 6 hours, and therefore breast-feeding need only be stopped for 24-48 hours. This is an exception to the radioactive contraindication to breast-feeding rule.

> **BAD BREAST**
>
> **Contraindications to breast-feeding**
>
> **B** Bad Bugs (TB)
> **A**ntithyroid Meds
> **D**iseases/Sexually Transmitted=HSV lesions on Breast and HIV
>
> **B**ad Bugs=CMV and TB too
> **R**adioactive and other Chemicals=Radioactive Meds and Chemotherapy
> **E**rrors of Metabolism, Galactosemia, PKU, Urea Cycle Defects (in the baby)
> **A**nti-Giardia (Meds like Flagyl®)
> **S**ulfonamides
> **T**etracycline

---

[7] Makes you wonder how they know this. Anyone drinking breast milk shouldn't be verbal enough to describe it!

Disorders that may interfere with breast-feeding

See the Bad Breast Sidebar. However, don't be fooled by the following:

 Don't be fooled into picking **candidiasis**, **contact dermatitis**, **fibrocystic breast disease**, or **mastitis**. Breast-feeding, if properly managed, *can* continue with each of these conditions.

However, inverted nipples can result in unsuccessful breast-feeding.

Breast Milk vs. Formula and Cow's Milk

They love to ask the differences that nobody remembers.[8] Keeping your curds and whey straight will keep the spider away.

	Human Milk	Cow Milk	Modified Cow Formula
Protein Concentration	0.9 g/dL	3.5 g/dL	1.4 g/dL
Whey: Casein Ratio	70% Whey 30% Casein MNEMONIC Human milk is WHEY better	20% Whey 80% Casein	Variable
Type of Whey Protein	Alpha lactalbumin	Beta lactalbumin	
Extra Goodies	The whey protein contains larger amounts of lactoferrin, lysozyme, and IgA These are digested more easily and promote gastric emptying		
Minerals (calcium, phosphorus, iron)	Lower		Higher
Calcium: Phosphorus Ratio	2:1		1.5: 1
Iron Absorption	Better		Worse
Vitamins ABC	Same		Same

---

[8] And this probably includes the drones writing the questions.

	Human Milk	Cow Milk	Modified Cow Formula
Vitamins DEK	Lower		Higher (clinically insignificant in mothers who picnic at the beach)[9]
Renal Solute load	Lower		Higher
Physiological advantages	More Lipase		

Iron

While *breast milk is lower in iron,* it has a higher "bioavailability"[10] during the first four months of life. Remember that iron stored during the fetal life compensates for any iron deficiency in breast milk, up until 4 months.

Watch how they ask the question. If they ask which contains more iron, the answer will be formula. However, if they ask which is a better source, or which results in better absorption, the answer will be breast milk.

Lactose and Calories

Both standard formula and breast milk are **lactose**-based and have the caloric content 20 kcal/oz = 20 kcal/30cc = 0.67 kcal/cc.

Protein

Cow's milk is higher in protein content (roughly 3% vs. 1%).

Although cow's milk contains more protein than human milk, this is a case of quality over quantity. The protein quality differs between cow and human milk, as outlined in the previous table.

The protein requirement of newborns is approximately 2.0-3.0 g/kg/day, whereas the protein requirement of preemies is approximately 3.0-4.0 g/kg/day.

Negative nitrogen balance in very low birthweight infants is to be avoided, since it causes weight loss. **Therefore, they need a lot of non-protein calories.**

Subtraction by Addition

Enhancing the caloric content of formula is not always good.

When mixing formula, adding more powder than is indicated will increase the protein load, which stresses the kidneys. Because of this, lipid and carbohydrate supplements are available.

Adding carbohydrate supplement can lead to diarrhea.

Adding lipid supplement may increase the risk for diarrhea or delay gastric emptying.

The bottom line is, anything that increases the caloric content beyond 30 kcal/oz will be incorrect.

---

[9] In other words mothers who have an adequate diet and get sunlight exposure.
[10] Iron in breast milk is absorbed better than iron in formula.

For very low birthweight infants, the goal is to prevent negative nitrogen balance.

 Whey is WAY better for infants and WEIGHS heavier in the protein content of human milk.

Fat Content

Cow's milk is roughly 3-4% fat, and human milk varies with Mom's diet (similar to cow's milk).

Antibody

High concentrations of IgA and other antibodies present in breast milk, protect against infectious disease, including local GI immunity.

Lactose-derived oligosaccharides inhibit bacterial adhesions to mucosal surfaces, therefore reducing the risk of bacterial infection. This is the case with both colostrum and mature milk.

 "Lactose" derived: picture bacteria that "lack toes" to adhere to mucosal surfaces.

Nutrition and Weight

Weight Gain/Full Term Newborn

After the initial weight loss during the first few days of life, the **average full-term newborn will gain 20-30 g/day.** If you are presented with a mother who complains that her child isn't growing, and the weight gain is in range (20-30 g/day), the answer will be, "reassure the mother." The caloric requirement for a newborn is close to 100 kcal/kg/day, and this is what you will use to assess whether a child is taking in adequate calories (should this be included in the question).

 They could give this information in pounds, so be prepared to divide by 2.2.

Weight Gain/Preemie

Preemies can be expected to gain 15-20 g/day on 120 kcal/kg/day.

Early Feeding of Solid Foods

You could be presented with a grandmother pushing for early introduction of solid foods,[11] while the mother is perfectly happy exclusively breast-feeding for the first 6 months of life. Aside from fueling the rivalry with grandma again, there are other good reasons for not introducing solid foods too early. Feeding solid foods such as cereals to breastfed infants before 6 months of age increases the likelihood of gastrointestinal infection. In addition, low amylase levels in the infant gut make it more difficult to digest solid foods.

Previously it had been believed that introducing solids early increased the chances of developing food allergies and obesity. This is now considered to be controversial.

The introduction of solid foods does not help an infant sleep through the night.

Weight/High and Low in Adolescent Females

If they present you with a case of an adolescent with a weight issue, the answer they want is to "ask her what she thinks about her weight".

Obesity

Overweight is defined as a BMI between the 85th and 95th percentiles for age.

Obesity has been defined as a BMI greater than the 95th percentile for age.

Severe Obesity is defined as a BMI greater than the 99th percentile for age.

A child who is **obese at age 6 has a 25% chance** of being obese as an adult, and a child who is **obese at age 12 has a 75% chance** of being obese as an adult.[12]

Obesity due to exogenous sources[13] does result in the teen being *tall* with advanced *bone age*. If they are "fat" due to hormonal/genetic (or **endogenous**) reasons, they are usually **short with delayed bone age**.

If no bone age is given, or other symptoms are described, consider Cushing syndrome as a possible explanation for obesity.

---

[11] "Back in my day, we started Hamburger Helper® at 2 weeks," is a common claim.

[12] A child who is obese at age 35 has a 100% chance of being an obese adult.

[13] Commonly known as overeating.

Medical Explanation

While there are medical explanations for obesity, a workup is not warranted if they describe a child who is obese with an unremarkable physical exam, normal linear growth, and normal developmental milestones.

The most common metabolic explanation would be hypothyroidism. However, overweight children who have an otherwise-normal physical exam and normal linear growth do not require routine testing.

If they present an obese child with small hands, hypogonadism, delayed developmental milestones, and/or cognitive deficits, they may be describing Prader-Willi syndrome or Bardet-Biedel syndrome.

Obesity and Fitting into Genes

When we see an obese child and obese parent, it isn't always the food they eat. **Genetics does play a role**.

Parental obesity makes it twice as likely that a child younger than 10 will be obese as an adult. This is the case even if the child isn't obese, but obesity in childhood certainly increases the risk. Biology seems to play an important role, since there is a correlation even in adopted children. Identical twins end up with similar weights, even when raised in different homes or even different states.

Despite this, *the most common cause of obesity is excessive food intake.*

Sweating to the Oldies and Treatment of Obesity

How many nutritionists does it take to change a light bulb? Answer: Just one, but the bulb has to want to be changed.

The same applies to the lifestyle changes needed to treat obesity. The child and the family have to recognize a problem and want to change.

It is a 3-pronged approach, including changing diet, increasing exercise, and modifying behavior.

Diet has to be changed without impacting growth. This may be easier if snacks and sugary drinks are eliminated first.

Exercise regimens are most effective when combined with dietary changes.

Modifying behavior includes support inside and outside the family.

Since "Sweatin' to the Oldies" with Richard Simmons will not be one of the answers, and fenfluramine (Fen-Phen) and dextro fenfluramine are no longer considered safe for adults, let alone children, these will not be the correct answers.

Since the roots of obesity can be found in childhood, **the best obesity therapy available for children is prevention**. For children, the only effective method is **behavior modification, along with diet and appropriate exercise**.

The Health Risks of Obesity

Obesity is not just a cosmetic issue. With obesity, there are loads of health risks involved. The list is long and includes such items as **depression, avascular necrosis of the hip, diabetes, hypertension, cardiac disease,** and **osteoarthritis** secondary to the strain on joints, especially those of the lower extremities.[14] While depression is associated with obesity, it is unclear if the obesity causes the depression or the depression causes the obesity.

Any child who is noted to be drinking a lot of diet sodas (high phosphoric acid content) is at high risk for osteopenia. If the child has been treated with steroids, the risk is even higher. The best way to reduce the risk for fractures would be vitamin D and calcium supplements.

Nutritional Deficiencies – Kwashiorkor and Marasmus

These are not common in the US, but are popular on the Boards, in refugee camps, and at communes everywhere. You will need to be able to distinguish the two.

Kwashiorkor

This is strictly a **protein** deficiency. That is why they will depict a child with a "pot belly" from starvation. Other physical signs may include pitting edema, rash, thin/frail hair, pallor, and overall thin appearance.

The edema part is easy enough, because low protein would result in less intravascular osmotic pressure, causing edema. As for

Vegan Wagon

Children placed on vegan diets are at risk for vitamin B12 deficiency. If you are presented with a child taking goat's milk, they are at risk for folate deficiency.

Breastfeeding mothers who are vegans should be taking prenatal vitamins with B12 to prevent deficiency in their infant.

Non-breastfed vegan infants should receive iron fortified soy (since milk is derived from animals and on the banned list for vegans) formula.

---

[14] Also known as the legs.

the name—kwashiorkor—think of it as **"squash-I-kor."** Squash is low in protein, so if that's all you ate, you would be protein-deficient.

Marasmus

This is a **general nutritional deficiency. Therefore, the hallmarks are muscle wasting without edema.** They are underweight and their **hair is normal**.

There can also be a combination of the two, but they will most likely expect you to recognize one or the other and that one is usually Kwashiorkor, since its features are the most distinctive.

NG Tube Feeding, What is NG (Not Good) About It?

Whenever possible, enteral feedings are preferable to parenteral feedings.

Parenteral feedings via a central line are indicated as follows:

When enteral or oral feedings cannot be administered for 7 days or more.

When partial oral feedings and standard peripheral IV either cannot meet nutritional requirements or will be needed for prolonged periods of time.

Regardless, in infants some enteral feedings should maintained unless contraindicated. Otherwise infants may lose the will and/or ability to feed orally. Prolonged periods without enteral nutrition also leave the GI mucosa more vulnerable to infection.

Here it is very important to read the question. If they ask what is the **most common complication** of nasogastric feeding, the answer is **diarrhea**. The second most common complication is GE reflux. If elemental formula is used, this risk is reduced considerably. **The diarrhea is rarely severe enough to cause dehydration**.

If they ask what the most **severe** complication is, the answer is **vomiting with aspiration**. This is why it is important to read the question and know the details cold. Also, remember **ostomy feedings** can result in **wound infections**.

Bolus or Continuous – Which is Better?

· **Infants who have gastroesophageal reflux** may respond better to continuous feeds and gain weight better. After a short period of continuous feeds, the vomiting and reflux may stop. They can then tolerate regular PO feedings.

· **Children with Crohn's disease** may need continuous NG feedings, which is helpful in reversing growth failure and inducing remission.

· **Children with malabsorption syndrome** also do better with continuous feedings.

· **Continuous is better for infants who have congenital heart disease.** These infants have increased nutritional demands, and often experience delayed gastric emptying and early satiety. Therefore, bolus feedings can lead to malnourishment and delay of corrective surgery. They need to get fattened up as quickly as possible.

Bolus is better for infants with oral motor discoordination, as long as there are no gut responses, gastric residuals, or evidence of malabsorption or dumping syndrome.

Nutrition in Specific Diseases

Liver Disease

Patients with liver disease have decreased delivery of bile acids, resulting in malabsorption of fat-soluble vitamins such as A,D,E, and K. This is especially the case with cholestatic disease. An example of the potential consequences could be an increased risk for rickets.

If ascites or portal hypertension is an issue, fluid restriction is in order. This means a more concentrated formula (and these formulas can be pretty repulsive), so sometimes NG or gastrostomy feedings are a necessary option. Maintaining adequate caloric intake is crucial to reduce the risk for growth failure.

Heart Failure

Patients with heart failure need to have their caloric intake increased while restricting fluids. The solution is to increase the concentration of the formula, which increases caloric density without increasing fluid, resulting (hopefully) in appropriate weight gain. These children are often also on diuretics to balance the tendency for fluid overload.

Renal disease

Patients in acute renal failure tend to be malnourished. In these children, 70% of calories should come from carbohydrates, and lipids should comprise less than 20%. Protein intake may be up to 0.5 – 2 g/kg/day. Infants in renal failure require low phosphorus formula.

Malignancies

Meeting the nutritional needs of children with malignancies is important to their response to treatment. Children with adequate nutrition at the onset of treatment may have reduced risk for infection and reduced severity of chemotherapy side effects.

Neurologically Impaired Patients

Neurologically impaired pediatric patients are at higher risk for GERD and are more prone to ill effects when fundoplication surgery is implemented.

Wound Healing

Adequate caloric intake, especially protein, is essential to wound healing. Vitamins C, A, zinc, and iron are especially important.

Food Allergies

Severe diet restriction in response to multiple food allergies will likely be the wrong answer, due to the nutritional hazards of diet restriction. In infants, for example, substituting rice milk for standard formula may result in vitamin D, calcium, protein, and fatty acid deficiency.

Calcium and vitamin D deficiency may occur in older children restricting dairy intake in response to lactose intolerance.

CASE STUDY You are evaluating a 5-year-old boy with a 3-day history of diarrhea and vomiting. He is now tolerating a small amount of fluids, although his vomiting is still intermittent. On physical examination, his mouth is pasty and he has good bounding pulses and a heart rate of 156 beats per minute.

What would be the most appropriate management in this patient?

THE DIVERSION You could be given several choices that will take advantage of clinical urban myths, including IV fluids in the ER, admission and bowel rest, and discharge on a bland "BRAT" diet especially since the child is experiencing "intermittent vomiting."

ANSWER REVEALED *The correct answer would be oral rehydration and discharge home with a regular diet as soon as it is tolerated. The BRAT diet lacks adequate nutrition. Diluting formula is also incorrect.* However, the decoy answer "get a serum bili" is not correct.

If the gut functions, it should be used. Whenever possible, enteral nutrition trumps parenteral nutrition

Food Additives

MYTH Artificial flavors and colors have not been proven to have any role in the development of ADHD. However, artificial flavors and colors may have a role in causing urticaria and angioedema.

Commercial Baby Foods vs. Home Prepared Foods

For home-prepared foods, several precautions are necessary:

- Foods should be cleaned and pureed so there are no solid chunks inadvertently left behind.
- Food should be fully cooked
- Served fresh or frozen for later
- No salt seasoning and, of course, no honey should be added

PERIL WARNING You might be tempted to believe that home prepared foods reduce the risk for food allergies, but once again, Grandma is wrong, and this is not the case.

Chapter 8

Preventive Pediatrics

Prevention is a big part of general pediatrics, so proper guidance and knowledge in this area is emphasized on the Boards. The nice part is that there are a few basic facts that are asked year after year.[1]

Lead Exposure

Lead levels should be drawn at **1 and 2 years of age, regardless of where the child is living.**

A sign of lead poisoning could be "**lead lines**" (calcification lines on bone x-ray). "**Basophilic stippling**" on CBC is another of the key words.

Lead levels as low as 10 mcg/dL can result in cognitive deficit, and should therefore be followed.

Lead levels at 45 mcg/dL or higher would require chelation therapy.

> **Leading the Way to Diagnosing Lead Poisoning**
>
> Symptoms and signs of lead poisoning include:
> - Headache
> - Irritability
> - Constipation
> - Lethargy
> - Microcytic anemia

Lead Levels	Signs and Symptoms	Intervention
10-20 mcg/dL	Mild cognitive delay	Education on lead exposure, environmental control measures, and continued lead level monitoring
Greater than 60mcg/dL	Severe toxicity / headaches, encephalopathy, lead lines on the gingiva, and/or anemia	Chelation

---

[1] For example, the most effective way to prevent drowning is a fence around the pool.

Lead levels are helpful in tracking recent exposure to lead, instead of chronic accumulation of lead.

While a capillary sample is adequate for screening purposes, it is not acceptable to base treatment on this. The lead level needs to be confirmed with a venous sample.

In addition to a **venous blood level** additional confirmation can be obtained with a

- FEP Level
- Abdominal film
- X-ray of Long bones

DTaP and Tdap and the end of Td

The DTaP vaccine is given at 2, 4, 6, and 15 months[2] and at the kindergarten visit. The most common adverse effects of DTaP are local erythema, mild fever, and irritability.

> ### Age Counts
>
> DTaP immunization is based on postnatal age, even for premies. Therefore, you do not adjust the immunization schedule for prematurity.

Take that Tdap

Just when you thought it was safe to memorize, the DTaP is not used in anyone older than age 7. They do not require the higher dose of diphtheria toxoid.

DTaP, Td, Tdap, and DT - sneaky! The rules and nomenclature have changed at dizzying rates.

The recommendations for adolescents and vaccination during wound management have changed. Many of these changes are due to the increased risk for pertussis both in older children and adults, and the young'uns they may infect.

Below you will find much of the important information in digest format.

Routine Immunization of Adolescents

Adolescents 11-18 years old should receive a single dose of Tdap if they have completed the DTaP immunization series in childhood. This should preferably be given between the ages of 11-12 years.

---

[2] The 4th dose can be given as early as 12 months of age, provided 6 months have elapsed since the 3rd dose was given.

This replaces the Td booster that was previously given. The commercial names for the licensed vaccines are Boostrix® and Adacel®. The two brands can be used interchangeably.

If given previously, a period of 5 years is recommended between the time they received the Td vaccine and the Tdap vaccine, to avoid local and systemic reactions to the vaccine.

Tdap and MCV4 can be given to adolescents during the same visit.

If you are catching up on vaccines, you must administer multiple doses of the same vaccine at least 6 weeks apart.

Wound Management

Clean wounds

TIG (tetanus immune globulin) would not be indicated for clean wounds under any circumstances.

If the immunization status is unknown or a child has received less than 3 tetanus vaccines, they need to receive a tetanus vaccine.

If more than **10 years** has passed since the last vaccine was given, then a booster is indicated.

Dirty wounds

If you are presented with a patient who sustained a "dirty wound" and they have received less than 3 tetanus vaccines or the history is unknown, then a tetanus vaccine and TIG are indicated.

If more than **5 years** has past since the last tetanus vaccine was given, a booster is indicated.

When tetanus toxoid is indicated, adolescents age 11-18 should receive a single dose of Tdap rather than Td. That is the preferred management if they have not received a previous Tdap.

However, if the adolescent received Tdap in the past or if Tdap is not available, then Td can be given instead. If TIG is indicated but not available, then IV immune globulin (IVIG) is given.

If a patient has not completed the primary series, then treatment of wounds should include tetanus toxoid-containing vaccination, as well as passive immunization with **tetanus immune globulin if the wound is dirty**. Dirty wounds would include those with risk of contamination from feces, dirt, or saliva or those resulting in severe injuries such as in the case of burns, frostbite, or crush injuries.

Catch-up Immunizations (diptheria, tetanus, and pertussis style)

You are expected to be familiar with appropriate catch-up immunizations in a variety of settings. This was complicated enough when the vaccines were a stationary target. They are even more complicated now. However, you should be able to keep up if you keep the following in mind:

- If the first dose of DTaP was given before **12 months of age, 4 doses** are needed (at least 4 weeks between doses 1, 2, and 3 and at least 6 months between doses 3 and 4).

- If the first dose was given **after 12 months of age**, only **3 doses** are needed (at least 4 weeks between doses 1 and 2, and at least 6 months between doses 2 and 3).

Children ages 7 – 18

- **Tdap** should be substituted for a **single dose** of Td in the catch-up series

- **Tdap** should be the booster for children aged 10 through18; use Td for other doses

Remember that the last two doses in the catch-up series should be given six months apart.

4 weeks are always required between doses 1 and 2.

These rules apply where the immunization status is truly known. If there is a possibility of prior immunization, then tetanus and diphtheria toxoid antibody concentrations can be measured, and no further immunization is necessary until adolescence (Tdap booster) if immunity is adequate.

DTaP is not indicated for children aged 7 or older. However, if DTaP were to be given to a child older than age 7 it **would** count as the adolescent Tdap booster. Bascially any doses of DTaP previously given can be counted as part of the Tdap/Td series.

DTaP starts with "D for Diapers"; Tdap starts with "T for Teens".

Precautions and Contraindications for Tdap

Contraindications

The following are contraindications to administering Tdap.

Serious allergic reaction (These cases should be referred to an allergist to confirm the allergy and to assess the need for possible desensitization).

Encephalopathy within 7 days of receiving pertussis-containing vaccine (not a contraindication for Td, however)

There must be no other identifiable cause for the reaction.

Precautions

The following are precautions to administering the Tdap and DTaP vaccines.

- **Guillain-Barré syndrome** 6 weeks or less after a previous tetanus toxoid vaccine (Tdap is preferred if absolutely necessary).
- **Progressive neurological disorder** – The primary concern is the pertussis component. Therefore, if absolutely necessary, then Td is preferred. If pertussis vaccination is necessary, then Tdap is still preferred.
- **Deferring the vaccine** – The following would be reasons to defer or postpone the vaccine.
  - Moderate or severe acute illness - defer until resolved
  - History of severe arthus hypersensitivity reaction after a previous dose- consider the implicated component (tetanus or diphtheria), and assess immunity if appropriate. Otherwise, defer until 10 years has passed since the previous dose.

Deceptively fine for giving Tdap and DTaP

THE DIVERSION

The following conditions might easily be misconstrued as contraindications or precautions for administering Tdap. However, there is no problem in administering this vaccine safely when indicated.

- History of **extensive limb swelling** (that was not part of an arthus reaction) after administering the vaccine
- **Stable neurological conditions,** including well-controlled seizures and cerebral palsy

---

Tap Dancing in Pregnancy

It is important to note that pregnancy is not a contraindication for Tdap or Td.

TAKE HOME MESSAGE

Therefore, if you are presented with a pregnant teenager on the exam, indications for Tdap and Td would be the same for every other teen they might present on the exam.

Close family contacts of newborns should be immunized if their immune status for pertussis is lacking or unknown.

· **Brachial neuritis**
· **Contact allergy to latex gloves**
· **Pregnancy/breast-feeding**
· **Immunosuppression**
· **Minor illnesses including antibiotic use**

History of an **anaphylactic reaction to latex would be a contraindication to the standard vaccine**. However, the single dose Boostrix® and Adacel® are latex-free.

History of Pertussis

If an adolescent between ages 11-18 years has a history of pertussis, he/she should still receive Tdap immunization.

Hib

The next time you are confronted with an anti-immunization groupie in real life or on the boards, remember these cold facts:

Before the introduction of the Hib vaccine

· 1 in 200 kids would develop invasive Hib disease before the age of 5
· Over half of these patients would have meningitis
· This was associated with a 5% mortality rate with an even higher morbidity rate

The Hib vaccine has greatly reduced the incidence of invasive disease caused by Hib, including meningitis and epiglottitis. [3]

Children are at risk for Hepatitis B at the following turning points:

1. Intrapartum

2. Early childhood (household contacts or group care facilities)

3. Adolescence (sexually transmitted and IV drug use)

Hepatitis B Vaccine

Hepatitis B infection is a major cause of liver disease, including **hepatocellular carcinoma**. To head the disease off at the pass, all children receive immunization against hepatitis B.

In 1/3 of cases of Hepatitis B, no identifiable risk factors are identified.

---

[3] Of course, the incidence of epiglottitis on the board exam is as high as it has ever been.

HOT TIP

In addition, children infected with hepatitis B virus have a much higher rate of long-term complications.

DEFINITION

The first dose is typically given at birth (prior to discharge from the nursery), the second dose at 1-2 months, and the third dose 6-18 months after the first dose.

HOT TIP

If you are presented with ANY child or adolescent who has not been completely immunized, you should begin or complete the 3-part series.

PERIL WARNING

The only absolute contraindication to Hepatitis B vaccination is severe allergic reaction to a prior dose. Being pregnant and/or having an autoimmune disease (e.g., SLE) are NOT contraindications, and these individuals can be vaccinated.

HOT TIP

If the mother is infected with hepatitis B (HBsAg positive) or has unknown hepatitis status, the newborn should also receive *hepatitis B immunoglobulin* in addition to the routine immunization.

Infants born to HBsAg positive mothers should have their post vaccination status verified by serologic testing. Other high risk groups should also have serologic testing done to confirm immunity after the Hep B vaccine series. These include immunocompromised patients, hemodialysis patients, and those whose jobs place them at high risk, such as health care workers and prostitutes. That is a curious linkage, to say the least.

> ## DTaP-HepB-IPV Combination
>
> Some important considerations for the combination vaccine are:
> - It cannot be used for those 7 years old or older. It is only approved for the primary series, and not to be used as the booster dose at kindergarten or later.
> - It cannot be used prior to 6 weeks of age, and therefore cannot be used for the birth dose of hepatitis B vaccine.

Hepatitis B vaccine in Preemies

It is recommended that preemies weighing less than 2 kg who have HBsAg negative mothers receive Hep B vaccine within 30 days or before discharge, whichever is first.

Preemies weighing less than 2 grams with HBsAg positive mother should receive Hep B vaccine **and HBIG** within 12 hours of delivery.

The same applies if the hepatitis status of the mother cannot be confirmed within 12 hours.

The birth vaccine in infants weighing less than 2 kg does not count toward completion of the series.

Hepatitis B Vaccination

You are expected to know the different indications for HBIG revaccination given various exposures. Follow these rules:

Hepatitis B Requirements in the Event of a Needle Stick

Infants and other unvaccinated folks	They get HBIG (just to be sure), and start the Hep B series.
If they received full series and are antibody positive (+)	They are fine and need nothing more.
If they received full series and are antibody negative (-)	Pretty much considered unvaccinated, so they are treated as such; they get **HBIG and full revaccination.**
Unknown	Pretty easy: test for antibody. If negative, give HBIG and start series.

Meningococcal Vaccine

Since 2005, the new kid on the block is the new and somewhat improved MCV4 vaccine against meningococcemia. The old vaccine was the MPSV 4, polysaccharide model.

The new and improved MCV4 is supposed to provide improved, longer lasting immunity than the old model and reduce the carrier state. However, it still provides protection against the same strains (A, C, Y and W-135).

More than half of meningococcal disease in infants is caused by the B subtype, for which the vaccine provides no protection. This has been asked on previous exams.

Think of **B** as the **B**ad strain of meningococcus, most common in **B**abies.

Routine Immunization for Meningococcemia

Routine immunization against meningococcemia with the **MCV4** vaccine is indicated for the following:

1) Pre-adolescents at the 11-12 year visit.

2) Adolescents at high school entry (or 15 years of age, whichever occurs first), if not previously immunized

3) Previously unvaccinated patients entering freshman college **dormitories**.

Special Considerations

Children with HIV infection

Children with HIV infection can receive the MCV4 vaccine if they are over the age of two.

Children 2-10 years at increased risk

This would include children with terminal complement deficiency, asplenia (including functional), or those who are traveling to regions where meningococcal disease is prevalent (take note if you are planning a trip to Burkina Faso). Prior receipt of MPSV4: These children should receive MCV4 if they are still at risk and it has been 3 years since receipt of MPSV4.

MCV4 is administered IM.
MPSV4 is administered SQ

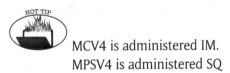

Human Papilloma Virus Vaccine

At the time of the publication of this book, the following are the recommendations for immunization of females against human papilloma virus.

Gardasil® is the trade name for the vaccine

The current recommended age for vaccination is females aged 11-12. However, the vaccine can be administered in girls as young as 9.

The HPV vaccine is now also recommended for males, since HPV is an STD; this provides protection against anal cancer.

Catch-up vaccination is recommended for females between the ages of 13-26 if they have not been previously vaccinated.

Vaccination is not considered to be a substitute for routine cervical cancer screening. Therefore, vaccinated females should go through cervical cancer screening according to recommended schedules.

MMR

Since the introduction of the MMR vaccine, the incidence of measles, mumps, and rubella have decreased by 99%! The vaccine is given between 12-15 months of age, with a booster at school entry. Vaccines given before age 12 months for travel or during an outbreak do not count toward completion of the series.

The following points are worth remembering:

- The second dose of MMR is given at age 4–6 years
- MMR can be given at any visit *as long as at least 4 weeks have elapsed since the first dose*
- Both doses must be given at 12 months of age or later
- If the 2nd dose is missing it should be given before age 11 or 12
- College students who received only 1 dose require a booster dose

Timing is everything

> **CASE STUDY**
>
> **If you are presented with a 7 month old infant who is exposed to measles, what should you do?**
>
> **THE DIVERSION**
>
> You could be presented with all sorts of choices. If you pick one of the diversions, you won't even get one "measly point" toward passing the boards! Here is the correct way to answer a question which tests your knowledge of this protocol.
>
> **ANSWER REVEALED**
>
> If given within 72 hours[4] of exposure, the measles vaccine will protect against infection. This rule applies to infants who are at least 6 months: therefore, a 7 month old infant falls into this category.
>
> If the exposure is greater than 72 hours but less than 6 days, measles immunoglobulin should be given.

In addition, it is important to note that any infant between ages 7 and 11 months traveling to a part of the world where measles is endemic would need to be immunized. This would be considered short term immunization, and they would need to resume the regular immunization schedule for MMR at the appropriate age (meaning that such an infant would receive three doses of MMR).

PERIL WARNING — After immune globulin is given, the child should still receive the MMR vaccine, **but not until 5-6 months after the after the immune globulin was given. The immune globulin would interfere with active immunity;** this is a biological case of passive aggression, where passive immunity blocks active immunity. MMR may not be given within 4 weeks of other live vaccines, including varicella and live intranasal influenza vaccines.

BUZZ WORDS — Up to 15% of kids who receive MMR will develop a high fever (>103) that occurs within 12 days after vaccine administration and lasts 1-2 days. 5% also will develop a rash during the same time frame. The correct answer will be "reassurance" if you should be presented with such a scenario on the exam.

---

4 Which to most of us is also known as 3 days, so put down the calculator, already!

Contraindications

The absolute contraindications to MMR administration are:

(1) Severe allergic reaction to a vaccine component

(2) Pregnancy

(3) Severely immunocompromised (e.g., chemotherapy, AIDS)

(4) History of life-threatening anaphylactic reactions to neomycin or gelatin would be contraindications to MMR vaccination

The following are NOT contraindications:

(1) Positive TB skin test

(2) Concurrent TB skin testing

(3) Pregnancy in the mother or other close contact

(4) Breast feeding

(5) Immunodeficiency in member of household

(6) Egg allergy

(7) Mild or asymptomatic HIV infection

(8) Non life threatening reaction to neomycin

(9) History of seizure (slightly increased risk for this, but not a contraindication)

Withholding the vaccine for mild reactions is a common myth.Don't fall for this trap on the exam..

MMR and PPD

A PPD can be placed **WITH MMR** with no mitigation of its effect. However, a PPD should not be placed within a 4-6 week period **AFTER** MMR has been given.

A positive PPD would not be a contraindication to MMR immunization. However, if a definitive diagnosis of TB is confirmed, then treatment should be started prior to administration of MMR (since the vaccine can worsen TB).

MMR and Varicella

MMR and varicella *can* be given together (and often are, at the 12 or 15 month visit).

Although there have been no documented cases of birth defects secondary to the vaccine, MMR *is* contraindicated in pregnant women; **however, therapeutic abortion is not medically indicated when the vaccine is given accidentally to a pregnant woman.**

MMR, Yellow Fever, Influenza Egg Allergy, and Avoiding Yellow Egg on your Face

MMR

The current MMR preparation does *not* contain enough egg cross-reacting proteins to be an issue.

Skin testing will not predict allergic reaction following vaccination, and will never be the correct answer. Withholding vaccination will not be correct either. Observation for 90 minutes after administration might be the correct answer, but this will not likely be among the choices given.

Yellow Fever / Influenza Immunization

Yellow fever and influenza vaccines, on the other hand, do have enough egg protein to worry about an allergic reaction, including anaphylaxis.

Penning Instructions for the Epi Pen

Some important facts on epi pens:

- Epi Pen Junior is for patients weighing 30 kg or less
- They can lose their potency within 6 months of the expiration date
- It should be administered in the outer thigh, not through clothes
- They should be kept at room temperature; therefore, they should not be stored in cars
- 3 pens should be prescribed: one for the child, one in an obvious place in the house, and one for the school or baby-sitter

---

Therefore, any child who has had a systemic allergic reaction to egg protein should be skin tested.

Systemic Allergic Reaction Skin Testing is indicated

Systemic Allergic Reaction: Urticaria, hypotension, airway distress

Immunization with egg protein	Skin testing with history of mild allergic reaction
MMR	No
Yellow Fever	**Yellow Yes**
Influenza	**Indeed Yes**

 In cases of a severe anaphylactic reaction to **eggs,** the influenza vaccine is contraindicated period. These patients should receive chemoprophylaxis instead, but not the vaccine.

Varicella Vaccine

Before widespread varicella vaccination, there were around 4 million cases per year, which led to around 11,000 hospitalizations and about 100 deaths. The CDC now recommends that all children entering daycare facilities or elementary schools have either received the vaccine or have demonstrated immunity.

The varicella vaccine is given routinely between ages 12 - 15 months. A 2nd booster vaccine is given upon entry into kindergarten between ages 4-6 years. Any older child who has not had chicken pox should also receive the vaccine series.

All children over 13 years of age require 2 doses of vaccine given at least 4 weeks apart.

HIV and Live Vaccines

Measles Vaccine

The following is the protocol for administering live vaccines in HIV positive patients

Measles Vaccine is indicated for those who are:

- **Symptomatic** but not severely immunocompromised

- **Asymptomatic**

Varicella Vaccine

Varicella vaccine is not routinely given to patients who are immunocompromised

One possible exception is children with ALL in full remission. There is a specific varicella vaccine available for this population.

The contraindications to varicella vaccination are:

(1) Pregnancy

(2) Prior allergic reaction to the vaccine

(3) Substantial suppression of cellular immunity (e.g., severe AIDS, bone marrow transplant, or solid organ transplant)

 According to the CDC, the following are NOT contraindications to varicella administration:

(1) Pregnancy in the recipient's mother or other household contacts

(2) Mild or asymptomatic HIV infection

(3) Immunodeficiency in household contact

VariZIG and Acyclovir

VariZIG and Acyclovir would be indicated in the following situations:

· **Immunocompromised children** (with no previous varicella infections or immunizations)

· **Pregnant women** without immunity

· **Premies later than 28 weeks** without evidence of maternal immunity

· **Preemies born before 28 weeks**, regardless of maternal immunity

· Full term infants if mother contracted varicella 5 days before or 2 days after birth

Pneumococcal Vaccine

 The CDC recommends that all children between 2-23 months of age receive the pneumococcal conjugate vaccine.[5]

The PCV-13 (Prevnar®) is now administered at 2, 4, 6, and 12 months.

The 23-valent (PPV-23) vaccine should be given to all kids over 2 who have a chronic illness or asplenia (functional or anatomic).

---

[5] PCV-13 = Prevnar®.

PCV, PPV, and Understanding Pneumo without blowing a Pneumothorax

· **The PCV-13** (Prevnar®) is given to all children according to the schedule outlined above

· **PPV-23** is suggested for all children over the age of 2 years if they have a chronic illness or asplenia

 The only contraindication for receiving pneumococcal vaccine is a serious allergic reaction to a component of the vaccine.

Rotavirus

After the previous form of rotavirus vaccine was caught in a scandalous relationship with intussusception, a new and improved more honest rotavirus vaccine has appeared on the scene. At press time, there is no link between the new vaccine and intussusception.

In February 2006 a bovine pentavalent rotavirus vaccine, the PRV RotaTeq®, was licensed for use in infants.

You are expected to know the following:

· Infants should routinely receive doses at 2, 4, and 6 months of age

· The first dose should be given between 6 and 14 weeks

· After the first dose, subsequent doses should be given at 4-10 weeks intervals

· Infants with transient mild illness, low grade fever, or infants who are breast feeding can be given the vaccine

· Infants with severe allergic reactions to previous vaccination should not receive the vaccine.

The first dose of the rotavirus vaccine should not be given after 15 weeks of age.

Once the series has been started, it needs to be completed by 8 months of age.

If the first dose is administered inadvertently after 15 weeks, then the remainder of the series should still be administered on schedule.

Special Considerations

Infants who have rotavirus gastroenteritis

Infants who get mild rotavirus gastroenteritis should still complete the 3-dose schedule. This is because initial infection only confers partial immunity.

However, infants with **moderate to severe** gastroenteritis should not get the vaccine until clinically improved.

Breeast feeding infants

Infants who are breastfeeding can get the vaccine.

Infants with mild illness

Children with mild illnesses or low grade fever can also get the vaccine.

Underlying GI disease

Infants with underlying GI disease who are not receiving immunosuppressive treatment should receive the vaccine.

Prematurity

Premature infants can receive the vaccine as long as they are at least 6 weeks of age and are to be discharged from the nursery. They also need to be "clinically stable."

Immunocompromised or pregnant household contacts

Immunocompromised household contacts would **not be** a contraindication to vaccine administration. Likewise, pregnant household contacts would **not be** a contraindication to vaccine administration.

Regurgitation of the vaccine

Infants who spit up or vomit the vaccine should just continue with the series. No re-administration is necessary.

Hospitalization after vaccination

If an infant receiving the vaccine has to be hospitalized, no precautions beyond universal precautions are necessary.

Contraindications

The rotavirus vaccine is contraindicated in infants who had a severe hypersensitivity reaction or allergic reaction to previously administered doses.

Immunocompromised infants

The benefits and risks should be weighed in determining whether the vaccine should be administered to immunocompromised infants.

Hepatitis A Vaccine

All children in the U.S. should receive the vaccine at age 1 year. The trade names are Havrix® and Vaqta®.

It is administered in 2 doses, dosed at least 6 months apart (preferably the same brand).

 Immunocompromising conditions are *not* a contraindication for receiving the hepatitis A vaccine.

Contraindications for Hepatitis A Vaccine

Contraindications to the Hepatitis A vaccine include hypersensitivity or allergic reaction to the vaccine components, including **aluminum hydroxide** and **phenoxyethanol**.

There are specific recommendations for children traveling to areas that are endemic for hepatitis A. If they are less than 1 year of age, they should receive passive immunization with immune globulin. If they are older than 12 months, they should receive the hepatitis A vaccine. This should be done four weeks prior to departure if possible (two weeks at the very least).

> **MNEMONIC**
>
> **CAPE:** Think of the influenza vaccine as providing a cape of protection for the following high risk groups.
>
> **C**hronic metabolic disorder or renal problems and **C**ardiac disease
> **A**sthma (**A**cquired immunosuppression)
> **P**ulmonary disorder
> **E**mpty bladder (renal problems)

Influenza

Annual immunization is indicated for:

· All children between 6 months and 18 years.

· Caregivers in or out of the house for children in this age group

· Children at higher risk of influenza or of complications (see below)

In the event of a vaccine shortage, priority would be given to the following high risk groups:

· Chronic Pulmonary Disease / Asthma

· Symptomatic Cardiac disease

· Immunosuppressed patients (from disease or medications)

· Sickle cell disease

· Conditions requiring long term aspirin therapy.

CASE STUDY **You could be presented with a list of conditions and asked to pick the one in which administering the influenza vaccine would not be indicated.**

THE DIVERSION The answer may not be so straightforward, since it may require you to know the treatment of the condition listed. For example, in the list they could include: asymptomatic heart murmur, JIA, Addison's disease, or history of Kawasaki Disease 3 months ago. You might mistakenly believe that the child with asymptomatic cardiac disease requires influenza immunization rather than the child with a previous history of Kawasaki disease.

ANSWER REVEALED The correct answer would be the patient with asymptomatic heart disease. The patient with Kawasaki is probably on long term aspirin therapy, the patient with Addison's disease is likely on chronic steroids (rendering them immunosuppressed), ditto for the patient with JIA.

HOT TIP Since infants cannot receive influenza immunizations until 6 months of age, the only way to protect them is to ensure that their caretakers and household contacts receive the influenza vaccine.

Getting through the Screen Door

Hypertension

When do you screen for hypertension?

Routine BP screening starts at age 3.

HOT TIP

Children with a diagnosis of ADHD who are taking Ritalin® (methylphenidate) and other stimulants need to have their blood pressure monitored.

When is a screen positive?

What *is* hypertension?

DEFINITION

Hypertension is a blood pressure that is greater than the 95th percentile for age and gender, taken *on at least 3 separate occasions, best done one month apart.*

Focusing on the underlined part is more important than the 95th percentile part (but don't focus too long or your eyes will glaze over).

> *CASE STUDY*
>
> **You are presented with a child who is noted to have high blood pressure. You won't have to know the definition of what that is, since they will clearly state that everything is normal except for the blood pressure. What is the next best step in the initial management?**
>
> *THE DIVERSION*
>
> Well, Well, Well – there could be all kinds of seemingly innocent non invasive choices, such as the "urinalysis" and "culture." Seemingly innocent, but if you pick these choices, you have overanalyzed yourself into picking the wrong answer.
>
> *ANSWER REVEALED*
>
> The correct answer could be to repeat the blood pressure two more times on two separate occasions. Remember to read the question and to remember the definition of hypertension. One elevated reading is not enough for any workup beyond confirming that the diagnosis is real.

Watch for clues in the question that you are dealing with the **wrong sized cuff**.

Hearing Screening

Conductive Hearing Loss

 Conductive hearing loss is due to anything which interferes with transmission of sound from the external to the middle ear.

 Watch for a description of a child who adjusts the volume on the TV to loud volumes.

Early intervention is needed to help facilitate language development in children with hearing loss.

If presented with choices, it is very important to read the wording of the question. For example:

· *Atresia of the ear canal* causes the *most severe degree* of conductive hearing loss.

· *Otitis media with effusion* is the *most common cause* of conductive hearing loss.

Patients with *cholesteatoma* often present with no hearing compromise. *Tympanosclerosis* is associated with little or no hearing loss despite its intimidating sounding name.

You will be expected to know that infants who fail the newborn hearing screen should be referred to an audiologist for evaluation before three months of age. One of the tests that may be done to further evaluate this concern is an ABR, or Auditory Brainstem Response. This test uses electroencephalographic waveforms to measure brainstem response to auditory stimuli.

Cholesterol Screening

Universal screening will, for now, always be the wrong answer. The following are the recommendations for screening children at risk for hypercholesterolemia.

This table outlines the American Heart Association Screening Guidelines

Clinical History	Definition	Recommended Lab Study	Management
Case A Parent with total cholesterol level > 240	Greater than 240. That simple.	Total *non fasting* cholesterol level	170 or higher, repeat and/or get fasting lipoprotein (see algorithm below)
Case B Children with the following risk factors: · Cigarette smokers · Hypertension · Physical inactivity · Diabetes · Obesity		Total *non fasting cholesterol* level, regardless of family history	170 or higher, repeat and/or get fasting lipoprotein (see algorithm below)
Case C Parent or grandparent with *coronary atherosclerosis*	Grandparent, first degree aunt or uncle who suffered from the following **before the age of 55:** · MI · Angina · Peripheral Vascular Disease · CVA · Sudden Cardiac Death · Documented atherosclerosis	Fasting lipoprotein	>110, repeat and consider diet, >160 after diet, may meet criteria for meds (see algorithm below)

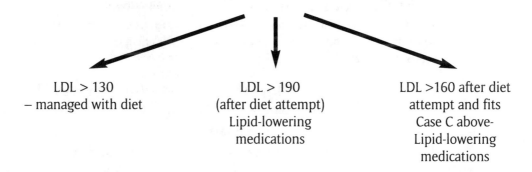

Child with parents cholesterol >240 and a non fasting cholesterol of > 170 will require *a fasting lipoprotein*

LDL > 130
– managed with diet

LDL > 190
(after diet attempt)
Lipid-lowering
medications

LDL >160 after diet
attempt and fits
Case C above-
Lipid-lowering
medications

Additional Risk Factors for Hypercholesterolemia

Additional Risk factors include

- Diet
- Steroid medications
- Anticonvulsants
- Beta blockers
- Alcohol
- Chronic diseases – liver, renal, hypothyroidism

Although it might seem counterintuitive, anorexia nervosa is a risk factor for hypercholesterolemia.

CASE STUDY

You are presented with a list of scenarios that are close to the criteria for cholesterol screening, but just missing the mark. They could ask in which of the following cases screening would be appropriate.

> **A mother with a cholesterol level of 230 at age 32**
>
> **A grandfather who had an MI at 63**
>
> **An uncle with angina at 55**
>
> **An uncle with a cholesterol level of 6.02×10^{23}**
>
> **A chain-smoking 16-year-old whose only activity is pushing the buttons of his PSP with his cigarette butts**

THE DIVERSION

There are several diversions here. Remember angina has to be present in a relative *before* the age of 55, so the uncle with angina at 55 doesn't count. The cholesterol greater than 240 has to be a parent. The uncle with Avogadro's number for cholesterol doesn't count, and neither does the child with a parent with cholesterol of 230 at age 32. This choice is a classic diversion for those who do not commit the details to memory. They are hoping that you will be confused on two fronts. By noting an age younger than 55, they are hoping you will be confused with the age criteria for cardiac disease in a parent; they are also hoping that you did not commit the number 240 to memory.

ANSWER REVEALED

The correct answer is the chain smoking video game addict, since he has two factors requiring cholesterol screening: physical inactivity and cigarette smoking.

This is why it is important to commit the above criteria to memory, focusing on the details. Doing so will give you at least one point on the exam, and this is the goal of studying.

Polycythemia

DEFINITION

Polycythemia must be from a venous sample. If they give you a capillary measurement, it is not valid and they are only trying to deceive you into working it up inappropriately.

Hyperviscosity Syndrome

Hyperviscosity syndrome is often a result of polycythemia.

 Consider hyperviscosity syndrome in any infant with history of twin to twin transfusion, delayed clamping of the cord, Down syndrome, or an infant of a diabetic mother.

Hyperbilirubinemia and *hypoglycemia* often occur with polycythemia

They might list complications that could occur with hyperviscosity syndrome, and among the choices may be hyperglycemia. Remember it is hypoglycemia that occurs with polycythemia.

To help remember hypoglycemia occurring with polycythemia, think of it as RBCs eating up all the glucose.

Vision Screening

Ophthalmologists, in addition to having the most frequently misspelled specialty, have a language that only they and Kenny from *South Park* understand.

First some definitions in the following table:

Ophthalmological Term	Language for the rest of the medical world
Amblyopia	The loss of visual acuity due to active **cortical suppression of the vision of one eye.** This can be the result of **deprivation amblyopia** which could occur due to ptosis, dense congenital cataract, or extended eye closure.
Esotropia	Inward turning eye (form of strabismus)
Exotropia	Outward turning eye (form of strabismus)
Esophoria	The tendency for inward deviation of the eye that typically is only found when an eye is covered and then uncovered.
Hyperopia	Eye alignment is difficult when significant focusing effort is required. Most children normally have mild hyperopia. This is the refractive state most likely to be seen in a 3 year old.

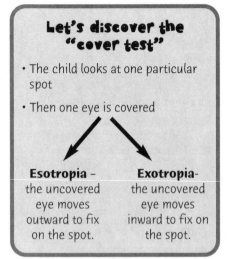

Let's discover the "cover test"

• The child looks at one particular spot

• Then one eye is covered

Esotropia – the uncovered eye moves outward to fix on the spot.

Exotropia- the uncovered eye moves inward to fix on the spot.

Cataracts – If a cataract is not picked up early with the red *reflex*, amblyopia ultimately results in the affected eye.

If the child is sitting for the cover test and one eye is abnormal and you attempt to cover the *good eye*, he will resist your doing so. This is ripe for a trick question.

Watch for the description of a child who is "clumsy," spills liquids more than the average child, and runs into objects. This is a sign of a faulty depth perception, as would be the case in a child with a cataract.

Through the eyes of a child: infant vision

You will be expected to be familiar with the visual capabilities of infants. The following will help you "track" these facts in order to keep them straight on the exam.

Optokinetic nystagmus – If you can spell this without vertical nystagmus and vertigo on flat land, you are almost there. This merely refers to the ability to see a moving target, follow it, and then return to the original gaze. This is one of the **earliest reflexes**; infants develop this in the first few months of life.

Ability to Fixate – begins at 6 weeks of age

 Infants can **Fix** at **Six** weeks of age

Color Perception develops at 2 months of age

Binocular vision with convergence ability develops at around 3 months of age.

 Picture a pair of binoculars that are a giant "3," which is the shape of binoculars.

Preference for patterns, including faces, occurs at 4 months of age.

 The visual acuity of a newborn is around 20/200. By 1 year of age, this improves to 20/30.

Tuberculosis Screening and Exposure

Induration of less than 5 mm usually is not significant. The same is true for induration of 5-10 mm with the exception of the following:

❑ Close contacts

❑ Positive X-ray findings

❑ Immunosuppression (e.g, HIV or chronic steroids)

Newborns/Mother with Active Disease

❑ If the infant's CXR is negative, the infant is treated with INH.

❑ If the infant's CXR is positive, the infant is treated with triple meds.

Newborn/Mother with Latent TB

Mothers with latent TB would have a positive PPD and a negative chest x-ray.

❑ Check PPD every 3 months

❑ If the infant's PPD is positive and CXR is negative, treat with INH for one year.

❑ If the infant's PPD is positive and CXR is positive, treat with triple meds.

The Bottom Line

❑ If at risk and CXR is negative, INH for one year is adequate with follow-up.

❑ If at risk and CXR is positive, triple meds are needed.

Ounce of Prevention:
When is Prophylactic Treatment Necessary?

Disease	Prophylactic Treatment
Meningococcus	Household contacts (especially children younger than 2 years) Daycare/preschool contacts (if exposed within 7 days of illness onset)
	Direct exposure to secretions (including doctors who intubate these children)
	Slept in same bed within 7 days
	Sat next to the patient on a plane for more than 8 hours
	Casual exposures (those not falling into the above categories) do not require prophylaxis. This includes doctors who had no exposure to secretions.
H. flu	**Household contacts** Households with: - Children who are younger than 4 and are incompletely immunized - Children who are immunocompromised *Daycare/preschool contacts should receive prophylaxis if there are 2 or more cases within 60 days
Tuberculosis	INH **Active TB:** (Not just a positive PPD) ❑ **Household contacts** should receive 3 months of INH regardless of test results. ❑ If the **PPD is positive**, then 9 months of treatment in children is warranted. ❑ **Negative Sputum for Acid Fast Bacilli is the key in determining infectivity, not the CXR.**
Hepatitis A	Children older than 12 months should receive the Hep A vaccine as prophylaxis within 2 weeks of the exposure. Children younger than 12 months should get immune globulin instead. Any children with immunocompromising conditions or chronic liver disease should receive immune globulin after exposure.

Injury and Illness Prevention

Anticipatory Guidance

Some important often tested points are:

Hot liquid burns are the most common burns. Remember, **sharp demarcation of burns increases suspicion of child abuse**.

Childproofing the home should be discussed. This is best done at the **6-month visit, before the child is mobile**. Water heaters should be set at 120 degrees F.

Eclipsing the Sun

The A and B of ultraviolet sunlight

Type of UV light	Timing of Risk	The Skinny
UV A	Constant throughout the day **A** is constant **A**ll day	· Drug induced photosensitivity reactions · Also contributes to the problems listed for UVB
UV B	Varies: Strongest from 10AM through 5PM **B** is strongest during **B**usiness hours	· Skin aging · Sunburn · Skin Cancer

80% of a person's sun exposure occurs before age 20, or the first 2 decades of life. Using sun screen in the pediatric population may reduce the risk by 80%.

Sunscreen Shots

· Sunscreen with an SPF of at least 15 should be used
· Physical sunscreens block out both UVA and UVB
· It should be applied 20 minutes before sun exposure
· Applying less than optimal amounts reduces the SPF rating

Dueling Airbags and Car Seats

You will need to know the appropriate car seat to use based on weight, height, and age.

Weight/Height/Age	Type of Car Seat	Where should it be facing?
Infants weighing less than 20 lbs and less than 2 years	nfant car seat or rear facing car seat	Rear facing in back seat
More than 20 lbs (toddler/preschool)	Convertible car seat with harness	Forward facing in back seat
School-age children (up to 4'9" tall, or until adult seat belt fits correctly)	Booster seat	Forward facing in back seat
Older Children (until at least 13 yr)	Standard Seat Belts	Back seat
More than 300 lbs	Portable StairMaster® and rowing machine	Whichever direction passenger is rowing or going

 The middle seat is the safest seat. Children should not be sitting in the front seat until at least age 13, regardless of weight.

Rear facing infant car seats should be positioned at a **45 degree angle.**

Bicycle Safety

Some important facts that you are expected to know regarding bicycle safety:

- Most bicycle deaths and injuries occur in children younger than 15 years
- Bicycle helmets are worn by less than 10% of children riding bicycles
- Bicycle helmets reduce serious injury by 85%
- 75% of deaths are due to head injuries
- Reflectors are required on pedals, tire sidewalls or rims, and the front and rear of the bicycle

CASE STUDY

You need to be familiar with bicycle safety facts in case you are asked a question that over or underestimates these facts. For example, they may ask you to pick the correct fact from a list of facts which all seem correct.

THE DIVERSION

They might, for instance, include in the list that bicycle helmets reduce serious injury by 65%, that 25% of bicycle fatalities are due to head injuries, that reflectors are required on bicycle tires, or some similar seemingly illogical statement.

ANSWER REVEALED

The correct answer in this case would be the simple statement regarding reflectors on tires. *When presented with a list of answers with percentages and numbers, look closely at the answer without the numbers. It could be the correct one.*

Firearms in the Home

Some important facts and statistics you are expected to know:

- Guns are present in 35% of US households.
- Safety mechanisms, including trigger locks, may reduce unintentional injury (although this is not proven).
- More than 90% of suicide attempts with a gun are fatal, thereby increasing the chances of suicide in those at risk.
- More than 75% of adolescent homicides are attributed to guns.
- Having a gun in the home increases the risk for adolescent suicide by 5 fold.

PERIL WARNING

Even though the official word is that trigger locks "may" reduce risk, choices that include definitive statements such as "handguns can be safely kept in the home as long as there is a trigger lock in place" will be incorrect. Locked and unloaded is the key (with ammunition stored and locked in a separate location). In addition, it is recommended that the gun have high trigger pressure to fire, in order to reduce the risk of a child firing a household gun.

Suicide Risk and Prevention

If you are asked,

"Which of the following groups is at highest risk for suicide?"

The correct answer will be "homosexual teenagers."

Drowning Prevention

Drowning is more common in **warm weather months**, especially where there is fresh water.
Peaks are at **preschool age** and **late teens**.

Age-dependent facts

· Infants are most likely to drown in a bathtub

· Children younger than 5 are most likely to drown in a residential pool

· Adolescents are most likely to drown in fresh water

· Above ground pools are less likely to cause drowning

· Drowning is higher among African American males

· Drowning is the most common cause of death of patients with epilepsy

· Males account for 75% of all drownings

· The ratio of near drowning to drowning is close to 1:1

The following is an important fact to commit to memory. The AAP recommends a **4-sided** fence around the pool, with a locked gate. This is the most effective preventive measure for preventing drowning in children.

A fence around the yard (with one side being the back door of the house) is NOT good enough, in real life or on the Boards.

Infant and toddler swimming lessons are fun social events, but **ineffective** when it comes to preventing drowning.

Floating Your Boat Safely

90% of boat-related drowning incidents occur in people not wearing life jackets.

The best way to prevent this is ... you guessed it... all children aboard a boat should be wearing a life jacket.

Additional causes of death and injury while boating include:

• Carbon monoxide poisioning

• Fractures and laceration

• Head injuries

Many of these accidents involve alcohol.

Preparing Families for International Adoption

You will be expected to be familiar with issues related to families adopting children from abroad. The following are some important points that may be tested on the exam:

1. There are no standards for oversight regarding issuing of visas for internationally adopted children, other than issuing an "orphan visa."

2. Children tend to lose 1 month of linear growth for every 3 months in an orphanage.

3. Microcephaly would be a red flag, indicating more serious medical conditions such as exposure to alcohol or perinatal brain injury.

4. You, as a pediatrician, should expect developmental milestones to match the child's linear growth.

5. Using standardized facial photographs or videos to quantify the risk for fetal alcohol syndrome is considered to be helpful, but has not been validated in international adoptees.

Cigarette Cessation in Adolescents

Some important points to be familiar with regarding tobacco use in teenagers are:

· Addiction occurs after exposure to a small amount of nicotine

· Certain respiratory sequelae may be seen in the teen years

· Up to 25% of low birthweight infant births are due to smoking during pregnancy

· Second hand smoke increases the risk for SIDS, otitis media, asthma, bronchiolitis, bronchitis, and pneumonia

· School-based education programs aimed at smoking prevention are effective if they focus on role playing refusal skills and provide information on the health impact

· Nicotine replacement therapy is not approved by the FDA for use in adolescents. Therefore, before using this treatment, you must first document that quitting is unlikely to be achieved without assistance, and you must feel confident that the adolescent will use it appropriately. Remember: first do no harm!

· If nicotine replacement fails to stop smoking, then bupropion when combined with counseling is an approved option

Other Respiratory Concerns:

Common exposures may cause breathing or respiratory problems in poorly-ventilated environments. This may include wood fires/stoves, cigarette smoke, hairspray, cooking spray, or other potentially harmful chemicals.

First Aid Considerations

The treatment of choice for a child experiencing an anaphylactic reaction is epinephrine. If the question asks for contraindications for epinephrine, there are none. After administration, the next stop is the ER.

You might be questioned on the correct technique for tick removal. This consists of grabbing the tick at the skin line with fine tweezers and removing with steady upward traction applied.

Chapter 9

Poisons and Environmental Toxins
Procedures and Acute Management

Risk of Toxicity in Children

You are expected to understand the increased risk to the fetus, infants, and young children compared to an equivalent toxic exposure in adults. Children of course place more non-food items in their mouths than most adults and are, therefore, at increased risk for exposure to toxic agents in the environment.

Children are also at increased risk for the manifestations of latent toxicity effects over the course of their lifetime as compared to adults.

Placenta Percenta

The placenta is not perfect at protecting the fetus from toxic substances. Specifically, it *blocks cadmium,* but *allows for the transfer of lead,* and even *enhances passage of mercury. PCB's* and *insecticides* can also *cross the placenta* easily due to their lipophilic nature and low molecular weight.

Drinking the Water

Even drinking water can be a culprit, especially on the boards. You are expected to know that drinking water can contain *E. coli, cryptosporidium, trichloroethylene,* and *perchloroethylene.*

> ### Syrup of Ipecac
> It is safe to assume that syrup of ipecac will ALWAYS be the incorrect treatment on the boards

Activated Charcoal

· The appropriate dosing is typically is 0.5 to 1 g/kg, up to an adult dose range of 25 to 100 g
· Cathartics, such as magnesium citrate and sorbitol, can be given to expedite exit of the ingested substance and to reduce enterohepatic excretion

When used in patients at risk for respiratory depression, such as those who have ingested phenobarbital, intubation should be done as well. The charcoal is then served with an NG tube and a wide variety of surgical tapes and Surgilube®.

While it may seem obvious, charcoal cannot be given with antidotes, because it would interfere with the absorption of the antidote. One exception to this is N-acetylcysteine, since it is given in such large quantities.

Remember the mnemonic CALM to remember those toxic substances which are "calmly" removed without charcoal.

Charcoal is a poor choice for:

- **C**yanide
- **A**lcohol
- **L**ithium
- Heavy **M**etals

Gastric Lavage

Gastric lavage is no longer recommended for most ingestions. The risks outweigh the benefits. Its use is reserved for potential life-threatening ingestions that have occurred within 60 minutes of seeking medical attention.

Foreign Body Ingestion

3 Coins in the Fountain

Coins are the most commonly ingested foreign bodies.

- 95% will pass within 4-6 days
- If they do not progress past the stomach within 24 hours they should be removed

This would be the case even if the child is asymptomatic, so do not be lulled into choosing no action if they note the child is asymptomatic.

Zincing Pennies and Button Batteries

Pennies that were minted after 1982 are not pure copper, and have significant zinc content. This can be corrosive on the esophagus. These should be removed quickly, and the patients should be referred for endoscopy.

Most children will not recall the year on the coin, or the coin itself for that matter; therefore, assume on the exam that any ingested penny should be removed quickly via endoscopy.

- All coins in the **proximal esophagus** should be removed by **endoscopy ASAP**

- All coins in the **middle - lower esophagus** should be observed for **12-24 hours** if asymptomatic, followed by endoscopy if the coin does not pass beyond that point

CASE STUDY A 3 year old who is completely asymptomatic is brought into your office. The baby-sitter noticed him chewing on a camera 3 days ago. She even brought the camera in to take a picture, but noticed that the camera does not work; the battery lid is open and there is no battery. What is the best next step in managing?

THE DIVERSION Since they emphasize that the child is asymptomatic, watching and waiting may seem to be the most logical choice vs. charcoal, repeat CXR in a week, or the seemingly gruesome chore of sifting through the stool until the battery is located (and then reinstalling it in the camera). All of these are incorrect.

ANSWER REVEALED In this case, the correct answer violates the least invasive rule. Here the correct answer will be endoscopy to remove the battery, since it has been more than 48 hours. If the battery is in the esophagus or has not passed the stomach, it must be removed.

Toxidromes

Acetaminophen Ingestion

The initial manifestations of acetaminophen toxicity include anorexia, nausea, and vomiting. This does not extend past the first 24 hours.

In cases of **significant toxicity**, the liver enzyme levels rise significantly during a latent phase that lasts 1-4 days.

In **severe toxicity**: following the latent phase, jaundice and liver tenderness will develop next.

The most important predictor of outcome regarding acetaminophen toxicity is the level taken 4 hours post ingestion.

- 150 or greater = *moderate* hepatoxicity
- 300 or greater = *severe* hepatoxicity

Everyone knows about hepatic toxicity, but *renal toxicity* is also a possibility. Even in cases of severe liver toxicity, LFT's can be normal for 2-3 days.

Treatment

It is very common to be asymptomatic **initially**, with liver toxicity presenting later on. Therefore, immediate discharge from the ER when the person is asymptomatic will always be the wrong answer.

Management:

- **First step** is to reduce absorption with activated charcoal.

- **Second step** -- Obtain an acetaminophen level 4 hours post ingestion, and plot level on the published nomogram to determine risk for hepatoxicity.

HOT TIP If it has been determined that more than 150 mg/kg has been ingested, then N-acetylcysteine can be given without obtaining levels (especially if it would delay initiation of treatment longer than 8 hours after ingestion).

PERIL WARNING However, if this is not the case, then the correct answer could very well be "hold off on administering antidote pending additional information."

N-acetylcysteine prevents the accumulation of toxic metabolites of acetaminophen.

CASE STUDY

A 17 yo female was seen in the ER 2 days ago for acetaminophen ingestion. Her acetaminophen level 4 hours post ingestion was 250 mcg/mL. She was given an appropriate dose of N-acetylcysteine. Her LFTs today were unremarkable. What is her prognosis?

THE DIVERSION

You might be deceived into believing that, even though the 4 hour levels were in the toxic range, the fact that the N-acetylcysteine was given immediately and that her LFT's are normal indicates that the patient is out of the woods. If you pick an answer based on this logic, both you and the patient will still be in the woods.

ANSWER REVEALED

Remember that the LFTs can be normal 2-3 days later, even in cases of severe overdose. The transaminase levels do not rise until 3-4 days after ingestion.

Salicylate Ingestion

Toxic ingestion of aspirin can include medications that contain salicylates, so look for clues in the question such as "wintergreen" odor on breath.

Management of Salicylate ingestion

- The initial treatment is activated charcoal
- Salicylate level 3-6 hours post ingestion
- Sodium bicarb (to alkalinize the urine) is required to correct metabolic acidosis. The acidosis is surprisingly not directly caused by salicylates, but typically by respiratory alkalosis and by buildup of organic acids as a result of salicylate action in cells.
- Ensure that hypokalemia is addressed and consider glucose even if not hypoglycemic.

Hyperpnea may then follow metabolic acidosis and could lead to *further respiratory alkalosis*. However, salicylates cause hyperpnea directly, so the picture is often mixed, starting with respiratory alkalosis and leading to worsening metabolic acidosis! To complicate it further, young children tend to lose the respiratory drive with salicylate toxicity, so they typically end up with a combined acidosis picture.

Remember to always calculate the anion gap when presented with acidosis and values for Sodium, Potassium, Chloride, and Bicarb. The formula is Sodium – (Chloride + Bicarb). *The anion gap would be elevated in salicylate poisoning.*

Fever is consistent with toxicity, so be careful not to follow the "sepsis" tree when they give other clues consistent with salicylate toxicity.

Ibuprofen Ingestion

Most children will be asymptomatic, but on the boards they will at least have *nausea* and *vomiting*.

Management of ibuprofen overdose is primarily supportive for GI upset (usually consisting of nausea and vomiting).

CASE STUDY You are presented with a teenager who has ingested a fistful of ibuprofen pills as a suicide gesture. Her vital signs are stable and she is otherwise fine physically. You are asked for the most appropriate next step in managing this patient.

THE DIVERSION Among the possible diversions could be the obligatory diversion of ipecac, which you should immediately avoid the way you would actually avoid ipecac itself; the same goes for gastric lavage. The most absurd diversion of all would be an ibuprofen level, which doesn't exist.

ANSWER REVEALED Of course, it is the "risk for co-ingestion tree" that you should be climbing. The correct answer will therefore be a level for another drug, such as salicylate or acetaminophen levels.

Ethanol Toxicity

BUZZ WORDS You might be presented with an adolescent who is having a seizure and who is hypoglycemic. Hypoglycemia is associated with ethyl alcohol ingestion.

The table below outlines blood alcohol levels, expected clinical consequences, and management strategies (mostly symptomatic).

Blood Alcohol Level	Clinical Presentation	Management
Mild < 0.1 g/dL	Euphoria, lowered inhibitions, and impaired coordination	Hide the car keys and the kitchen spoons and forks, and follow closely to the bathroom
Moderate 0.1-0.2	Slurred speech, ataxia, impaired judgement, and mood swings	Monitor until sober or until given a series on the Fox network, whichever comes first
Severe > 0.3	Confusion and stupor	Hospital administrator
Greater than 0.4	Coma, respiratory depression and death	Aim for hospital admission before getting to confusion and stupor
Beyond 0.45	Charlie Sheen	Currently on tour

If presented with a patient with ethanol toxicity, monitoring for hypoglycemia and electrolyte imbalance is important. You should also be aware that ethanol intoxication can mask the toxicity of other drugs.

The presentation of ethanol toxicity might not be obvious. Remember, ethyl alcohol might be present in items other than a liter of Absolut Citron®. Ethyl alcohol is also present in mouthwash, cough and cold preparations, elixirs, and even colognes and perfumes.

Methanol Toxicity

Once upon a time, rubbing alcohol consisted of methanol. However, it also exists in the board world as well as the real world in the form of windshield washer fluid, cooking fuel, perfumes, and antifreeze for your car.

There might not be immediate signs of toxicity (as in the case of a child acting drunk after ingesting ethanol). However, do not be fooled by the innocent presentation in the history. This is a Trojan horse toxicity. Methanol gets broken down to formic acid and formaldehyde, which can wreak havoc, especially on the liver and the optic nerve (leading to blindness).

Clinical presentation could include *acidosis, increased anion gap*, and *CNS depression.*

This is one of the rare cases where administration of ethanol to a minor might be appropriate. In this case, ethanol serves as an alcohol dehydrogenase antagonist, slowing the conversion of methanol to formaldehyde. Another agent that accomplishes the same thing with less toxicity would be **4-methypyrazole (4-MP)**. However, as of this printing it has only been approved in Europe (but if it does make its way to the exam, it will likely be a correct choice).

Additional treatment would include sodium bicarbonate to help counter formic acid

Narcotic and Opiate Toxicity

The typical presentation of opiate toxicity would be a teenager in the ER who is responsive to painful stimuli, with pinpoint but reactive pupils, cyanosis, and respiratory depression. Additional "depressions" include bradycardia, hypotension, and low temperature.

"Comatose, shallow breathing, and miotic pupils," along with a decreased respiratory rate and decreased heart rate.

Pinpoint pupils are also known as miotic pupils. This is easy to distinguish from mydriasis by envisioning the **o** in mi**o**sis as a pinpoint pupil.

Other conditions with decreased levels of consciousness, and how they differ from opiate toxicity:

Conditions with depressed level of consciousness	How it differs from opiate toxicity
DKA	Dehydrated with **rapid** deep breathing, pupils are not constricted
Organophosphate toxicity	Does have constricted pupils; however, also presents with *profuse sweating, tearing, abdominal pain, wheezing, and respiratory distress*
Major head trauma	Dilated pupils, which are nonreactive

Propoxyphene, a narcotic analgesic, also presents with ventricular arrhythmias, seizures, and/or pulmonary edema.

Treatment of opiate toxicity consists of the antagonist **naloxone**, which helps treat and make the diagnosis.

PCP

They will likely describe someone who is wide-eyed (mydriatic) and violent. Unless Charlie Sheen is one of the choices, PCP ingestion will be the correct answer. PCP would also result in anasarca and asymmetric pupils.

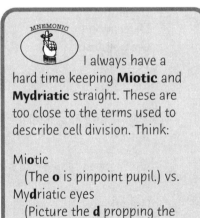 I always have a hard time keeping **Miotic** and **Mydriatic** straight. These are too close to the terms used to describe cell division. Think:

Mi**o**tic
(The **o** is pinpoint pupil.) vs.
My**d**riatic eyes
(Picture the **d** propping the pupil open. Also, note that my**d**riatic and **d**ilated have a **D** in them.)

Organophosphates

A typical presentation would be a toddler who is lethargic, in respiratory distress, and is *sweating and wheezing*. They often hint at exposure to insecticides by mentioning that the child was in a backyard shed.

Think of an overstimulated person playing the organ (organophosphate): muscles twitching, salivary secretions, urination, and GI cramps from moving so much.

In addition to ingestion, organophosphates can also be *inhaled* and *absorbed through the skin*.

The mechanism of action is by inhibiting acetylcholinesterase, and therefore the effect is due to acetylcholine overload.

The classic mnemonic is **SLUDGE:**

Salivation
Lacrimation
Urination
Defecation or Diarrhea
Gastrointestinal
Emesis

These all are related to the "fight or flight" mode. That is to say, you would be in a rush, creating slush = sludge.

Alternatively, you could memorize **DUMBBELS:** (notice the incorrect spelling of the word)

Diarrhea
Urination
Miosis
Bronchospasm
Bradycardia
Emesis
Lacrimation
Salivation

Insecticides can be insidious in the environment and can have a long term impact on children's health, particularly on brain development. Unwashed fruits and vegetables would be one important source. In addition, children are more likely to be exposed in general due to behavioral factors.

Cholinergic effects are broken down into 2 categories, **muscarinic** and **nicotinic**. You need to know how each is managed.

Muscarinic effects

The muscarinic effects are primarily *pulmonary*, including bronchospasm and increased pulmonary secretions.

Administration of *atropine* is key to countering the muscarinic effects.

Nicotinic effects

The nicotinic effects are primarily *neuromuscular*, and are treated with *pralidoxime*.

Tricyclic Antidepressants (TCA)

Many of the presenting signs are *anticholinergic* including mydriasis, dry mouth, urinary retention, and constipation. Sedation is also a risk. Medications with anticholinergic side effects include tricyclic antidepressants (TCAs), mydriatic agents, and antispasmodics. Watch for a clinical history of a member of the household taking one of these medications. If they give you a toddler presenting with clinical signs consistent with anticholinergic ingestion, watch for a history of a household contact that is on tricyclic antidepressant therapy.

Here the key will be "anticholinergic signs" (like dry mouth, dry mucous membranes) and mydriasis (which you now know is dilated pupils). The same symptoms for antihistamine overdose are "blind as a bat," "red as a beet," "hot as a hare," "dry as a bone," and "mad as a hatter."[1] The bowel and "bladder lose their tone," and the "heart runs alone."

If they present a patient suspected of ingesting TCAs, with the anticholinergic signs described above, then you need to know that *within 24 hours* they may develop **dysrhythmias. Tachycardia and hypertension are other diagnostic signs.**

---

[1] How mad is a hatter anyway?

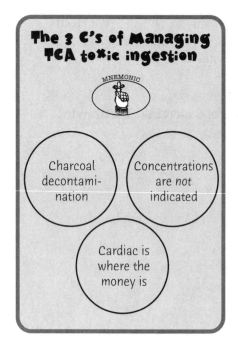

The 3 C's of Managing TCA toxic ingestion

MNEMONIC

- Charcoal decontamination
- Concentrations are *not* indicated
- Cardiac is where the money is

PERIL WARNING The dysrhythmias do not typically lead to V fib, and should not be treated with cardiac medications. The only intervention is *alkalinization of urine.*

PERIL WARNING Measurement of TCA levels is not clinically useful.

HOT TIP The most important parameter to measure is EKG monitoring for widened QRS complex.

TREATMENT **Activated charcoal is the method of choice for decontamination.** Widening QRS complex is treated with sodium bicarbonate boluses. Repeat until the QRS duration is less than 100 msec.

CASE STUDY **You are presented with a patient who is getting allergy testing and casually mentions that "he is on no medications other than a tricyclic antidepressants." They will note that all allergy testing is negative. Does the child have significant allergies?**

THE DIVERSION **Pay particular attention when they say "no medications other than (Fill in the blank)." They are telling you about this medication for a reason.**

ANSWER REVEALED Tricyclics render allergy testing unreliable, since they can interfere with the histamine response. They want you to know that the test is not valid.

Beta Blocker Ingestion

A child who has ingested a beta blocker will present with a *depressed sensorium* and bradycardia, as well as hypotension, and perhaps diaphoresis.

A child suspected of ingesting a beta blocker would need to be observed on a monitor.

Hydrocarbon Ingestion

Symptomatic patients might present with non-specific signs, including nausea and vomiting. Specific signs include a history of choking and/or gagging, with a persistent cough and/or tachypnea. They will likely provide or show labs consistent with hypoxemia and describe or show a film with *diffuse bilateral infiltrates.* This will be your clue.

Hydrocarbon ingestion can lead to ARDS, which is Acute Respiratory Distress Syndrome.[2] Symptomatic patients might require oxygen, bronchodilators and other supportive care.

Patients who are asymptomatic do not require any intervention other than observation for 6 hours. A chest x-ray wouldn't be necessary. Treatment is largely supportive, including oxygen saturation assessment, as well as intubation when indicated.

If the patient is stable, there is no evidence that early intubation or PEEP will have any role. Asymptomatic patients can, in fact, be discharged.

---

[2] Formerly known as Adult Respiratory Distress Syndrome. I guess they changed the name to acute when they realized it occurs in children and is seen on the pediatric board exam.

Carbon Monoxide Toxicity

BUZZ WORDS

The key is "flu-like symptoms in a patient who is **afebrile**, with a **supple neck**." They may describe symptoms in other family members, including the family pet. Hopefully you won't also be expected to know how to treat the family pet. The signs and symptoms are very vague, and include fatigue, headache, dizziness, nausea, dyspnea, weakness, and confusion. It is either someone in a coma in the last row of Grand Rounds, or it is carbon monoxide intoxication.

HOT TIP

Think of carbon monoxide poisoning when they describe depressed sensorium, drowsiness, and supple neck *in an afebrile patient.*

BUZZ WORDS

They might give you some signs such as "singed nasal hairs," "charcoal-stained clothes," and "carbonaceous sputum," or hacking and heaving like Keith Richards on the Rolling Stones tour bus.

PERIL WARNING

Although obtaining carboxyhemoglobin levels is a crucial initial first step, symptoms do not always correlate with carboxyhemoglobin levels. In addition, cherry red mucous membranes was previously believed to be a key factor in making the diagnosis, but it is now considered to be too insensitive a sign. Make sure this is not one of the choices you select when asked about important diagnostic criteria. **Oxygen saturations are completely unreliable in this setting.** Oxygen saturation does not distinguish between carboxyhemoglobin and oxygenated hemoglobin.

Hyperbaric Chamber

Hyperbaric oxygen was once the darling of treatment. It is now reserved for severe cases, which would include the following situations:

1. Pregnancy
2. Acidosis
3. Signs of cardiac involvement
4. Signs of neurologic involvement

In routine cases, administering high flow oxygen through a nonrebreather mask would be the correct answer.

CASE STUDY

You are presented with a patient who is lethargic, confused, and in distress, emphasizing a *normal pulse oximetry reading*. What is the best treatment ?

THE DIVERSION

You may be thrown by the normal pulse oximetry reading and believe that administering 100% oxygen is not the correct answer. You better check your own pulse, since this would be another question you would be answering incorrectly if you fell for this trick.

ANSWER REVEALED

If they describe a patient suffering from carbon monoxide poisoning, then 100 % oxygen would be the correct answer indeed. Pulse oximetry may be normal even in severe CO poisoning. Don't be fooled by a normal pulse oximeter reading.

EITHER OR CHOICES

If there is no improvement with 100% O_2, then carbon monoxide poisoning is not the correct answer. Consider cyanide poisoning (not for you, as a diagnosis) when there is no improvement with administration of 100% oxygen.

Cyanide Poisoning

Cyanide poisoning presents in a similar fashion to CO poisoning with a failure to respond to O_2.

Any smoke exposure can cause cyanide poisoning.

TREATMENT

The most recently FDA-approved treatment for cyanide poisoning is hydroxocobalamin. However, previously sodium thiosulfate or nitrate were used, so if those show up on boards they may be correct choices as well.

Acid Base Ingestion and Alkaloids

Chlorine

Ingestion of chlorine may not require much intervention, and discharge from the ER can be the correct answer since the concentration of hypochlorous acid is low.

Ethylene Glycol

Ethylene glycol toxicity occurs in 3 phases.

Patient presents with a drunken appearance, with no odor of alcohol on the breath, large anion gap, and **oxalate crystals on urinalysis**.

Phase 1: Nausea, vomiting, tachycardia, hypertension, metabolic acidosis, calcium oxalate crystals leading to hypocalcemia

Phase 2: Coma and cardiorespiratory failure, due to acidosis and hypocalcemia

Phase 3: 1- 3 days, renal failure due to acute tubular necrosis, with the patient needing dialysis

> **CASE STUDY**
>
> **You are presented with a patient who is lethargic, ataxic, and has vomited. Lab values will include a low serum bicarb level and an elevated anion gap.[3] At this point, you will have to decide if it is ethanol or ethylene glycol toxicity.**
>
> **THE DIVERSION**
>
> They drop confusing hints in the question to trick you into believing that ethanol is the culprit.
>
> **ANSWER REVEALED**
>
> The key is to look for clues in the question, such as the child being seen alone in the garage. Assuming there isn't a fully stocked bar in the garage, ethylene glycol is the likely culprit. If they throw in something about crystals in the urine, then there really is no diversion at all.

---

[3] Remember to calculate the anion gap each time you are presented with a serum sodium, bicarb, and chloride.

Iron Ingestion

Toxic ingestion occurs at doses of 40mg/kg of elemental iron. The toxicity is primarily *GI-related, but also can be due to free iron* systemically.

Ingestion of less than 40 mg/kg of elemental iron in an asymptomatic patient is not significant. These patients can be observed at home.

Phase 1: Vague GI – within 6 hours, vomiting (often hemorrhagic), diarrhea, and abdominal pain. Any patient who is symptomatic within 6 hours of ingestion should be brought to medical attention. *This is the case even if the estimated ingestion is less than the 40mg/kg threshold.*

Phase 2: Decreased GI symptoms and deceptive improvement, 6-24 hours

Phase 3: Multisystem effects

- Metabolic acidosis
- Coagulopathy
- Cardiovascular collapse

Phase 4: GI obstruction due to scarring and strictures

 Management consists of serum iron levels **4 hours post ingestion**

Serum iron > 350, WBC > 15, and glucose > 150 would be considered significant.

In a symptomatic patient, an abdominal film should be done to identify iron tablets which have not yet been absorbed. Elevated WBC and/or hyperglycemia would also correlate with severe iron ingestion. Additional lab studies should include electrolytes, aminotransferases, CBC, and coagulation studies.

 Appropriate treatment includes:

Chelation Treatment

Indications for chelation treatment would include severe symptoms, as well as the following findings:

- anion gap acidosis,
- serum iron concentrations of greater than 500 mcg/dL (89.5 mcmol/L),
- a significant number of pills visible on abdominal film

With deferoxamine chelation treatment, the urine turns a pink-red color when the serum iron level exceeds the serum iron binding capacity. Treatment can be stopped when there is adequate clinical improvement and/or the urine is no longer pink.[4]

Activated charcoal absorbs iron poorly, and is not indicated for iron ingestion. Syrup of ipecac is no longer indicated either.

The Masquerade Party of Toxicology: Managing Unknown and Multiple Agents

You are expected to know specific points in managing patients who might have ingested multiple agents and/or situations where the agent is unknown.

- First steps (as always) are the ABC's of patient stabilization, before anything else.
- Look in the history for hints of environmental exposures, such as family members taking medications that could explain the presenting symptoms.
- **Labs**, in addition to drug testing, would focus on acid/base status, glucose concentration, and anion gap
- **Acetaminophen** and **salicylate** levels should be obtained when multiple agents are suspected or unknown. This would include intentional ingestion.

Caustic Substances

Initial symptoms following ingestion of a caustic substance include *coughing, crying, drooling, difficulty swallowing,* and *chest pain.*

The ingestion of crystalline substances isn't as alarming, since the child will often spit it out ASAP.

Esophageal burns can present *without any oropharyngeal lesions.* In addition, the presence or absence of oral lesions does not correlate with the severity of esophageal burns. Therefore, endoscopy within 48 hours is indicated in any case where ingestion of a caustic substance is suspected.

Gastric lavage is contraindicated with caustic substance ingestion.

---

[4] Fill in your own Rose Wine joke.

Alkali substances

Alkali substances tend to injure the esophagus and may even lead to esophageal perforation.

Acidic substances

In addition to the esophagus, acidic substances can injure the stomach, since they are not neutralized as alkali substances are.

Dishwasher Detergent

Typically with ingestion of dishwasher detergent or drain cleaner, the impact is immediate, leading to burns of exposed tissue, or oral/esophageal burns. These patients typically present with *drooling, dysphagia, or emesis.*

This leads to deep liquefaction necrosis of the affected tissues, leading to ulceration and perforation as potential complications

Additional findings could include vomiting (with hematemesis), as well as stridor or wheezing. Watch for signs of burns on the face, hands, or chest.

This is why even small amounts of alkali substance can cause significant damage. The toxicity is primarily via direct contact with skin and mucosa; systemic signs will rarely be part of the presentation on the boards.

If you are presented with a patient who is symptomatic after ingesting a caustic substance, endoscopy should be implemented in less than 24 hours to determine the presence and severity of esophageal burns.

The presence or absence of oral lesions also is not predictive of esophageal injury.

Activated charcoal is not indicated; it will not absorb alkali, and will inhibit endoscopic examination.

"Whipped Oven Cleaner"

Watch for the description of a child who was exposed to a common household cleaning substance that could be mistaken by a child as food, i.e., scented floor cleaners or foam oven cleaner spray bottles that could be confused with whipped cream or edible cheese in a can. Although it would be debatable how appetizing the latter would be to a child.

Endoscopy End Game

Even though esophageal burns can be present in an asymptomatic patient, endoscopy is not indicated in these patients, especially on the boards. However, observation for 6 hours to await presentation of symptoms would be appropriate. If asymptomatic after 6 hours, endoscopy would not be indicated.

If they present you with a patient who has wheezing or stridor in this setting, airway stabilization and/or protection would be indicated as well.

Lead Exposure

> **CASE STUDY**
>
> **A 15-month-old presents with an elevated lead level. The parents have been doing kitchen, bathroom, and home equity loan renovations. What is the most likely cause of the child's lead poisoning?**
>
> **THE DIVERSION**
>
> You will be tempted to pick choices like "pica" or "lead plumbing," especially since the kitchen and bathroom have plumbing that will be exposed. That is the decoy, because if you pick lead plumbing your score will plummet like a lead sinker on a fishing trip.
>
> **ANSWER REVEALED**
>
> The correct answer is *household dust*. Lead can be absorbed both through the GI and respiratory tracts; therefore, children are at high risk for absorption of lead through household dust during home renovations.

 Watch for home remedies, such as *amarcon* or *greta,* both of which can lead to elevated serum lead levels.

Mercury

Even though thermometers no longer contain mercury, children are still at risk for environmental exposure. Mercury can be inhaled or ingested, primarily through consumption of fish.

Mercury exposure is **not** a high risk during home renovations.

PCBs

PCBs are synthetic hydrocarbons that are pervasive in the environment and can be concentrated in certain foods.

 High exposure to *PCB's during fetal development can lead to low birthweight*, dark pigmentation of the skin, early eruption of teeth, acneiform rash, and can ultimately be fatal.

PCB can cause **P**igmentation and rash, **C**utting teeth prematurely, and **B**irthweight that is low.

There are also long term neurodevelopmental consequences.

Bioterrorism

Varicella vs. Smallpox lesions

Not only do most of you feel terrorized just taking the boards, but elements of bioterrorism are starting to creep their way onto the boards as well. They expect you to distinguish between varicella and smallpox lesions.

Smallpox lesions begin in the face and extremities, whereas varicella begins centrally and spreads peripherally. Varicella lesions rarely leave scars, while smallpox usually does result in scarring. Smallpox lesions tend to all be in the same stage of development; varicella lesions are in varying stages of development.

Cutaneous Anthrax

Virtually all cases are the cutaneous form of anthrax, which is all you need to know for the boards. The incubation period is less than 2 weeks.

The lesion starts out as a pruritic papule, similar to a routine insect bite, that progresses to a central bullous lesion that becomes necrotic, forming an central black painless eschar. This is classic for anthrax, and should be easy to identify if a lesion is described as such on the exam. The surrounding tissue is swollen and red. There is no associated tenderness. The eschar falls off in 1- 2 weeks.

Systemic signs including adenopathy, fever, malaise, and headache also may be present. However, these are vague symptoms; the key to answering questions related to anthrax correctly will be the cutaneous signs outlined above.

Chapter 10

Born Yesterday: Fetus and Newborn

Neonatal medicine involves virtually every other area of Pediatrics, including Genetics, GI, Neurology, and Infectious Disease. This chapter focuses on areas that are primarily manifested or dealt with during the neonatal period.

Apnea

Apnea

 Apnea is defined as no breath for greater than 20 seconds. Less than that would be considered *periodic breathing*.

The causes of apnea include:

- **Metabolic** (hypoglycemia, hypocalcemia, maternal medications)
- **Infectious** (sepsis, pneumonia)
- **Neurological** (seizures, intracranial hemorrhage)
- **Cardiac** (PDA)
- **GI** (GE Reflux)

Remember the mnemonic APNEA: A = Apnea, **P** = PDA, **N** = Neuro, **E** = External (infection, external meds) and Electrolytes, **A** = Any infectious process. And just remember that GE reflux is a common cause.

Apnea of prematurity is often successfully treated with theophylline or caffeine.[1] There is a two-fold increased risk of SIDS in premature infants diagnosed with apnea of prematurity.

Treatment rarely reduces the risk for SIDS in this population.

---

[1] Oddly enough, caffeine is also how "boredom secondary to reading about apnea" is treated.

Primary vs. Secondary

Primary Apnea

Primary apnea can be reversed with tactile stimulation.

The post delivery pattern of primary apnea is gasping, with increased depth and rate of respiration, followed by apnea. At this point, if oxygen and stimulation are given, there should be a good response.

Most infants will begin breathing independently by 1 minute of age. If the infant is not breathing or responding to stimulation due to primary apnea, he/she will usually respond to bag and mask ventilation.

Secondary Apnea

With no resuscitation, there will be another round of "gasping," followed by apnea. This is secondary apnea. **Oxygen and stimulation won't work in this case**. *Positive pressure ventilation is needed.*

Unfortunately, **primary apnea can occur in utero,** and it is difficult to determine if the newborn is experiencing primary or secondary apnea. Therefore, all apneic newborns who fail to respond to tactile stimulation and remain apneic 30 seconds after delivery, require positive pressure ventilation, under the assumption that you are dealing with secondary apnea.

Transient Tachypnea of the Newborn

TTN is a diagnosis of exclusion, presenting within the first few hours with, of course, tachypnea, retractions, and grunting. Respiratory rate is greater than 60. It typically resolves within 72 hours.

If associated with increased work of breathing, grunting, nasal flaring, and/or retractions, NPO status and close monitoring are in order.

Once these signs are resolving and x-ray is otherwise uncomplicated, feedings can be started (as long as the respiratory rate is below 80 breaths/minute). *Feedings should be advanced slowly until the respiratory rate falls below 60 beats/minute.*

Assessing Comatose and Lethargic Infants Without Becoming Lethargic

The most common causes of coma and lethargy in infants are sepsis, metabolic disturbances, and asphyxia. You can distinguish these on the exam by looking for signs in the history they present to you.

Galactosemia

Galactosemia in and of itself can cause lethargy. However, infants with galactosemia are also at increased risk for sepsis.

Therefore, the *presence of galactosemia does not rule out sepsis as the cause of lethargy* in an infant.

Organic Acidemias

The infant could be described as having a normal delivery. Symptoms develop a bit later. You can expect increased anion gap metabolic acidosis and thrombocytopenia. Elevated urine ketones can be expected with propionic acidemia, as well as elevated serum ammonia levels. Propionic acidemia is also an increased risk for sepsis.

Citrullinemia

Newborns with citrullinemia could present with *poor feeding, lethargy, emesis,* and *coma,* which is pretty non-specific. They have hyperammonemia. Throw in elevated serum glutamic-oxaloacetic transaminase and glutamic-pyruvic transaminase levels and elevated PT/PTT levels as well, and you have the lab picture. Elevated citrulline levels will probably not be included, since the answer would then be too obvious, wouldn't it?

Respiratory alkalosis is common in citrullinemia. *Metabolic acidosis is not.*

Neonatal hypoxic-ischemic encephalopathy (HIE)

Neonatal hypoxic-ischemic encephalopathy (HIE) would have to include a history of a complicated delivery. Added features could include metabolic disturbances such as elevated serum ammonia, lactic acidosis, hypoglycemia, hypocalcemia, and hyponatremia.

Anion gap would be normal.

Transient hyperammonemia

Transient hyperammonemia would typically be seen in a premie with pulmonary disease. They might present an infant with coma and a seizure within the first 24 hours of life.

Antenatal Screening

Alpha-fetoprotein

Elevated AFP

Remember, AFP measurement is only a screen, which may need additional studies, including ultrasound, to confirm suspected findings.

"Incorrect dates" could be the correct explanation for elevated AFP; therefore, consider incorrect dates as the potential answer.

To help remember some of the associations with increased AFP, think of the word **RAIN** (rain elevates the levels of reservoirs, including the AFP reservoir).

> **R**enal (Nephrosis, Renal Agenesis, Polycystic Kidney Disease)
> **A**bdominal Wall Defects
> **I**ncorrect Dating/Multiple Pregnancy
> **N**euro (Anencephaly and Spina Bifida)

Low AFP

This is mainly associated with chromosomal abnormalities like **Trisomy 21** or **Trisomy 18**.

Biophysical Profile

The biophysical profile, in addition to the non stress test, includes an ultrasound evaluation of the following:[2]

- ❏ Fetal Movement
- ❏ Reactive HR
- ❏ Breathing
- ❏ Tone
- ❏ Volume of Amnionic Fluid

Non Stress Test

The non stress test measures spontaneous fetal movements and heart rate activity.

The non stress test measures heart rate activity. It **therefore measures fetal *autonomic nervous system integrity*.**

Contraction Stress Test

The Boards are stressful tests, but the "Contraction Stress Test" measures fetal heart rate in response to uterine contraction. **Therefore, the stress test measures uteroplacental insufficiency and tolerance of labor.**[3]

Normal (no late or significant decelerations) would be reassuring, and positive (late decelerations after 50% of contractions) would require further investigation.

Fetal Heartbreaks

Note that 1% of fetuses may experience arrhythmias. Most of the them are benign.

The most common cause of bradycardia is heart block, which may be seen with maternal lupus.

Supraventricular tachycardia with heart rates exceeding 240 beats per minute require treatment. Treatment consists of giving the antiarrhythmic medication to the mother.

This is to avoid congestive heart failure and hydrops in the fetus.

Respiratory Distress Syndrome (RDS)

RDS is a result of deficient surfactant in the lining of the alveoli. Surfactant levels gradually increase until 33-36 weeks gestation, after which there is a surge. If an infant is born prior to this point, he/she will be surfactant deficient and therefore suffer from RDS.[4]

---

[2] You would think this would be on the OB boards but indeed you are expected to be familiar with this on the exam.

[3] Once again, you would think they would be asking this on the OB boards, not the pediatric boards.

[4] Surfactant is needed to keep the alveoli opened during expiration. Imagine trying to breathe in and out of a balloon that collapsed each time you took a breath rather than remaining partially inflated.

RDS is also known as **"Hyaline Membrane Disease"** because the cellular debris that covers the terminal bronchioles in RDS forms a hyaline membrane — whatever that might be!

Distinguishing RDS from GBS Pneumonia in a Preemie

As you know, the CXR will be of no help. They are indistinguishable. Likewise, non-specific clinical signs like tachypnea, grunting, and respiratory distress are no help. One reliable sign of sepsis in the newborn period is the ratio of bands to total neutrophils; if greater than 0.2, sepsis or pneumonia is more likely. Remember to consider calculating this ratio when the CBC values are given.

The typical presentation of RDS would include **tachypnea, nasal flaring, and expiratory grunting,** as well as **retractions. Cyanosis could be a part of the picture as well.**

Chest x-ray would include *"granular opacifications,"* and *"air bronchograms,"* with obscure heart and/or diaphragm borders. The classic description is a *"ground glass"* appearance. Be sure to look at an atlas to compare this symmetric appearance with the asymmetries seen in meconium aspiration.

If symptoms persist beyond 3 days, a **PDA** could be a complicating factor. In addition, the x-ray findings of **pneumonia secondary to Group B Strep** are often indistinguishable. Therefore, they will have to note something in the history, such as prolonged and progressively worsening symptoms despite respiratory assistance.

Other coexistent conditions can **worsen RDS.** These may include hypoglycemia, hypocalcemia, anemia, and acidosis. Extremes of temperature can be complicating factors in the history as well. In addition, **hypoglycemia** can mimic RDS.

When **hyperbilirubinemia** co-exists with RDS, the threshold for *kernicterus is lowered.*

Risk for RDS

The risk for RDS **is increased** with:
- Infants of diabetic mothers
- C-section delivery
- Birth asphyxia

The risk for RDS **is decreased** with:
- *Prolonged rupture of membranes*
- *Prenatally administered steroids*

Seeing it Coming/Prenatal Tests

An L:S[5] Ratio greater than 2.0 suggests low risk for RDS. If enough time is available before delivery, *prenatal steroids* can help decrease the risk for RDS in premature infants.

---

[5] Lecithin: Sphingomyelin ratio.

Maternal diabetes can interfere with the accuracy of the L:S ratio.

Venting and other treatments for RDS

Mechanical ventilation is usually indicated for a pH lower than 7.2 and PCO_2 greater than 60 in infants with RDS (and/or other signs of respiratory failure). Air leaks are common in infants on a vent.

Exogenous surfactant, high frequency ventilators and ECMO[6] are also used when indicated. The goal of treatment is to maintain PO_2 between 50-70 mm Hg.

Exogenous Surfactant

Once a diagnosis of RDS is made, administration of surfactant is implemented. However, if the baby is <30 weeks, or is otherwise at risk for RDS, therapy should be prophylactic (just after delivery), or early (within two hours of delivery). Once a diagnosis has been made, surfactant administration is termed "rescue."

Clinical improvement is expected as follows:

- · Decreased oxygen requirement
- · Reduced inspiratory pressure
- · Improved lung compliance

Make sure you read the question carefully: *decreased* pulmonary compliance and increased inspiratory pressure would not be an expected improvement with surfactant. *Decreased* inspiratory pressure and *increased* pulmonary compliance would be.

Pulmonary interstitial emphysema (PIE) can account for some deterioration in infants with RDS on ventilators. This is essentially air leaking into the interstitium, and often precedes a full-blown pneumothorax.

BPD Graduates from RDS

BPD is **chronic lung disease** (CLD), commonly seen in infants on prolonged ventilator support. It is due to both *prolonged oxygen exposure and barotrauma.* Infants with RDS that require prolonged ventilator support are at risk for **bronchopulmonary dysplasia** (BPD).[7]

> ### Twins
>
> In general, monozygotic twins are at higher risk for complications because they share a chorion AND an amnion.
>
> B twins are at higher risk for developing respiratory problems than are A twins.

---

[6] Extracorporeal membrane oxygenation; essentially temporary heart lung bypass.

[7] For psychiatrists, BPD is borderline personality disorder.

BPD is treated with diuretics. Infants with BPD are at r*isk for hypocalcemia* as a side effect of diuretic use.

The typical chest x-ray description in an infant with BPD is "diffuse opacities" as well as "cystic areas with streaky infiltrates," and "ground glass appearance."

> ### ECMO Okay
>
> You are expected to know the eligibility criteria for ECMO or extracorporeal membrane oxygenation. ECMO is primarily for infants with reversible lung disease of less than 10-14 days duration, with failure of other methods. In addition, the infant cannot have any systemic or intracranial bleeding or congenital heart disease.

Wilson–Mikity[8] **syndrome** is another chronic lung disease of the newborn. It is different from BPD in that there is often **no history of RDS and there is no history of prolonged oxygen exposure or ventilator support**. The x-ray findings are small cystic changes *as well as fine lacy infiltrates.*

BPD is associated with inflammatory changes in the lung tissue, whereas Wilson–Mikity is not.

In Wilson–Mikity, the changes in the lung often *precede the presentation of symptoms.*

Sepsis

Remember all that is lethargic and floppy with "out of whack" labs is not sepsis. **Remember to consider:**

- ❏ Congenital Adrenal Hyperplasia
- ❏ Inborn Errors of Metabolism

Group B Strep

Early Onset Facts

Group B strep infection typically manifests as pneumonia, meningitis, and/or sepsis.

The empirical treatment of suspected neonatal sepsis, like the format of filling in tiny circles with a number two pencil, has not changed in over 25 years.[9]

---

8 Not to be confused with musician Wilson Picket. OK, yes, I know I'm dating myself but, man, was he good.

9 Fortunately, the use of number 2 pencils on the recertification exam at least has gone to the wayside.

That treatment is still *ampicillin* and *gentamicin* (until you have an exclusive diagnosis of GBS AND clinical improvement, then it's OK to narrow to Pen G). Don't be fooled into choosing ampicillin and cefotaxime. The latter is responsible for outbreaks of drug resistant *Enterobacter* and *serratia*.

Late Onset Facts

Late onset occurs within the **first month.**

The incidence of late onset group B strep infection is NOT increased with prematurity.

While pneumonia and other focal infections do occur, meningitis occurs more commonly with late onset group B strep sepsis.

> *Listeria* infection is associated with a history of maternal flu-like symptoms during pregnancy

Of course, premature rupture of membranes increases the risk for sepsis in newborns.

Toxoplasmosis *(Toxoplasma Gondii)*

With toxoplasmosis occurring **early in pregnancy**, there is a **lower chance of fetal infection**, but when infection does occur, the **consequences are more severe**. The opposite is true later in pregnancy—**there is a greater chance of infection, but the sequelae are less severe.**

> Recognize that the majority of newborn infants with congenital toxoplasmosis are asymptomatic in the neonatal period.

Most affected pregnant women show no clinical signs, and when they do, lymphadenopathy may be the sole symptom.

Signs at Birth

When symptoms are present at birth, common findings include microcephaly, hydrocephaly, chorioretinitis, cerebral calcifications, jaundice, and hepatosplenomegaly.

Diagnosis is made by **immunofluorescence (IFA).**

MRI is used to diagnose encephalitis. Look for *"ring-enhancing" lesions.*

CMV vs. Toxo: Cerebral calcifications in CMV are periventricular. With toxoplasmosis, they are diffuse.

CMV has a **V** in it to remind you that the calcifications are periVentricular. Or consider, in CMV, calcifications, Circu**MV**ent, or hand around, the ventricles.

 GONDII The following are associated with congenital toxoplasmosis:

Greatly Reduced Head
On the Brain/Water (hydrocephalus)
Nothing (asymptomatic)
Diffuse Calcifications
I (=**E**yes/ chorioretinitis)
Icteric and hepatosplenomegaly

Later Signs/When Asymptomatic at Birth

❑ Deafness

❑ Impaired vision

❑ Seizures

❑ Mental retardation

❑ Learning disabilities

❑ Cognitive deficits

 Remember TOXO:

Tremors (seizures)
O (zero hearing)
X (Optic chiasm, blindness)
O (zero or impaired intelligence) Not the best, but still easier than rote memory, eh?

50/50 Rule

50% of infected pregnant women will pass the infection on to the fetus, and 50% of these fetuses will be born asymptomatic. Once again, an infection occurring later in pregnancy means a greater chance of the infant being asymptomatic.

In addition to affected neonates, toxoplasmosis infection causes severe disease in immunocompromised hosts, such as those with HIV or those receiving chemotherapy.

Treatment is with *pyrimethamine, sulfadiazine,* and *folinic acid.*

Toxoplasmosis is why we tell pregnant women that they can get out of changing the kitty litter while they are pregnant – this is a mode of transmission for toxoplasmosis.

Birth Trauma

Clavicular Fracture

In most cases, watchful observation is all that is necessary, and you can expect the callus to recede within 2 years.

 Watch for this if you are presented with a neonatal CXR. It is easy to miss the clavicular forest while focusing on the Lung and GI trees.

 Erb's Palsy and Phrenic Nerve Palsy can occur with a clavicular fracture.

Brachial Plexus Injury

You will need to be familiar with the 2 classic types of brachial plexus injury and distinguish them based on their clinical presentations or their appearances on the picture section. These occur in less than a **half a percent of deliveries**, but occur in a much *larger percentage of deliveries on the Boards.*

Erb's Palsy

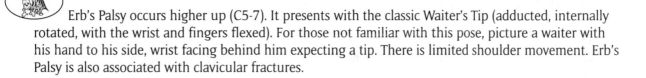 Erb's Palsy occurs higher up (C5-7). It presents with the classic Waiter's Tip (adducted, internally rotated, with the wrist and fingers flexed). For those not familiar with this pose, picture a waiter with his hand to his side, wrist facing behind him expecting a tip. There is limited shoulder movement. Erb's Palsy is also associated with clavicular fractures.

Erb's Palsy is more common than Klumpke palsy. With Erb's Palsy the nerve is stretched, not broken, and the ability to grasp is preserved. *Therefore, the grasp reflex remains intact.*

 Picture a **waiter** getting a big "**Herb Plant**" instead of a tip.

 Phrenic Nerve paralysis leading to respiratory distress can occur with Erb's Palsy as well. Watch for this in the history.

Klumpke Palsy

Klumpke Palsy occurs much lower down (C8, T1). It affects the muscles of the hand, resulting in the **claw hand**.

 Picture someone being born grabbing a "Klump" of sand.

 They may also lose the ability to grasp with Klumpke Palsy, despite this initial presentation.

It can be associated with **Horner syndrome**, so keep this in mind if this is noted in the history.

Cord Issues

Clingy Cord

The umbilical cord should **fall off by the 2-week visit**. Keep this in mind if they present you with an anxious grandmother who is concerned that the cord has not fallen off on time. Why grandmother is still having babies though, is a matter for another time.

If it stays attached beyond **one month**, think LAD (Leukocyte Adhesion Deficiency) or low WBC count.

It is important to note that, for the purpose of the boards, all that is needed for umbilical stump care is washing with soap and water and pat dry. There is no decreased infection risk by applying alcohol to the stump. Cultural remedies are okay, provided they do no harm (e.g., applying mercurochrome, which contains mercury). [10]

Single Umbilical Artery

In the real world, most incidences of a single umbilical artery are **not** associated with renal disease. However, it must be considered, especially on the exam!

When presented with a newborn with a single umbilical artery, you are expected to know that a renal ultrasound is indicated.

Bloody Cord

Yes, the baby should be kept below the cord before clamping, for around 30 seconds, to prevent decreased red cell volume.

 However, the obstetrician should not "milk" the cord toward the baby. This could lead to polycythemia.

Cath Business

Umbilical artery and vein catheter placement carry with them certain complications. To help remember some of the more common complications, think: **"NEO CATH."**

> **N**ecrosis
> **E**mbolization (liver)
> **O**mphalitis/Infection
>
> **C**ompromised Femoral Pulse
> **A**ccidental Hemorrhage
> **T**raumatic Perforation Thrombosis (Renal Artery and Aorta)
> **H**epatic (dysfunction)

Witch's Milk

Breast hypertrophy in a newborn is usually a benign finding. This is the case even if milk is produced. This has been called witch's milk.

The correct answer is to leave it alone. Expressing the milk by squeezing it out will be the wrong answer. In fact, this will make it worse, since this stimulates prolactin and oxytocin secretion and will prolong it. It also increases the risk for mastitis.

---

[10] Mercurochrome is no longer available in the US, but is readily available on the boards.

Facts and definitions to Watch Out For

Definitions

Strict definitions of terms are important because they might describe something, or imply a disorder or problem, that does not meet the criterion for the "definition." If you fall into the trap you will get the question wrong.

LGA/SGA

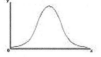

The Boards can present you with a small baby an imply it is SGA.. Unless you know the definition, you will be fooled. **An SGA baby is in the lower 10th percentile, and an LGA baby is in the upper 10th percentile for weight for gestational age.** If they tell you the baby is in the upper 15th percentile, it is not LGA.

In addition, LGA is greater than 3900g and SGA less than 2500g. SGA babies have a higher morbidity and mortality risk than AGA babies. In the short term, they are at higher risk for temperature instability, polycythemia, and fasting hypoglycemia.

SGA and IUGR

An SGA baby is small for gestational age, adjusted for the gestational age. SGA and IUGR may go hand in hand. However, preemies won't be SGA if their weight is appropriate for their gestational age. IUGR babies tend to have more difficulty tolerating labor, and therefore IUGR is often associated with perinatal asphyxia.

Infants of mothers with chronic illness are at higher risk for being SGA. Teenage mothers are at higher risk for delivering SGA babies.

Growth in SGA babies, especially in those with IUGR, does not usually begin to catch up until age 2 years. Babies who are small for dates are at higher risk for developing neurodevelopmental disabilities.

Full Term

This is defined as 40 weeks plus or minus 2 weeks. Any baby born in the range of 38-42 weeks is considered to be full term; thus, a 42 week baby is actually considered term.

Post Term (Prolonged pregnancy)

Sometimes too much is too much. Babies born post term, i.e., more than 2 weeks post dates, also present with problems.

Post term newborns may be described as having dry skin that is peeling, long fingernails, and decreased lanugo on the back. The ears will have strong recoil.

Fetal Deaths/Causes

The most **common causes of fetal demise are chromosomal abnormalities and congenital malformations.**

The normal arterial blood gas values for a newborn infant is a pO2 60 – 90 mmHg and a pCO2 35-45 mmHg.

Scalping pHs

They may present you with a scalp pH of 7.29 and ask you for the most appropriate next step.

You might be tricked by all of the diversionary choices that involve the beginning of an extensive workup.

In the end, nothing but reassurance is necessary, since a **normal scalp pH is 7.25 or higher.** Remember this, because they can present you with a normal one and imply in the question that it is abnormal. However, less than 7.2 is a bad sign.

The Passing of the Meconium

If meconium has not been passed in the first 48 hours, this should be looked into.

The possible causes of delayed passing of meconium in an infant are:

- Meconium plug syndrome
- Hirschsprung's disease
- Imperforate anus

Hirschsprung's Disease (Congenital Aganglionic Megacolon)

Hirschsprung's Disease (Congenital Aganglionic Megacolon) is due to the absence of parasympathetic innervation of the internal anal sphincter.[11] The affected segment is contracted, resulting in constipation. *Hirschsprung's Disease is limited to the recto-sigmoid colon.*

Hirschsprung's Disease is due to a segment of bowel that is aganglionic. The region proximal to the aganglionic segment then becomes distended.

No passage of meconium in the first 48 hours is the classic presentation. However, infants can present with abdominal distention alternating with periods of diarrhea. **Diagnosis is by biopsy.**

Hirschsprung's Disease is also associated with **Down** syndrome.

Meconium/To Tube or Not to Tube

We all go to mec deliveries, but, for the purpose of the Boards, intubation is not necessary if the baby is vigorous. With a floppy baby, suction the oropharynx (at delivery), then intubate and suction below the cords. If the baby is vigorous, visualization is okay. Remember not to stimulate the baby first, like you would normally do!

Careful observation is still required, since you can still have no meconium at the cord level with meconium deeper in the bronchial tree.

Based on prior research, suctioning at the perineum before the shoulders are delivered was felt to be critical. A recent rigorous study has shown no difference in outcome between suctioning on the perineum and no suctioning prior to delivery of the shoulders.

It may be initially difficult to distinguish congenital heart disease from pulmonary hypertension without meconium.

Meconium Aspiration/Meconium Ileus

Meconium ileus can, of course, be seen with cystic fibrosis. On the picture section they might even show some calcifications in the bowel.

First Breath

In the event they present you with a case of bona fide mec aspiration syndrome, persistent pulmonary hypertension is the most likely complication they will be describing.

Around **60 mm Hg pressure** is needed to inflate the lungs with the first breath.

Clonus Bonus

Remember that **bilateral ankle clonus** can be a **normal** finding in an **infant**, so don't assume it is an abnormal finding.

---

[11] Yeah, you probably have to read that one over a couple of times to know what it means clinically, but (or shall we say butt) you never know when that sort of detail might pop (or poop) up on the exam.

Special Delivery

HOT TIP

Newborns are at risk for heat loss because of the high surface-area-to-body-mass ratio. Heat loss is reduced by the use of a *radiant warmer* and drying with warm blankets. Ultimately, the best source of warmth is skin to skin contact with the mother (which has emotional benefits as well). Cold stress should be avoided because it can lead to depletion of fat and glycogen stores.

The one exception to the radiant heat warmer answer is extreme premies, or ELGANs[12] as they are now known, who weigh less than1 kg. Placing these tiny babies in an open air radiant heat warmer can result in too much evaporative fluid loss. Therefore, a closed humidified environment is required for usually at least the first 24-72 hours of life. Basically, an isolette is better than open air radiant heat, even though access for procedures is less convenient.

Apgar

Although Virginia Apgar was an anesthesiologist, her work is the domain of the pediatric boards. Know that the 1-minute Apgar does not reflect long term problems if the 5-minute Apgar is fine. This is because the 1 minute Apgar reflects life in the uterus and his/her endurance of the delivery process to the harsh life outside the uterus. The 5 minute Apgar reflects transition and adjustment to the new world. A 5 minute Apgar of 7 or less is reflective of difficult adjustment. We are assuming that anyone reading this is familiar with the Apgar measurement, having attended scores of deliveries by the time this book has reached your eyes.

Very Low Birthweight (VLBW) Infants and Apgars

PERIL WARNING

Due to neurological immaturity, including poor tone, an Apgar greater than 6 cannot be expected in these tiny infants.

No Time to Wait

PERIL WARNING

You do not use Apgar results to make decisions regarding administration of CPR, since you would never "wait one minute" before making a decision.

However, you are expected to know that positive pressure ventilation is required in the presence of bradycardia and impaired ventilatory efforts.

> ### Placental Weight
>
> It might seem trivial, but a question on this topic could appear on the exam.
>
> *DEFINITION*
>
> Know that the Fetal/Placental weight ratio increases progressively during pregnancy. If it does not, it is evidence of decreased fetal growth. The ratio at birth is normally 6.5 – 7.0 at term (think of a tall basketball player[13] in the normal uterus).

> ### Be Mechanical Fanatical
>
> Often the key to the answer is mechanical failure (e.g., an overheated child on the warmer, "the probe fell off the baby"), which might lead to sudden deterioration of an infant on a ventilator.
>
> - Is the tube blocked?
> - Did the O_2 tubing fall off the wall?
>
> Choices involving "mechanical failure" are often the correct information buried in the question in a can of red herrings.

---

[12] Extremely low gestational age newborn.
[13] Who are typically 6'5" – 7' tall.

If despite adequate ventilation with oxygen, the heart rate remains below 60 bpm, chest compressions are to be implemented.[14]

In the neonate, compressions should be given at a rate of 100 per minute, with one ventilation per 3 compressions.

Home Deliveries

If you see the phrase "home delivery," highlight it because it's there for a reason. Ultimately, **hemorrhage, sepsis, or bleeding secondary to vitamin K deficiency**[15] will be the key to the answer they are seeking.

They could describe an infant that has been treated with antibiotics, which removes the normal GI flora, resulting in decreased absorption of vitamin K.

The Eyes Have It

Silver nitrate solution is not effective in preventing neonatal *chlamydial* conjunctivitis. It only protects against conjunctivitis secondary to gonorrhea. Therefore, if given a choice between silver nitrate and erythromycin, erythromycin would be the *correct* choice.

Anuric Infants

If they ask you to evaluate an anuric[16] infant, the following stepwise approach would be in order

1) Recheck the plumbing by evaluating the abdomen and genitalia
2) Make sure fluid intake has been adequate
3) Obtain a cath urine specimen for analysis
4) BUN and Creatinine
5) Renal ultrasound
6) If you do all this and the results are normal and then the baby starts to pee, you can stop now.
7) If anything comes up positive and/or the baby still hasn't been convinced to pee, then you can call in the urologist, even on the boards, but only once you have done all of the above.

Preemie Dreamy

Some important points about preemies can, and will, be held against you. If you know the basics, you should be able to answer these questions with ease.

---

[14] Since the protocols are updated fairly frequenlty,we suggest you refer to the most recent CPR guidelines to confirm the latest recommendations.

[15] IM vitamin K would not be a part of the home delivery of course.

[16] No urine output for 24 hours.

Very Low Birth Weight Infants (VLBW)

What exactly is a very low birth weight infant? Any infant weighing less than 1500 grams should be considered to be VLBW.

VLBW infants require D10 in order to provide sufficient glucose without fluid overload.

Factors which impact **prognosis** include the following:

· Gestational age (the most important factor)
· Morbidity while in the NICU
· Intracranial hemorrhage

VLBW and Sepsis

In the absence of another explanation such as pre-eclampsia or placenta previa, infection must be considered as a trigger for premature delivery. Sepsis has to be ruled out in the VLBW infant unless an alternative cause of the preterm birth seems clear.

Coverage for common bacteria would be accomplished with the old standbys, ampicillin and gentamicin.

If the infant presents with vesicular lesions, neonatal herpes is likely, and treatment with acyclovir would be a correct choice. Thrombocytopenia, or even a bloody spinal tap, could be another sign of neonatal herpes. Do NOT let the fact that the mom has no history of herpes throw you off the herpes diagnostic trail.

> ### Premie Pressure
>
> While there are no set norms for blood pressure in preemies, use the following if a question on this pops up on the exam.
>
> The preterm baby's mean arterial blood pressure should not be less than the corrected gestational age in weeks. Therefore, a 28 week premie should not have a mean arterial blood pressure less than 28.

Catch up Growth

· Catch up growth in preemies occurs during the *first 2 years*.
· They should attain *normal height at age 2* and beyond.

Preemies and Calcium

Preemies are **at risk for rickets** because of inadequate intake and absorption of calcium and phosphorus.

Caloric Requirements for Preemies

For your favorite preemie, caloric requirement is **120 kcal/kg/day.**

Preemie Chow/or Formula

Here are some facts to "chew on."

❏ The optimal **whey/casein ratio** is 60/40.
❏ Glucose polymers are better absorbed than lactose
❏ MCT's (Medium Chain Triglycerides) are therefore needed in preemie formula
❏ Contains higher calcium and phosphorus
❏ Contains 24 kcal/oz

Preemie Breast Milk

It contains higher amounts of everything than full term breast milk, with the exception of carbohydrates.

Lytes and Bytes, Sweets and Treats

Necrotizing Enterocolitis (NEC)

The following are some important points to remember about Necrotizing Enterocolitis (NEC).

NEC is associated with:

· **Hypoxic Injury** – RDS, birth asphyxia, and/or prolonged apnea, among other conditions
· **Bacterial Infection**

Blood cultures are often positive, and pneumatosis intestinalis is a common finding on x-ray. It is best to keep them NPO for at least 3 weeks after an episode of NEC.

Some of the typical findings associated with NEC are general, such as lethargy, apnea, and poor feeding, while others are more specific, such as **bloody stools, erythema of the abdominal wall,** and **thrombocytopenia.**

Pneumatosis intestinalis, in and of itself, is not diagnostic, because it can occur with other disorders. However, on the Boards it should be present, and they will probably show you a film that also shows **air in the biliary tree**. The combination of these two findings would be sufficient for an assumption of a diagnosis of NEC and a slam-dunk for you.

The long term complication of NEC that you need to be aware of is *intestinal strictures.*

Management of NEC should include an NG tube to intermittent suction, IV fluids and antibiotics, CBC, lytes, coagulation studies, as well as serial abdominal films as indicated.

Surgical intervention is required up to half the time.

Jaundice (Neonatal)

Questions on this are certainly fair game. In addition to the basic garden-variety presentations like breast-fed and physiological jaundice, they will throw in some Yellow Zebras as well.

Facts

- A bilirubin up to 12.4 within the first 24 hours can be normal in a full term newborn.

- Visual diagnosis is generally unreliable, even more so in darker skinned infants.

- Near term infants 35-38 weeks are at higher risk for jaundice.

- Frequent breastfeeding decreases the risk for jaundice.

- Screen for a prior history of breast feeding difficulties, which increases the risk for hyperbilirubinemia.

- Infants of East Asian decent are at higher risk for hyperbilirubinemia.

ABO Incompatibility

Remember, even with a "setup,"[17] only **a small percentage will actually result in significant hemolysis leading to jaundice**.

ABO incompatibility may cause anemia in a **first-born child**. However, Rh incompatibility does not usually cause anemia in a first born child, unless they were to mention a previous miscarriage.

The anemias of both ABO incompatibility and Rh incompatibility can be severe and can occur at 1 -2 months of age.

Breast Feeding vs. Breast Milk Jaundice

Believe it or not, there is a difference between the terms. If you are confronted with the two in a multiple-choice situation, don't be fooled.

Breast fed jaundice occurs during the first days of life, and is due to decreased caloric intake and dehydration. Withholding breast milk is not appropriate in "breast fed jaundice."

Breast milk jaundice occurs after the first week of life and is due to inherent factors too complicated and boring to get into here. Suffice it to say that holding breast milk for one day and having the mother pump is the answer they are looking for.

Phototherapy is **contraindicated treatment** with an elevated **direct (conjugated) bilirubin** or a **family history of light sensitive porphyria**. With elevated direct, they might describe the "**Bronze Baby Syndrome**" in a child started on phototherapy that did not first have a direct level checked. Phototherapy would be what caused the Bronze Baby Syndrome.

Physiologic Jaundice

Physiologic jaundice is hyperbilirubinemia that occurs on Day 2 through Day 5, in an otherwise healthy infant with no other pathological explanation. It is a diagnosis of exclusion, but very common.

An elevated bilirubin that occurs during the first 24 hours is abnormal. It cannot by definition be called "physiologic jaundice."

If they ask what would be the "first step," it would be to check a total and direct bili (checking direct bilirubin is important before starting phototherapy).

---

[17] E.g., mother with blood type O and baby with A or B.

The incidence of neonatal jaundice is reduced with maternal heroin use.[18] It is also reduced with smoking, alcohol, and the double P's: Phenobarb/Phenytoin.

A Jaundiced view of Neonatal Jaundice (Factors that can worsen neonatal Jaundice)

Any medication such as sulfonamides, which compete for space on albumin, can increase the levels of bilirubin. **Severe acidosis** can have a similar effect.

In these conditions, since much of the bilirubin is not bound to albumin, kernicterus can result at lower levels.

A **PDA** can result in blood being shunted from the liver, resulting in decreased metabolism of bilirubin and increased indirect bilirubin.

The term "YELLOW" is pretty relevant but some of the mnemonic is a stretch. Here is an alternate mnemonic that brings to mind a friend's term for preemies on an oscillator and bili lights (you guessed it, "Shake and Bake"). The alternate mnemonic is **"LIE and GLOW"** – easy to remember if you think of your favorite orange youngster under those pretty blue lights. The point is that the more relevant and the more outrageous, the more chance you will remember. I continue to encourage you to personalize stories or mnemonics for anything you find difficult to remember.

> ### What are the Causes of Indirect Hyperbilirubinemia? YELLOW
>
> **Y**ou Never Know: Gilbert Disease, Gilbert Goes Yellow
>
> **E**ndocrine: (Hypothyroid - Hypopituitarism); Enterohepatic Circulation Increased (Obstruction, Pyloric Stenosis, Meconium Ileus, Ileus, Hirschsprung's Disease)
>
> **L**ucy Driscoll Syndrome: I don't even know what this is, but you never know, they could ask.
>
> **L**ysed Blood Cells: Hemolytic Disease, Defects of Red Cell Metabolism, Isoimmunization
>
> **O**verdrive: Some are both Direct and Indirect. Galactosemia, Tyrosinosis, Hypermethionemia (Cystic Fibrosis)
>
> **W**asted Blood: Petechiae, Hematomas, Hemorrhages anywhere, Cephalohematomas, Swallowed maternal blood

Lysed blood cells: Hemolytic Disease, Defects of Red Cell Metabolism, Isoimmunization

Increased

Enterohepatic circulation: Obstruction, Pyloric Stenosis, Meconium Ileus, Ileus, Hirschsprung's Disease (and Endocrine: Hypothyroid – Hypopituitarism)

Gilbert Disease

Lucy Driscoll Syndrome: I still don't know what this is, but you never know, they could ask.

b**O**th Direct and Indirect: Galactosemia, Tyrosinosis, Hypermethioninemia, Cystic Fibrosis

Wasted Blood: Petechiae, Hematomas, Hemorrhages anywhere, Cephalohematomas, Swallowed maternal blood

---

[18] However, this does not mean one should encourage heroin use!

Exchange Transfusion

Sometimes an exchange transfusion will be necessary. The complications of exchange transfusion can easily be remembered with Transfusion imPaCT NO!: Thrombocytopenia, Potassium high, Calcium low, No! volume.

 Transfusion im**PaCT NO**!

P otassium high

C alcium low

T hrombocytopenia

Volume **No**! (hypovolemia)

And it rhymes to boot!

De×tro Strip Deceptions

 Blood samples contaminated with IV solution containing glucose can result in a falsely elevated result on the Dextrostix. In addition, shortened **time** on the strip will result in a **lower level**.

Remember the "d" sticks are not totally accurate and, therefore, if that is the only value provided in the question, the "next" step is to **verify the result with serum glucose**.

Metabolic Issues of the Newborn

Sugar Babies / Hypoglycemia

Hypoglycemia is serum glucose less than 25 in a preemie and less than 35 in a full term newborn. In practice, it's less than 40. The Boards won't split such sweet hairs.

The very low birth weight infant is at risk for hypoglycemia due to small muscle mass and low glycogen stores. This, along with maintaining good body temperature, is the most important step for initial management and board questions.

Hypoglycemia can present in any number of ways such as the classic jitteriness, lethargy and apnea, as well as *cyanosis and seizures.*

Management

Hypoglycemia is managed with a 2 -3 mL/kg D10 bolus. Glucagon IM could be another option. However, this is rarely successful with low birth weight infants. Low muscle mass means low stores, and you can't tap sugar out of a low muscle mass stone.

"A mother who has had tocolytics to arrest labor" could be the tip-off; these agents can stimulate fetal insulin, resulting in hypoglycemia.

Remember: **tachypnea can be a sign of hypoglycemia**, and in fact it can be the only sign of hypoglycemia that they give you on the exam.

Sugar and Spice/ Infants of Diabetic Mothers

Like all questions, they are not likely to test your knowledge of the obvious, in this case LGA babies and hypoglycemia. Another manifestation of infants of diabetic mothers is **polycythemia**, possibly due to increased erythropoietin. Another risk is **hypoplastic left colon**.

As fetuses, infants of diabetic mothers are exposed to high glucose levels, and as result produce a lot of insulin. After delivery, insulin levels remain high despite being cut off from their sugar source. Therefore, these infants often develop hypoglycemia for several hours after delivery. The increased insulin also promotes growth, which explains why they are typically LGA.

Remember **L**arge Body, small **L**eft Colon.

Hypocalcemia

Hypocalcemia = Ionized calcium lower than 4.5 mg/dL (1 mmol/L) and a total calcium lower than 8.5 mg/dL.

Late Hypocalcemia

Late hypocalcemia occurs in an infant mistakenly given cow's milk. Hypocalcemia is due to the "high phosphate" load on the kidneys.

Signs of Hypocalcemia include jitteriness, **Chvostek's sign** (facial muscle twitching on tapping plus cheek shake sign) and **Trousseau's sign** (carpopedal spasm). A **prolonged QT Interval** can be seen on the EKG with hypocalcemia.

To help remember what Trousseau's sign actually is, think: "To Row" – you need your wrist to row, making this easy to remember that it is *carpopedal spasm.*

CASE STUDY An infant with hypocalcemia has been receiving calcium replacement and continues to show signs of hypocalcemia. What is the best next step?

THE DIVERSION Among the choices will be to continue to administer calcium or get a repeat value of calcium. However, these would be incorrect.

ANSWER REVEALED The correct next step would be to administer magnesium, because serum Mg and Ca levels are directly correlated. An elevated Mg will decrease PTH secretion. Hypomagnesemia can result in intractable hypocalcemia that won't respond to calcium replacement until you correct the magnesium.

Treatment

TREATMENT Treatment of hypocalcemia is pretty straightforward: increase calcium in the IV or bolus with calcium gluconate. In both hypocalcemia and hypoglycemia, jitteriness will have no long-term consequences. However, when a seizure results, there can be long-term CNS consequences.

HOT TIP Consider hypocalcemia in any infant born to a mother on **Mg sulfate**. A **magnesium level** is also indicated, especially if there is no response to calcium administration.

Blue on Blue

Peripheral cyanosis in an otherwise healthy full term infant is another example where they will imply a problem when there is none.

PERIL WARNING Acrocyanosis cyanosis in and of itself requires no treatment other than routine placement in the warmer.

Heme Dreams/Neonatal Hematology Issues

Anemia

At birth, 50% Hgb is Fetal HgbF. For a full term infant, Hgb less than 13 at birth is considered anemia.

The **Kleihauer Betke Test** detects for the presence of fetal cells in the mother's blood. It is used to evaluate neonatal anemia.

Polycythemia

Polycythemia is a **central venous HCT** of 65 or higher. The key phrase is *central venous*, since a heel stick might be hemoconcentrated.

Treatment is indicated when the hematocrit is greater than 70. Polycythemia will often lead to *hypoglycemia, hyperbilirubinemia,* and/or *thrombocytopenia.* Treatment for symptomatic polycythemia is a partial exchange transfusion.

If the value they give you is from a capillary blood sample or heel stick, then the answer will be to obtain a central venous value, especially in an acidotic hypotensive baby.[19]

Polycythemia Arena

We know that **polycythemia leads to elevated bilirubin levels**. Remember that it also can lead to **hypoglycemia**.

Remember yellow bananas aren't very sweet; i.e., jaundiced kids can have hypoglycemia.

Hyperviscosity Syndrome

Hyperviscosity syndrome results from polycythemia. This syndrome can result in *lethargy, hypotonia, and irritability.*

Anemia in Preemies vs. Full Term Infants

Of course, pre-term infants have lower hematocrit values than full-term infants. Therefore, the bottoming out levels of "physiologic" anemia are lower and occur earlier in pre-term infants than in term newborns. In FT infants, the Hgb can fall to as low as 11 or even 9. Pre-term infants often go as low as 7 to 8. FT infants reach their "nadir" at 2 - 3 months; preemies can reach it in 1 - 2 months. The main point to remember is that in preemies the initial Hct is lower, and they bottom out earlier.

---

[19] Or house officer.

Apt Test

The Apt Test tests blood in the neonate's gastric aspirate to determine if it is actually maternal blood. For example, if they ask you what you would do about a neonate that is being gavage fed, and there is blood in the residuals, "Apt Test" would be the correct answer.

Thrombocytopenia

Thrombocytopenia is a platelet count lower than 100,000. Maternal ITP is one of the main causes, and it can last several weeks until the mother's IgG is cleared out.

Coagulation

A prolonged PTT can be a normal finding in neonates until 9 months.

Hemorrhagic Disease of the Newborn

Hemorrhagic Disease of the Newborn can be Early or Late onset.

Early Onset/Hemorrhagic Disease

Early onset is within 3 days in newborns who are breast-fed exclusively and not given IM vitamin K.[20] This will manifest with bleeding at circumcision or from the umbilical cord.

Late Onset/Hemorrhagic Disease

Late onset can occur **up to 3 months of age**.

A typical scenario would be an infant who is breast-fed and develops diarrhea. Another scenario might be a baby who did not receive IM vitamin K or only received the oral form.

Oral vitamin K is insufficient for preventing hemorrhagic disease of the newborn.

---

[20] And delivered at home, a favorite scenario on the Boards.

The latest unproven buzz is that the rapidly increased use of immunizations and the administration of vitamin K at birth have resulted in an increase in autoimmune diseases and cancer. None of this has been proven to be true, and it would be an incorrect assumption on the exam.

Maternal medications can also increase the risk for hemorrhagic disease in the newborn.

Logically, if there is a history of the mother taking anticoagulants, this will increase the risk

Anticonvulsants can induce liver microsomal activity and also contribute to hemorrhagic disease of the newborn.

However, they might note the mother was taking antibiotics during pregnancy. You may not realize that there is an increased risk for hemorrhagic disease, but there is. Common culprits are the quinolones, cephalosporins, and meds used to treat tuberculosis.

Nephrology

Acute tubular necrosis is a possibility in the newborn period, manifesting as proteinuria and hematuria. Renal ultrasound would be the most appropriate test to order (following the "least invasive test" rule).

Seizing the moment (Neonatal Seizures)

Seizure in the DR

If a neonatal seizure occurs within 24 hours of birth, it is likely to be secondary to birth asphyxia. Often there will be a hint of this in the history presented.

Most neonatal seizures are subtle.

Typical descriptions of neonatal seizures include "staring spells," "decreased motor activity," lip smacking, and/or other abnormal facial movements.

Most full-term newborn infants who have neonatal seizures secondary to asphyxia *will not have any long-term neurodevelopmental sequelae.* This is indeed worth noting.

Neonatal encephalopathy and hypoxic-ischemic encephalopathy (HIE) are the most frequent causes of neonatal seizures in the full term infant. However, metabolic causes have to be ruled out first.

Once the common metabolic causes have been ruled out, **phenobarbital** will be the correct treatment.

In the case of neonatal asphyxia, remember that the brain isn't the only organ involved. Indeed, intrapartum asphyxiation can lead to multiple organ system failure. For example, the intestine, kidney, lung, liver, and heart can all be affected.

Full term newborn infants presenting with seizures due to asphyxia do not usually manifest long-term neurodevelopmental problems. However, when infants with hypoxic ischemic injury develop seizures, there is more concern for impaired neurodevelopmental outcome. Nearly half of these infants may have abnormal outcomes, manifested by cognitive problems, motor problems, and/or epilepsy.

Hyperalimentation (HAL) [21]

An important point to remember is that HAL-induced cholestasis is due primarily to protein intake, and this should be limited to 2 g/kg/day. If all else fails, phenobarbital can be used to stimulate bile secretion and decrease serum bili levels.

Cleft Lip/Palate

Cleft Lip/Palate is frequently part of a variety of syndromes. Therefore, watch for descriptions of other anomalies.

To help remember some of the syndromes associated with Cleft Lip/Palate, consider the following mnemonic:

CAT: picture a Giant Lip, parting like a Curtain and a CAT appearing. **CAT** stands for:

> **C**rouzon Syndrome
> **A**pert
> **T**reacher Collins Syndrome *(Dominant: picture a dominant "teacher" carrying a whip)*

Initially, special nipples are required for feeding. Surgical correction for this problem is done around 6 months. Children with Cleft Lip/Palate are also at risk for ear infections.

---

[21] Which is not to be confused with HAL, the rebellious robot in *2001: A Space Odyssey*.

Abdominal Wall Defects

Omphalocele

 An omphalocele is a protrusion of the bowel through the umbilicus.

With an **omphalocele,** the bowel contents will be **covered with a membrane**. The presence of the membranous cover is the key to distinguishing an *omphalocele* from *gastroschisis* in the picture section.

Omphalocele is often associated with other anomalies including **Beckwith Wiedemann syndrome** (macroglossia, macrosomia, and hypoglycemia).

To help remember some of the features associated with Beckwith Wiedemann syndrome, think Big Width Wiedemann syndrome: picture a big man **eating M and M's** (**M**acroglossia and **M**acrosomia) with his "big tongue" and "big body," getting so large that he ends up with an eviscerated bowel covered with a membrane. Hypoglycemia is the driving force behind this ferocious appetite.

Chromosomal abnormalities are common with omphalocele.

Gastroschisis

 Gastroschisis is the herniation of bowel through a defect in the abdominal musculature *near the umbilicus.*

Whereas omphalocele can involve intestines and other organs (e.g., liver), gastroschisis is usually **limited to intestinal contents,** and is **not covered with a membrane**. In addition, gastroschisis tends to be located on the right *near the umbilicus*, and herniation of other organs is rare. With omphalocele, the defect is through the umbilicus, the liver can also be involved, and chromosomal anomalies are common.

Picture the O in Omphalocele as the membrane cover. Picture the membrane being made out of DNA strands to remind you that this can be associated with *chromosomal defects*.

The most important **initial management** is to keep the bowel contents moist. In addition, NG tube placement is important.

Tracheoesophageal Fistula

TE fistula commonly includes esophageal atresia. Esophageal atresia may be diagnosed/suspected by the inability to pass an OG/NG tube, and may be confirmed on x-ray.

They will likely describe a history of polyhydramnios. Intermittent cyanosis can be a finding, due to excess secretions pooling and causing airway obstruction.

You could be asked for further studies, and you will need to know that you should be ruling out other associated findings common with VACTERL syndrome.

Until surgical intervention takes place, the airway needs to be protected from secretions via 1) frequent suctioning and 2) placing the infant in a position that elevates the head.

Diaphragmatic Hernia

If you hear the terms "scaphoid abdomen" with "decreased breath sounds on the **left side**," look no further; you have been given a gift.

Imperforate Anus

These can present with anything from a thin membrane obstructing the anus to full blown atresia. **Low obstructions** typically present with the anus displaced anteriorly and connected to the rectum via a fistula. **High obstructions** typically present with a fistula connecting into the vagina or the urinary tract. Note this when the history is consistent with these findings.

In addition, imperforate anus is associated with VACTERL syndrome.

Intraventricular hemorrhage

Intraventricular hemorrhage (IVH), as with any intracerebral hemorrhage, should be managed like any other potentially unstable situation. Begin with the ABCs before anything else. If imaging is needed in an unstable newborn, it should be done by cranial ultrasound at the bedside. If the patient is stable and a subarachnoid or subdural hemorrhage is suspected, then a head CT would be indicated.

Many times IVH will be asymptomatic, but, if present, clinical signs may include anemia, hyperglycemia, thrombocytopenia, hyponatremia, and/or acidemia. IVH usually occurs within the first 96 hours of life for preemies.

Grading IVH

Should they ask about grading:
Grade 1 is Germinal Matrix
Grade 2 is IVH without Dilation
Grade 3 is IVH with Dilation
Grade 4 is all this plus parenchymal involvement

> **Caput Succedaneum** crosses the suture lines and will be described as "soft, boggy pitting."
>
> A **Cephalohematoma** is more localized and will be described as firm and tense.

MNEMONIC
Cephalohematoma has a pH in the word to help remember that it is "phirm" and an "L" to help remember that it is localized. Remember that it is unilateral and does not cross. It is also slower to heal.

Maternal Medication Machinations

Beta Adrenergics

Beta adrenergics such as *terbutaline* can be used for short-term tocolysis. However, neonatal hyperinsulinism resulting in hypoglycemia is a risk factor.

General anaesthesia

General anaesthesia is considered to carry little risk to the newborn.

Corticosteroids

A single one-time use of corticosteroids imparts a *reduced risk* of intraventricular hemorrhage, necrotizing enterocolitis, and RDS.

Repeated corticosteroid use carries an increased risk for growth impairment of the head, although the long-term significance of this and other possible risks are unknown at this time.

Prenatal use of *dexamethasone* may carry some increased risk, but this is not clear currently.

Narcan® Agent

Narcan® is used to reverse the respiratory depression that can be seen when the mother received narcotic-based analgesics during delivery.

Remember: it should not be used when the mother is addicted to drugs, because it might cause seizures (rapid withdrawal symptoms). In addition, the half-life of Narcan® is shorter than that of narcotics; therefore, monitoring after administration is important.

Neonatal Abstinence syndrome

Neonatal abstinence syndrome refers to the postnatal withdrawal effects in an infant after drug exposure in-utero. This used to just refer to opioid withdrawal, but it has been expanded. You are expected to distinguish between drug effects and withdrawal effects. The withdrawal effects vary from drug to drug.

Early discharge is not an option for an infant who has been exposed to drug use in utero. A urine drug screen from the infant should be obtained within 24 hours of delivery.

The table below outlines several drugs and their withdrawal profile.

Drug	Withdrawal profile and Association
Alcohol	Hyperactivity, irritability Hypoglycemia can be seen in alcohol withdrawal as well *See Fetal Alcohol Syndrome in Genetics Chapter.*
Cocaine	**No official withdrawal or abstinence syndrome exists.** However, while there is no known official withdrawal syndrome or teratogenic effects, these children are at increased risk for anomalies due to vascular constriction. This includes *cerebral infarctions, limb anomalies,* and *urogenital defects.* There is also an increased risk for *placental abruption.*
Marijuana	Maternal marijuana use has not been definitively shown to be associated with any specific infant features or developmental issues at this time. A few studies have *low fetal growth* concerns, but this is unconfirmed. There has been suggestion of abnormal vision response to light and/or infant tremulousness, but this probably won't be tested on the exam.
Amphetamine	Although there is no established withdrawal syndrome, children exposed to amphetamines in-utero are *irritable* and easily agitated with routine environmental stimulation. They often experience IUGR, and are prone to developmental and cognitive impairment.
Barbiturates	*Hyperactivity, hyperphagia, irritability, crying* and *poor suck swallow coordination.*
Opioid	*Hyperirritability, tremors, jitteriness, hypertonia, loose stools, emesis* and *feeding difficulties.* *Seizure activity* would also be consistent with opioid withdrawal. Methadone and/or oral morphine may be needed to manage withdrawal.
Tobacco	Cigarette smoking is associated with increased risk for *low birthweight, miscarriage, IUGR, and prematurity.* Increased risk for *cleft lip/palate* has been shown and could creep up on the exam. There is an increased risk for *SIDS.* In addition there is an increased risk for *asthma and other respiratory ailments even in the absence of post-natal exposure to smoke.*

Phenobarb is not Yellow

Infants exposed to phenobarbital in-utero are often *jittery* and *irritable*. However, they are at lower risk for hyperbilirubinemia.

Honorable Discharge

Most newborns are stable enough to be discharged within 48 hours after a vaginal delivery, or 72 hours after a c-section.

Early discharge may be okay after an uncomplicated vaginal delivery if the newborn has been feeding well and has voided and stooled. In addition, they need to be assessed for jaundice prior to discharge, and of course the family has to be deemed reliable to followup.

Watch for signs in the question that would make the infant ineligible for early discharge.

Even though there is no "official" withdrawal syndrome, cocaine and amphetamine are harmful to the developing brain. They also impair uteroplacental circulation.

Screening for PKU

It is important to note that most infants with a positive PKU screen do not have PKU. The positive screen only indicates elevated phenylalanine levels.

This can represent delayed enzyme maturation, hyperphenylalaninemia, or biopterin deficiency, rather than PKU.

Chapter 11

Fluids and Lytes, and Everything Nice

Most Board candidates would rather appear on *Are You Smarter Than a 5th Grader?* and get all the questions wrong than study Fluids and Lytes. In fact, we dread editing this chapter.

This is a chapter that really doesn't lend itself to rote memory, and requires a clear understanding of the underlying principles. Some time invested in learning the logic can result in a clean sweep of this material, which comprises a large section of the exam.

You need to know a lot of the normal values, the abnormal ones, and the tricks they play to fool you. This can be a recurring dream or nightmare.[1] Follow the bouncing jokes and you will recognize the tricks and answer the questions correctly.

Acid Base Metabolism

In determining the cause of an acid base disturbance, the following systematic approach should be helpful (technically, it is not acidemia until the pH is <7.36 or alkalemia until the pH is >7.44, but these are general guidelines):

Step 1: **Look at the pH**

- If the pH is > 7.40, you are dealing with alkalosis
- If the pH is <7.40, you are dealing with acidosis

Step 2: **Look at the Bicarb**

- If the bicarb is >25, you are dealing with a metabolic alkalosis
- If the bicarb is < 25, you are dealing with a metabolic acidosis

Calculating Osmolality

You will be expected to be able to calculate serum osmolality using the following equation, which you should commit to memory.

Make a habit of calculating this each time you are presented with the electrolytes in the question.

$$2*Na\ (mEq/L) + [BUN\ (mg/dL)/2.8] + [Glucose\ (mg/dL)/18]$$

The Basics of The Happy Twins - Acid and Base

Acid and Base both work together to make pH happy, that is, H+ and HCO3. However, if acidosis is corrected too rapidly, the inside of the cell gets confused and becomes acidotic.

DEFINITION
The formula to correct metabolic acidosis is sodium bicarb = Weight x 0.3 x the Base Deficit.

DEFINITION
Infants have lower baseline bicarb levels than adults do. In fact, up to age 16 months, children have an average bicarb level of 22. It is closer to 25 in older children and adults.

---

[1] Like the ones you still have about forgetting to study for a final scheduled in one hour.

Step 3: **Look at the PCO$_2$**

　　　· If the PCO$_2$ is > 40, you are dealing with a respiratory acidosis

　　　· If the PCO$_2$ is < 40, you are dealing with a respiratory alkalosis

These are general rules, since infants have lower bicarb levels than adults. The renal threshold for bicarb in term neonates is 21 mEq/L. Remember that their kidneys are not yet fully developed.

Whenever you are presented with an arterial blood gas, circle the components and write down whether each value would result in alkalosis or acidosis. This will go a long way toward understanding the clinical acid-base scenario you are facing.

Respiratory Acidosis

In this case, **hypoventilation is the primary cause of the acidosis,** so you would expect to see an elevated PCO2; for example, **pH 7.15** and a **PCO$_2$ 75.**

CNS dysfunction would be an example where respiratory drive is blunted, resulting in hypoventilation.

Respiratory Alkalosis

In this case, **hyperventilation is the primary cause of the alkalosis** so you would expect to see a low PCO$_2$ and an elevated pH; for example, **pH 7.55** and PCO$_2$ **25.**

Metabolic Alkalosis

In metabolic alkalosis, you are dealing with a bicarb >25 and a pH greater than 7.40.

Loop diuretics such as furosemide and thiazide diuretics such as metolazone and hydrochlorothiazide can be associated with and cause metabolic alkalosis.

Compensatory Mechanisms

The body will try to buffer to minimize any changes in the pH. However, **compensatory mechanisms are incomplete.**

- **Metabolic Alkalosis** – Here the respiratory system will try to compensate by holding onto CO_2, and this is done via **hypoventilation.**

Compensated Metabolic Acidosis

Metabolic acidosis results in poor delivery of oxygen to peripheral tissue. If the patient is breathing spontaneously, then hyperventilation will result in compensatory hypocarbia.

Compensated metabolic acidosis will result in a low pH and a lowered PCO_2 in an attempt to compensate; for example, **pH 7.20** and **PCO_2 25.**

Septic shock (for example, secondary to meningococcemia) would be a clinical scenario where this may be seen.

In addition to administering isotonic fluids (start with 20 mL/kg of normal saline or equivalent), in cases of severe metabolic acidosis (e.g., pH less than 7.10), administration of 1 mEq/kg sodium bicarbonate may be indicated to raise the pH above 7.20.

However, establishing adequate ventilation would be necessary (of course), in order to make sure CO_2 is efficiently eliminated.

Compensated Metabolic Alkalosis

Compensated metabolic alkalosis will result in an elevated pH and an elevated PCO_2 in an attempt to compensate; for example, **pH 7.55** and a **PCO_2 of 55. Bicarb** will be elevated as well, around **48.**

A classic example of metabolic alkalosis is an infant with **pyloric stenosis.** The steps leading to **hypochloremic metabolic alkalosis** are as follows: *barfed his acid*

· Projectile vomiting ⟶ Loss of hydrogen ions ➜ Alkalosis

Loss of chloride ions ➜ Hypochloremia

· Contraction of
extracellular fluid ⟶ Increased bicarb reabsorption in
the kidneys ➜ worsening alkalosis

Remember, the respiratory response to this metabolic alkalosis would be "hypoventilation" to retain CO_2. But this is also known as "not breathing," so hypoventilation can never adequately compensate for metabolic alkalosis.

Compensated Respiratory Alkalosis

Compensated respiratory alkalosis will result in an elevated pH and low serum bicarb in an attempt to compensate. For example, a **pH 7.48** and a **PCO$_2$ of 20. Bicarb of 15** would be the attempted compensation.

This would occur if a child moved to **Colorado** and was breathing rapidly because of the thin air. In this case, **hypoxia** would trigger **hyperventilation, leading to respiratory alkalosis.** Compensation is accomplished by **increased excretion of bicarb by the kidneys.**

Metabolic Acidosis

Fall into the Gap

Diuretics and Metabolic Acidosis

Acetazolamide and potassium-sparing agents such as **spironolactone** can lead to metabolic acidosis.

Some folks shop at the *Gap*®, some folks visit the Delaware Water Gap, and others look at David Letterman's grin and obsessively focus on the distracting gap in his teeth. All of this is for later; right now we have to focus on the Anion Gap.

The first thing you should do when you either have a patient with *acidosis* or you are given the patient's serum *sodium, chloride,* and *bicarbonate* is to calculate the *anion gap* as follows:

Serum Sodium – (Chloride + Bicarbonate)

Whenever you are presented with serum sodium, chloride, and bicarbonate, you should calculate the anion gap as reflexively as your accountant calculating tax deductions on April 14th.

The anion gap measures ions that are not accounted for in routine labs, including such delicacies as *protein, organic acids, phosphate, sulfate*, and *lactic acid*. **A normal anion gap is between 8-12 mEq/L.**

Normal Anion Gap

With **a normal anion gap,** the **serum chloride will be elevated.**

Acidosis with a normal anion gap is caused by either:

· Loss of bicarbonate

· Kidney dysfunction

· Diarrhea

· Addition of hydrochloric acid

· Renal tubular dysfunction

Diarrhea is the most common cause of a non-gap metabolic acidosis in children.

> ### Normal Anion Gap Acidosis/Buying a Used Carp
>
> These causes can be referred to by the mnemonic device USEDCARP, which represents the following:
>
> - **U**reterostomy
> - **S**mall bowel fistula
> - **E**xtra chloride
> - **D**iarrhea
> - **C**arbonic anhydrase inhibitor use
> - **A**drenal insufficiency
> - **R**enal tubular acidosis
> - **P**ancreatic fistula

Renal Tubular Acidosis

Renal tubular acidosis results in an ***increased chloride*** and is, therefore, a **normal anion gap acidosis.** But just when you thought you had it all figured out, there is **distal** and **proximal** renal tubular acidosis.

Follow the bouncing anion and you will see a foolproof way to get the question right once you narrow your choices down to distal and proximal renal tubular acidosis. **In fact, if you see these as two of the choices you can pretty much assume one of them is the correct answer.**

$$Na - (Cl + Bicarb)$$
$$8-12$$

Pick Up Distal Tubular Acidosis

In **distal tubular acidosis,** the proximal tubule is fine and it keeps all the bicarb it needs to. However, if the distal tubule is not doing its job, then H+ is not shown the door, and the **urine will have a high pH and cannot be acidified. Therefore, the kidneys keep too much H+.**

 Renal (Distal) Tubular Acidosis Type 1 is caused by the inability of the distal renal tubule to acidify urine. Therefore, the urine pH will always be greater than 5.5.

Distal RTA is also associated with increased calciuria.

Boxing Bicarb and Arranging Acid / All Else Falls into Place

Remember that the kidney is the key to acid-base metabolism, more than breathing is.

The **Proximal** Tubule **B**oxes and takes **B**icarb **B**ack in.

The **Distal** Tubule **A**rranges for H/**A**cid to leave the building.

Any breakdown in one of these sites has obvious consequences.

RTA Imitators

RTA (Distal) Type I may be mimicked by use of potassium-sparing drugs like spironolactone.

RTA (Proximal) Type II is mimicked by use of carbonic anhydrase inhibitors like acetazolamide.

Proximal Renal Tubular Acidosis (Type 2)

This is a result of the proximal tubule's *inability to absorb bicarb*. Bicarb is lost. However, the distal tubule is fine and it continues its job of showing H+ the door.

Renal (Proximal) Tubular Acidosis Type 2 is caused by the inability of the proximal tubule to take back its bicarb, resulting in excessive bicarb in the urine. *However the kidneys can acidify the urine and the urine pH is less than 5.5*

If you are questioned on the following specific facts, use the following to guide you to the correct answer.

· **Secretion of hydrogen** ion occurs at the **collecting duct**
· **Reabsorption of bicarb** occurs at the **proximal tubule**

Rental Tubular Acidosis Type 3

Type 3 is rarely used as a classifiation today because it is now thought to be a combination of type 1 and type 2.

Renal Tubular Acidosis Type 4

Type 4 RTA is due to resistance to aldosterone (or to aldosterone deficiency); therefore, you can expect to see **hyperkalemia**.

Both RTA Type 2 and 4 can present with a urine pH > 5.5, but only Type 4 presents with hyperkalemia. RTA Type 1 will have a high urine pH.

Widening the Gap /Elevated Anion Gap

Acidosis with an elevated anion gap is usually due either to:

· Overproduction of organic acids

· Ingestion

· Inability to excrete acid, as in renal failure

With an **elevated anion gap,** the **serum chloride will be normal.**

> **MUD PILES**
>
> The classic mnemonic for conditions that are associated with an elevated anion gap is **MUDPILES:**
> • **M**ethanol
> • **U**remia
> • **D**iabetic ketoacidosis
> • **P**araldehyde
> • **I**ngestion - Iron / Isoniazid (INH)
> • **L**actic acid
> • **E**thanol / Ethylene glycol
> • **S**alicylates

Inborn Errors of Metabolism

Passing the exam isn't as simple as just memorizing MUDPILES. One of the more important etiologies to consider is **organic acidemia,** including **propionic** or **methylmalonic acidemia in an infant.**

The typical presentation will be an infant who **appears healthy at birth** but later develops *lethargy, poor feeding,* and *seizures.* Lab values might include *low WBC and platelets* as well as *elevated serum ammonia.* Elevated blood pressure might be part of the history as well.

It is important to note other metabolic derangements that present in the newborn period which would not result in elevated anion gap metabolic acidosis.

· **Urea Cycle Defects** present with hyperammonemia but no metabolic acidosis.

Non-specific signs such as lethargy, vomiting, and, ultimately, failure to thrive can be mistaken for **sepsis.** With compensated metabolic acidosis one would expect to find a low pCO_2 (in the mid 20's). The patient will be afebrile with a normal WBC.

Sold on Sodium

Sodium is important because it is the big name in town that maintains osmolality, and if it shifts, it impacts the brain, resulting in a big ego for everyone (brain swelling) or injured ego (brain contraction).

 The daily requirement for sodium = 2-3 mEq/kg/day.

Hypernatremia

Extracellular fluid in hypernatremia

Extracellular fluid as a percentage of total body weight decreases with age. In other words, we shrink and look more and more like Grandpa Simpson from *The Simpsons*.

 When will you see hypernatremia? In two situations:

1. Sodium Excess: Too much sodium taken in

    a. Improper mixing of formula (not enough water, sugar instead of salt)

    b. Ingestion of sea saltwater

    c. Excessive sodium bicarb after resuscitation

    d. Breast milk with excessive sodium

    e. Iatrogenic [3]

Water deficit

· Diabetes insipidus

· Diarrhea (both sodium and water are lost, but water more than sodium in this case)

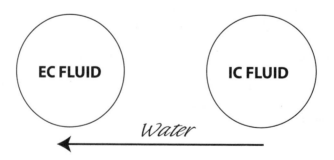

---

[3] Greek for "whoops!"

Extracellular fluid is maintained in hypernatremia. Remember, water chases sodium like a long lost lover. Wherever sodium excess is, water wants to go. Therefore, if there is hypernatremia, water is drawn out of the intracellular compartment. **This results in increased extracellular volume,** which can result in **pulmonary edema.**

Diabetes Insipidus

Kids with diabetes insipidus are urinating a lot. There is a deficiency of ADH; low "Anti" diuretic hormone, so there is diuresis.

 Diabetes "I am Sipping and Sipping this" – because you would sip and sip if you were peeing all the time.

 Look for "**a child that is urinating profusely but has no sugar in the urine.**"

Labs will **show a high serum osmolality with inappropriately dilute urine.**

Treatment of DI consists of drinking water (based on thirst) and DDAVP.

Nephrogenic Diabetes Insipidus

This is an **X-linked** disorder, and is therefore **only found in males.** The kidney does not respond to the vasopressin, resulting in **dilute urine and hypernatremic dehydration.**

Nephrogenic DI will fail to respond to **exogenous vasopressin,** and central DI will respond. Beware: if they describe a **familial DDAVP pattern among males, nephrogenic DI is your answer.**

Hyponatremia

Hyponatremia is serum sodium less than 130 mEq/L. There are 3 categories of hyponatremia:

1. Hypovolemic
2. Euvolemic
3. Hypervolemic

The best study to order to determine the type of hyponatremia you are dealing with is **urinary fractional excretion of sodium (FENa).**

With a sodium < **120,** the patient may present with lethargy and seizures.

Hyponatremia

Hyponatremia is the result of one of two mechanisms:

1) Loss of sodium

2) Increased water (diluted)

    ❑ Too much taken on board: **Polydipsia**

    ❑ Too little let out: **SIADH**

Sometimes, while sodium and water are both lost, more sodium is lost than water. The result, however, is still hyponatremia (3rd space losses post op, for example).

GI Losses ➡ Hyponatremia

The following is important to remember:

With hyponatremia secondary to GI losses, the kidneys will hold on to sodium, resulting in **low urine sodium (< 10).**

Increased Urinary Excretion of Sodium ➡ Hyponatremia

SIADH

No matter how well you know something, it is very easy to get confused in the heat of the battle, especially when a question asks, "are all true *except.*" Intelligent folks have missed questions like this by not being careful.

Remember, SIADH results in *diminished urine output.*

You can remember this logically as "ANTI - Diuretic" – the opposite of a Diuretic. Or think of it as "**S**yndrome of **I A**m **D**efinitely **H**ydrated (cause I ain't peeing)."

"Appropriate ADH"

Now that we know all about the inappropriate ADH, we should know when it is appropriate. Whenever there is **high serum osmolality,** you will want to retain fluid, and this results in concentrated urine secondary to "appropriate ADH."

Causes of SIADH

First, translate the labs into English. They might describe some **cerebral injury or insult** (trauma, tumor, etc.) Since the pituitary produces ADH, trauma or infection involving the brain can result in SIADH. In addition, certain **pulmonary or endocrine disorders can trigger SIADH.**

With SIADH, the serum labs will include evidence of **hyponatremia,** coupled with an inappropriately normal or high urine osmolality (300 or higher). Urine sodium should be greater than 25. **Remember, renal and other functions will be normal.**

Remember **SIADH:**

> **S**urgery
> **I**nfection
> **A**xon (neurological such as Guillain Barré, Brain Tumor)
> **D** (Day After, Post Op, of any kind)
> **H** (Head and Hemorrhage)

SIADH presents with hyponatremia; however, the underlying problem is **fluid retention, not excretion of sodium.** SIADH also presents with **normal serum potassium, elevated urine sodium > 25mEq/L (25 mmol/L).** *Plasma volume is increased in SIADH.*

The lab values expected in SIADH are as follows:

- **Low serum sodium** − 124 mEq/L
- **Low BUN** − 2 mg/dL
- **Elevated BP**
- **Decreased urine output** - < 1cc/kg/day

The **urine** in patients with SIADH will have **high osmolality** and **high sodium concentration.**

The preferred **treatment** is **fluid restriction.**

This may be difficult in infants and — no matter what — correction will be slow. SIADH is a diagnosis of exclusion, so you may need to rule out other disorders leading to hyponatremia before choosing fluid restriction.

If fluid restriction alone does not work, the use of furosemide and hypertonic saline is an option. **Demeclocycline** blocks the effects of ADH on the kidney. However, since it is a derivative of doxycycline, it is only indicated in children 8 years of age or older. **Lithium** also blocks the effects of ADH, but it is not usually recommended due to its side effect profile. However, it is still important to know in case it comes up on the exam.

3% sodium chloride would be indicated if the serum sodium is less than 120 mEq/L.

Thiazide diuretics would be incorrect in the treatment of SIADH, since they can lower sodium further.

CASE STUDY

You could be presented with a patient with a head injury or meningitis. They will either imply or come right out and tell you the patient has SIADH. You will then be asked to decide on a treatment. They will have to note that there are no neurological symptoms.

THE DIVERSION

Among the choices will be obvious ones that are incorrect, including maintenance, twice maintenance, and 1.5 times maintenance. Even if you realize that the correct answer is 2/3 maintenance and that 0.66 maintenance is the same thing (without pulling out a calculator), answering the question correctly may not be that easy. You will be expected to know when to use demeclocycline, which inhibits ADH secretion from the kidneys.

ANSWER REVEALED

Demeclocycline would be indicated if there is no clinical improvement with appropriate fluid restriction.

Renal Failure

BUZZ WORDS A patient with diminished urine output who is taking in fluid in excess of urine volume will develop hyponatremia. They will also have to present you with a clue that renal disease is present, i.e., **elevated creatinine.** The patient will likely also present with **edema** and **urine sodium > 20 mEq/L.**

PERIL WARNING If you are presented with a patient who is oliguric and hemodynamically unstable, the correct initial treatment is with 20 mL/kg of isotonic solution (e.g., normal saline, packed RBC, or albumin).

Once hemodynamically stable, adjustments would be based on the urine output, weight, and other symptoms included in the question, including the presence of pulmonary edema or other conditions.

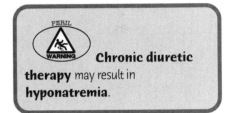

> ### Calculating Fluid Maintenance
>
> Okay, we all know the 100 mL/kg/day, 50 mL/kg/day, and 20 mL/kg/day calculation; well, the quick version to calculate the hourly fluid rate is:
>
> 4 mL/kg/hr (for the first 10 kg) PLUS
>
> 2 mL/kg/hr (for the next 10 kg) PLUS
>
> 1 mL/kg/hr (for each additional kg)

Hypervolemic Hyponatremia

Medications that cause hyponatremia

The table below outlines medications that can cause hyponatremia.

> **PERIL WARNING** **Chronic diuretic therapy** may result in **hyponatremia**.

Agent	Mechanism
Vincristine	SIADH
Cyclophosphamide	Diminishes water excretion
Chlorpropamide (oral hypoglycemic)	Stimulates vasopressin release
Thiazide diuretics	Blocks renal sodium and chloride reabsorption, decreasing the kidney's ability to produce dilute urine
Metolazone	Blocks renal sodium and chloride reabsorption, decreasing the kidney's ability to produce dilute urine

Dilutional hyponatremia

HOT TIP

· Dilutional hyponatremia is due to *water intoxication*

· **Total body sodium is normal**

· There are no signs of intravascular volume depletion

· Seizures occur due to <u>cerebral swelling</u>

· **Urine sodium concentration is increased**

 It is important to note that the total body sodium is normal in dilutional hyponatremia. Remembering this is worth at least one point on the exam.

You may need to distinguish dilutional hyponatremia from other similar clinical scenarios.

· **Third spacing of fluid** may occur after extensive surgery, due to either **1) endothelial damage and/or leakage** or **2) hypoalbuminemia** and **low oncotic pressure.** It also occurs in *nephrotic syndrome.* In this case, urine sodium concentration is low (less than 10 mEq/L). **Edema** is an important feature.

· **Renal salt wasting** would also present as hyponatremia, but hypovolemia would also be a feature.

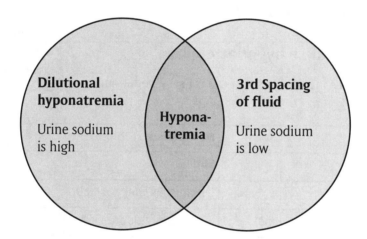

Pseudohyponatremia

This is one of the favorite tricky Board questions. They give you a **low sodium value** and then ask you if the **total body sodium** is normal, low, or elevated. Of course, the answer is not the obvious. Follow the logic arc here and you will slam-dunk this trick at least once and maybe twice on the same exam day.

> Remember: with "low water" for a given circulatory volume, the lab will report "low sodium."

Step 1

They will describe a situation where there are **elevated triglycerides** and/or **plasma proteins**. A typical example would be **nephrotic syndrome**.

Step 2

TG's take up a lot of room, so there is **less "water," but the "volume" is the same.**

Labs report sodium per volume, not sodium per water. The sodium level will be reported low, since water is the only part that actually contains sodium. Therefore, the sodium level in *circulation* really is normal.

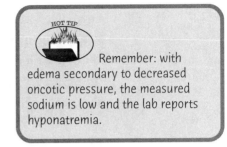

HOT TIP

Remember: with edema secondary to decreased oncotic pressure, the measured sodium is low and the lab reports hyponatremia.

Step 3

There is lots of water outside circulation in conditions of edema. In fact, there is more water than usual and all this water *does contain sodium. Therefore, **the Total Body Sodium** is elevated.*

Potassium

DEFINITION

The daily requirement for potassium = 1-2 mEq/kg/day

Hypokalemia

DEFINITION

Hypokalemia is serum potassium less than 3.5 mEq/L.

BUZZ WORDS

A typical scenario would be a child with a history of diarrhea presenting with muscle pain and weakness. Hypokalemia can also present as **"weakness and paralysis," "constipation and ileus,"** or "polyuria."

PERIL

WARNING

Hypokalemia can be *caused by* diarrhea and *result in* constipation.

Causes of Hypokalemia

❑ Poor Intake (Anorexia Nervosa)
❑ Loss
  · **GI**/Vomiting /Diarrhea
  · **Renal**/(i.e. diuretics, renal tubular disorders, or excess aldosterone)

EKG Changes

The EKG changes one would expect with hypokalemia are:

- **Flattening of T waves**
- **ST depression**
- **Premature ventricular beats**

In extreme cases, there may also be a **U wave** that appears just after the T wave.

CASE STUDY

You are presented with a boy who has a 2-3 day history of vomiting and diarrhea. He has taken water and juice, but has become progressively weaker and has difficulty sitting or standing without support. You are then asked for the explanation for his weakness.

THE DIVERSION

You will be presented with several diversionary electrolyte-based explanations for the child's weakness. Dehydration will be tempting, as will be hyponatremia. However, the question will specifically ask for the explanation for his weakness.

ANSWER REVEALED

In any question asking for a specific explanation for weakness in the face of vomiting and dehydration, the answer will be hypokalemia.

Emergency Treatment of hypokalemia

TREATMENT

In emergency situations, potassium is replaced using KCl 0.5 -1.0 mEq/L per kg over an hour. The maximum would be 40 mEq/L.

However, this is only in emergency/urgent situations.

You must remember the following caveats:

- In mild cases, oral replacement of potassium is appropriate.
- If the hypokalemia is due to dehydration, then fluid replacement with added potassium is all that is needed.
- If **acidosis** is a factor, potassium **acetate** is used. That should be easy to remember phonetically.
- If hypophosphatemia is an issue, then potassium phosphate is used.

EKG monitoring is required during IV infusion of KCl.

 There are other electrolyte abnormalities that can present with weakness and EKG changes:

- **Hypocalcemia** can present with muscle weakness and *prolonged QT interval.*
- **Hypomagnesemia** can occur in patients with diarrhea, as well as a *prolonged PR or QT interval.*
- **Hypoglycemia** will present with muscle weakness but no EKG changes
- **Hyponatremia** will present with muscle weakness but no EKG changes

Hyperkalemia

Causes of hyperkalemia

- ❏ Excess intake
- ❏ Not enough out (renal failure, HypO aldosteronism)
- ❏ *Redistribution* - Acidosis (H goes into the cell, K goes out of the cell)
- ❏ Cell breakdown (pseudohyperkalemia)

The initial EKG findings seen with hyperkalemia include **peaked T waves.** However, at substantially higher potassium levels, i.e. 10 or greater, you are likely to see the **absence of P waves** and **widened QRS complex.** This is associated with **electromechanical dissociation (EMD).**

The widened QRS complex can be misinterpreted as **idiopathic bundle branch block (IBBB) or ventricular tachycardia.** However, they would not describe muffled heart sounds or absence of pulses in IBBB. A pulseless state is possible with ventricular tachycardia at rates 200 or greater, but you would not have muffled heart sounds. Bottom line: read the question carefully.

> **CASE STUDY** You are presented with an infant with an abdominal mass who becomes hypotensive. The physical exam is noteworthy for non-palpable pulses and distant heart sounds. The EKG shows a wide QRS complex. What is the appropriate *immediate* treatment?
>
> **THE DIVERSION** You might be tempted to pick a diversion, like a normal saline bolus to treat shock. Or perhaps you guessed correctly that the patient's abdominal mass is due to an adrenal tumor and the patient is experiencing hypovolemic shock; based on this, you might pick hydrocortisone IV, or maybe a pressor like dobutamine. But if you did, you might become pulseless yourself when you realize the correct answer.
>
> **ANSWER REVEALED** In this case, it is adrenal failure that has resulted in hyperkalemia. This has resulted in **electromagnetic dissociation (EMD)**. The most appropriate *immediate treatment* would be IV **calcium chloride**.

Emergency Treatment of Hyperkalemia

If you are presented with a patient with potassium greater than 10 who is showing signs of EMD, then the correct treatment is **IV calcium chloride.**

Milder cases of hyperkalemia may be treated with:

- Glucose and insulin
- Sodium bicarbonate
- Inhaled albuterol
- IV furosemide (Lasix®)
- Oral polystyrene resin

Potassium Acid/Base Montage

Few things strike more fear in mice and hens than this. However, it is also one of the most logical to keep straight. Here goes:

Alkalosis and Potassium

Step 1: Alkalosis ➜ High pH ➜ *Very little H in the EC Fluid*

Step 2: The H's in the cells move out to help out their Cation brethren ➜ *H Moves from IC to EC* ➜

Step 3: To replace the "H Cats" leaving the cell, the K Cats move from the ECF into the ICF ➜

Step 4: Therefore, **during alkalosis**, K heads in the house, resulting in ➜ *lower measured potassium levels*.

Summary: **During alkalosis, K moves to the IC fluid and H moves out, resulting in lower measured serum potassium.**

Acidosis and Potassium

The opposite occurs:

Step 1: Acidosis ➜ Low pH ➜ Lots of H floating around the EC Fluid.

Step 2: There are just too many H's running around the EC with too much time on their hands.

Step 3: They begin to "squat" where they don't belong by moving into the IC.

Step 4: And because there is only room for one positive ion for each seat, the weaker K gets kicked out of the ICF, and now there is increased K in the EC fluid with acidosis.

Summary: **Acidosis ➜ H moves in and K moves out, resulting in high measured serum potassium.**

Suspected diuretic abuse

If you are presented with a patient suspected of loop diuretic abuse to lose weight, the key abnormality to look for, in addition to hypokalemia, is **alkalosis.**

HOT TIP

The most effective way to determine loop diuretic use is via measurement of urine and serum electrolytes. Hopefully, knowing this fact will be sufficient when they ask for the best way to determine loop diuretic abuse or use. In case they want you to know the equation, here it is — but first I suggest you slug down a double espresso to remain awake:

$$\left.\frac{\text{Urine Sodium / Serum Sodium}}{\text{Urine Creatinine / Plasma Creatinine}}\right\} = \text{FeNa}$$

A low value – (<1.5) – Low urinary sodium loss.

A high value – (> 2.5) – High urinary sodium loss.

This formula is also of value in determining if a patient is experiencing pre- or post- renal azotemia. A low value would correlate with pre-renal azotemia.

Tonic for your Dehydration

Isotonic Dehydration

Isotonic dehydration would be dehydration with serum sodium between 135-150.

In this case, fluid replacement should be **20 mL/kg of normal saline.**

While sodium and water are lost proportionately, more ECF than ICF fluid is lost, resulting in a symptomatic patient.

Hyponatremic Dehydration

Hypotonic dehydration would be dehydration and serum sodium **less than 135**.

If the question mentions or hints at a dehydrated child that was **fed "tea" or "water" by a grandmother, think hyponatremic dehydration**. In addition, they may mention a **seizure** or poor skin turgor. It is usually due to GI losses, such as diarrhea. Additional findings could include prolonged capillary refill.

Because fluid moves from the ECF to the ICF, it is this form of dehydration that causes the greatest circulatory disturbances, and the **patients are more symptomatic on presentation.**

CNS Effects

Free water moves into CNS cells with a serum Na of 125, and this is the reason for the seizure.

Treatment

Initial treatment is with normal saline boluses. If that doesn't work, then hypertonic 3% saline in the ICU would be correct. **Hypertonic saline is not indicated as the initial treatment.**

> **Free Water? Okay. When?**
>
> HOT TIP
>
> In the case of the exercising adolescent (or even older child), replacement fluids should be sports drinks designed to replace electrolytes (specifically, significant amounts of sodium may be lost in sweat). Previously plain water was recommended, but this has changed.

Treatment of Hyponatremic Dehydration

In this case, in addition to correcting the fluid part of dehydration (see below), you need to replace some of the sodium.

(Desired sodium - measured sodium) X weight X 0.6 = **A**

Maintenance sodium = 3 mEq/kg/day

Add maintenance to the A, and you have the amount of sodium you need to replace over 24 hours. You can **use 3% saline solution to replace sodium if rapid correction is needed**.

Hypernatremic Dehydration

Hypertonic dehydration is dehydration with a serum sodium greater than 145. It is due to **water** loss or **sodium** gain. The **end result is a lot of sodium in the ECF.** Severe hypernatremic dehydration is defined as **170** or greater.

Infants with hypernatremic dehydration will often have a history of being fed **improperly mixed formula** (at least on the boards this will be the case). They may be *irritable, lethargic, with doughy skin and a high-pitched cry.* Eventually **seizures** can result.

> **Dehydration Estimation**
>
> Since intravascular volume is preserved, there is a tendency to underestimate fluid loss. Therefore, assume 10% dehydration in hypernatremic dehydration.

Looks Aren't Everything!

With **hypernatremic dehydration**, water tends to go into the ECF, and this diminishes the clinical signs of dehydration; therefore, **assume 10% dehydration** regardless of clinical presentation. Due to osmotic pressures, fluid is drawn out of the intracellular compartment into the extracellular compartment; therefore, there is less *circulatory disturbance,* and it takes longer for symptoms to present for a given level of dehydration. **It can also result in acidosis, due to the release of hydrogen ions secondary to cellular destruction.**

Remember, **hyponatremic dehydration** causes pontine damage. That is easy to remember because hyp**o**natremic dehydration and p**o**ntine both have an "**o**" in them.

In **hypernatremic dehydration,** the clinical picture is deceptively good, so do not be misled by a rosy clinical picture.

Because of the **intracellular dehydration** that results from the mass water exodus heading out to the sodium, the shrinkage of brain cells can result in **tearing of bridging blood vessels** and **intracranial hemorrhage.**

Occasionally, however, the brain cells get smart, and with the water chasing its sodium mate, the brain cells take on a new lover, **idiogenic osmoles,** to lure the water back.

Idiogenic osmoles develop over 1-2 days, and do not go away so quickly either. Therefore the dehydration should be corrected slowly over 2-3 days in order to avoid cerebral edema as the water rushes in like an anxious lover to meet the new and improved mate-the idiogenic osmole.

The sodium should be decreased more quickly than 10-12 mEq/L per day in order to avoid this mad rush of water into the brain cells.

Altered Mental Status

Remember: one of the ways the body deals with this is "extreme thirst." An unconscious patient, infant, or somebody who is psychotic will not act on the thirst mechanism and, therefore, **will likely have hypernatremic dehydration** (keep this is in mind in case you see one of those types of patients mentioned in the question).

The treatment goal for hypernatremic dehydration is to correct the sodium concentration as well as circulating volume.

If the dehydration is chronic, sodium is reduced slowly at the rate of 0.5 mEq/L per hour.

Severe hypernatremia (170 or greater) should be corrected over 48-72 hours using 0.5 or 0.25 normal saline.

If there are signs of overcorrection, hypertonic solution should be used as a brake to slow the train down.

Potassium should be held until urine output is established.

Degree of Dehydration

At some point on the exam, you will be called upon to calculate fluids and to assess degree of dehydration. This really is a simple calculation with simple answers. The amount of rehydration will depend on the level of dehydration.

5% Dehydration

Tachycardia with "decreased tear production" may be descriptions you'll see. Decreased urinary output and increased urine concentration would be other signs of 5% dehydration.

Taking care of business:

- ❏ **5%** means the child is "short" **50 mL/kg**.
- ❏ You simply add this to the maintenance fluid = the total fluid the child should receive over 24 hours.
- ❏ **Half of this total is given over the first 8 hours**.
- ❏ **Half is given over the next 16 hours**. Hopefully, you and the child can then both go home.

10% Dehydration

Look for "tachycardia" plus poor tear production, **sunken eyes, poor skin turgor, and sunken fontanelle.**

- ❏ Taking care of business once again:
- ❏ **10%** means the child is "short" **100 cc/kg**.
- ❏ Over 24 hours, this would be **maintenance plus 100 cc/kg**.
- ❏ **Emergency phase** – This will be approximately **20 cc/kg over an hour**. Take whatever is left over and **give half over the next 7 hours** and the **other half over the remaining 16 hours**.

> ### Signs of Dehydration
>
> Hypotension is a later sign of dehydration. Tachycardia is an earlier sign.
>
> In addition to hypotension, decreased skin turgor and bounding pulses would also be later signs of dehydration.

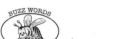 With **hypernatremic dehydration**, maintenance fluid and correction should be calculated for 24 hours. Also, the emergency phase is not necessary, since the ECF volume is maintained nicely even in the face of 10% dehydration.

Never drop the sodium by more than 10-12 in a 24-hour period, or you risk cerebral swelling.

15% Dehydration

The same clinical signs you see with 10%, plus signs of **shock**, including **delayed cap refill time**.

Really taking care of business:
- ❏ Here the child is short a good **150 cc/kg**.
- ❏ Over 24 hours, you need to give **maintenance plus the 150 cc/kg**.
- ❏ In this case, you keep giving **20 cc/kg boluses until you see some clinical improvement**.
- ❏ Then you can give **half of what is left over during the next 7 hours and the remaining half over the next 16 hours**.

Of course, now with the availability of PDA applications that do the calculations for you, the ability and necessity of learning these formulas has gone to the dustbin of history (along with the ability to spell, write cursive, and sit still for long periods of time).[4]

If you are presented with a patient in **septic shock**, they may require up to 3 boluses of 20 mL/kg normal saline which adds up to... hmm... let's see here... oh yes, a total of 60 mL/kg total.

If one of the choices is "the total amount is based on findings on frequent reassessment," this would be the correct answer.

Best Oral Replacement Fluid

All oral rehydration fluids must contain glucose. In order to cross the microvillus membrane of the GI tract, sodium molecules must be accompanied by a glucose molecule. Sodium is not permitted entry unless accompanied by a paid club member in the form of glucose.

When you are treating a patient with moderate to severe dehydration, i.e., a patient with tachycardia and delayed cap refill, you need to use **oral rehydration fluid**, which contains **75 mEq/L of sodium**. The rate should be 50 mL/kg over 1-4 hours, even if administered with a dropper.

---

4 If you don't know what a dust bin is, I rest my case.

In cases of **mild dehydration**, you can use standard **maintenance hydration fluids**, which contain **50 mEq/L**. This solution can also be used once cap refill is normalized in cases of severe dehydration.

Standard formula is the wrong answer if you are presented with an infant with moderate to severe dehydration.

The BRAT diet is not part of AAP recommendations, and therefore is not the correct answer on the exam for managing acute gastroenteritis.

CASE STUDY

You are presented with a toddler who has had 2-3 days of vomiting and diarrhea. He is tolerating some clear liquids. He has dry mucous membranes and mild tachycardia. What is the best management of this patient?

THE DIVERSION

You might be tempted to go straight for the bolus of isotonic fluids. You might also follow the herd and pick the answer that suggests a BRAT diet. They might also offer "give diluted formula" if the patient is an infant.

ANSWER REVEALED

However, the correct answer would be to institute oral rehydration therapy, followed by a regular diet consisting of complex carbohydrates, fruits, and vegetables. Infants should be given usual formula at full strength.

Fluids and Lytes in Specific Clinical Conditions

Pyloric Stenosis

This is a classic example of **metabolic alkalosis.** Metabolic alkalosis may also be present in a patient with an **NG tube.**

The infant will be hungry immediately after a vomiting episode. In fact, this diagnosis can be very difficult to suspect in preemies, so they may try to trip you up with that. The loss of hydrogen chloride leads to *hypochloremic* **hypokalemic metabolic alkalosis.**

It is important to note that *initially* the vomiting will be *non-projectile.*

K⁺ and the Kidney

In addition, there is total body potassium depletion *even if the serum potassium levels are normal.* The persistent vomiting causes a loss of HCl from the stomach. The kidneys, as a result, try to retain hydrogen at the expense of potassium, causing hypokalemia. The alkalosis results in potassium and hydrogen exchanging places across cell membranes, with potassium going into the cells and hydrogen ions being driven out. This causes further drop in potassium levels.

Because emesis contains chloride, the kidneys try to retain chloride. Therefore **urine chloride should be low, < 10.**

You are presented with a patient with pyloric stenosis, given a bunch of labs, and then you have to pick the one that is inconsistent with the diagnosis.

While this type of question may seem straightforward, it is not always so simple.

- First, it is crucial to write down in the margins the adjective description of the lab values, since this is how you have been studying. For example, a bicarb of 35 should be written down as "alkalosis."

- Second, when picking a lab which is *inconsistent with a diagnosis*, it is best to step back and *first cross off the ones which are consistent with the diagnosis*. Remember this, because on more than one occasion they have given a bunch of lab values and you had to choose the *one* that was inconsistent with pyloric stenosis. Remember: it is hypochloremic metabolic alkalosis, and there is low chloride, H+, and sodium.

Just remember that pyloric stenosis is associated with a **hypochloremic metabolic alkalosis**. Therefore, you would expect:

- High pH
- Low serum chloride
- Low serum sodium
- Low or normal serum potassium
- **Hyperbilirubinemia may also be present**

High serum potassium would be inconsistent with a diagnosis of pyloric stenosis. Of course, a heel stick sample could have a high potassium level, but it would be due to hemolysis, not underlying pathology. It is highly doubtful that they would get that petty on the exam. Bottom line: understand the classic lab findings consistent with pyloric stenosis.

Cystic Fibrosis

Because cystic fibrosis is associated with an increased loss of sodium and chloride in sweat, it can lead to **hypochloremic hyponatremic metabolic alkalosis with dehydration**.

Acute Renal Failure

A patient in renal failure who is volume-depleted still needs to be hydrated. Therefore, if you are presented with a patient who is volume-depleted because of gastroenteritis or a pyelonephritis with renal failure, they want you to know that giving fluids is the best option available. This concept is very likely to be tested on the exam.

The bottom line: **coexisting volume depletion should be corrected in patients with acute renal failure.**

Post Op Fluid Management

There is a risk for increased ADH secretion: therefore, fluid restriction is important, since the most important complication to monitor for is over hydration (and subsequent hyponatremia).

Babbling Tower of Tables

If past exams are any indication, it is very likely that you will get a table of lab values (on this and many other subjects) from which you will have to pick the correct diagnosis. This may include 6-10 questions that can be the difference between passing and failing. No pressure!

However, if you keep a cool head, this can be an easy 6-10 points for you to pick up on the exam.

Diagnosis	Sodium	Potassium	Chloride	BUN	Glucose	Urine Specific Gravity	Abnormal Labs
Hyponatremic Dehydration	125	4.0	85	25	90	1.025	Decreased sodium and chloride Increased BUN and specific gravity
Hypernatremic Dehydration	152	4.0	120	25	90	1.025	Increased sodium, chloride, BUN and spec. gravity
Pseudohypo-natremia	120	4.0	108	15	650	1.015	Decreased sodium Markedly elevated glucose
SIADH	120	4.0	85	5	90	1.025	Decreased sodium, chloride and BUN Increased spec. gravity
Diabetes Insipidus	152	4.0	120	25	90	1.002	Increased sodium, chloride, BUN Decreased spec. gravity
Lab Error	120	4.0	108	15	90	1.010	Sodium is decreased and chloride is normal

CASE STUDY

You are presented with a patient who is post op for resection of a craniopharyngioma. The patient is noted to have hyponatremia and an elevated serum creatinine. Urine output is increased, and urine sodium is greater than 100 mEq/L with a urine osmolality of 350.

What is the diagnosis and what is the treatment?

THE DIVERSION

This is a very tricky question. When presented with a patient with a cranial lesion, especially a craniopharyngioma, it is easy to immediately assume a diagnosis of SIADH. Those who write board questions know this.

If you picked SIADH and fluid restriction as the treatment of choice, you will be suffering from SIAQI or "Syndrome of Inappropriately Answering the Question Incorrectly."

ANSWER REVEALED

Read the question carefully and you won't go wrong. With SIADH or "Syndrome of I Am Definitely Hydrated," urine output will be low and urine sodium concentration will also be low. Hypervolemia is the result, and fluid restriction is the correct management. The patient in this vignette, however, has elevated urine output and elevated urine sodium. Therefore, the correct diagnosis is **cerebral salt wasting**, and the correct treatment is replacement of fluid and sodium losses.

Chapter 12

Genetics: Everyone Into the (Gene) Pool

Chromosomes and Genetics

Frequently Tested Genetic Disorders

Turner Syndrome

Turner syndrome is associated with **webbed neck, delayed secondary sexual characteristics**, and **left-sided congenital heart defects such as bicuspid aortic valve** or **coarctation of the aorta.**

In adolescents, presenting features could include **short stature, minimal or no breast development**, and **primary amenorrhea.**

Infants may present with **short 4th and 5th metacarpal bones, widely spaced nipples,** and/or **lymphedema of the hands and feet.**

They could also describe a child with a "wide carrying angle of the elbows," as well as chronic otitis media.

Additional features include hyperconvex nails, low hairline, small mandible, high arched palate, and the ever-popular low-set ears seen in lots of other syndromes.

In addition to the phenotypical features outlined above, there must be a full or partial X chromosome deletion. Turner syndrome can only be diagnosed in a female.

If you are presented with a male, turn left at the corner; Turner syndrome will be incorrect.

Turner Not Trisomy

Since it is not a Trisomy, **Turner syndrome is NOT associated with advanced maternal age.** On the other hand Klinefelter Syndrome does involve a 3rd chromosome, so it, and all the trisomies, **ARE** associated with advanced maternal age. But remember: most kids with these disorders are born to younger moms – they are the ones having kids, after all.

Turner syndrome is the most common chromosomal defect discovered in spontaneous abortions. 45XO is the most common form.

Buccal smear is woefully inaccurate for diagnosing Turner syndrome. A karyotype is necessary for definitive diagnosis.

Some girls who have Turner syndrome may have mosaicism. If you are "fishing" for Turner and initial chromosome analysis is normal, then turn to a FISH study to look for mosaicism. If you wish to carry this "fish story" further, then remember that elevated FSH can also be a feature of Turner syndrome.

Growth hormone has been used effectively to treat short stature in Turner syndrome.

Noonan Syndrome (Moon Man Syndrome)

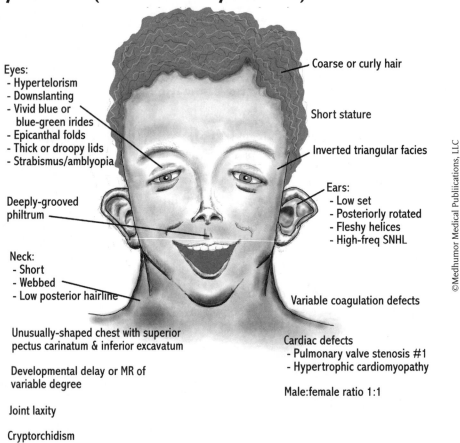

Eyes:
- Hypertelorism
- Downslanting
- Vivid blue or blue-green irides
- Epicanthal folds
- Thick or droopy lids
- Strabismus/amblyopia

Deeply-grooved philtrum

Neck:
- Short
- Webbed
- Low posterior hairline

Unusually-shaped chest with superior pectus carinatum & inferior excavatum

Developmental delay or MR of variable degree

Joint laxity

Cryptorchidism

Coarse or curly hair

Short stature

Inverted triangular facies

Ears:
- Low set
- Posteriorly rotated
- Fleshy helices
- High-freq SNHL

Variable coagulation defects

Cardiac defects
- Pulmonary valve stenosis #1
- Hypertrophic cardiomyopathy

Male:female ratio 1:1

©Medhumor Medical Publications, LLC

Noonan Syndrome used to be known as "Male Turner syndrome," but it is not a male version of Turner. It **can** occur in **females,** so don't be fooled if they present the classic features in a female patient. These features include **pectus excavatum**, **webbed neck**, **low set ears**, and **pulmonic stenosis**. The karyotype is normal.[1]

 Envision:

- ❑ **A Moon Man** pulling a **web neck** and

- ❑ Grabbing the Moon and **placing it on his chest,** snugly on the **Pectus Excavatum**.

- ❑ The Moon changes the tide on his chest and **pulls down the ears**, and also exerts pressure on the heart, resulting in **Pul"moonic" Stenosis**

Cri Du Chat Syndrome

"Cry of the Cat" is easy to remember because this is what these children may sound like. It is the result of a deletion on the short arm of chromosome 5.

 Picture a cat with 5 instead of 9 lives.

Apert Syndrome

The main characteristic is premature closure of the cranial sutures, resulting in **craniosynostosis**. There is also **syndactyly**.

Both Apert syndrome and Crouzon syndrome present with craniosynostosis. However, only Apert presents with syndactyly.

Picture **premature closure of the fingers** and the **cranial sutures**.

---

[1] Technically speaking, genetics does play a role in Noonan syndrome; however, unlike in Turner syndrome, there are no identifiable genetic patterns on karyotyping.

There is an Apert syndrome, an Alpers syndrome, and an Alport syndrome. Follow the table below to avoid confusion.

Alpers	Apert	Alport
Alpers is associated with ataxia, partial seizures, intellectual disability, and liver disease	Apert is associated with choanal atresia, craniosynostosis, syndactyly, and/or intellectual disability	Alport is associated with renal disease, sensorineural hearing loss, and cataracts

Duchenne Muscular Dystrophy

If they show you large calves, it's not an Olympic skater; it is "pseudo" hypertrophy in a child with DMD.

Fanconi's syndrome

Fanconi's syndrome is a rare disorder of the kidneys. The cause of the disease is the loss of minerals in the urine, leading to failure to thrive.

It is easy to confuse Fanconi's syndrome and Fanconi's anemia. Fanconi's syndrome is described above. However, while **Fanconi's Anemia** is a syndrome that can affect the kidneys, it has many more associations, including bony abnormalities and, of course, anemia.

Crouzon syndrome (Cruisin)

The main features of Crouzon Syndrome (AKA craniofacial dysostosis) are craniosynostosis, a high prominent forehead, shallow orbits resulting in proptosis (prominent eyes), and a "beak nose."

You need **prominent eyes and forehead to cruise** through the test. It is also autosomal dominant, and if you are wealthy enough to be "Cruisin" around the world on your yacht, you are clearly assertive and "dominant."

Klinefelter syndrome (47 XXY)

This is typically described as a teen that is **infertile** with **small testes**, but is otherwise normal. They can be described as being **socially awkward, with normal intelligence**.

Watch for key buzz words such as **delayed speech, poor self image,** or **mild motor delay.**

> **CASE STUDY**
>
> **You are presented with a patient who is noted to have delayed motor and language development. On physical examination, he is quite tall, with legs and arms longer than expected for his height. You also note 4 café-au-lait spots measuring between 4 and 5 mm each. His parents state that in school he is a bit of a loner. You note that he has a very calm demeanor. What would be the next most appropriate diagnostic step?**
>
> **THE DIVERSION**
>
> Here you are being diverted into suspecting neurofibromatosis because of the café-au-lait spots. In addition, the long arms and legs will divert you into believing this is Marfan syndrome.
>
> **ANSWER REVEALED**
>
> The history is most consistent with Klinefelter syndrome, and the next most appropriate diagnostic step would be chromosome analysis. The café au lait spots are a true diversion, both in size and number. Six or more café-au-lait spots measuring at least 5 mm would be consistent with neurofibromatosis.

 Weight and head circumference should be normal. *Height can be well above average.*

 The word in German for small is *Klein.* That is a good way to remember the small testicles in "Klein-felter" syndrome.

Treatment may include testosterone supplementation.

Trisomies

HOT TIP The incidence of **all trisomies** increases with advancing maternal age. Trisomies are the only genetic disorders that increase with advancing maternal age.

Trisomy 21 (Down syndrome)

Genetic Variations

There are no phenotypic differences between a child with Down syndrome due to translocation or due to a regular trisomy. The genetic implications, however, are quite different. In the case of trisomy without translocation (due to nondisjunction), there is an empiric 1% risk plus the age-related risk for recurrence. Cases involving translocations have a higher risk of recurrence.

Translocation

If the carrier is identified with a *full* translocation (21q 21q), there is a 100% chance of Down syndrome recurring. However, this is extremely rare. With a *partial* translocation, the risk is closer to 15%.

HOT TIP If the infant has a translocation, chromosomal studies of the parents are crucial. If the partial translocation is from the mother, the chances of recurrence are higher than if it is from the father.

Risk for Recurrence

The risk for recurrence equals the overall risk for the general population (1%) plus the mother's age-related risk. At age 40, the age-related risk is 1/90. At age 22, it is 1/1,500.

Clinical Associations

Children with Down syndrome are at increased risk for **leukemia, duodenal atresia,** and **cardiac disease**, especially **AV canal (endocardial cushion defect).**

CASE STUDY Any question dealing with the risk of giving birth to a child with Down syndrome requires you to pause, take a breath, and read the question carefully. In addition to casually mentioning that a given child has Down syndrome due to translocation or to trisomy, they could also plant other deceptive features in the wording of the question.

THE DIVERSION They could ask you which age group gives birth to more infants with Down syndrome.

Or

They could ask you which age group is at greater risk for having a child with Down syndrome.

These are very different questions.

ANSWER REVEALED More children with Down syndrome are born to mothers in their twenties, since more women in their twenties have children, period. In addition, women in their twenties are less likely to have prenatal screening. Therefore, women in their 20's give birth to more babies with Down syndrome.

However, women in their 40's are at greater risk for having babies with Down syndrome.

HOT TIP The most **common** abnormality seen in Down syndrome is **hypotonia**, which is seen in 80% of cases. This may play a role in the feeding difficulties and constipation commonly seen in Down syndrome.

TAKE HOME MESSAGE Children with Down syndrome are at particular risk for *atlantoaxial instability*. If you are asked what you should be concerned about when doing a sports physical on a patient with Down syndrome who wants to participate in Special Olympics, **atlantoaxial instability is your answer**.

Physical features of Trisomy 21 include the following, most of which can be identified in the newborn period. These can be remembered with the word "**Down syndrome:**"

Dysplasia of the Middle Phalanx of the 5th Finger
Ouch! Cardiac Disease (Not a stretch – picture it – it works)
Wide Gap between the 1st and 2nd toe
Neck has excess skin in the back

Spots (Brushfield Spots in the eye)
Y – Use the letter Y to remind you of the protruding tongue
Nice Simian Crease (I think I have one; it can occur in the general population too.)
Duodenal Atresia (Remember the association with Hirschsprung disease)
Really extensible joints
Oncology/leukemia risk
Moro reflex is incomplete
Ears are small and anomalous

They are sometimes missing their 12th rib. This is easy to remember since 12 is 21 backwards and you can picture a #21 chromosome in place of a 12th rib (which is as good as missing).

Should they present you with a child with Down syndrome with any neurological findings, think of **atlantoaxial instability** as the cause, and work from there.

Remember that the AV Canal (endocardial cushion defect) throws off the axis in the EKG reading.

Trisomy 13

Just focus on a few classic features and you will recognize this on the exam. They will likely show **punched-out scalp lesions.**

Since the #13 is considered bad luck, you can remember the features of trisomy 13 with the word "**BAD LUCK**"

Brain (Holoprosencephaly and Microcephaly and Mid Scalp Lesions)
Airs (Low Set Ears)
Digits (Extra Digits = Polydactyly)

Leukocytes (unique nuclear projections in the neutrophils)
Uterus (Bicornuate Uterus and Hypoplastic Ovaries)
Cleft Lip and Palate (Bilateral)
Kidneys (Cystic)

Trisomy 18

Be prepared to see this in an infant in the picture section. Remember the following features and you will recognize it easily.

 I remember the features as follows:

- ❑ I picture an "**18** year old" at a rock concert. I then picture a "**clenched fist**"[2] and the "**rocker bottom feet.**"

- ❑ The fist has been clenched for days, resulting in "**hypoplastic nails.**"

- ❑ Such a person would be drinking a lot and too busy rocking back and forth to notice he is banging his head on the wall. This results in a "**prominent occiput**" and the "**low set ears.**"

- ❑ He also would be too busy to go to the bathroom, resulting in the kidneys getting bent out of shape turning into "**horseshoes**" = Horseshoe Kidneys.

> Remember that **birth of any trisomy increases the risk of having another child with other anomalies.** Therefore, genetic testing is indicated after the birth of any child with trisomy #X.

Holt Oram Syndrome

Children with Holt Oram Syndrome have **ASD and upper limb**[3] **defects**. In particular, they may have **three-jointed thumbs**.

 "Hold Your Arm" syndrome: "Hold your arm" by a 3-jointed thumb. This will help you remember the upper limb defects, and the 3-jointed thumb. ASD has 3 letters to help with the 3-jointed thumb association.

Or you can simply remember it as **"Heart Arm"** syndrome.

Lesch Nyhan Syndrome

Lesch Nyhan Syndrome typically presents as a child with evidence of **self-mutilation,** usually in the form of bite marks. **Intellectual disability** and **choreiform movements** are the other hallmarks.

"Elevated uric acid levels" is another clue.

---

2 They can also describe an overlapping of the index finger over the 3rd, 4th, or 5th digits.

3 Also known as the "arm".

McCune Albright Syndrome

Diagnostic signs are café au lait spots, abnormal bones (fibrous dysplasia) AND a child going through **precocious puberty**.

McCunE AlBright where the CEAB would stand for **C**afé **A**u lait spots, **E**arly puberty, **A**bnormal **B**ones.

Contiguous Gene Malformations

Prader-Willi Syndrome

Guess which celebrity? Hint: **Slick Willy Syndrome**. Features are: floppy baby, intellectual deficits, obese later in life, **talks a lot but with little content, testicles and hands are small, and has a large appetite**.

Much of the morbidity and mortality in kids with Prader-Willi syndrome comes as a result of complications of obesity (diabetes, sleep apnea, slipped capital femoral epiphysis).

Prader-Willi syndrome is one where you might need to know a little genetics. It is one of only a few disorders that are known to result from *imprinting*.

The following 2 possibilities occur in Prader- Willi syndrome

· A deletion of the **father's chromosome 15**

· **Maternal disomy (2 copies of chromosome 15 from the mother)**

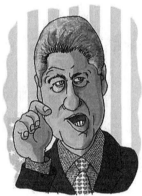

"I did not have dinner with that man ... Dr. Silverstein."

Prader-Willi vs. Laurence-Moon-Biedl Syndrome

Laurence-Moon Syndrome (LMBBS)[4] is an autosomal recessive genetic disorder characterized by progressive CNS, ophthalmologic, and endocrine problems.[5]

Distinguishing PWS from LMBBS on the basis of a picture alone can be tricky. Kids with LMBBS tend to have more anomalies such as syndactyly and retinal dystrophy. Both will be obese and have hypogonadism.

---

[4] Also known as Laurence-Moon-Bardet-Biedl Syndrome, not to be confused with John-Jacob-Jingle-Heimer-Schmidt Syndrome.

[5] Just to confuse you more, LMBBS has recently been split into Laurence-Moon syndrome and Bardet-Biedl syndrome, but for the purposes of the exam, they should consider these as a single grouping (hey, this is not the Genetic Boards!)

Watch out for "pseudo hypogonadism" where the genitalia are normal-sized but the body is big in comparison. The tip-off might be **significant gynecomastia.**

Angelman Syndrome

Genetically, the following 2 possibilities result in Angelman syndrome
- A deletion of the **mother's chromosome 15**[6]
- **Paternal disomy (2 copies of chromosome 15 from the father)**

Kids with Angelman syndrome are usually diagnosed between 3 and 7 years of age. All kids with this disorder will have severe developmental delay, profound speech impairment, ataxia and other movement disorders, and behavioral anomalies such as frequent laughter, easy excitability, or short attention span. Many kids have microcephaly and seizures. This combination of laughing and abnormal jerky movements led to Dr. Angelman calling these kids "puppet children."

Beckwith Wiedemann Syndrome

Important features of Beckwith Wiedemann syndrome include:
- Hypospadias
- Omphalocele
- Macroglossia
- Macrosomia
- Hypoglycemia
- Hemihypertrophy

DiGeorge Syndrome[7]

Thymic and hypoparathyroid hypoplasia result in **hypocalcemia** and **immune deficiencies.** In addition, there are **cardiac outflow abnormalities**.

DiGeorge syndrome is a microdeletion syndrome. Therefore, routine chromosomal analysis won't pick it up. For this, fluorescent in situ hybridization studies are needed.

---

[6] 15q11-q13 if you must know.
[7] DiGeorge syndrome is covered in greater detail in Chapter 15 Allergy and Immunology.

Patterns of Inheritance

Understanding the inheritance patterns will enable you to eliminate 2-3 choices immediately. Knowing how to navigate the information in the question will allow you to instantly eliminate the incorrect choices deceptively left there for you.

X-Linked Recessive Disorders

Males are affected and females are carriers. If they describe **ANY female relatives with the disorder**, then it is **not X-linked recessive**. There is **no male-to-male transmission**.

HOT TIP If they "casually" mention in the question that "he had two uncles who had a similar problem," you know that only males are affected and they are pointing you towards an X-linked recessive disorder.

Linking the x-Linked recessives

X-linked recessive disorders frequently involve an **enzyme deficiency.** The following disorders are x-linked recessive

- ❑ **Hemophilia A/B** – These are Factor 8 and 9 **enzyme deficiencies**
- ❑ **Glucose-6-phosphate dehydrogenase (G6PD) Deficiency** – An enzyme deficiency, and remember it as G**X**PD deficiency.
- ❑ **Chronic Granulomatous Disease** – Here the enzyme to break down bacterial cells in the neutrophil is defective, so again it is an enzyme deficiency. Also remember it as C**X**GD.
- ❑ **Duchenne Muscular Dystrophy** – Remember it as Du**X**chenne.
- ❑ **Nephrogenic Diabetes Insipidus** – Again, this is an enzyme deficiency. Think of it as Ne**X**rogenic.
- ❑ **Retinitis Pigmentosa** – Also an enzyme deficiency, and you can remember it as retinitis pigmen**X**osa.

Androgen Insensitivity

PERIL *WARNING* The patient described in the question will be phenotypically female but genetically male, so don't be fooled, it is still an X-linked recessive disorder.

- ❑ **Androgen Insensitivity (formerly known as testicular feminization)** – Again the enzyme is defective, and you can remember that it has *testicular in the name of the disorder so it has to be X-linked* even though it presents in phenotypical females.
- ❑ **Wiskott Aldrich Syndrome** –To remember this change the name to "Whiskey All Rich" syndrome, so picture a bunch of "guys" sitting around drinking to help remember that it is X-linked recessive and affects males mostly.

CASE STUDY Make sure you read the question carefully. They can present you with a scenario where the mother is a known carrier of an X-linked recessive disorder, and can then ask you one of two questions:

1. What are the chances of having an *affected male* child
2. What are the chances of having an *affected child*

THE DIVERSION This question can be a slam dunk, but if you do not pay attention in the moment, you can easily miss the question. Highlight the word *male* or *child* and you won't be tricked with X-linked recessive disorders.

ANSWER REVEALED The table that follows provides the logical conclusion to any question dealing with the chances of having a child with an x-linked recessive disorder when the mother is a carrier.

MALES	FEMALES	CHILDREN
50% will be affected 50% will not be affected	50% will be carriers 50% will not be carriers	25% will be carriers 25% will have disease 50% will be normal

X-Linked Dominant

There aren't that many X-linked dominant disorders. Just in case, here's how it works.

Because the disorder is on the X, fathers have only one X to give their daughters; therefore, ALL of their daughters will have the disorder. For the same reason, none of their sons will have the disorder.

If mom has the chromosome, then 50% of all children will have it and 50% of children won't. **There are no carriers of a dominant trait. This is the same pattern for autosomal dominant**, making it difficult to distinguish and therefore a very unlikely question.

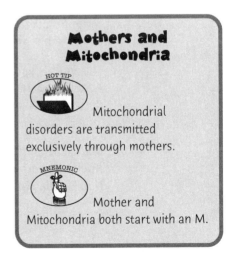

Mothers and Mitochondria

HOT TIP Mitochondrial disorders are transmitted exclusively through mothers.

MNEMONIC Mother and Mitochondria both start with an M.

Aicardi syndrome

In addition to **macrocephaly, seizures**, and **ocular abnormalities**, a key feature of Aicardi syndrome is the **absence of the corpus callosum**.

"A-Card-e" syndrome. Picture **a card replacing the corpus callosum**. The **card** blocks your view.

Because it is X-linked dominant, male children of affected males do not inherit this syndrome from their fathers.

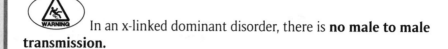 In an x-linked dominant disorder, there is **no male to male transmission**.

Specific X- Linked Dominant

There aren't too many of these out there, and **they will most likely not ask you to pick this up from the question**. But in case they do, the disorders to consider are:

- ❏ X-linked hypophosphatemic rickets[8]
- ❏ Pseudohyperparathyroidism
- ❏ Aicardi syndrome
- ❏ Alport syndrome

Autosomal Dominant

 Autosomal dominant disorders can be transmitted from father to son.

In addition, autosomal dominant disorders have the following characteristics:

- · Variable expressivity
- · Possible reduced penetrance
- · High risk for spontaneous mutation with prior family history.

Specific Autosomal Dominants

Here the phrase to link these disorders is **TAR MAN**. Envision a MAN going around "TAR"ring people, which would make him the dominant man in town.

> **T**uberous Sclerosis
> **A**chondroplasia
> **R**etinoblastoma
>
> **M**arfan syndrome
> **A**pert, **A**ll porphyrias (and, just to confuse you, occasionally Alport syndrome)
> **N**ail Patella Syndrome and **N**eurofibromatosis[9]

---

8 See Endocrinology chapter for ongoing revised and often confusing changed nomenclature for this disorder.
9 Neurofibromatosis can have variable expressivity with a high spontaneous mutation rate.

The Autosomal Dominant Disorders are rounded out by:

- ❑ **Waardenburg Syndrome** (A War Dominates everyBODY = Autosomal)
- ❑ **Huntington's Chorea** (A ton of hunters would mean a large BODY of hunters in Korea)
- ❑ **Peutz-Jeghers Syndrome** (Mick Jagger certainly is a "dominant BODY")
- ❑ **Von Willebrand Disease**
- ❑ **Gardner Syndrome**

Autosomal Recessive

 Vertical transmission through 3 generations **rules out an autosomal recessive** disorder.

This will be a bit of a stretch, but it is far better than **randomly memorizing** the autosomal recessives, so follow along. Picture yourself **REC**eding because you go to get **GAS** from a guy wearing a **HAT** but he gives you a **WAK** on the hand with a pickax.

Galactosemia
Alpha 1- Anti Trypsin Deficiency
Sickle Cell and Thalassemia

Hurler Syndrome
Ataxia Telangiectasia
Tay Sachs Disease

Wilson Disease
Adrenogenital Syndrome (and Alpers Syndrome)
Kartagener Syndrome

Pickax = **PKU**

> **Heme Beam**
>
> Factor 8 and 9 deficiencies as well as sickle cell disease can all be diagnosed prenatally.

Prenatal Screening

In Utero Testing

· **Chorionic villus sampling** can be done at **12 weeks.**

· **Amniocentesis** can be done at **16 weeks**.

CASE STUDY **You are asked to decide among several choices which is the best in predicting fetal lung maturity.**

THE DIVERSION You will be presented with several choices, which will include *surfactant* or *surfactant protein* A, sphingomyelin, alpha-fetoprotein, and phosphatidylglycerol.

ANSWER REVEALED Surfactant will be very tempting, but you know the answer could never be that simple. The correct answer is **phosphatidylglycerol**, which is an important component of surfactant and is absent prior to 35 weeks gestation. This would be the best substance to measure in predicting fetal lung maturity.

PERIL WARNING If this question were regarding a *mother with diabetes*, the correct answer would be *total surfactant activity*. This is because other parameters including phosphatidylglycerol aren't as reliable in that setting.

Fetal Ultrasound

Fetal ultrasound is used to track intrauterine growth over time. Structural anamolies (such as myelomeningocele) are best detected on ultrasound between 12 and 24 weeks gestation.

PERIL WARNING Maternal obesity, if stated outright in the question, can be a complicating factor that blunts the accuracy of ultrasound findings.

Teratogens

Fetal Alcohol Syndrome

The features include **prenatal** and **postnatal growth delay** and **neurological developmental deficits**.

 Typical clues include: **flat philtrum** (that thing in the middle of your upper lip), **thin upper lip, small 5ᵗʰ fingernail, midface hypoplasia, and short palpebral fissures.**

Picture a **child drinking alcohol:**
- ❑ From having the bottle in his mouth so often, it forms a mark on the middle of his face (**midface hypoplasia**) and **thins out his upper lip and philtrum**.

FAS and intellectual disability

Fetal alcohol syndrome (FAS) is the most common *preventable* cause of intellectual disability. In addition to intellectual disability, children with FAS can also have behavioral and psychiatric disorders (even in the absence of intellectual disability).

 In addition to FAS, Fragile X syndrome and Down syndrome are the other most common *identifiable* causes of intellectual disability.

> **Maternal Smoking**
>
> Maternal smoking results in low birth weight infants, higher miscarriage rates, IUGR, and prematurity.
>
> In addition, maternal smoking is associated with cleft lip/palate.
>
> Smoking during pregnancy is associated with asthma, wheezing and other respiratory ailments, independent of maternal smoking after delivery.
>
> Maternal smoking is associated with SIDS as well.

Anticonvulsants

You will need to know the general and specific teratogenic effects of **phenytoin, phenobarbital,** and **carbamazepine.** Exposure to these meds is associated with an increased risk for **microcephaly, intrauterine growth retardation,** and other major malformations, such as the "**anticonvulsant face**" and "**fingernail hypoplasia.**"

In addition, **cardiac** defects, **cleft lip, hypospadias** with **cryptorchidism,** and **clubfoot deformity** are associated with anticonvulsant use during pregnancy. With carbamazepine exposure, there is an increased risk for spina bifida.

Change "carbamazepine" to "**Car-Bam**" and picture an auto accident resulting in "**spinal**" problems and "**facial deformities.**"

Phenytoin exposure results in a specific profile that includes **finger stiffness** and **severe nail hypoplasia**.

Instead of phenytoin, think of "**Funny Toe'n**" and picture **funny toes** instead of fingers. **Cardiac, skeletal,** and **ophthalmological anomalies** may occur as well.

By the way, "**anticonvulsant face**" is obvious by the broad bridge of the nose, small anteverted nostrils, and a long upper lip.

Valproic Acid can result in a neural tube defect. Easy to picture the V in Valproic Acid as a defective neural tube (not to be confused with the "Y" in Down sYndrome to remember the protruding tongue).

Lithium/Pregnancy

Folic acid supplementation prior to conception can decrease the incidence of neural tube defects by **more than 50%**.

Cardiac defects such as **Ebstein's anomaly** are the most common.

However, lithium is felt to be a much weaker teratogen than previously believed.

Lithium use during pregnancy is reserved for those mothers at greatest risk for relapse if they are not taking lithium.

Isotretinoin

The classic features of isotretinoin embryopathy simply need to be memorized.

The classic features of isotretinoin embryopathy are as follows:
- Microcephaly
- Microphthalmia
- Hypoplastic ears
- Truncus arteriosis
- Absent thymus

Remember: isotretinoin not only shrinks pimples but also shrinks the head, the eyes, and the ears. It also takes away the thymus and, for good measure, throws in truncus arteriosis.

Anticoagulants

In particular, you need to be aware of **warfarin embryopathy**.

The important features to remember, in addition to *depressed nasal bridge* and *short nose,* are **hypoplastic distal phalanges** and **stippled epiphyses.**

ACE Inhibitors

ACE inhibitors should not be used during pregnancy.

Findings with ACE inhibitor exposure include anuria, oligohydramnios, hypoplasia of the skull, and fetal hypotension.

Malformations

It is important to define the following to avoid confusion and getting a question wrong due to a technicality:

A **sequence** is the result of a localized abnormality early in fetal development. An example would be Potter syndrome (Oligohydramnios Sequence), whose effects all stem from oligohydramnios. Pierre Robin sequence is another example.

An **association** is the clustering of anomalies that cannot be explained by chance. Examples would be CHARGE and VATER associations.

CHARGE

The **CHARGE association** stands for the following:

Coloboma/cognitive deficits
Heart disease
Atresia (choanal)
Retarded growth and development
GU abnormalities (genital hypoplasia)
Ear anomalies (hearing loss)

You will need to recognize this on the exam.

 Intelligence is below normal. Think of it as a "**charge card,**" where the syndrome **costs you your intelligence**.

VACTER-L

This syndrome has gone through a variety of incarnations. You will be asked to recognize it.

Vertebral Defects
Anal Atresia
Cardiac Defects/ VSD
TE Fistula
Radial Hypoplasia and **R**enal Abnormalities

Limb abnormalities

It often presents with a "single umbilical artery." **Intelligence is normal.**

Craniosynostosis

Craniosynostosis can be easily corrected, **but it must be recognized before five months of age**, since treatment is more successful when done prior to the period of greatest head growth. Neurological complications, such as hydrocephalus and increased intracranial pressure, are more likely to occur when two or more sutures close prematurely.

Positional plagiocephaly is of lesser concern since it usually resolves spontaneously or may be managed with a helmet, preferably prior to 9 months of age.

On the other hand, coronal suture synostosis is often associated with other anomalies. Therefore, at the very least a good family history should be obtained.

You may be expected to distinguish between the closure of cranial sutures secondary to slow brain growth (which would result in a small, symmetrical head) and premature closure of a single cranial suture. The latter would present with an asymmetrically-shaped head, and the former with a small but normally-shaped head.

Cleft Lip and Palate

The chance of recurrence doubles when two children have this.

Oligohydramnios sequence (Potter syndrome)

Potter syndrome is now known as oligohydramnios sequence. This is due to the associated characteristics being caused by oligohydramnios.

The important features of oligohydramnios sequence include:

1- Typical facies described as "pugilistic"
2- Hypoplastic lungs
3- Limb malformation
4- Renal agenesis
5- IUGR

They may describe the following: **club feet**, **pulmonary hypoplasia**, and "**glove-like**" excess skin on the hands, in addition to **fetal membranes being covered** by **yellowish nodules** (or the word **amnion nodosum**).

Oligohydramnios can occur in the absence of renal agenesis. Anything that causes low amnionic fluid volume can result in oligohydramnios sequence.

Genitourinary anomalies are an important part of the workup. Kids with Potter syndrome **ultimately die of pulmonary complications**.

Rubinstein-Taybi Syndrome (Thumby)

The key phrase or picture they will show is a "**broad thumb.**" This is easy to remember by changing the name of the syndrome to "**Rubinstein Thumby**" syndrome. They also have **cryptorchidism**.

 It is difficult to bring down an undescended testicle with a broad-based thumb.

 In Pfeiffer syndrome, the thumbs and great toes are also short and broad; however, the eyes are prominent and widely spaced, just as they are in Crouzon syndrome. Therefore, a child who looks like a cross between Crouzon and Rubinstein-Taby would likely have Pfeiffer syndrome.

Russell Silver Syndrome (Wrestle Silver Syndrome)

Features include **triangle face** (small chin) and **growth retardation**. These children are very small.

 Picture a **small (growth retarded) wrestler** with a **triangle face made of silver**.

Prune Belly Syndrome

This will be obvious; lack of abdominal muscle development leads to the prune belly appearance. What else do you need to know? Let's go to the chalkboard.

It is also associated with **bladder outlet obstruction**, which leads to **oligohydramnios**. The oligohydramnios results in **pulmonary hypoplasia** — and while we are down there, the **testes are undescended** (well, picture it as a pit of the prune that never came down).

Treacher Collins (Teacher Calling)

The picture is very distinctive. One good look in the atlas and you will see it clearly. **Conductive hearing loss, a small jaw, ear abnormalities, and lower eyelid abnormalities** are part of the picture; **intellectual disability** is **not**.

 You can't be a teacher, or a Treacher, with abnormal intelligence.

Since it is a dominant trait, picture a "dominating" teacher in control of a class. It occurs in several family members. In the picture section, they might show a family portrait in which several members have the same dysmorphic features. **One or more family members with a hearing aid could be the tip-off.**

Tuberous Sclerosis

"Child with seizures and intellectual disability," with a past history of infantile spasms should make you think of tuberous sclerosis.

Syndactyly refers to the union of two or more fingers or toes. This typically only involves a skin connection between the two; however, it can also include fusion of bones.

Clinodactyly is permanent deviation of one or more fingers, usually the 5th finger (pinky).

Celebrity Dysmorphology

It is quite a challenge to remember the details of clinical syndromes and know the fine differences between them. For example, you will be expected to distinguish which syndromes are "autosomal dominant," which ones are associated with "sensorineural hearing loss," and which ones are associated with both.

When you have actually taken care of a patient with a given syndrome, it is easier to know this information cold. However, during the course of training and practice it is virtually impossible to "see" every syndrome. By associating them with well-known, popular and historical figures, you have essentially "seen the case" (See Prader-Willi above).

Disclaimer and Explanation

We are not in any way trying to disparage children who suffer from any syndrome or their families. We are merely providing a memory aide for pediatricians to remember the syndromes.

Achondroplasia

Children (and adults) who have achondroplasia have the classic look of the "Munchkins" in the *Wizard of Oz* movie. They have **large heads** and **very short extremities**, which made for the "cute look" that the casting directors were after.

This is why it is also known as "short-limbed dwarfism," especially of the proximal portion of the limb. This is called **rhizomelic shortening.** They also have **frontal bossing**. Folks with achondroplasia have genu varum ("bowlegs").

Lumbar lordosis gives them that puffed out chest appearance, and they also have small foramen magna, which can result in **nerve root compression.**

There are frequent respiratory problems – over 3/4 of kids with achondroplasia have significant sleep apnea.

Intelligence is normal.

Hurler's Syndrome

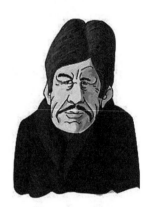

Hurler's syndrome is an example of a "mucopolysaccharidosis" or MPS (thank goodness for the medical spellchecker). Hurler's syndrome is MPS type I, for those of you keeping track at home. These folks have **"coarse facies," "corneal clouding,"** and **"thick skulls."** I think of *Death Wish* star Charles Bronson.

In addition, these kids have severe intellectual disability, as well as other neurologic deficits.

Picture a coarse-faced Charles Bronson, blinded by rage (**corneal clouding**) in *Death Wish 2* "hurling" someone from a building. He isn't the brightest character, and you can now remember the **"thick skull."**

The other mucopolysaccharidoses are similar, but they each have distinguishing features that will be obvious in the description.

Hunter's syndrome does NOT have corneal clouding and it is X-linked recessive.[10] Other differences from Hurler's are that kids with Hunter's syndrome **are short and have skeletal abnormalities**. BOTH Hunter's and Hurler's syndromes have hepatosplenomegaly and progressive deafness.

To remember that it is X-linked, picture a hunter with a bow and arrow. The tips of the arrows have giant X's. Their short stature and skeletal abnormalities help them get around while hunting without being seen. You can also remember that Hunter's syndrome is not associated with corneal clouding because you need to "see in order to hunt."

In addition, focus on the following **H** pattern. **H**unter's and **H**urler's syndromes are associated with **H**epatosplenomegaly and **H**earing deficits.

---

[10] This is MPS Type II, for those with the micro-grid scorecard.

Williams Syndrome
(Robin Williams as a Zany Character)

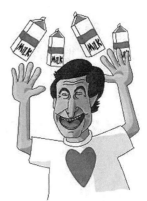

Think of Robin Williams as a zany character: **elfin facies** with **wide spaced teeth** and an **upturned nose**. Kids with Williams syndrome usually have mild intellectual disability. They are also known to have a "cocktail party" personality because they are typically very friendly.

Hypercalcemia: Picture Robin Williams throwing milk containers around the room, eventually "**winning the hearts**" of everyone. You can think of the calcium as causing "**supravalvular aortic stenosis.**"[11]

Fragile X Syndrome

This is the most common (known) inherited cause of intellectual disability.

Clues include: "**male,**" "**mild intellectual disability,**" and a **positive family history of uncles** and other males who are "weird."

Celebrity: long face, large ears, weird behavior, and macroorchidism—think of **Prince Charles**.

Sometimes they can go esoteric and mention the specific problem on the X chromosome that makes it "Fragile." This would be a *repeat of the CGG trinucleotide* on the X chromosome..

More women than men *carry* the abnormal X chromosome, but they are less likely to be affected. Twice as many males exhibit Fragile X syndrome as females. **It is the most common cause of *inherited* intellectual disability. Fragile X is overall the second most common cause of *genetic* intellectual disability, after Down syndrome.**

Remember that Down syndrome is genetic, but rarely inherited

While Fragile X syndrome typically presents in boys, it *can* manifest in females. This would be very unlikely on the exam, but worth considering if presented with such a case.

---

[11] It is not physiologically accurate, but it is one way of looking at it.

If you are given a choice between karyotype and DNA testing in working up a kid who has intellectual disability, choose DNA testing, as it is much more sensitive in diagnosing Fragile X.

Rett Syndrome

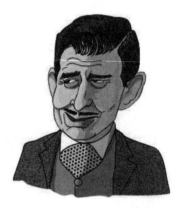

They will describe a **girl around 1-2 years of age** who has lost developmental milestones. Look for "**autistic-like behavior,**" "**wringing hands,**" and regression of developmental milestones.

These girls have normal development at first, but around 4 months of age their head growth decelerates. They then enter a period where they do not continue their development (stagnation - usually from age 6-18 months), followed by a loss of their milestones (regression - usually from 1-4 years of age). After this, there is usually no further decline. These children usually survive into adulthood, although they may not gain/regain purposeful hand use or functional speech.

Celebrity: Rhett Butler (Clark Gable) from *Gone with the Wind*. Picture him **walking backwards**, wringing his hands, saying: "Frankly my dear, I don't give a damn, which is why I am **backing out** of the deal."

Hallermann Streiff Syndrome

These kids really look like hockey great Wayne Gretzky.

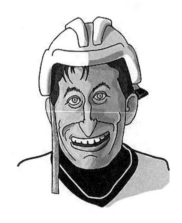

"**Pointed nose,**" "**bird-like face, including small eyes.**"

"**Hollering Star Syndrome:**" when a doctor and hockey fanatic like me sees a kid like this, at first glance he thinks it is Wayne Gretzky and he starts "hollering," resulting in small teeth just like a hockey player.

Peutz-Jeghers Syndrome

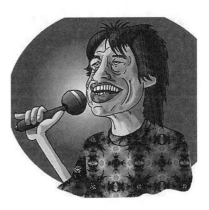

"**Mucosal pigmentation of lips and gums,**" in addition to "**hamartomatous polyps of the intestine.**"

Treatment consists of **removing any polyps.**

It is inherited in an autosomal dominant fashion. Cancer is the major cause of mortality with this syndrome.

This looks like Mick Jagger. To remember that this is an **autosomal dominant** trait, remember that **Mick Jagger has "dominated" the rock music industry** for close to 50 years. He has been accused in the past of being "hammered" (hamartomatous polyps).

Pierre Robin Sequence

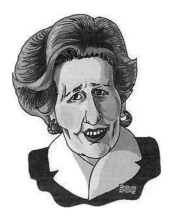

These patients have **small chins** relative to their tongues, and cleft palate with micrognathia. They look like Margaret Thatcher.

Children with Pierre Robin sequence might also be described as having posterior positioning of their tongues.

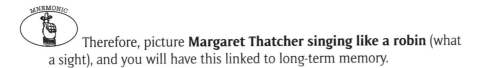

Therefore, picture **Margaret Thatcher singing like a robin** (what a sight), and you will have this linked to long-term memory.

Kids with Pierre Robin sequence have glossoptosis (tongue sticks out) – not because they have big tongues, but because their tongue is relatively large compared to their small chin. This is an important distinction, and not knowing it could cost you on the exam.

In addition, extremity anomalies are quite common, including syndactyly, clinodactyly, hip and knee anomalies, and spinal deformities like kyphosis and scoliosis. About half the kids have some sort of CNS involvement, including language delay, seizures, and developmental delay.

Upper airway obstruction caused by glossoptosis can lead to **cor pulmonale.**

Sturge Weber Syndrome

Affects the eyes, skin, and CNS.

Characteristics are:

- ❏ Port wine stain (AKA nevus flammeus)[12]
- ❏ Developmental delay (former Soviet Union)
- ❏ Seizure (of power)
- ❏ Hemiplegia (half as powerful as before)
- ❏ Vision problems/calcification
- ❏ Think of Mikhail Gorbachev and the old Soviet empire.

Glaucoma is on the same side as the lesion. The focal seizures occur on the contralateral side.

As soon as you suspect this is the diagnosis (i.e., if they note the port-wine stain), the child needs **a referral to an ophthalmologist** to rule out glaucoma and other associated urgent eye problems.

---

[12] Which is a lot more fun to say.

Chapter 13

Allergy and Immunology

Prevention

Breast-feeding

Breast-feeding for the first 6 months of life (or using hypoallergenic formula) delays the onset of eczema.

· Breast-feeding does not eliminate the risk, it only delays the onset. The risk for development of eczema beyond age 2 is the same.

· **Breast-feeding or hypoallergenic formula does not reduce the risk for** asthma, **allergic rhinitis, allergic conjunctivitis, or allergic gastroenteritis.**

Elimination diet during pregnancy (as a means of reducing risk for allergic disease) is not the correct answer.

Latex Fruit Syndrome

You could be asked to choose which fruits somebody with latex allergy should avoid.

The following fruits are examples of those that should be avoided:

Papaya, avocado, banana, chestnut, passion fruit, fig, melon, mango, kiwi, pineapple, peach, and tomato.

CASE STUDY

You are presented with a toddler with moderate to severe atopic dermatitis and are asked to determine which foods could be triggering it. You are presented with several choices.

THE DIVERSION

You will be tempted to go for several choices. Since you already know that milk, eggs, soy, wheat, and peanuts represent 90% of the foods that can cause atopic dermatis, eliminating these from the diet would seem to be the most logical answer. Logically illogical that is!

ANSWER REVEALED

Randomly eliminating multiple foods without evidence of a correlation will be the wrong answer. Allergy shots will be incorrect. The correct answer will be food allergy testing, in order to specify any food allergies triggering the atopic dermatitis.

Genetics and Atopy

The following are symptoms of atopy, and they are linked. Children with one are at risk for another:

1. Allergic rhinitis
2. Eczema
3. Asthma
4. Food Allergy

The most important component is a **parental history of atopy.**

One parent with atopy ➜ 50% risk for allergic disease

Two parents with atopy ➜ 70% risk for allergic disease

However, genetics is not the only contributing factor. There are environmental influences/exposures (including diet) that may increase or decrease risk.

Maternal diet does not play as important a role in subsequent development of atopy as previously believed. Therefore, if you are questioned on this concept on the exam, the correct choice would be for the mother to have a regular healthy diet without specific dietary limitations.

Delaying the introduction of solid foods past 4-6 months does not prevent the development of atopic disease. Therefore, holding off on fish, eggs, or peanut butter exposure will not prevent allergies to these food items.

Allergic Rhinitis

Allergic rhinitis presents in an older child (i.e., age 10-12 or older) with, in addition to *runny nose, sneezing,* and *itching,* **eye symptoms** such as **itchy, swollen, or watery eyes. Eosinophils** will be present in nasal secretions.

Perennial allergic rhinitis is due to exposure to indoor allergens such as dust mites, animal dander and annoying older brothers.

In fact, if they tell you that a nasal smear was obtained, you can pretty much be sure that allergic rhinitis is the diagnosis, since other forms of rhinitis aren't diagnosed this way.

One exception: non-allergic rhinitis with eosinophilia syndrome (NARES), which can present with eosinophils on nasal smear. However, with NARES the skin test would be negative and serum IgE levels would not be elevated.

Treatment of allergic rhinitis

The first step in treating allergic rhinitis is to identify and eliminate the offending allergen, followed by medication if necessary.

Nasal steroids are the first line treatment for allergic rhinitis. However, oral antihistamines or antihistamine-containing eye drops may be used when indicated.

Oral Allergy Syndrome

Oral allergy syndrome is caused when certain allergens come in contact with the oral mucosa.

This will typically be presented in a child with allergic rhinitis who complains of a tingling sensation in the mouth when eating a specific food, typically a raw fruit or vegetable. Certain fruits or vegetables may contain proteins similar to airborne allergens. Patients who are allergic to an airborne allergen may be at risk of developing reactions to the similar food protein. If the same food is eaten cooked, the same symptoms will *not* be seen. Affected individuals typically only need to avoid that specific food in its uncooked form.

Not all noses that run are allergic rhinitis. You will be expected to distinguish conditions with similar presentations as follows:

- **Infectious rhinitis** presents in **younger children** with nasal congestion that is **worse in the winter**

- **Vasomotor rhinitis** presents with *congestion, rhinorrhea,* and **post-nasal drainage, unrelated to any specific triggering or infectious agent.** It can, however, be triggered by **emotions, pollution, cold drafts, rapid temperature changes, or changes in humidity.** This is probably where the old wives' tale regarding wearing a hat to avoid "catching cold" came from.

> ### Signs of Sinusitis
>
> Children with allergic rhinitis are at risk for sinusitis, which is often underdiagnosed. Watch for signs of sinusitis if you are presented with a patient with chronic allergic rhinitis. These patients are also at increased risk for otitis media.

> ### Asthma Matters
>
> Viruses can also trigger wheezing and "reactive airway"
>
> HOT TIP
>
> If you are presented with a child with asthma, before selecting treatment with antibiotics you must be presented with clear documentation of a bacterial infection. X-ray findings consistent with atelectasis alone would be a diversion. For example, pie (wedge) shaped densities would be atelectasis, and thinking this is pneumonia will result in pie in your face. Likewise, chest PT would not be helpful.

· **Rhinitis medicamentosa** is a rebound reaction to **adrenergic nose drops,** resulting in severe nasal congestion.

Beware of the history if you are being led to believe that a child is allergic to pollen, especially if they throw in the word "hay fever" in quotes. **Pollen requires repeated exposure over years, and is usually not seen before age 3.** The most likely diagnosis is **recurrent upper respiratory tract infection** in a child younger than 3 presenting with recurrent rhinorrhea.

Urticaria, Angioedema, and Anaphylaxis

Anaphylaxis

A typical anaphylactic reaction will be categorized as **respiratory distress, urticaria,** and **general discomfort.** Children will often describe a **sense of doom.** Additional signs could include **angioedema of the lips and eyelids** and, of course, **wheezing, respiratory distress,** and/or **cough.**

The primary causes of anaphylaxis in children include foods, stings, vaccines, and medications. These are also important causes of urticaria and angioedema.

- The most common food allergens in the pediatric population are:
    · cow milk
    · eggs
    · peanuts
    · tree nuts
    · soy
    · wheat

Milk, egg, and soy allergies are often outgrown by 5 years of age.

Allergies to peanuts, tree nuts, and seafood typically are not outgrown.

When a 5 year old makes a **MES** it can be cleaned up, **M**ilk **E**ggs **S**oy.

Hot pressed peanut oils typically do not contain sufficient proteins that bind IgE. Therefore, avoiding all hot pressed peanut oil is not necessary. Likewise, **sunflower oil** is okay with peanut-allergic kids.

The sooner epinephrine is given, the lower the mortality. All of the symptoms may not develop until 2 hours after ingestion. The dosing for epinephrine is 0.30 mg for patients weighing 30 Kg or more, and 0.15mg for those weighing less than 30 kg. A late phase reaction can occur up to 24 hours after the initial exposure.

The dosing of epinephrine is easy to remember. A child weighing **30 kg** or greater gets a **0.30 mg** dose.

You receive a call from a school nurse who has a 6 yo girl in her office. Other than a history of milk allergy, there is no other significant history. After eating lunch, which was prepared at home by the father, she was sent to the nurse because she didn't feel well and complained of a stomach ache. The nurse noted no rash or respiratory distress. Other than giving her something to settle her stomach she would like to know what else to do. Your advice?

Of course, with such mild symptoms you must choose from several choices that seem equally correct. Sending her back to class, sending her home, or having her sit in the nurse's office all seem reasonable for a child who only seems to have indigestion, with no rash or respiratory distress. Giving subcutaneous epinephrine would be over the top, wouldn't it?

The only thing over the top about giving epinephrine to this patient would be that choosing this answer could be the one question putting you over the top to a passing grade. Abdominal pain and general discomfort could be the only sign of an anaphylactic reaction, and giving epinephrine to a child with a history of a food allergy with this presentation would be absolutely correct.

You are expected to be able to distinguish the abdominal discomfort of "food poisoning" or "food sensitivities" from an anaphylactic reaction.

If abdominal discomfort is caused by an anaphylactic reaction, they will also have to describe generalized discomfort and a previous history of food allergy.

Specific food sensitivities include:

· Spicy foods ➡ abdominal discomfort
· Beans ➡ abdominal discomfort and flatus

Watch for these specific foods and symptoms (in the absence of a history of food allergy), and food sensitivity will be the correct answer, not anaphylaxis.

Antihistamines may diminish symptoms when given to a child experiencing an anaphylactic reaction. However, this would only serve to give a false sense of security, and it will always be the wrong choice in a question on treatment of anaphylaxis.

> **Eosinophilia**
>
> In addition to being associated with allergic disorders, this can be a tip-off to parasitic diseases. Envision a giant E becoming a worm (with legs if you prefer).

Chronic Urticaria

Urticaria is considered chronic if it lasts longer than 6 weeks; less than that it is considered acute.

The most likely cause of chronic urticaria is food.

The most appropriate **long-term** treatment of chronic urticaria is 2nd or 3rd generation antihistamines such as **fexofenadine** (Allegra®), loratadine (Claritin®), and cetirizine (Zyrtec®).

First generation antihistamines, such as diphenhydramine and hydroxyzine, can be used for break-through exacerbations.

Steroids are rarely necessary in the treatment of chronic urticaria. Allergy testing has no role in identifying a trigger for chronic urticaria.

A positive skin test for an allergen in a patient with chronic urticaria does not necessarily mean that allergen is the cause of the chronic urticaria.

Contrast Media

Contrast reactions are not IgE-mediated. They are an **osmolality- hypertonicity reaction that triggers degranulation of mast cells and basophils with release of mediators, which then cause the reactions.**

This is why pretreatment with antihistamines (like diphenhydramine) and/or prednisone work when indicated.

CASE STUDY

A 5 year old boy who has experienced a severe allergic reaction to shrimp in the past needs a CT scan with IV and oral contrast. What precautions should you take?

THE DIVERSION

You will be given several choices including pre-treatment with antihistamines and prednisone. This will be a tempting choice, since you have been given the red herring allergy to shrimp.

ANSWER REVEALED

The correct answer will be reassurance, since the risk of a reaction is negligible. The association of shellfish allergy to radiocontrast material (presumably because of the iodine content) is a myth.

The only time pretreatment with prednisone and diphenhydramine would be indicated is with a documented history of an adverse reaction to radiocontrast media.

Hymenoptera Stings

The Sting of Age

BUZZ WORDS

One presentation of a local reaction would be a child sustaining a bee sting, and the following morning local erythema has spread dramatically. However, to distinguish this reaction from cellulitis they will note that the child is afebrile and the swelling is non-tender.

Any child with a systemic reaction to a bee sting requires a **referral to an allergist.**

Any child with a life threatening reaction to a bee sting requires **venom immunotherapy,**[1] which is *98% effective in preventing future reactions.*

If chronis urticaria is due to a chronic exposure, they will give you clues in the question, and in such cases an **acute** allergic reaction is not likely.

Ragweed

Other words to look for are "**sneezing, wheezing, and squeezing**" (tight chest) plus "**teary eyes.**"

Ragweed and Respiratory both begin with **R's.**

Allergic Reactions

The Mt. Rushmore of Allergic Reactions: Types 1-4

The following will help you remember the four types:

Type 1	IgE Mediated = Anaphylactic Reaction	**Anaphylactic = A = Type 1**
Type 2	Mediated by Antibodies	**Body (Anti) = B = Type 2**
Type 3	Immune Complex/Arthus	1 Plus 2 = **3/ Complex**
Type 4	Delayed Hypersensitivity = Poison IV	**Poison IV** = Roman numeral 4 = **IV**

---

[1] Immunotherapy is allergy shots.

Skin Testing

Immediate skin testing would be indicated under certain circumstances, which would include the need to identify a specific allergen. Here are some conditions when this could be indicated:

- Severe atopic dermatitis
- Allergic rhinitis unresponsive to routine treatment
- Food allergy
- Asthma triggered by airborne allergens
- Insect sting allergy
- Vaccine or drug allergy
- Latex allergy

Antibiotic Allergies

The only antibiotic reaction that can be "skin IgE tested" is penicillin allergy. Should they get specific, the IgE mediated reaction is one that begins **within 24 hours of exposure**. If the reaction occurs later, then it is not IgE mediated and not verifiable by skin testing.

Milk Allergies

Severe Allergic Reaction to Cow Milk Based Formula

If they describe an infant around 3-4 months of age who develops an **urticarial rash** after an initial, or soon after exposure to milk, the correct management is **referral to a pediatric allergist.** This is in contrast to development of an **eczematous rash,** which can occur as a result of milk ingestion but is thought to be T-cell related.

In Vitro Allergy Testing

In vitro allergy testing would be indicated in a patient who experienced a life threatening allergic reaction

HOT TIP

Regarding insect sting allergy, there is a 25% false negative rate for both skin testing and in vitro testing, which renders false test results marginally reliable. Therefore, if in vitro is negative, skin testing is done and vice versa. The testing must be done 4-6 weeks after the reaction to be reliable. Allergy testing with insect bites is limited to those experiencing reactions beyond simple local inflammation. When testing is done, it should be general, not for a specific insect.

Skin Testing/ False Negatives

Look in the question for any hint of antihistamine use. This WILL interfere with the results of skin testing. Sometime they can be tricky, e.g., antidepressants or other medications that have antihistaminic effects will interfere with some testing. Here is another example of the importance of highlighting something seemingly irrelevant in the question.

A **False Positive** can result because of poor administration— e.g., trauma can result in an inflammatory reaction. It is best not to have former professional wrestlers administer the testing.

Penicillin Rash

In order for a rash to qualify as a bona fide IgE-mediated reaction, the rash will have to appear within 1 day of taking penicillin. If the rash appears days into therapy, it is most likely a non-IgE mediated reaction and could even be a viral exanthem.

Pets and Allergies

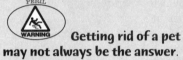

Getting rid of a pet may not always be the answer. When it is the clear cause of an exacerbation of symptoms, taking steps to reduce the exposure is usually the answer. This is because of the emotional attachment children have to their pets. At the very least the pet should be kept out of the child's bedroom at all times.

The Rast Test

RAST Fast and ELISA

· **RAST is done in vitro.** **ELISA** is a variation on this theme.
· **RAST Testing** is **not impacted by antihistamine treatment** like skin testing.
· RAST testing carries no risk for an anaphylactic reaction (unlike skin testing which, obviously, is in vivo).
· It can also be indicated in a child with extensive atopic dermatitis, which limits skin surface area for testing.

Skin testing, however, is generally thought to be **more sensitive** and it is **less expensive**.

Immunodeficiencies

The Significance of Efficiency in the Deficiencies

There are a variety of immunodeficiencies you need to know for the exam. It is a well-represented topic on the exam and is worth taking the time to learn. The core information to focus on is as follows.

You will almost certainly be presented with a patient whose parents are concerned over the number of infections their child has. It is important to note that the typical child can have one "infection" a month with "reassurance" being the correct answer. This is especially the case if all they have are self-limited GI and respiratory ailments.

Failure to thrive and limits in linear growth,[2] coupled with recurrent infections, would be a clue that they are presenting a child with a potential immunodeficiency. In addition, if they present a child

---

[2] This is also known as being "short" by the rest of the world.

with a recurrent infection in one location, i.e., recurrent UTI's, this would be a tip-off that further investigation is indicated.

Some other associations are as follows:

- **B Cell (antibody) dysfunction** – recurrent, pyogenic infections
- **T Cell function** – chronic or recurrent candida infections (i.e., nails, scalp, or mouth)
- **Wiskott-Aldrich Syndrome** – eczema and petechiae (due to thrombocytopenia)
- **Severe combined immunodeficiency** – absence of lymphoid tissue

> ### Adaptive Immunity
>
> The key component in adaptive immunity is antigen-presenting cells.

HOT TIP A low lymphocyte count would correlate with T cell dysfunction, since the majority of circulating lymphocytes are T Cells.

Cellular Immune Deficiencies

Ataxia Telangiectasia

BUZZ WORDS If they describe the following combination - "ataxia" with discoloration of the conjunctiva, as well as frequent sinus infections - unwrap your gift.

DiGeorge syndrome

Di George anomaly is part of the group of disorders caused by deletions on the long arm of chromosome 22. Known by the mnemonic CATCH-22, the disorders include **C**ardiac defects, **A**bnormal facies, **T**hymic hypoplasia, **C**left palate, and **H**ypocalcemia.

BUZZ WORDS DiGeorge syndrome may be characterized by neonatal tetany, congenital heart disease, and abnormal T cell function. In the history, they may describe dysmorphic facies (low set ears), loud murmur, and tetany (secondary to hypocalcemia).

The holosystolic murmur may be heard best at the left sternal border. There is no parathyroid and a small or absent thymus (due to poor development of the pharyngeal pouches).

Infection may be the major presenting problem - these kids can present like SCID, depending on the degree of thymic hypoplasia. In addition, parathyroid deficiency can lead to diarrhea and hypocalcemia, which leads to tetany.

Treatment is aimed at the underlying problems (hypocalcemia, infection, cardiac defects). In general, the prognosis is poor, and children may die from sepsis. The **best therapeutic approach (for complete DiGeorge syndrome)** would be **thymic transplantation**.

Think of the character "George" on *Seinfeld*. Even when he "murmured" he was loud. He was also dysmorphic, and always frozen with fear (tetany).

Severe Combined Immunodeficiency

SCID is caused by a severe defect in B and T cell functions. This leads to dermatitis, diarrhea, failure to thrive, and life-threatening infections. Kids usually present in the first 3 months of life with otitis and thrush, as well as diarrhea and dermatitis. Other than these findings, the physical exam may be normal in most infants.

Most kids have a low white count, but it can be normal or elevated. Despite the "severe combined" in the name, the **B cell count can be normal**.

No matter what the white count is, there will be a complete absence of T cell function. The diagnosis is made by fluorometric analysis of T, B, and NK cell subsets.

Treatment is initially supportive, with care aimed at the underlying infections. Bone marrow transplant is essential and curative. Left untreated, children with SCID may die before their first birthday.

The **Bubble Boy** had a form of this – **ADA deficiency** (adenosine deaminase, if you must know), which results in dysfunctional B and T Cells.[3]

For fans of *Seinfeld*, the Bubble Boy made an appearance, and a catch phrase from the show was "yada, yada, yada" = easy to remember **ADA**. Just don't get carried away and yada yada yada the whole exam.

---

[3] It can also be associated with abnormality of HLA antigen expression, and abnormal assembly of the cytokine receptors. However, this is way too boring for the main text of this book and even for those who write Board questions, so stop reading this stuff and get back to the material that actually matters.

Wiskott – Aldrich Syndrome

WAS is an X-linked immunodeficiency that usually involves low levels of IgM and, invariably, thrombocytopenia. In its most severe form, kids have small platelets, humoral and cellular immunodeficiency, eczema, autoimmune disease, and a tendency for hematologic malignancies.

The typical presentation is a **male** infant with unusual bleeding (bloody diarrhea, bruising, and/or bleeding from circumcision). The majority of kids have severe eczema, and sometimes they have secondary infections such as recurrent otitis media and pneumonia.

Treatment involves management of bleeding and infections. Bone marrow transplantation can be curative.

Humoral Immune Abnormalities

Bruton's Disease

Bruton's Disease is also known as X-linked agammaglobulinemia (XLA) and primarily affects B cells. **The T cell count is often elevated.**

In addition to a lack of B cells, there is an absence or decrease in lymphoid tissue such as tonsils, adenoids, Peyer's patches, and peripheral lymph nodes, as well as the spleen. The most common way that kids present is with recurrent infections with encapsulated pyogenic bacteria such as *Pseudomonas*, *Strep pneumo*, or *H. flu*.

Since it is X-linked, typically only male offspring are affected. Female carriers are asymptomatic. Males usually present under 1 year of age with recurrent pneumonia or ear infections. Older kids may get sinusitis.

Pretty simple to follow: **B** as in **B**ruton's. Remember it as "**BruXon's**" disease to recall that it is X-linked.

Diagnosis is made by first measuring immunoglobulin levels. When they are all found to be low, confirmation is made by measuring B and T cell subsets.

Children with Bruton's Disease require IVIG to protect them from recurrent bacterial infections. They are at risk for bronchiectasis and chronic pulmonary insufficiency.

Common Variable Immunodeficiency

CVID is the most common of the primary immunodeficiencies and is characterized by a defective antibody response. The B-lymphocytes do not differentiate into plasma cells, so there is a deficiency of the immunoglobulin subtypes. In addition, most patients have a T cell defect as well.

Kids are susceptible to recurrent infections of the upper and lower respiratory tract. In addition, recurrent herpes and zoster infections are common.

There is a frequent association with autoimmune diseases such as rheumatoid arthritis, cytopenias, or thyroid abnormalities. There is also a greatly increased risk of lymphoma, usually EBV-associated.

Like children with Bruton's Disease, these kids require IVIG to protect them from recurrent bacterial infections.

X-Linked Hyper IgM Syndrome

X-linked immunodeficiency with Hyperimmunoglobulin M is an X-linked disorder caused by absence of CD40 ligand, leading to disruption of B cell differentiation.

Affected individuals have frequent otitis and sinopulmonary infections, as well as diarrhea. There is also a high incidence of opportunistic infections. Lab studies show low levels of IgG, IgA, and IgE, with high levels of IgM. Males usually present between ages 6 months and one year with the signs and symptoms described above.

Treatment is with Ig replacement.

Hyper IgM Syndrome would explain the **presence of *Pneumocystis carinii* in the absence of HIV infection**. It is a **T cell abnormality that prevents conversion of IgM to IgG**.

If you are asked for the immunodeficiency for which Ig replacement is most appropriate, the answer will be X-linked hyper-IgM syndrome.

IgA Deficiency

Selective IgA deficiency is one of the most common immunodeficiencies. Over 80% are asymptomatic. Recurrent sinopulmonary infections are the most frequent manifestations of IgA deficiency.

Job Syndrome = Hyper IgE

Hyper **E** can easily be remembered as 3 **E**'s: **E**osinophilia, **E**czema, (don't forget recurrent skin infections), and elevated Ig**E** (picture a giant **E** on the nose, and you will remember **recurrent sinopulmonary infections** as well).

Infections are usually with Staph aureus. Kids also get chronic thrush as well as multiple fractures and other skeletal abnormalities.

Hyper IgE is often mistaken for atopic dermatitis, but in the latter there will be no skeletal abnormalities or abnormal facies like in Hyper IgE.

Boys with Wiskott-Aldrich typically have a milder rash than Hyper IgE, and have bleeding problems from the thrombocytopenia — a problem not seen in Hyper IgE.

Treatment is with antibiotics and steroids.

Transient Hypogammaglobulinemia of Infancy

Unlike Bruton's or CVID, there is no intrinsic B cell deficiency. Instead, decreased T-helper function leads to lower than normal amounts of IgG and IgA. The disease usually begins to manifest itself by age 6 months or so (as the infant breaks down more and more of the mother's immunoglobulins). Kids tend to outgrow it by 3-6 years of age.

Laboratory exam shows a severely low IgG level. IgA may also be low, but IgM is usually normal.

Innate Immune Defects

Chronic Granulomatous Disease

Chronic Granulomatous Disease is a disorder of *phagocytic function.* The defective phagocytes cannot undergo the "respiratory burst" needed to kill ingested bacteria and fungi, leading to life-threatening infections with these pathogens. About two-thirds of CGD is X-linked, and the remainder is autosomal recessive.

 Most kids present within the first 5 years of life. To remember which organs are most commonly involved, think of which ones are barriers to infection: skin, GI tract, lungs, liver, lymph nodes, and spleen. In addition to infection, patients often have granulomas of the skin, GI tract, and GU tract.

They can present with multiple episodes of abscesses caused by *Staph aureus.* UTIs due to organisms such as *Serratia marcescens* would be another sign.

The diagnostic test is the nitroblue tetrazolium (NBT) test, which assays the phagocytic oxidase activity. Believe it or not, you may be expected to know this.

 Treatment is aggressive antibiotics and interferon-gamma.

LAD

LAD stands for "leukocyte adhesion deficiency," and it is a defect in chemotaxis, which is essentially a problem with the white blood cells getting where they have to go and staying there.

 These kids may have a high white blood count (20,000) and infections such as a perirectal abscess, indolent skin infections, and omphalitis. The infected areas have no pus and minimal inflammation (because of the poor chemotaxis). Wound healing is delayed.

LAD typically results in recurrent infections in the skin, mucosa, and respiratory tract.

Although not usually the presentation in real life, on the Boards, LAD may have a history of delayed umbilical separation.

 Bone marrow transplantation can be curative.

Complement Deficiency

All of the described components of the complement pathway are associated with clinically significant deficiencies.

A history of recurrent or overwhelming infection with meningococci should make you consider complement deficiency.

Most complement deficiencies are inherited as autosomal recessive. Properdin deficiency is the only X-linked complement deficiency.

Secondary Immunodeficiency

HIV

Any kid with a vague history of fevers, weight loss, night sweats, and malaise should make you think of HIV infection (in addition to malignancy and TB).

HIV is a lentivirus and has an affinity for the C4 T lymphocyte. In general, HIV is transmitted mainly by heterosexual sex, but the primary mode of transmission in kids is vertical.

The main feature is a **decreased C4 count** (Remember, 4 = H = Helper). Also, remember that during the first year, HIV can present as **elevated immunoglobulins**.

Like chemotherapy patients, kids with HIV must receive prophylaxis against PCP, usually with Bactrim®.

Ratios/Cells

CD4/CD8 count is fair game for the test. Just know that the number 4 is similar to the letter H (Helper) and the number 8 is similar to S (Suppressor). That's a good way to remember T4/T8 ratios.

HIV Medications

A few HIV drugs you might want to know:

· Zidovudine: A nucleoside analog reverse-transcriptase inhibitor (NRTI)

· Nevirapine: A non-nucleoside reverse transcriptase inhibitor (NNRTI)
· Indinavir: A protease inhibitor

TREATMENT

Treatment often involves two nucleoside analog reverse-transcriptase inhibitors and either a protease inhibitor or a non-nucleoside reverse transcriptase inhibitor.

Testing the Immune System

The following table outlines which lab tests are used to measure the efficacy of a given component of the immune system.

Test	Component of Immune System
NBT (Nitroblue Tetrazolium)	Tests neutrophil activity (not number). Normal turns blue, abnormal stays colorless. **Chronic granulomatous disease** reflects this deficiency.
CH50	Tests the **complement system**. You order this if they describe **repeated serious bacterial infections**.
TB/Candida Skin Test	Tests for cell-mediated immunity associated with T-cell defects such as AIDS.
Immunoglobulin Levels	Tests the "**humoral system**," whose defects usually manifest as recurrent "less serious" infections (therefore, more "humorous," humoral, get it?) It is rarely seen before 6 months of age (because of the presence of Mom's antibodies). BUZZ WORDS Look for the words "healthy until 6 months" in the question.
Specific Antibody Tests	IgG levels may be normal. If a humoral defect is still suspected, check for subclasses from vaccination (e.g., tetanus, rubella, pneumococcus, etc.)
Rebuck Skin Window	Tests the ability of the cells to migrate in LAD.

Subclass

HOT TIP

There are also subclass IgG deficiencies. Here the total IG count is normal, and specific subclass testing has to be done to make the diagnosis.

HOT TIP

With perinatal HIV, while antibodies in the first year are high, they are actually dysfunctional, and later on they are low. Often this is the only clue they will give you to HIV being the answer.

Chapter 14

You Give Me Fever:
Infectious Diseases

Bacterial Infections

Bacteremia and Septicemia

Bacteremia

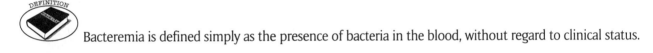 Bacteremia is defined simply as the presence of bacteria in the blood, without regard to clinical status.

Occult bacteremia presents without signs other than fever. We worry about this typically in the case of fever without an obvious source.

Despite the routine administration of the pneumococcal conjugate vaccine, one of the primary causes of occult bacteremia is *Streptococcus pneumoniae.* Hopefully, someday soon this will be a thing of the past. Regardless, it will be something you need to consider on board exams for years to come.

Septicemia

 Septicemia is the presence of bacteria in the blood along with *severe illness.*

The rules for the ages

The etiology of septicemia can be broken down by age as follows:

Age	Etiology of Septicemia
Neonates (<1 month)	Group B strep, *E. coli, Streptococcus pneumoniae* (pneumococcus), and *Staph aureus*
Infants (1-12 months)	Group B strep, *E. coli, Streptococcus pneumoniae* (pneumococcus), *Staph aureus*, and *salmonella*
Immunocompromised patients	Gram-negative bacilli are the main cause, including *Pseudomonas, E. coli*, and *Klebsiella. Staph* can also be a cause
Asplenic patients[1]	*Streptococcus pneumoniae*

Less than one month

 Infants one month old or less with a fever greater than 100.4 F need a full septic workup, including blood cultures, urine culture, and a lumbar puncture. They need to be admitted to the hospital. Infants with respiratory symptoms also need a chest X ray.

 There are no exceptions to this rule – in real life or on the Boards.

One – two months

Provided they meet certain criteria, febrile infants between 1-2 months old can be treated as outpatients after blood cultures and parenteral[2] antibiotic administration.

Appropriate antibiotic treatment in a neonate would consist of **ampicillin** and **cefotaxim**e or **gentamicin**.

Vancomycin is rarely used in neonates.

Older than 2 months

The treatment of febrile infants over two months old is dependent on additional factors.

---

[1] They will simply note a condition where functional asplenia is common, i.e., sickle cell disease, without coming right out and telling you that asplenia is a factor.

[2] Latin for IV or IM.

When presented with a febrile infant, take close note of the parent's account, in addition to the medical history of the baby. Look for terms like *"inconsolability"* or *"lethargic."* These words should make you reach for the choice that includes a spinal needle.

Treatment of infants older than 3 months would consist of **vancomycin** and **ceftriaxone**.

The Septic Newborn

Think about:

❏ Group B Strep

❏ *Listeria monocytogenes*

> **CASE STUDY**
>
> **You are presented with an infant with classic signs of sepsis. They note that the pregnancy and labor/delivery history were unremarkable, except for the mother having a slight fever and flulike symptoms. Also, the placenta had what can be best described as white nodules. What is the best treatment?**
>
> **THE DIVERSION**
>
> This is classic neonatal sepsis and how can you go wrong using the classic treatment with the dynamic duo of Ampicillin/Cefotaxime?
>
> **ANSWER REVEALED**
>
> Well, this is classic *Listeria infection*, and the correct choice would be Amp/Gent.

Because both can present with preterm labor, treatment is the same. **Microabscesses** (described as white nodules on internal organs) are seen in the infant with *Listeria monocytogenes* only. **Amp and gent, not cefotaxime**, is the treatment of choice for ***Listeria monocytogenes***.

If the mother was described as ***asymptomatic* during pregnancy, Group B Strep is most likely**. If she is symptomatic (flu-like symptoms), then *Listeria* is the most likely etiology.

The Skinny on Infections

Several infections reveal themselves in the dermatological sense, aka skin lesions. Therefore, the following graph outlines some of the associations that should serve as dead giveaways on the exam.

Infection etiology	BUZZ WORDS Dermatological manifestation
Neisseria meningitidis	Petechiae or purpura. Pay particular attention if you are given a patient with a "non blanching rash." PERIL WARNING If you are told the patient received the meningococcal vaccine, this does not confer 100% immunity and meningococcemia is still a possible diagnosis.
Staph aureus	Pustules
Neisseria gonorrhea	Lesions
Pseudomonas	**Ecthyma gangrenosum,** which are large pustules on an indurated inflamed base
Salmonella typhosa	**Rose spots**

Septic Shock

Septic shock is due to the hypoperfusion of vital organs, typically due to a toxin released by the bacteria. This leads to *metabolic acidosis.*

DEFINITION *Therefore,* septic shock is defined as end-organ failure. Look for *hypotension* or *decreased urine output,* in addition to liver failure and decreased cardiac output.

DIC to the ICU

When endothelial cells are damaged, it creates an environment for thrombus formation, with platelets adhering and fibrin deposited. This is the beginning of DIC, which of course stands for *disseminated intravascular coagulation.* Both complement pathways are then activated.

BUZZ WORDS

In order to realize that you are being presented with a case involving DIC, think of all the clotting factors being used up. The platelet count falls and the fibrinogen is used up. **D-dimers rise** as a result of fibrin degradation.

HOT TIP

Meningococcemia is an important etiology to keep in mind for septic shock. **Monotherapy** would be inappropriate in a critically ill child. **Vancomycin** and **ceftriaxone** would be the appropriate choice.

BUZZ WORDS

Neisseria meningitidis presents with mild non-specific symptoms, including runny nose, headache, lethargy, myalgias, and/or joint pain. This quickly evolves to a petechial/purpuric rash. Patients may also present with signs of meningeal irritation.

HOT TIP

Additional specific treatment of DIC is controversial, and you should not be tested on this.

Meningococcemia Prophylaxemia

The following would be considered indications for prophylaxis:

All persons that have had contact with the patient's oral secretions or have examined the patient's throat.

All household contacts and those with close contact outside the house.

TREATMENT

Rifampin is the drug of choice for prophylaxis in children.

For those older than 18: rifampin, ceftriaxone, ciprofloxacin, or azithromycin may be appropriate.

PERIL WARNING

Remember: rifampin turns your secretions electric orange, including urine and tears. This may not help you on the boards, but it certainly is cool. If it is included as a finding, it should not be of concern.

CASE STUDY

You are presented with a case where you are either told the child is in septic shock, or it is obvious by the description. You are then called upon to answer 1-2 questions on this case scenario.

- **You might be asked to pick which labs will help you identify the diagnosis.**
- **You might be asked for the correct treatment of a child in DIC.**

THE DIVERSION

Among the choices regarding diagnosis will be a PT/PTT. Among the treatment choices will be to administer clotting factors and/or platelets. This will be particularly tempting if the bleeding aspect is emphasized.

ANSWER REVEALED

Obtaining a PT/PTT would not be the correct answer since PT and PTT are UNPREDICTABLE and of little use in diagnosing and monitoring DIC.

Consider DIC in a sick (septic) patient who develops a bleeding problem and one or more of the above lab abnormalities. The first step would be treatment of the underlying problem (i.e. antibiotics) if you are dealing with septic shock. The second step would be replacement of clotting factors and platelets.

Thrombocytopenia is almost always present, as are elevated fibrin degradation products (FDPs). Elevated D-dimer (above 2000 ng/ml) is a good test, because it checks for fibrin degradation products specifically involved with thrombin. D-dimer is more specific to DIC than just FDPs.

Meningitis

You need to be aware of causes of meningitis according to age as follows:

Age	Cause
Neonatal	-Usually bacterial -Sometimes enteroviral infection, especially in the spring or summer -Most common bacteria are Group B strep, *Listeria monocytogenes*, and *E. Coli.*
Young Children	*Streptococcus pneumoniae, Neisseria meningitidis, enteroviruses, Neisseria meningitidis, Borrelia burgdorferi, Rickettsia rickettsii*

Complications of meningitis

Neurological complications

Neurological sequelae include seizures as well as focal deficits (including aphasia, visual field deficits, and hemiparesis). A subdural hematoma must be considered; however, in the absence of increased intracranial pressure, management is only supportive.

SIADH

Because of the risk of SIADH, urine output and serum electrolytes and osmolality need to be monitored closely.

 If there are focal signs, a CT must be obtained before doing an LP.

Peritonitis

Primary (Spontaneous) Peritonitis

 Primary peritonitis occurs without an obvious intraabdominal source. It occurs in a patient with:

- Nephrotic syndrome
- Cirrhosis of the liver

In children with nephrotic syndrome, it will usually be due to an encapsulated organism, such as **pneumococcus** due to the loss of IgG.

 Treatment is with a *third generation cephalosporin* <u>and</u> an *aminoglycoside*

Secondary Peritonitis

Secondary peritonitis is usually the result of a perforated bowel, i.e., ruptured appendicitis, incarcerated hernia.

A typical presentation would be a child on peritoneal dialysis presenting with fever, abdominal pain, and a high WBC on CBC or in peritoneal fluid.

Typical infections are due to *gram negative organisms* and *anaerobes.*

Peritonitis due to Dialysis

This is the most common complication in chronic peritoneal dialysis, with the most common pathogen being *Staph epidermidis.*

Do not carelessly choose *Staph aureus* as the most likely organism causing peritonitis in a dialysis patient.

Likewise, *Staph epidermidis* is the most common cause of VP shunt infection.

Just the Facts (Things Worth Noting)

Latex Agglutination (The Truth About It)

BINS: To remember the organisms for which latex agglutination can test, picture a bunch of latex gloves available in a giant bin next to the Empire State building.

B (Group B Strep)
Influenza/H *(Haemophilus influenza type b)*
Neisseria meningitidis
Strep Pneumo = pneumococcus

False positives are frequent, especially in children who recently received the Hib vaccine.

Certain species of *E. coli* cross-react with *N. meningitidis*.

> Latex agglutination would only be helpful with partially treated infections when culture results are not as reliable.

Developing Nations

With any child from a developing **country**, look for either something that **U.S. kids are immunized against,** a **chronic condition** that was not diagnosed previously, or infectious diseases that are more common in the "developing world."

TB, HIV, pertussis, invasive *H. flu infection,* and *sickle cell disease* would be examples of diseases they might describe in children from developing countries.

Respiratory and GI Flora

Due to over-treatment of respiratory infections, resistant strains of pneumococcus are on the rise. Liberal use of antibiotics can alter normal colonization in the GI tract. This results in infection with pathogenic strains such as *Clostridium difficile, Staph,* and *Salmonella. For more information on Clostridium difficile, see the entry on pseudomembranous colitis later in this chapter.*

Opportunistic Infections

Pneumocystis jiroveci (carinii) Pneumonia (PCP)

PCP and HIV go hand in hand. It occurs **early** and is often **fatal. They won't mention a history of HIV infection. Trimethoprim/ sulfamethoxazole (Bactrim®)** is used prophylactically as soon as the diagnosis is made.

> ### Neutropenia and Fever
>
> When they present you with an immunocompromised child with fever and /or neutropenia, you need broad-spectrum antibiotics, especially for gram-negative organisms. Zosyn® (piperacillin-tazobactam) plus an aminoglycoside or ceftazidime monotherapy are reasonable choices.
>
> A first- or second-generation cephalosporin as monotherapy will never be the answer in treating an immunocompromised child with fever and neutropenia.

Look for the buzzword "ground-glass appearance" if they describe an x-ray. They could also describe general perihilar infiltrates that can evolve to interstitial infiltrates.

PCP pneumonia is also common in cancer/bone marrow transplant patients, which is why they also receive Bactrim® prophylaxis.

Cryptosporidium

While Cryptosporidium primarily occurs in immunocompromised patients, this is not exclusively the case. *It can also occur as a self-limiting illness in healthy children,* and when it does, it typically lasts around 10 days.

Cryptosporidium diarrhea typically presents as severe, *non-bloody, watery diarrhea* similar to viral gastroenteritis, except it lasts a lot longer.

Nitazoxanide oral suspension can be used to treat children older than one year of age with diarrhea due to cryptosporidiosis as well as *Giardia intestinalis.*

In immunocompromised patients with cryptosporidiosis, believe it or not, oral administration of Human Immune Globulin or bovine colostrum has been beneficial. Doesn't sound very appetizing, but is certainly something you are expected to know.

Azithromycin is not effective treatment.

TB

- **TB** is also considered an opportunistic infection in patients with HIV.
- **Atypical TB** is also common in children with HIV.

Chlamydia Pneumonia (Clam Eyelid-a)

If they describe a newborn (first 2 months of life) with an **afebrile "staccato cough"** and tachypnea with or without eye discharge, think of chlamydia. **"Intracytoplasmic inclusion bodies"** in the scrapings is another phrase to look out for.

Definitive diagnosis of *Chlamydia trachomatis* is by PCR. *Chlamydia pneumoniae* is best diagnosed via the microimmunofluorescent antibody test.

Chlamydia conjunctivitis is treated with oral erythromycin, or sulfonamides if erythromycin is not tolerated. **Topical treatment will be the wrong choice.**

Chlamydia pneumonia is either treated with azithromycin for 5 days or erythromycin for 14 days.

For uncomplicated **chlamydia genital infections**, doxycycline for 7 days or azithromycin in a single 1gram PO dose are acceptable.

Erythromycin, ofloxacin, or levofloxacin for 7 days are also acceptable alternatives for uncomplicated genital infection.

Picture "clams" instead of eyes with discharge, coughing. **Cold clams have no fever.** If you put the eye drops in there, **they gobble it up and the rest of the body gets none** (therefore, systemic antibiotics are needed). Lab findings could also include **E**osinophilia. Treatment is with **E**rythromycin. Both begin with an **E.**

The 4 C's of Chlamydia are Cough, **C**onjunctivitis, **C**hlamydia, and **C**ixteen weeks of age.

The most common adverse reaction associated with **macrolide antibiotics,** such as erythromycin, clarithromycin and azithromycin, is diarrhea. Other GI adverse reactions, including dyspepsia, abdominal pain, and nausea, are less common.

Chlamydia Pneumonia in Adolescents Too

They could very well throw you an adolescent with pneumonia. They will present you with a teen with a low-grade fever and infiltrates. Mycoplasma won't be one of the choices. In that case, chlamydia pneumonia will be the answer.

Diagnosed with "immunofluorescent" antibodies. Picture "glow-in-the-dark clams".

Rickettsial Diseases

Rocky Mountain Spotted Fever

Rocky Mountain Spotted Fever (RMSF) is the most common fatal tick-borne disease in the US.

Rickettsia rickettsii is the bacteria which causes RMSF. This disease is characterized by fevers, myalgias, headache, and a petechial rash. The peak times for infection are May and June.

The rash is "**mac pap**" or "**purpuric macular rash,**" which becomes **petechial**. They will always describe the **headache.** Keep in mind that the rash starts on the wrists and ankles and spreads centrally.

Around one quarter of affected individuals will have CNS symptoms, mainly confusion and lethargy.

Picture the patient being held prisoner in the Rocky Mountains, bound at the hands and ankles, to help remember this.

If they present symptoms during the winter, it is unlikely to be RMSF. Despite its name, the disease only rarely occurs in the Rocky Mountain states (less than 2% of all cases).

Think of a **Rocky Mountain climber** who develops a rash on his **hands and feet** from climbing the Rocky Mountains. His hands come in contact with tiny microscopic stones, which form tiny **red dots (petechiae).**

You may be presented with a patient with the classic signs of Rocky Mountain Spotted Fever (RMSF), with a trip to Long Island thrown in to throw off those expecting to see a trip to the Rocky Mountains mentioned.[3] Sometimes you will read through the entire one page vignette written in 0.5 Helvetica font and the last sentence tells you the diagnosis. You may then be asked several questions:

- What is the most important immediate step?
- What is the treatment?

Among the choices will be *direct immunofluorescence of a skin biopsy*. After all, isn't documentation of a diagnosis important before treatment? Among the choices of treatment will be *doxycycline*, which everyone knows can't be used in a child younger than 8, so you go ahead and cross out this diversionary answer.

Well this is a disease that has 2 exceptions to these rules. During the acute phase, the only reliable test is direct immunofluorescence of a skin biopsy. *This test is not very sensitive*, and patients should receive treatment if the index of suspicion is high. In other words, "treat first and ask questions later." *Waiting for test result is never going to be the correct answer when Rocky Mountain Spotted Fever is suspected.* Despite treatment, the mortality rate is still around 4%. Quick diagnosis based on acute clinical assessment is key.

Chloramphenicol used to be the treatment of choice; however, the current preferred treatment is **doxycycline**, even in a child younger than 8, as the risk of teeth staining from a single course is actually quite low.

Treatment is for at least 7 days or until the fever has resolved for at least 3 days.

---

[3] A trip to the Rocky Mountains would never be included.

Human Ehrlichiosis

Human ehrlichiosis can be clinically indistinguishable from Rocky Mountain Spotted Fever. Symptoms may include fever, headache, and myalgias.

While both Rocky Mountain Spotted Fever and erlichiosis can present with thrombocytopenia and hyponatremia, human ehrlichiosis is more likely to present with leukopenia and elevated liver function tests.

Q Fever

Q Fever results in **pneumonia, but no rash**, and is spread by inhalation of infected particles, not a tick bite. There is no test during the acute phase. Serologic testing can be helpful later on in the course. Treatment is with doxycycline.

Patients usually start with flu-like symptoms, followed 5 days later by respiratory symptoms.

Picture someone holding a letter Q as a giant eraser and going over the patient from head to toe **"erasing any traces of a rash."** The **eraser scrapings** that are left behind get inhaled, **resulting in pneumonia**. In addition, you may think of Q fever as "Quiet Fever," that is, it does not announce itself with a rash.

Q Fever is considered to be self-limited, requiring nothing beyond supportive care. However, treatment with doxycycline can speed up recovery. The same caveat that applies to Rocky Mountain Spotted Fever applies here: the benefits of treatment, when indicated, outweigh the potential for dental staining.

Cat Scratch Disease

CASE STUDY

You may be presented with a patient who has a draining lymph node that was preceded by a bite from a cat. The patient has no other underlying disorders. You will be asked to pick the most effective treatment.

THE DIVERSION

This is an excellent question that has successfully diverted many a board candidate from the correct answer. After all, you have a draining lymph node following an episode where the skin integrity was breached. Must be a staph infection! What about trimethoprim-sulfamethoxazole (Bactrim®), cephalosporins, or doxycycline? What about penicillin, amoxicillin, or nafcillin? If you pick any of these diversions in an _otherwise healthy child_ and if remaining on the hospital staff is pinned to your passing the boards, you took a step in the wrong direction.

ANSWER REVEALED

Despite the presence of malaise and anorexia, cat scratch disease is a self-limited disease that only requires supportive treatment. See below for the correct treatment in an _immunocompromised patient_.

BUZZ WORDS

Following a scratch or bite from a cat (or sometimes a dog), the regional draining lymph node can become swollen and tender – this is cat scratch disease, a self-limiting illness that also causes anorexia and malaise. The disease can be serious in AIDS and other immunocompromised patients.

The diagnosis can be confirmed by serologic testing with enzyme immunoassay (EIA) or the immunofluorescent antibody (IFA) test.

Treatment

TREATMENT

The etiology is **_Bartonella henselae,_** and the treatment of choice is supportive. However, **treatment** would be indicated for hepatosplenomegaly, large painful adenopathy, and with immunocompromised hosts.

The following antibiotics are appropriate when clinically indicated:

· Azithromycin

· Erythromycin

· Ciprofloxacin

· Trimethoprim-sulfamethoxazole

· Rifampin.

Ciprofloxacin would, of course, only be indicated in children older than 18 for the most part.

INEFFECTIVE antibiotic treatment for Cat Scratch Disease includes penicillin, amoxicillin, and nafcillin.

Painful suppurative nodes may be treated with needle aspiration for relief of symptoms.

Incision & drainage and surgical excision are to be avoided.

> **You are asked to evaluate a child who sustained a cat bite the day before. He presents with tenderness and swelling of his right index finger. The patient is penicillin allergic and you are asked to pick the appropriate treatment.**
>
> Included in the choices will be amoxicillin, penicillin, and/or amoxicillin/clavulanate. These should be easy to eliminate since they mention the patient is penicillin allergic. However, you might also be fooled into believing this is Cat Scratch Disease and pick "supportive care only" or "surgical excision." If you do, you will be scratching your head while petting your cat when you realize you got this question wrong.
>
> If you are presented with a patient who develops cellulitis at the site of an animal bit within 24 hours, the likely etiology is *Pasteurella multocida.* You must cover for *Staph* as well as *Pasteurella multocida.* If the patient weren't penicillin allergic, amoxicillin/clavulanate would be appropriate. In this case, the appropriate medications include cefuroxime, cefpodoxime, doxycycline, azithromycin, or trimethoprim-sulfamethoxazole. If age appropriate, fluoroquinolones would be a correct choice to cover *Pasteurella.* If you choose one of these answers, you will be well on your way to "pasteurelling the boards."

pen allergic Bite

Haemophilus Influenzae

The advent of the Hib vaccine has dramatically decreased the amount of *H. flu*, type B meningitis and invasive disease in kids under 5.

Therefore, *Haemophilus influenzae (H. flu)* is another example of a disease that is seen less and less frequently in clinical practice, but remains a popular Boards topic. It is also another blow against the theory that "just reviewing the cases you have seen in residency will mean that you pass the Boards."

H. Flu type B causes neonatal sepsis, childhood meningitis, and epiglottitis. The mortality and morbidity rates from these infections are high.

A typical presentation is a child coming from *(fill in the developing country)*. The implication is that a serious *H. flu* infection developed because of the lack of immunization. Docs who write Board questions are one jingoistic[4] lot indeed. If you are presented with a patient who has not received immunization or immunization status is unknown, the signs of invasive *H. flu* infection could include periorbital cellulitis, pyogenic arthritis, epiglottitis, or bacterial meningitis.

Remember, *H. flu* is a "**gram-negative pleomorphic organism,**" which may also be included in the description.

Treatment

Watching and waiting is **not** appropriate, because it is an aggressive organism. **Ceftriaxone or cefotaxime** are the treatments of choice. Alternatives include meropenem or chloramphenicol.

The vaccine does **not** provide protection from **non-typeable *H. flu*,** which is a cause of otitis media in kids and pneumonia in older patients.

Along with *Strep pneumo* and *Neisseria meningitidis*, *H. flu* is an encapsulated organism. Remember these three when thinking about splenectomized patients.

---

4 Extreme nationalism

Chemoprophylaxis following *H. flu* infection

Household Contact

If there is at least 1 household contact younger than 4 who is incompletely immunized, then rifampin prophylaxis would be indicated for all household contacts, regardless of age.

If there is one immunocompromised child in the household, then all members of the household need to be given rifampin prophylaxis.

Chemoprophylaxis is not recommended for occupants of households where all members are immunocompetent and have been fully immunized.

If the index case has non-typeable *H. flu,* then it is a trick and nobody needs rifampin.

Childcare and Nursery exposure

If there are 2 or more cases of invasive *H. flu* infection occurring within 60 days, all unimmunized or immunocompromised children need to be treated with rifampin prophylaxis.

Prophylaxis is not necessary for nursery school or childcare children older than 2 who have only been exposed to one index case.

Pertussis

The typical catarrhal stage presents as an indistinguishable common cold progressing to paroxysms of coughing, with inspiratory whooping and possibly posttussive emesis. Typically the patient is **afebrile**.

In **infants**, the presentation can be atypical, with a very short catarrhal stage. Watch for a description of an infant who is gasping, gagging, or experiencing apnea. Infants younger than 6 months of age are at the greatest risk for complications.

The typical duration of pertussis can last up to 10 weeks.

It might help if you remember that pertussis in the olden days was known as "the 100 day cough".

In the past, if an infant had bona-fide documented pertussis, he or she did not need to be immunized. However, this is not necessarily the case anymore. The duration of immunity following clinical disease is unknown. The correct answer will now most likely be that such children should go through the full series.

Adults and teenagers with atypical presentation are an important source of pertussis to infants. It is transmitted via close contact or via aerosolized droplets.

Pertussis has three phases:

> 1. Catarrhal
>
> 2. Paroxysmal
>
> 3. Recovery
>
> One week prior to the catarrhal stage is an asymptomatic incubation period.

Culture is the gold standard for confirming diagnosis, but it is often not practical since many factors can affect growth of the organism. PCR is now the method of choice for diagnosis.

not!

Direct immunofluorescent assay (DFA) is no longer in common use and will therefore be the incorrect choice.

Treatment

Appropriate treatment is with **erythromycin**, **clarithromycin**, or **azithromycin.** Bactrim® is an alternative. Treatment will only **shorten** the *catarrhal stage* (the first 1-2 weeks when URI, not cough, is the major symptom). This is not helpful for the most severe manifestation, because the classic "whoop" hasn't presented yet.

If given **during the paroxysmal stage** (the actual whoop and cough stage), it **decreases the period of communicability, but does NOT shorten the coughing stage.**

Prophylaxis after Exposure

Anyone exposed to someone with pertussis, regardless of immunization status, needs to be **treated prophylactically with erythromycin, azithromycin, or clarithromycin** in order to **prevent the spread**. Exposure would include all household contacts and close contacts in child care.

If you see a **WBC count of 20-40K** with increased **lymphocytes,** and a cough described in a preschooler, think of pertussis. Again, they will imply lack of immunization; for example, parents who are against immunization, recent immigrants, etc.

Immunity to pertussis wanes over time. Many adults with protracted "colds" with cough may actually have pertussis, and pass it on to an unimmunized neonate. Look for this in the history. In fact, pertussis vaccine booster is now recommended for all teenagers and all adult household contacts of newborn infants.

Salmonella Diarrhea

Chickens and humans are the carriers. *Salmonella* can be contracted from foods such as poultry or eggs, contaminated unwashed vegetables, contaminated medical instruments, or reptiles such as pet turtles.

If they describe a group on a **picnic** in the **summer,** and then **1-2 days later** several attendees present with **watery loose stools** with **vomiting** and **fever**, think of *Salmonella*. Diagnosis is made from identification in the stool.

Treating *Salmonella*

You are presented with an otherwise healthy patient with a classic history for *Salmonella* diarrhea, including the picnic and undercooked chicken salad made with mayonnaise that sat out in the sun for 8 hours. What is the correct treatment?

You will be provided with a smorgasbord of antibiotic delights, all there for your culinary and diversionary pleasure.

Pick any of these other than supportive care and you have taken a step to studying for the boards in the hot sun next summer right next to the baking mayonnaise.

Remember, treatment for *uncomplicated (non-invasive) Salmonella* gastroenteritis is not necessary. In fact, it may lead to the carrier state.

Treatment is indicated in infants younger than 3 months of age and anyone else at risk for invasive disease. This list would include those with malignancies, severe colitis, or anyone who is immunocompromised.

Cefotaxime or ceftriaxone are appropriate initial treatment choices pending culture and sensitivity confirmation.

Typhoid Fever

You could be presented with a patient infected with the Typhi serotype of *Salmonella* who has general systemic signs, including malaise, fever, and poor appetite.

Additional signs would include hepatosplenomegaly, as well as "red" or "rose" spots.

Constipation rather than diarrhea could be an early presenting sign.

Non-typhoidal *Salmonella* would present as diarrhea, abdominal cramps, and fever.

Treatment with broad-spectrum cephalosporins would be indicated for patients with invasive typhoid fever.

Pseudomonas

Pseudomonas may cause **osteomyelitis/osteochondritis** as a result of **puncture wounds**. Often, they will describe it after a nail goes through a shoe.

Pseudomonas is also the cause of **otitis externa** (Swimmer's Ear) and infections from **mechanical ventilators**. Water is the common denominator.

Pseudomonas aeruginosa is a major cause of sepsis and pneumonia and has a very high mortality rate. *Pseudomonas cepacia* is a major cause of pneumonia and death in kids with cystic fibrosis.

> ### Pseudomonas/ Leukemia and Cystic Fibrosis
>
> Here is another example where you need to know two diseases that have something in common. It might come in handy on a Match Question.

Cancer patients, especially those experiencing neutropenia, are at risk for *pseudomonas* infections.

Piperacillin/tazobactam and gentamicin are effective against *pseudomonas* infection. Carbapenems (imipenem and meropenem) and ceftazidime can be used for pulmonary infection.

Ciprofloxacin and levofloxacin are the only quinolones that are effective against *pseudomonas*.

Ceftaz is the "Tazmanian Devil" of cephalosporins and can treat *pseudomonas*.

Brucellosis

Picture a COW going BRUUUUCE instead of MOOOOO.

This is often transmitted with milk and dairy products. While the history and physical findings are generally nonspecific, i.e., patients have fever and malaise, they will always note exposure to an affected animal within the preceding 2 months.

A typical description is a child **on a dairy farm with fevers and myalgias**. Because you know that cows go "Bruuuce," your memory will be jogged when you see brucellosis among the choices.

Blood cultures are not particularly helpful. Antibody testing is best.

The key to successful treatment in prolonged treatment with tetracycline **or** trimethoprim/sulfamethoxazole **and** rifampin.

Generally, relapses are not due to resistance. Relapses are due to premature discontinuation of therapy. Monotherapy is associated with a high rate of relapse; **combination therapy is recommended**.

Treatment is with **T**etracycline or **T**rimethoprim/sulfamethoxazole (depending upon age).

Think of a cow being milked. Milk is delivered through the cow's **teat** (yes that's how it is spelled by farmers). Cow Teat ➜ **T** = Teat ➜ **T** = Treatment ➜ **T** = Tetracycline[5] ➜ **T** = Trimethoprim/ sulfamethoxazole.

Doxy

Pseudomembranous Colitis

This is a severe form of diarrhea that develops after a course of **clindamycin OR ANY antibiotic including penicillins or cephalosporins.** Think of this when they describe **diarrhea** and **make it a point to mention a recent course of antibiotics**.

Heme positive stools will often be in the question. The most common preceding antibiotic used to be clindamycin (in fact, *C. difficile* colitis used to be called Clindamycin Colitis). But any antibiotic use can lead to this diarrhea-causing infection, and common things being common, the most common antecedent antibiotics are now cephalosporins.

In the clinical description they will describe "bloody mucous diarrhea" and they will mention **a recent antibiotic course.**

The diarrhea does not have to be grossly bloody – they may mention that the stool was "heme positive" or "guaiac positive."

You are presented with a patient with classic pseudomembranous colitis and are asked to pick the most appropriate first line treatment.

Capitalizing on the _previously correct treatment,_ vancomycin will be sitting right there as the pseudo-correct treatment for pseudomembranous colitis.

The correct treatment today for most patients is metronidazole, not vancomycin, as explained below.

---

[5] More specifically, doxycycline.

Treatment is **with oral metronidazole (Flagyl®).** Vancomycin PO would be the alternative drug in patients who do not respond to metronidazole.

Vancomycin is no longer the initial treatment because of concerns of promoting vancomycin-resistant organisms.

Strep

Streptococcus pneumoniae

Penicillins and cephalosporins are generally effective against *Streptococcus pneumoniae*.

The exception would be meningitis, where a combination of vancomycin and cefotaxime/ceftriaxone would be necessary. Rifampin would be an appropriate alternative in the case of cephalosporin allergy.

Susceptibility testing would be indicated to tailor antibiotic treatment appropriately.

Group A strep

Strep Pharyngitis

Strep pharyngitis will present as sore throat as well as fever, headache, and sometimes abdominal pain. It could be described as erythema and edema of the posterior pharynx.

Scarlet fever could be described with an associated rash that blanches easily and spares the face, palms, and soles. Watch for the description of **Pastia lines**, which are red lines in the skin folds of the neck, axilla, groin, elbows, and knees. They could describe the typical sandpaper rash as well as perioral pallor.

"Strep throat" is caused by Group A streptococcal bacteria, which also goes by the name *Streptococcus pyogenes*. Transmission is from person to person. Cough is usually absent. **Exudate is usually associated with viruses.** Macules and vesicles are *not* associated with Group A strep pharyngitis. A positive standard rapid strep test is reliable; however, a culture would be required for a negative test to rule out false negatives.

ASO (antibodies to streptolysin O) would be used to confirm a recent infection but not a current infection.

The preferred treatment for strep throat is penicillin or amoxicillin. Those allergic to penicillin should be treated with erythromycin, azithromycin, clindamycin, or a first generation cephalosporin. Asymptomatic contacts do not have to be treated, unless they become symptomatic by developing fever, pharyngitis, abdominal pain, or pain with swallowing.

Treatment for strep throat is to prevent rheumatic fever. It does not prevent poststreptococcal glomerulonephritis.

Strep Cellulitis

Strep cellulitis could be described as rapidly growing inflammation and red skin, with fever and chills. They could describe red streaks associated with lymphangitis. This is also called erysipelas.

Necrotizing fasciitis

Watch for the start of infection with a relatively minor trauma, which rapidly evolves to erythema, marked inflammation, and bullous formation.

Toxic Shock Syndrome

It starts out as fever, nausea, and vomiting, as well as diarrhea. This then evolves to shock and organ failure.

It may also be caused by strains of Staph, EB virus, coxsackievirus, and adenovirus.

Group B Strep

Risk factors for Group B Strep include:

- Low socioeconomic status
- Multiple sex partners
- Hx of STDs and young maternal age
- Rupture of membranes greater than 18 hours
- The use of any instrument that breaks skin (such as fetal scalp monitor)

On the exam they won't note anything in the history to let you know an infant is at risk for group B strep, except perhaps some of the factors listed above.

Early Infection will present the usual signs of sepsis, in the *first week* of life.

Late Infection will present with **a more focal infection** at 1-3 months of age.

Group B Strep prophylaxis

The CDC (and therefore the doctors who write Board questions) currently recommends screening for GBS colonization between 35 and 37 weeks gestation, and recommends that prophylaxis be given to women who meet one or more of the following criteria:

(1) have had a previous infant with invasive GBS disease

(2) have had GBS bacteriuria during the current pregnancy

(3) have a positive GBS screen during the current pregnancy

(4) have unknown GBS status and either gestation less than 37 weeks, ROM more than 18 hours, or intrapartum fever over 38.0 C

Women having C-sections without labor or rupture of membranes do NOT need GBS prophylaxis — no matter what their GBS status.

Botulism

There are three important types of botulism:

(1) Food-borne botulism – from ingestion of improperly packaged or incorrectly stored food

(2) Wound botulism – from systemic spread of the organism from an infected wound

(3) Infantile botulism – from intestinal colonization in infants, as their intestinal flora is too underdeveloped to prevent infection

In the infantile form, **spores are ingested and they germinate after ingestion.** Then toxin is produced and absorbed in the GI tract. Picture an infant eating a jar of honey, which then expands in the GI tract.

For botulism, think **4 D**'s in a bottle:

> **D**iplopia
> **D**ysphagia
> **D**ysarthria
> **D**ying to pee (urinary retention)

You can also picture **4 D's** as if they were 4 bees **buzzing around in a bottle of honey.**

An infant, *younger than 6 months of age,* **with "poor sucking or feeding,"** "hypotonia greatest in the upper extremities," "descending paralysis," and **"ptosis"** are the typical buzzwords. Additional findings could include weak cry, poor gag reflex, and constipation. **Don't look for a history of honey intake** because it won't be there. Still, botulism will be the correct answer.

Infants often have several days of constipation before other symptoms present.

Mechanism of Action/Botulism

This may seem trivial, but it is precisely the kind of information they will test you on. In the **adult form** of botulism (from poorly canned goods), preformed **botulism toxin is ingested**. This makes sense; this is why your mother told you (or she should have) to never eat from a can that is expanded.

Botulism is diagnosed by the presence of *Clostridium botulinum* toxin and/or organisms in stool or serum.

PCR is *not* used in the diagnosis of infantile botulism.

They DO expect you to know the pathophysiology of the botulism toxin. It will also come in handy when you are rounding with a toxicologist.

The toxin blocks the release of acetylcholine into the synapse. Picture a GIANT bottle of honey sitting in the way of "a little Colleen."

CASE STUDY You are presented with an infant with infantile botulism and are asked for the *most appropriate treatment*.

THE DIVERSION Of course, 4 out of the 5 choices are antibiotics and none of them will be correct, especially the aminoglycoside as explained below.

ANSWER REVEALED _Supportive care_ will be the correct answer. However, presented with _antitoxin_ as an option for treatment, it would probably be the correct choice.

Antibiotics are **not** to be used because they can result in the lysis of spores and the release of additional neurotoxins.

PERIL WARNING Aminoglycosides can potentiate the toxin. Any antibiotic will be the wrong answer, especially aminoglycosides-mentioned twice for emphasis.

Most cases of infant botulism progress to complete respiratory failure, sometimes requiring 2-3 weeks of ventilation.

MNEMONIC Picture a giant pencil poking around the bottle and picking out the buzzing D's from the jar and saving the day.

EITHER OR CHOICES **Myasthenia gravis** can present similarly. With myasthenia gravis, the Tensilon test will be positive and onset is more gradual. With botulism, Tensilon won't be positive.

Syphilis/Mother and Newborn

Titers are of IgG, which crosses the placenta. Therefore, if the mother has been identified as "properly treated" and the infant **has lower titers than the mother,** there is no need for treatment. You need to follow the infant to document decreasing titers over a few months.

Picture a paper-thin P (for Penicillin) passing through the placenta.

If they describe a "macular papular rash," or "hepatosplenomegaly and peeling skin" in a newborn, think syphilis.

Remember, the FTA-ABS[6] remains positive for life, but VDRL eventually goes down. VDRL and RPR are nonspecific non-treponemal antibody tests. They are merely screens that need to be verified with treponemal tests such as the fluorescent treponemal antibody absorption test (FTA-ABS) or microhemagglutination assay for antibodies to *T. pallidum* (MHA-TP). Non-treponemal tests (VDRL and RPR) may result in false positives due to a variety of viral illnesses, including EB virus, varicella, and hepatitis.

FTA-ABS is **F**orever.

> ## Syphilis in the Newborn?
>
> If the mother was treated during the pregnancy, do you need to treat the infant?
>
> ❏ No, if she was treated more than a month before delivery
>
> ❏ Yes, if she was treated within the last month of pregnancy
>
> ❏ Yes, if she was treated with erythromycin. (It does not cross the placenta)
>
> ❏ Yes, if the baby's titers are higher than the mother's titers

Syphilis (Congenital)

Congenital syphilis is often not picked up at birth.

In addition to non-specific signs, look for "**sniffles**," "**bullous lesions**," and "**osteochondritis**" of the joints. They may also describe "poor feeding." Affected infants will also have hepatomegaly. Additional associations include include hydrops fetalis, intrauterine growth restriction, hepatosplenomegaly, hemolytic anemia, jaundice, and a maculopapular rash.

Treatment of congenital syphilis is with penicillin.

---

6 FTA-ABS is "fluorescent treponemal antibody absorption".

CASE STUDY **You may be presented with an infant born with congenital syphilis. They note that the mother was treated with erythromycin 2 months prior to delivery. What treatment should the infant receive?**

THE DIVERSION "Well," you say to yourself, as you embark on a long diversionary journey to the incorrect answer, "They are testing me to see if I know that if the mother was treated more than one month prior to delivery, then no treatment is necessary." And there sitting for you, all made up in attractive diversionary clothing is "no further treatment."

ANSWER REVEALED Well, they actually are assuming you know that no treatment is needed if the mother was treated more than one month prior to delivery. What they were testing you on is whether you knew that *erythromycin doesn't cross the placenta*, and therefore treatment with penicillin is the actual correct answer.

Hemolytic Uremic Syndrome

BUZZ WORDS "Low **H**CT," "low platelets," "**H**ematuria," "elevated BUN/Creatinine," and "decreased urine output with bloody diarrhea" are your clues.

Because it is often contracted from contaminated food or water (***E. coli***), exposure to **poorly cooked meat** or **spoiled milk** may be included in the question.

EITHER OR CHOICES Sometimes these kids can be mistaken for new leukemias. They will be anemic with low platelets. The white count is variable. An elevated BUN/Creatinine can also be seen in new onset leukemia, so look to your history for more clues. Your main clue to HUS will be the presence of diarrhea and hematuria.

Campylobacter Infections

Campylobacter Fetus

Campylobacter fetus is a systemic infection seen in neonates or immunocompromised children. It is treated with broad spectrum cephalosporins or gentamicin.

Campylobacter jejuni

Can present as fever, abdominal pain, and/or bloody diarrhea

Azithromycin can shorten the course of illness.

Tularemia (Rabbits)

Tularemia is caused by the gram-negative bacteria *Francisella tularensis*.

Fevers, hepatosplenomegaly, and rash are common features. Regional lymphadenopathy is also frequent.

One of the ways you can get this infection is by eating **rabbit meat.** Treatment is with **gentamicin**. Other acceptable antibiotics are **streptomycin**, **tetracycline,** and **ciprofloxacin**. The latter two are age dependent.

Rabbits are **gentle** animals; therefore, it takes a **gentle antibiotic** = **"Gentle-mycin."**

Bubonic Plague

Bubonic plague is caused by *Yersinia pestis*.

Yes, bubonic plague still exists, and if you are not familiar with its manifestations and treatments it can become the plague of your existence if you have to take the exam again. And by the way, if you don't believe that the plague still exists, take a nice long trip to India. Be sure to drink tap water and eat all the street food you can get your hands on.

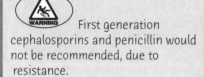 The physical findings include "buboes." What's that, you ask? Buboes are swollen painful lymph nodes, usually inguinal. They can also involve the cervical and axillary nodes. The history will likely include exposure to or handling of dead animals.

It comes in 3 varieties

· **Septicemia** – with signs of shock
· **Pneumonic form** – primarily pulmonary manifestations[7]
· **Meningeal form**

The best treatment is streptomycin and gentamicin. Since streptomycin is about as easy to find as a consultant familiar with bubonic plague, gentamicin is the drug of choice.

Other options include doxycycline, chloramphenicol, and tetracycline.

Staph aureus

Methicillin **sensitive** *Staph aureus* (MSSA) infection is treated with beta lactamase-resistant agents such as oxacillin/nafcillin, which may be more effective than cephalosporins or vancomycin (especially for certain infection sites).

For more invasive infections such as endocarditis, bacteremia, or meningitis, gentamicin or rifampin may be used as well.

Coagulase-negative infections typically occur as a result of indwelling IVs and catheters. *S. epidermidis* is coagulase negative.

MRSA in the USA

You can expect to be tested on Methicillin resistant *Staph aureus* infection (MRSA). The following are specific points regarding hospital acquired MRSA and community acquired MRSA.

Yersinia Enterocolitica Not Appendicitica

Enterocolitis due to *Yersinia enterocolitica* can be mistaken for acute appendicitis.

Watch for a history of ingestion of unpasteurized milk or raw meat, typically in a child younger than 5.

It can present with bloody diarrhea, along with the typical signs seen with appendicitis, including RLQ pain and elevated WBC.

In otherwise uncomplicated cases, no intervention is needed. Complications would include an immunocompromised patient and involvement beyond the GI tract. In those cases, treatment would include trimethoprim-sulfa, cefotaxime, aminoglycosides, and fluoroquinolones in patients older than 18.

First generation cephalosporins and penicillin would not be recommended, due to resistance.

---

[7] This is not to be confused with mnemonic devices frequently misspelled as pneumonic.

Hospital Acquired MRSA

Hospital acquired MRSA infections account for over 50% of hospital acquired *Staph aureus* infections. These strains are resistant to all beta-lactamase antibiotics and cephalosporins.

Nasal and skin carriage is the primary source for *S. aureus*, and therefore this is the highest risk factor for developing hospital acquired infection. The nasal carrier state can persist for years.

Hospital acquired MRSA infection is usually multidrug resistant. If you are presented with a case of hospital acquired MRSA, you should assume that it is susceptible only to vancomycin.

Community Acquired MRSA

Community acquired MRSA infection usually involves skin and soft tissue. However, more invasive disease such as pneumonia can also occur.

Although community acquired MRSA is also resistant to all beta-lactam antimicrobials, its resistance is not as widespread. Community acquired infection is often susceptible to several antibiotics, including trimethoprim-sulfamethoxazole, gentamicin, and doxycycline.

When treating carbuncles/furuncles from MRSA: If a furuncle is less than 5 cm due to community acquired MRSA, all that is required is incision and drainage.

Antibiotic Antics

Aminoglycosides

Unlike other antibiotics, effectiveness is dependent on high peak levels. Toxicity (such as ototoxicity) is associated with high trough levels.

Peak levels are measured 30 minutes after the dose is given. Trough levels are measured 30 minutes before the next dose.

Penicillin

Penicillins work by interfering with cell wall synthesis. Beta lactamase producing bacteria produce penicillinases, which cleave penicillin. Penicillinase-resistant antibiotics are required for these organisms, including *Staph* organisms.

Ampicillin/amoxicillin

High dose amoxicillin would be indicated for penicillin-resistant pneumococcal ear or sinus infection. In addition, it is indicated for routine OM, sinusitis, pneumonia, and initial treatment of UTIs. It would not be indicated for "highly resistant" strains.

For "intermediate" resistant strains, 80-90 mg/kg/day would be indicated. Specifically, this would be indicated if you were presented with a child younger than 2 years of age attending daycare who received antibiotics in the preceding 3 months.

Ampicillin with or without gentamicin would be the treatment of choice for *Listeria monocytogenes* infection.

MRSA infections are resistant to methicillin because of interference with the penicillin binding proteins, which are required to attach to the organism.

It is not due to a penicillinase.

Cephalosporins

Like Star Trek® and its spinoffs, we have several generations to track and contend with.

First generation

First generation cephalosporins are effective against gram positive cocci. This includes methicillin sensitive *Staph aureus*. They are not effective against methicillin resistant *Staph aureus*. Read the question carefully, at first blush these can be confused with each other.

First generation does not penetrate CSF well and should not be used to treat meningitis. They are also not effective against *Listeria* or enterococcus.

Second Generation

2nd generation cephalosporins are the forgotten middle child of the cephalosporin family.

Second generations are best against beta lactamase producing gram negatives, including *Enterobacteriaceae, H. influenzae,* and *Moraxella catarrhalis* (however, they are generally not as good at this as the 3rd generation).

They have some effectiveness against gram positives, but not as good as first generation.

Third Generation

Third generation cephalosporins have excellent CSF penetration and cover a broad spectrum. They are, therefore, a good choice for meningitis.

Cefpodoxime and cefdinir are effective oral medications for otitis media and sinusitis, as well as group A beta hemolytic strep.

Ceftibuten and cefixime are effective against urinary tract infections or respiratory infections.

Warning: Extensive use of cephalosporins has lead to resistant strains of *Klebsiella, E. coli, Proteus mirabilis,* and *Pseudomonas aeruginosa.*

Fourth Generation

Cefepime is a fourth generation cephalosporin. It is a broad-spectrum agent that may be used for gram negatives such as *pseudomonas.* It also has good activity against gram positives such as *S. aureus.*

Clindamycin

Clindamycin is active against the following

- **Aerobic gram positive cocci:** streptococcus, staphylococcus, and *Corynebacterium diphtheriae*
- **Anaerobic gram positive cocci:** *Peptostreptococcus* sp, gram-positive non spore-forming bacilli (*Actinomyces* sp, *Propionibacterium* sp), clostridia except for *C. difficile,* and a significant percentage of some non perfringens clostridial species.
- **Anaerobic gram negative cocci:** *Bacteroides, Prevotella, Fusobacterium* sp
- **Chlamydia:** *Chlamydia trachomatis*
- **Protozoa:** *Plasmodium sp, Pneumocystis (jiroveci) carinii, Toxoplasma gondii,* and *Babesia* sp.

Macrolides

Macrolides would be indicated for *Mycoplasma, Moraxella catarrhalis, H.flu S, pyogenes, Strep viridans, Chlamydia,* pertussis, and *Legionella pneumophila,* as well as nontuberculous mycobacteria.

Azithromycin and clarithromycin are as effective as erythromycin, with fewer GI side effects. Therefore, erythromycin is rarely a first line medication.

Rifampin

Rifampin would be appropriate prophylaxis when indicated for meningococcal exposure (ceftriaxone or ciprofloxacin would also be appropriate). Indications for prophylaxis would include those who were exposed to secretions (including health professionals who examined the patient's throat), or those in the same household or otherwise close contact.

Rifampin is also indicated for invasive and/or resistant *Staph* infection, including osteomyelitis and endocarditis. It would be indicated for treatment of tuberculosis in combination with other medications.

 If presented with a pregnant patient, rifampin is absolutely contraindicated in pregnancy because of its potential for teratogenicity.

Quinolones

Fluoroquinolones are restricted to diseases where there is multiresistance with no safe alternatives. Primarily this includes diseases caused by *Pseudomonas aeruginosa*, such as UTIs, GI and respiratory diseases, as well as osteomyelitis. Anthrax would be another indication.

 If you are presented with a child on fluoroquinolones, note that antacids with aluminum, magnesium, or calcium can interfere with absorption.

NSAIDs may increase the CNS effects of fluoroquinolones. Quinolones may increase the risk for cardiac arrhythmias.

Tetracyclines

Tetracyclines are contraindicated in children younger than 8, except for those with Rocky Mountain Spotted Fever, in which it is indicated regardless of the age.

Trimethoprim with sulfamethoxazole

Trimethoprim with sulfamethoxazole can be used to treat acute UTI, inflammatory bowel disease, burns, umbilical cord care, and *Chlamydia* urethritis. T-S is also very useful against minor MRSA infections.

It would be indicated for GI infection due to *Salmonella* or *Shigella*. It can be a 2nd line treatment for otitis media and sinusitis.

 Side effects include Stevens Johnson Syndrome, as well as rash and neutropenia.

Vancomycin

Vancomycin would be indicated for MRSA infection in patients who cannot tolerate other medications. It is also used to treat endocarditis.

Vancomycin would be treatment of choice for resistant corynebacteria and resistant pneumococcus.

 An important side effect is reddening of the skin due to histamine release (Red Man Syndrome).

You need to be familiar with VREC which is vancomycin resistant enterococcus. Enterococcus is resistant to ALL cephalosporins. Enterococcus typically responds to ampicillin and vancomycin, but resistance to vancomycin is increasing and is a subject that could be tested on the exam.

Metronidazole   *Flagyl*

Metronidazole is appropriate treatment for *Trichomonas vaginalis*, *Treponema pallidum* (aka syphilis), *Gardnerella vaginalis*, and *Helicobacter pylori*.

Disease Entity	Antibiotics of Choice
Complications of Pneumonia or Sinusitis (such as Pleural Empyema or Orbital Cellulitis)	Either cefotaxime or ceftriaxone plus either clindamycin or vancomycin
Meningitis	Newborn: Cefotaxime and ampicillin Beyond newborn: Vancomycin plus cefotaxime or ceftriaxone
Recurrent OM 2nd line	Ceftriaxone 50 mg/kg per dose in up to 3 doses over 1-5 days
Neisseria gonorrhea infection	Ceftriaxone 125 mg IM once or Cefixime 400 mg PO once
Pseudomonas (foot puncture, fever with neutropenia,[8] CF exacerbation, or meningitis[9])	Cefepime or ceftazidime

---

[8] Fever with neutropenia would also require gram positive coverage with vancomycin or oxacillin.

[9] *Pseudomonas* meningitis would require an aminoglycoside as well.

Viral Infections

EBV/Infectious Mono

 Infectious mono can present with high fever, tonsillitis, and enlarged lymph nodes, as well hepatosplenomegaly. Red throat will often present with white exudate.

Presence of heterophile antibody confirms the diagnosis. If the heterophile is negative, serum IgM is a secondary test to confirm the diagnosis. This is especially important to note if you are presented with a patient younger than 4. The heterophile false negative rate is much higher in children younger than 4.

EBV infections can evolve to lymphoma in immunocompromised hosts.

Steroids may be indicated for pending airway compromise or thrombocytopenia.

A rash can develop following ampicillin treatment in patients who have infectious mono. This is not necessarily an allergic reaction, especially if they specifically state the patient was diagnosed with mono.

CMV (Cyto-Megalo-Virus)

CMV is one of the most important causes of congenital infection. It may lead to intellectual disability and other disabilities such as hearing loss.

Congenital CMV nfection is usually clinically silent. However, some infants with silent congenital infection, are later found to have hearing loss or learning disability."

If you are presented with a patient who is seropositive for CMV, as a chronic carrier, it is important to know that he or she may shed the virus in urine, saliva, or genital secretions. CMV may cause serious disease in immunocompromised patients.

Diagnosing CMV

A **urine culture for CMV within the first 3-4 weeks of life** is the definitive diagnostic study.[10]

---

[10] The "shell-vial assay" is an adaptation of tissue culture, which is more rapid than standard cultures.

CMV, think **5 C's**: **C**horioretinitis, **C**erebral, **C**alcifications (Periventricular = **C**enter) with diagnosis confirmed with urine **C**ulture and the potential for **C**ensorineural hearing loss (Sensorineural hearing loss). These babies can get thrombocytopenia with subsequent petechiae and purpura ("*blueberry muffin baby*").

You can also remember this as in **CMV**: the calcifications Circu**MV**ent the ventricles.

Additional findings would include **hepatosplenomegaly, jaundice,** SGA and microcephaly. Neurological findings would include seizures, hypotonia, and weak suck.

Acquired CMV/Older Children

CMV can present with a clinical picture **much like mono**. If mono is described and EBV is not an option, CMV is the answer.

Treatment

Ganciclovir is the treatment of choice. Its main side effect is marrow suppression.

Picture a "**gang of cyclists**" whose **whipping chains destroy bone marrow**.

Infections with Transfusion

With any transfusion-related infection, especially pneumonia, think CMV. With any child with mono-like symptoms who is negative for **Epstein-Barr virus**, **think CMV** as well**.**

If you can recall all the "CMV Negative" blood you ordered for your oncology patients, you'll remember that CMV is a common infection transmitted by transfusion.

There is the possibility of HIV eluding screening if testing occurs during the "window period" soon after infection, during which a blood donor is infectious but screening results are negative.

Arbovirus

Arboviruses can cause encephalitis in the late spring and early summer months. The viruses are transmitted by ticks and mosquitos. Disease is best prevented by tick and mosquito control.

Arboviruses include:

- St. Louis encephalitis
- La Crosse Encephalitis
- Western and Eastern equine encephalitis
- California encephalitis
- West Nile encephalitis
- Colorado tick fever
- Dengue fever

Typical presentation includes fever, irritability, change in mental status, and headache. CSF findings include mild pleocytosis and elevated protein, along with normal glucose concentration. Most resolve within a couple of weeks.

The diagnosis is confirmed with virus specific IgM in the CSF or serum. A four-fold elevation in serum IgG taken during acute infection and during convalescence is another accepted method to confirm diagnosis.

Enterovirus

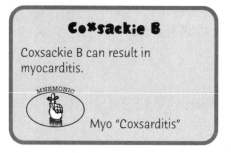

Coxsackie B

Coxsackie B can result in myocarditis.

Myo "Coxsarditis"

"High fever," "rash," and perhaps signs of "viral meningitis" **in the summer**.

You will most likely be presented a patient younger than 5. They typically present with vague symptoms inducing malaise, fever, and vomiting. Additional findings would include pharyngitis and/or conjunctivitis.

Coxsackie virus falls in this category.

Neonates can develop severe disseminated infection if exposed at birth. This may be indistinguishable from sepsis due to a bacteria.

Enteroviruses can be identified via PCR within 24 hours.

Mumps

Mumps is another example of a disease that is rarely seen in clinical practice. Mumps virus is a paramyxovirus.

General symptoms of mumps are fever, headache, malaise, and muscle ache. If described, swelling of the **parotid gland** and/or **testicles** will be what gives it away. In addition, children with mumps can be described with unilateral facial swelling anterior to the ear, with difficulty opening the mouth. There will be no abnormalities noted in the oral cavity.

Complications may include parotitis, meningitis/encephalitis, orchitis, or pancreatitis (look for abdominal pain in the description).

To remember complications of **MUMPS:**

> **M**eningitis
> **U**nderwear (orchitis)
> **M**uscle Aches
> **P**ancreatitis (pain in the belly)
> **S**welling of the parotid gland

Orchitis is a rare complication. However, infertility is NOT a common result.

Bumped by Mumps

Even though many of you have never had or treated mumps, you may be expected to manage a mumps outbreak at a school located on the boards.

What to do?

- Children who are fully immunized can remain in school
- Children who have not received their 2nd booster dose need to receive the booster before returning
- Children who never received it need to receive the vaccine before returning
- Children whose parents refuse to immunize based on religion or other reasons must wait 26 days after the last person in the class developed parotitis due to mumps virus.
- The child who has mumps can return to school 9 days after the onset of parotitis

---

Differentiating Mumps from Viral Parotitis and other Imitators

CASE STUDY

You are presented with a child with a *high fever* who is *toxic appearing* and is *fully immunized*. Physical exam is noteworthy for unilateral preauricular submandibular swelling. What is the diagnosis?

THE DIVERSION

The diversionary choice sitting right there will be mumps. However, if you are specifically being told that the patient is fully immunized, then mumps will <u>not</u> be the correct answer.

ANSWER REVEALED

The combination of low-grade fever and toxic appearance makes for a diagnosis of *bacterial parotitis*. Mumps is associated with low-grade fever and a non-toxic appearance.

EITHER OR CHOICES

A **stone in the salivary gland** will likely cause **"intermittent swelling."** This will be the buzzword to watch for.

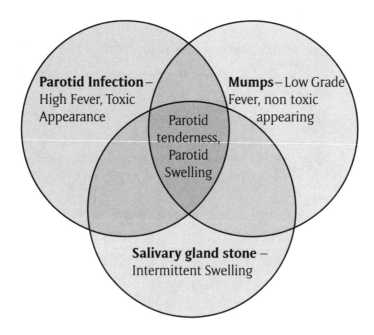

You may be presented with a teenage boy with a typical clinical presentation of mumps, including parotitis. They might even just come right out and tell you the patient has mumps. You are then asked for the most likely additional manifestation.

Of course, you will be dazzled by choices like orchitis, pancreatitis and encephalitis.

Although mild subclinical pancreatitis can occur, it is rare. While pleocytosis can be seen in one half of patients with mumps, encephalitis is a rare complication. Orchitis is a common manifestation. However, infertility is a rare manifestation if you are presented with both choices.

Roseola (Roses)

The formal name is **human herpesvirus type 6 (HHV-6).** It is also known as roseola infantum and exanthem subitum.

This will likely be the choice you have when this is described clinically in the question.

"3-5 days of high fever." *After the fever passes,* **"mac-pap rash" will appear**. It is not uncommon to have a **febrile seizure** with the fevers.

Think of the rash as a dozen roses being presented AFTER the fever to say goodbye; thus, Roses = Roseola.

Seizure is not an uncommon occurrence with roseola infection. They could present you with a classic clinical scenario of roseola followed by a seizure, and ask you for the most likely cause. Of course the correct answer will be human herpesvirus type 6.

German Measles (Rubella)

Rubella really is only a mild viral illness. It only becomes important when an expectant mother is infected, leading to congenital rubella syndrome. 50% of infants infected during their first trimester are affected – most commonly with ophthalmologic problems.

They will never use the terms "German Measles" or even "Measles." They will use the more formal terms. Therefore, it is important to keep **rubella** and **rubeola** straight, in a way that you won't forget in the heat of the battle.

For rubella think of **BELL** in the middle of the word.

Rubella is German measles: picture a "bell" ringing in Germany during Oktoberfest and the image is with you.

Cataracts and **PDA** are associated with rubella.

Picture the bell (rubella). The bell has a white eye on it (the cataract).

Pregnant women should NOT be vaccinated.

> **CASE STUDY**
>
> **You are asked to evaluate a boy who was recently adopted with unknown immunization status. He presents with a low grade fever, generalized maculopapular rash and enlarged occipital and preauricular lymph nodes. He does not appear to be toxic. Which of the following is the most likely diagnosis?**
>
> **THE DIVERSION**
>
> You will be presented with several diversionary choices, including EBV infection, rubeola, HIV infection, and TB.
>
> **ANSWER REVEALED**
>
> The key to answering this question of course is the uncertain immunization status. The maculopapular rash, low grade fever, and subacute clinical picture are consistent with rubella. Rubeola, or measles, would also present with a maculopapular rash. However, the clinical description would include cough, coryza, and conjunctivitis. Likewise, EBV virus would present with higher fever and a more toxic clinical presentation.

RubeOLa (Measles)

The typical buzzwords for rubeola are **confluent macular papular rash**, **Koplik spots**, and **conjunctivitis** in a miserable kid who is coughing.

Measles is **transmitted by droplets** or airborne with an incubation period of 8-12 days. Humans are the only natural hosts.

Symptoms consist of **FCC**: **F**ever, **C**ough, **C**oryza (think of the FCC[11] in charge of airborne messages). This, along with the mac pap rash and conjunctivitis, will be the keys to recognizing this in the picture section. They can also have fever and photophobia.

They could ask when they are most contagious. The answer is 5 days before to 5 days after the rash appears. Therefore, **exposure BEFORE the rash appears is still a problem**.

The sequence of signs and symptoms can be confusing. Here is the roadmap:

  · The prodrome is on the first two days.

  · Koplik spots appear shortly after.

  · Then the rash comes around day 5.

  · The rash is worst after about a week and begins to resolve around day 10.

Isolation isn't enough to protect immunocompromised patients. They would also require immunization and immunoglobulin.

If they describe a *preschool* age child from a developing country with FCC as the presentation, think measles (preschool because hand-washing practices are lacking in this group). Because immunization rates are less than 100%, there ARE measles outbreaks in the US. Therefore, arriving from another country is not a prerequisite for a child with measles.

If you are presented with a patient with coryza and cough, along with vomiting and diarrhea, the most likely diagnosis is influenza, not measles. This would be best diagnosed via enzyme immunoassay antigen detection.

The preferred method for diagnosing measles infection is serum IgM, which remains elevated for over a month after the onset of rash.

---

[11] FCC= Federal Communications Commission.

Post Exposure Management for Susceptible Contacts

Persons exposed to measles who are not completely immunized, including infants 6 to 12 months of age, should receive the measles vaccine, alone or as MMR. If exposure has been within 6 days, immune globulin should also be given, especially to infants under 12 months, pregnant women, and immunocompromised individuals.

MMR is given **within 3 days of exposure** might help prevent the onset of disease.

M has 3 down strokes; therefore, remember 3 days for MMR.

Any infants who receive the MMR vaccine **before age 1** will need to be revaccinated after their 1st birthday**.**

Revaccination must occur **5 months after the IM immunoglobulin was given**, provided the child is at least 12 months of age.

Therefore, patients with mild or asymptomatic HIV should be given the MMR vaccine even though it is a live vaccine. The morbidity and risk associated with **measles** is far worse than the risk associated with the vaccine.

Fifth Disease (Erythema Infectiosum)

They will rarely use the term "Fifth Disease." They prefer **parvovirus B19** (if in doubt, choose this for any question of what causes hydrops fetalis, aplastic crisis in sickle cell disease, and, I believe, the Major League Baseball Steroid Scandal and all of the most recent major hurricanes raging through the Gulf Coast).

Fifth Disease is spread by respiratory droplets. The prodrome is non-specific, with fevers, sore throat, runny nose, headache, and malaise. This is followed by the classic "slapped-cheek" rash. Over the next few days, the rash occurs on the extremities, favoring the extensor surfaces. Polyarthropathy may also develop. It is especially concerning if contracted by a pregnant mother; this may lead to fetal hydrops.

Herpes Simplex

HSV in the Newborn Period

 Any seizure in the newborn period should have you considering a herpes infection. This is especially the case if they describe a **temporal lobe** seizure. The **mother will be described as asymptomatic** because there is usually "no history" of herpes documented when an infant presents with systemic HSV, despite our best efforts at eliciting one. Most invasive neonatal herpes infections are caused by Type 2 HSV.

The typical presentation is an infant in the neonatal period (first 28 days) with signs of **sepsis, meningitis, and seizures**. In addition, they may tip you off by telling you the **gram stain on CSF is negative**.

Rapid diagnosis of HSV meningitis can be made by PCR, especially in CSF. CSF culture is not the method of choice because of false negatives.

Direct fluorescent antibody staining is a reliable method to identify HSV in vesicle scrapings. In general, viral cultures are obtained in serious illness, with fever of unknown origin, when biopsies are obtained, or when bacterial cultures are negative.

If you are presented with a prepubertal patient with a genital herpes simplex type 2 infection, sexual abuse should be suspected.

HSV in Childhood

In older children, HSV typically causes a localized infection or viral meningitis.

Herpes can also be transmitted as an ascending infection through the infected birth canal **(even with intact membranes); therefore, delivery via c-section does not rule out transmission of perinatal infection.**

Neonatal infection can also be transmitted postnatally from an adult with a cutaneous or oral lesion.

Acyclovir

Acyclovir is used for primary genital and mucocutaneous HSV infections for prophylaxis and treatment in immunocompetent patients. IV acyclovir would also be indicated in immunocompromised patients with varicella or disseminated zoster, as well as to treat HSV encephalitis in any patient.

Acyclovir is not routinely used in children with varicella infection. However, it would be indicated in patients who are immunocompromised, taking chronic steroids, and/or children older than 12 years in general.

Neonates with skin or mucous membrane manifestations of herpes are initially treated with IV acyclovir, followed by extended PO treatment.

HIV

Chronic non-specific symptoms in a child or neonate should make you consider HIV infection. These include weight loss, fevers, or night sweats. A history of *recurrent* or *persistent* thrush may be a clue.

The most sensitive test for HIV in children younger than 18 months is PCR for HIV DNA. The presence of HIV antibody up to 18 months after birth is an unreliable indicator of congenital HIV, since this can and often does reflect transplacental transmission of maternal IgG.

Perinatal

Vertical transmission of HIV during delivery is the most common mode of transmission in kids. Breast feeding is another important mode of transmission.

Since vertical transmission can be reduced dramatically through the administration of medications such as *zidovudine* and *nevirapine,* routine prenatal HIV screening is now recommended for all women. There are now rapid HIV detection tests available in many centers for women who are in labor and have unknown HIV status. Administration of zidovudine during the perinatal period can drastically reduce the mother-to-baby transmission of HIV.

The following are buzzwords for HIV in children: "recurrent bacterial infections," "hepatosplenomegaly," "failure to thrive," "developmental delay," and "cognitive impairment." You can remember this with the following memory aid:

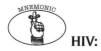 **HIV:**

Hepatosplenomegaly
Intellectual delay
Very poor antibodies (and bacterial infections)

Exposure

If somebody is going to **seroconvert**, it will occur during the **first 6 months of exposure**. **Testing** and **tracking** should be done **at time of exposure, 6 weeks, 12 weeks, and 6 months**. This would apply to any form of exposure, including child abuse.

The use of antiretroviral (ARV) agents is limited to needle sticks where there is a strong likelyhoood of HIV transmission. ARV agents are not administered routinely for all needle sticks, especially where there is low risk of disease transmission.

Neonatal Testing/Maternal Antibody Scorecard

Because maternal antibody to HIV is an IgG (free ride across the placenta), **serologic testing in the infant is unreliable. Therefore, polymerase chain reaction (PCR) is the gold standard for HIV testing in the neonatal period.**

In infants screening is done at:

❑ Birth
❑ 2 months
❑ 4 months
❑ 6 months

HIV Manifestations/First Year of Life

One presentation is a clinical description consistent with ***Pneumocystis*** *jiroveci* (formerly known as *Pneumocystis **carinii**)*[12] with no history of AIDS or HIV exposure. Remember that your buzzword for PCP on CXR is "ground glass appearance."

---

[12] Somehow PJP doesn't have the same ring to it as PCP.

Foscarnet

Foscarnet is a medication used to treat:

- **CMV retinitis** (induction and maintenance) in immunocompromised patients

- Severe **mucocutaneous disease** caused by acyclovir resistant HSV

- **Zoster** caused by acyclovir-resistant varicella zoster virus

 Foscarnet is not indicated for the treatment of CMV gastroenteritis. It is also not indicated for the treatment of EBV infection, HSV encephalitis, or HSV mucocutaneous infection as a first line treatment (acyclovir must be tried first).

Follow the Zoster

Zoster (shingles) is the secondary infection of varicella, caused by reactivation of VZV from latency.

Children with zoster can return to school if the lesions can be covered or once they are crusted.

The **recurrent bacterial infections** during the first year of life are due to an **increased** production of **nonfunctional antibodies**. The developmental delay is likely due to **encephalitis**.

Vaccines and HIV

HIV positive children receive ALL routine vaccines, with the exception of the measles and varicella vaccines, which are contraindicated in children who are severely immunocompromised (CD4+ counts less than 15% of normal for age). They also receive the inactivated rather than the live influenza vaccine.

Chicken Pox (Varicella)

Varicella (chicken pox) infection is becoming as rare as the NY Mets playoffs appearances, and, pretty soon, as rare as a NY Islander playoff appearance. However, all three are fair game on the Boards.

Remember that kids are contagious from several days before they have their rash until all the lesions are crusted over. Anyone around a child during this period should be considered "exposed." An immunocompromised child exposed during this period would need to receive varicella zoster immune globulin (VZIG) to help prevent infection.

Most children who contract chicken pox do fine. The most common complication is superinfection with *Staph aureus* involving skin. In more severe cases, invasive infections may lead to pneumonia and osteomyelitis. However, immunocompromised kids (chemotherapy, AIDS) are much more susceptible to disseminated varicella, and can develop viremia, pneumonia, encephalitis, or other complications.

Newborns

VZIG is the treatment of choice for a newborn exposed to chickenpox. What constitutes exposure? If the mother develops chickenpox between **5 days before delivering through 2 days after delivering**, then the infant is at risk. VZIG is considered to be a preventive measure rather than treatment, and it needs to be administered within 96 hours of exposure.

Now how do you keep that straight? In the heat of the battle, you could find yourself asking (put on your best Clint Eastwood voice) **"Did he say 5 days before and 2 days after or is it the other way around? Huh, Punk!?"**

Well, there is no need to be concerned. Just remember the following and it will be impossible to forget. The Roman numeral for 5 is **V**. V is in the beginning of the word **V**aricella so it is 5 days **before** delivery. There are 2 **L**'s at the end of the word, so it is 2 days **after** delivery. Therefore, normal infants older the 2 days who were exposed to varicella do **not** need to receive VZIG.

VARICELLA	
FiVe days before	**2** days after (LL)

Adenovirus

CASE STUDY

You are presented with a patient who has a combination of conjunctivitis, pharyngitis, and otitis media. They casually mention that this is during the summer.

THE DIVERSION

The diversion is the expectation that you are to treat with antibiotics.

ANSWER REVEALED

However, the correct answer will be supportive measures only. Remember that the combination of conjunctivitis and pharyngitis is often the way adenovirus is presented on the exam, especially if the patient presents during the summer.

BUZZ WORDS

Adenovirus can cause **conjunctivitis**, **pharyngitis**, **adenopathy**, and even **intussusception**. Pay special attention if they mention **summer** in the question. It is seen more frequently in the late winter, spring, and early summer.

Enteric adenovirus and norovirus can cause diarrhea.

Consider norovirus if presented with a child with diarrhea who recently went on a cruise ship. It is often transmitted by infected food handlers.

Bronchiolitis

Typical presentation is a young infant 1-6 months old with URI symptoms, including rhonchi and fever. Treatment is supportive.

RSV Infection

The clinical description will likely be an "**infant**" with "**expiratory wheeze,**" "retractions," "tachypnea," and the nonspecific description of fever and URI symptoms.

The CXR will have "**diffuse infiltrates**" and hyperinflation. Diagnosis is best confirmed with rapid diagnostic assay via antigen testing.

Confirmation is not necessary for management.

Diagnosis: Immunofluorescence is how it is confirmed. Picture a "**R**eally **S**hiny **V**irus" because it lights up.

If they ask how healthcare providers can **BEST** prevent the spread of RSV, the answer is "**good hand washing.**"

Pure RSV bronchiolitis may not respond to albuterol therapy. Since there is often a reactive component, response to beta agonist therapy does not necessarily rule out RSV bronchiolitis.

Influenza

Influenza presents differently depending on the age of the patient you are presented with.

Infants may present with a croup-like cough or URI symptoms.

Older children may present with a simple URI and low grade fever. They can also present with cough, sore throat, or rhinitis, as well as vomiting and diarrhea.

Teenagers present with a more adult-like presentation, including sudden onset of high fever, myalgia/malaise, headache, non-productive cough, chills, and sore throat.

Rapid antigen screen is the quickest and most useful method to identify influenza.

Supportive therapy is indicated for most uncomplicated cases.

Antiviral medications would be indicated for severe disease or those patients at risk for complications or who have close family contacts at risk.

Sensitivity to antiviral agents is variable and far too convoluted to go into here (especially for anyone who has to drive soon after reading this book).

Rotavirus

The words to look for are: "1-2 day history of fever," "several episodes of watery stools," and "intermittent vomiting." Evidence of dehydration will also be described.

Diagnosis is done by Rotazyme antigen testing of the stool (of course). There is a 1 to 3 day incubation period.

There is no specific treatment for rotavirus, but many small infants need to be hospitalized because of dehydration.

Rabies Virus

If you are bitten by a rabid board question about rabies, here are your guidelines.

Rabies prophylaxis is indicated if the immune status of the attacking animal is unknown and/or the animal cannot be isolated and watched.

Bats can transmit rabies to humans even without known bites. Therefore, if you are presented with a patient who wakes up in a room with a bat, treatment for rabies would be indicated , even in the absence of a known bite taking place.

Rabies immunoglobulin (RIG) is given within 7 days of exposure in conjunction with rabies vaccine.

Parasitic Infections

Ascaris Lumbricoides (A Scary Lumbar-Coilee)

BUZZ WORDS

They will describe someone visiting or returning from a faraway place where ascaris is endemic, presenting with symptoms consistent with obstruction or abdominal pain.

CASE STUDY

You might be presented with a child with signs of acute abdominal obstruction, with the implication of appendicitis or other surgical cause. Buried in the question will be a history of immigration from or travel to a tropical region.

THE DIVERSION

The diversion will be the signs of obstruction, which will be emphasized in the question, with the risk for parasitic infection barely mentioned or certainly not emphasized.

ANSWER REVEALED

If you read the question carefully, you will realize that the obstruction is due to *ascaris lumbricoides* infestation, and pick the correct diagnosis and treatment if there is a second followup question.

MNEMONIC

"A Scary Lumbar Coilee:" picture a scary coil tangled up in the lumbar spine causing abdominal pain and obstruction.

TREATMENT

The following would be appropriate treatment for asymptomatic or symptomatic *Ascaris lumbricoides.*

- Albendazole in a single dose
- Mebendazole for 3 days
- Ivermectin in a single dose

Entamoeba Histolytica

E. Histolytica causes amebiasis.

Amebic dysentery (acute amebic colitis) starts with 1-2 weeks of belly pain, diarrhea, and tenesmus (painful but ineffectual urge to defecate). Stools are liquid, consisting mainly of water, blood, and mucus.[13]

Clinical course can range from asymptomatic to minor or severe GI effects, as well as liver and brain abscesses or lung disease. Only about 10% of *E. histolytica* infections cause invasive disease - the rest are asymptomatic.

Stool exam will identify hematophagous trophozoites. Stool cultures are usually positive. Blood is invariably present in the stool. Abdominal ultrasound is also a minimally invasive and cost-effective diagnostic tool.

Enter amoeba "hysterical:" picture a crazy, hysterical amoeba playing tennis (tenesmus) in your bowels causing bloody mucous diarrhea.

Don't forget! Amebiasis can cause a liver abscess. Drug of choice for amebiasis is Flagyl® (metronidazole).

The following regimens are recommended:

· **Asymptomatic cyst excreters (intraluminal infections)** can be treated with luminal amebicide, such as iodoquinol, paromomycin, or diloxanide.

· **Patients with mild to moderate or severe intestinal symptoms or extraintestinal disease (including liver abscess)** should be treated with metronidazole (or tinidazole), followed by a therapeutic course of a luminal amebicide (iodoquinol or paromomycin).

Corticosteroids and antimotility drugs administered to people with **amebiasis** can worsen symptoms and the disease process.

---

[13] Apologies from the editors if you were studying while eating your lunch.

Toxocariasis

BUZZ WORDS

Toxocariasis is due to a roundworm that goes by the name of *toxocara canis*, a Board classic. It can present with **GI symptoms** (hepatomegaly and abdominal pain) and respiratory symptoms (wheezing). This is because it **"migrates" everywhere**. **Exposure to dogs and cats** is the risk factor and they might tip you off with "**eosinophilia.**" Look for the **preschooler who has been eating dirt**.

There are 3 clinical manifestations of toxocariasis:

1) **Visceral larval migrans** – these patients present with fever, hepatomegaly, and wheezing.

2) **Ocular larval migrans** – as you can guess, these patients present with visual disturbances.

3) **Covert toxocariasis** – patients with covert toxocariasis may present with GI symptoms as well as pruritus and a rash.

CASE STUDY

You could be presented with a patient with abdominal pain and wheezing, with the casual mention of exposure to cats and dogs thrown in to further throw you off. They casually note eosinophilia and bury hepatomegaly in the cascade of physical findings. They might note that the child was seen eating dirt while playing. You will be asked to make the diagnosis.

THE DIVERSION

This is an excellent method to throw you off on several diversionary paths. The combination of abdominal pain and wheezing suggest pneumonia. The exposure to cats suggests asthma and allergies. The presence of eosinophilia further substantiates this diversionary path. Treatment and steps to address each of these issues will be there for your diversionary pleasure.

ANSWER REVEALED

The key to separating the correct answer from the diversions will be the hepatomegaly, which again will be buried in the physical findings, but not to those who tease it out with a highlighter (or other methods for those taking the electronic recertification exam). If they mention the child eating dirt, it should also help pull you away from the diversionary choices and help you identify the correct answer: visceral larva migrans. If the question asks for the most appropriate test to make the diagnosis and the correct treatment, we have this information below.

ELISA is the test to diagnose VLM. In order to rule out other parasitic infections, stool cultures should still be done.

Treatment is with *mebendazole* or *thiabendazole.*

You can remember this with the "L" links. **L**onghaired cats and **L**icking dogs cause **L**arval disease in the **L**ungs and the **L**iver.

Parasite Treatment

Parasite	Treatment	
Giardia lamblia	Metronidazole (Flagyl®), Tinidazole, and Nitazoxanide are effective against *Giardia.* Furazolidone is an alternative	Picture a giant lamb (Gigantia Lamb Ya) riding the train (Metro). It also works against Hysterical Amoeba, which calms down in the subway (metro)
Trichomonas vaginalis	Flagyl®	
Schistosomal/Liver Fluke/Tapeworm	Praziquantel	Picture a crazy tall can (Crazy-Can-Tall) pulling in the tapeworm.
Strongyloidiasis	Thiabendazole	Picture a "strong guy" loitering. The only way to stop him is with somebody strong enough to bend his thighs (Thigh Bender Zole).
Enterobius vermicularis	Mebendazole, pyrantel pamoate, or albendazole – one time dose, repeated in 2 weeks.	The whole family is treated in the presence of recurrent infection. Routine treatment of whole family would be correct as well.

Mebendazole

 Mebendazole is used to treat worms of varying shapes and sizes, including pinworms, roundworms, hookworms, and whipworms. Other options for worms include pyrantel pamoate or albendazole.

Permethrin

Permethrin 5% is the first line to treat scabies. It is safe for use in infants and young children.

Permethrin 1% is used for head lice, but is too weak to treat scabies.

Lindane is no longer used.

Anti Malarial Medication

If you are presented with a patient traveling to a spot where there is no known chloroquine resistance:

Travelers should take chloroquine weekly starting one week before departing, then weekly during the trip, and then weekly for 4 weeks upon returning.

If you are presented with a patient traveling to a spot where *P. falciparum* resistant to chloroquine exists:

Atovaquone-proguanil, doxycycline, or mefloquine would be indicated.

Fungal Infections

Candidiasis

The most likely cause of **a *mild* Candidal** infection is **antibiotic use.** With **"systemic candidiasis,"** **immunosuppression** is the most likely cause, e.g., bone marrow/organ transplant, malignancy, or corticosteroids.

To remember the most likely causes of **systemic candidiasis**, try the following (**YEAST**):

Y (Widespread immunosuppression)
Extensive Burns
Antibiotics
Suppressed Immunity
TPN use

Cryptococcosis

Cryptococcus neoformans is an encapsulated yeast. It causes both pulmonary disease as well as meningitis/meningoencephalitis. It is most commonly associated with AIDS.

Look for a history of exposure to **bird droppings (e.g., pigeons)**.

Picture someone **stuck with a pigeon** in a **giant CRYPT**. There is no air and he is getting a **headache** so severe it feels like **meningitis**.

Amphotericin B, in combination with oral flucytosine or fluconazole, is indicated as initial therapy for meningitis and other serious cryptococcal infections.

The only way to recover is to be **taken from the crypt into a giant open amphitheater** in the mountains.

Flucytosine (5-FC) is indicated for resistant infections. **It is always used in combination with Amphotericin B or fluconazole.**

There is a **liposomal** formulation of Amphotericin B which should be used in patients with renal impairment.

Coccidioidomycosis

These patients present with **vague influenza-like symptoms**. They often will tip you off by mentioning recent travel to **California, Arizona, or Texas**. Symptoms develop within a month of exposure, and patients usually present with vague complaints, including fevers, night sweats, headaches, chest pains, and muscle aches.

CAT: California, **A**rizona, **T**exas. Change the disease name to **CAT CITY –oido-Mycosis** and you'll have this memorized.

Treatment is with amphotericin B, fluconazole, or ketoconazole.

Again, you have to be in the open air. **The CAT has to go to an open-air amphitheater** (preferably in large states like California, Arizona, and Texas.)

Aspergillosis and Asthma

Think of **aspergillosis** when they present an **"asthmatic" with worsening symptoms, despite treatment**. There are increased **eosinophils** and **infiltrates** noted on CXR. Invasive aspergillosis only occurs in immunocompromised patients.

In the past, allergic bronchopulmonary **aspergillosis** has been treated with corticosteroids. More recently, antifungal therapy has been recommended.

Voriconazole or **amphotericin B** in high doses are the drugs of choice for invasive **aspergillosis.**

Histoplasmosis

Histoplasmosis is found throughout the Ohio, Missouri, and Mississippi river valleys. Most people infected remain asymptomatic, and those who get sick are usually immunocompromised.

They will describe general **influenza-like symptoms**, which could be anything.

Hepatosplenomegaly in the clinical description (which you highlighted) is the key to choosing this as the correct answer.

 Remember, **H**istoplasmosis, **H**epatosplenomegaly.

 Like crypto, histoplasmosis is also obtained from bird droppings. **Hepatosplenomegaly will help confirm the diagnosis of histoplasmosis.**

 Immunocompetent children with uncomplicated disease only require supportive care.

For disseminated disease, especially in immunocompromised patients, Amphotericin B is recommended. It is found to be more effective than the azoles. If necessary, fluconazole would be the most appropriate azole.

 Histoplasmosis, **H**epatosplenomegaly, **H**elp yourself (self-limited).

Sporotrichosis

Sporotrichosis is caused by *Sporothrix schenckii* resulting in a subacute or chronic fungal infection. It usually involves both superficial and deep tissues.

It typically occurs in floral nursery or tree farm workers. Watch for a history of children working or visiting such places. **Lymphocutaneous manifestations** are the most common. This will be presented as an ulcer on the finger, or perhaps the wrist, along with a chain of nodules parallel to the draining lymphatic channel. Bones and joints can also become involved, with the knee being the most commonly affected joint.

Antifungals

Amphotericin B

Amphotericin B is used to treat a variety of fungi, including *Candida, Aspergillus, Zygomycetes, Histoplasma,* and *Coccoides immitis.*

Side effects include febrile reactions, hypokalemia, and nephrotoxicity.

If you are presented with an immunocompromised patient who is not responding to antibiotics and has a low neutrophil count, they are at risk for disseminated fungal infection. Treatment with amphotericin B could be appropriate in this situation.

Fluconazole

Fluconazole is most effective against *Candida albicans*. *Aspergillus* and other *Candida* strains are often resistant. If placed on long term fluconazole treatment, monitoring of LFTs would be appropriate.

Infants younger than 6 months of age who have recurrent oral thrush due to *Candida* could be experiencing maternal breast colonization. Once a day fluconazole is superior to oral nystatin for resistant oral thrush.

Modes of Transmission

You will be expected to be familiar with the mode of transmission of a variety of infectious agents, as well as the precautions necessary to prevent spread.

Droplet Transmission

Infections spread by droplet transmission, primarily by sneezing and coughing. These do not remain suspended for prolonged periods of time. Therefore, the only precautions are covering your mouth when sneezing or coughing. They do not require any special air ventilation systems to prevent spread.

Examples of organisms transmitted by droplet transmission include **mumps, rubella,** and **pertussis**.

Airborne Transmission

These are organisms that can remain airborne for prolonged periods of time. Therefore they can spread through the hospital ventilation system. Special air handling units are needed to prevent spread.

Examples include **aspergillosis, tuberculosis, measles, varicella, and disseminated zoster.**

Picture an **ATM** as a hospital air conditioning system delivering **V's** and **Z's** as droplets to remember that the hospital ventilation system can spread these organisms.

Legionella pneumophila, Candida parapsilosis, and *Pseudomonas aeruginosa* do not spread through the hospital ventilation system and therefore only require standard precautions.

Direct contact

RSV virus is an example of organism transmitted by direct contact. Therefore, handwashing is the best method of preventing transmission.

Chapter 15

Inborn Errors
of Metabolism

Inborn Errors of Metabolism: A diverse and confusing collection of disorders, including organic acidemias, urea cycle defects, fatty acid metabolism defects, and storage disorders. Basically, in anything metabolic you can think of, something can go wrong. *Don't worry, we'll break it down for you so you don't have a breakdown.*

Inborn errors of metabolism should come to mind in any infant that has a *sudden onset of lethargy, vomiting, tachypnea, apnea, irritability, or seizures.* Pay particular attention to antecedent events they describe, no matter how inconsequential they may seem, i.e., feeding. This is often the crucial clue to getting the correct answer.

This can be presented to you on the exam in several forms. The more challenging form will be the "Best Answer" format where you need to diagnose a **classic "septic" infant that is not septic, or perhaps a repeat case of "Reye Syndrome."**

Many of these disorders are quite similar. This is another example where focusing on the "specific differences" between disorders will pay handsome dividends. **However, a logical approach to the question is something you cannot memorize.** If you use the step-by-step approach outlined below, the questions themselves will help you make the right diagnosis and get a series of questions correct.

> **Remember:** A metabolic disorder will often have the following in the description: **lethargy, vomiting, poor feeding, and depressed CNS. In some cases, they will describe "coma," "seizure," or "apnea."**

Approaching Inborn Errors of Metabolism

Given that all **metabolic disorders present with vomiting and lethargy, distinguishing the fine differences between them can be a challenge.** *Key phrases* and wording are what distinguish one disorder from another. In fact, paying close attention to the fine differences between various disorders can help you score points on enough questions to push you over the top.

Despite thorough screening (see the screen door below), metabolic disorders can still present frequently; that is, on the board exam, where it counts for the moment.

The Screen Door

The trend is to screen for most metabolic disorders so future generations of pediatricians will have no first-hand knowledge of or experience with them. You will still need to know them for the Boards. Remember that newborn screening to identify infants in the United States who have phenylketonuria (PKU) or hypothyroidism is conducted in every state and Puerto Rico.

In addition, many states also screen for galactosemia, hemoglobinopathies, congenital adrenal hyperplasia, biotinidase deficiency, maple syrup urine disease (MSUD), and homocystinuria.

Step 1: Afebrile

If they emphasize that the infant is *afebrile*, that is an indication that they are letting you know the **ID tree is the wrong tree**. Look for other clues in the question that this is not an infection.

Step 2: Serum NH$_4$ (Ammonia)/ABG

ABG	Elevated Serum NH$_4$	Normal Serum NH$_4$[1]
Metabolic Acidosis	Propionic Acidemia Methylmalonic Acidemia Fatty acid oxidation defects	MSUD, some organic acidemias
ABG Normal	Urea Cycle Defect Transient hyperammonemia	· Aminoacidopathy · Galactosemia[2] · Non-ketotic hyperglycinemia

Metabolic Disorders Presenting with Acidosis

Organic Acidemias

Important features include
- **Elevated Ammonia (in many, but not all)**
- **Acidotic**
- **High Anion Gap**

---

[1] Normal serum ammonia value in a newborn is below 110mcmol/ L.

[2] And just to make it more confusing — there may be an acidosis from sepsis.

Sepsis can also present with a metabolic acidosis.

Organic acidemias typically present with a "drunk-like" intoxicated picture, but the disease is life threatening. Important lab findings include **elevated serum ammonia levels (in many, but not all organic acidemias)** and **ketonuria.** Organic acidemias often present in the first 2 days after the **introduction of protein in the diet.**

The most important **initial step** after diagnosing one of these disorders is **hydration,** to maintain good urine output. After that appropriate diet is indicated.

If you are presented with an infant who is **1-2 days of age, acidotic, ketotic,** has an **elevated serum ammonia level,** the most important laboratory study will be measurement of **urine organic acid levels.**

In general, when they present you with an infant with a septic appearance with sepsis ruled out, a metabolic cause is likely; obtaining a **serum ammonia level** will often be the correct answer they are seeking.

Additional correct choices might include a serum **lactic acid level, serum pyruvate, total and free carnitine, and/or acetylcarnitine.**

Since metabolic acidosis can suppress bone marrow, granulocytopenia and **thrombocytopenia** may occur with organic acidemias. Therefore, do not dismiss the possibility of a metabolic disorder if you are given a history consistent with organic acidemia **and** a low platelet and WBC count.

Some organic acidemias respond to **biotin.**

Organic Acidemias

Think of organic acids as **very powerful alcoholic drinks**, because a child with this disorder will present as someone who is drunk. Examples include methylmalonic and propionic acidemia and biotinidase deficiency.

"Decreased appetite," "falling down frequently," "delayed developmental milestones," with no overt physical abnormalities or dysmorphology are all clues.

Of course, a **brain tumor** could present with balance problems and vomiting, but somewhere in the question will be the hint that the **symptoms have been progressively worse if it is a brain tumor.** They might also mention morning headaches and visual disturbances to indicate a brain tumor.

Isovaleric Acidemia

Isovaleric Acidemia also presents with lethargy and poor feeding. They might also mention a **seizure** and **high incidence of infections**. *Odor of sweaty feet* is another feature, so make sure nobody has tossed off their shoes after a bad night on call before jumping to diagnostic conclusions.

Treatment is with *protein restriction.*

Propionic Acidemia

Like the others, it too presents in the newborn period with tachypnea, poor feeding, and lethargy.

Methylmalonic Acidemia

Methylmalonic acidemia is another possibility that presents in much the same way as propionic acidemia. Remember that the **anion gap will be elevated**.

Methylmalonic acidemia may **respond to vitamin B12**.

Defects in Fatty Acid Metabolism

Fatty acid oxidation defects are inherited in an autosomal *recessive* pattern. Examples are Medium, Long, and Very Long Chain Acyl-CoA Dehydrogenase Deficiencies (MCAD, LCAD, VLCAD).

An infant who has a defect in fatty acid metabolism, in addition to **hypoglycemia,** may also present with **hepatomegaly.** [3] Watch for signs of a preceding benign illness, during which oral intake was decreased. This could occur in a toddler, since many of the *signs of fatty acid oxidation defects present with fasting.* In between episodes, the child is fine.

Note the <u>absence of reducing substances</u> and <u>ketones</u> in the urine as well as <u>normal serum amino acids</u>.

Definitive diagnosis is via the **plasma acylcarnitine profile.**

---

[3] Fatty acid oxidation defects may or may not have hepatomegaly; however, it may be part of the presentation on the boards.

Urea Cycle Defects

Urea cycle defects present with **hyperammonemia** in the **absence of acidosis.** In addition, look for a **symptom-free period, followed by hypotonia** and **coma.**

Respiratory alkalosis may be present, as well as **lactic acidosis.**

Hyperammonemia will result in symptoms consistent with encephalopathy (vomiting, lethargy and ultimately coma).

Treatment is to reduce the serum NH4 by **reducing protein intake and increasing glucose intake by IV**. Dialysis might be needed on a PRN, usually acute, basis.

Ketonuria does not occur with urea cycle defects. If you are presented with an infant with elevated serum ammonia and hypotonia, ketonuria rules out urea cycle defects and leaves open the possibility of **organic acidemias. Zellweger syndrome** may also present with hypotonia as well as *dysmorphic features,* but elevated serum ammonia will *not* be a feature.

Note that several metabolic disorders can also present with hypoglycemia, but they will *not present with hepatomegaly.* This includes organic acid defects, hyperinsulinism, and urea cycle defects.

Some urea cycle defects improve with **arginine**.

Hypoglycemia in Infants

Disorders of Carbohydrate Metabolism

Galactosemia

Infants with galactosemia will appear *normal at birth.* However, that is until they are given their first meal containing lactose, which would include both items on the expected first menu: *formula* or *breast milk.* They then will present with non-specific findings, including poor feeding and failure to thrive.

More specific findings would include:
- *Abdominal distension*
- Hypoglycemia
- Gram negative sepsis
- Non-glucose reducing substances in the urine

Watch for a history of infection with gram negative organisms including *E. coli.* In addition, the test for reducing substances in the urine must be for non-glucose reducing substances.

 The disease is due to the deficiency of galactose-1-phosphate uridyltransferase (friends refer to him as *GALT).* The definitive diagnosis is made by measuring GALT in RBCs.

Treatment is with a galactose-free diet. Failure to treat may result in **cataracts, intellectual disability** and/or **liver disease.**

Cataracts are reversible with diet change.

Infants of Diabetic Mothers

Because of exposure to higher than normal serum glucose in utero, IDM's have their insulin production going strong. Therefore, they are at risk for **hypoglycemia** and **jitteriness**. They can also present with *seizures*. Checking serum glucose is crucial.

Hypoglycemia can be the cause of **tremors, apnea, cyanosis,** and **lethargy.** Remember, **tachypnea** can also be due to hypoglycemia. Infants of diabetic mothers are also at risk for hypocalcemia, hyperbilirubinemia, and polycythemia.

Inherited Fructose Intolerance

The key clue in the description is **"seizures just after a meal,"** and a child who "stays away from sweets" (now THAT should get anyone's attention).

 Treatment is "avoidance of fructose."

Screen the Screen

There is something called the Duarte variant that occurs in infants who have half the normal amount of GALT; however, they do not require treatment. *Therefore, infants who are positive on routine screening measures of enzyme activity require more specific testing before treatment is implemented.*

Several glycogen storage diseases also present with *hepatosplenomegaly.* However, the mere mentioning of *positive reducing substances* in the urine should point you toward galactosemia.

Differential Diagnosis:

- **Lactose Intolerance** – presents later in childhood and is much more benign

- **Maple Syrup Urine Disease** – presents with *hypoglycemia,* but also presents with *acidosis, increased tone,* and as the name implies, the odor of maple syrup in the urine – yum! Seizures are also seen in MSUD.

- **Urea Cycle Defects** – in addition to *lethargy* and *poor feeding, urea cycle defects* present with *coma* and *hyperammonemia.*

You are presented with an icteric 4 day old newborn with lethargy and hepatomegaly. As a part of the septic workup, a lumbar puncture is done and is positive for *gram negative organisms.* What is the BEST additional study to obtain?

Well, well, well, what do you know – you have a newborn with a classic picture of sepsis confirmed with a positive gram stain of the CSF? Slam Dunk! The next study to perform is a culture of the CSF. You scratch your head, and say "What can be more straightforward than that?" You can continue scratching your head wondering why you got this one wrong.

While you don't want to over think every question on the exam, if something seems so obvious that even the members of the engineering staff who have listened to morning report would know the answer, it cannot be that simple.

They note that the patient has hepatomegaly, and that is for a reason. You would need to realize that hepatomegaly and risk for gram-negative sepsis is the hallmark of galactosemia. However, even knowing this would not be enough – you would also need to know how galactosemia is diagnosed. It is diagnosed by measuring **galactose-1-phosphate activity in RBCs,** or as they can be alternatively described on the exam, **erythrocytes.**

Take home message: when you are presented with an infant with a sepsis-like picture, with hepatomegaly and positive culture for gram-negative organisms, think of galactosemia lurking in the erythrocyte.

This must be coupled with knowing *all the associated findings of galactosemia.*

If they ask for the correct treatment, in addition to antibiotics, diet restriction would also be required.

If they ask for an associated finding, the answer might be *reducing substances in the urine.*

Hyperinsulinism

A typical presentation would include an **afebrile infant** presenting with **generalized seizures.** An important part of the presentation will be **hypoglycemia,** remedied with an **injection of glucagon.**

Height, weight and head circumference will all be in the upper limits of normal, typically in the 95th percentile for all parameters.

Keep in mind the differential diagnosis in order to avoid picking the wrong answer on a technicality.

- **Beckwith-Wiedemann syndrome** – while this too presents with *macrosomia, watch for* **microcephaly** *rather than macrocephaly.* Additional findings include macroglossia, visceromegaly, and omphalocele

- **Adrenal Insufficiency** – also presents with *hypoglycemia.* However, in this case they will need to let you know about **ketonuria.** If they note the absence of ketones in the urine, they are ruling adrenal insufficiency out for you.

- **Hereditary Fructose intolerance** – While this, like adrenal insufficiency, also presents with *ketonuria,* they will have to note the **onset of vomiting after ingestion of a fructose containing food product.**

- **Galactosemia** – While this presents with hypoglycemia, it also presents with vomiting, failure to thrive, hepatomegaly, and, most importantly, non-glucose reducing substances in the urine.

In **Beckwith-Wiedemann syndrome,** the hypoglycemia is due to **islet cell hyperplasia.**

CASE STUDY You are presented with a full term infant who is hypoglycemic. The serum insulin levels are noted to be elevated. Despite receiving a glucose IV infusion, the infant remains hypoglycemic. What do you do next? Which medication would be MOST appropriate to solve the problem?

THE DIVERSION This is a description of an infant with *refractory hypoglycemia* and you might be tempted to pick glucagon, which will be sitting right there diverting you away from the correct answer. Well, you say, "Isn't insulin inappropriately high in this patient? Isn't calcium required to squeeze out insulin from the pancreas?" Yes! Therefore, wouldn't calcium channel blockers help solve the problem? Good thought! However, it would be the wrong answer, since calcium channel blockers rarely help with refractory hypoglycemia in infants.

ANSWER REVEALED The correct answer, believe it or not, is **diazoxide**, which decreases insulin secretion *and* stimulates cortisol release. This is a bit unfair, but who said this is fair. Just remember that diazoxide will be the drug of choice in *refractory hypoglycemia in infants*.

Inborn Errors of Metabolism that Defy Categorization

Biotinidase Deficiency

BUZZ WORDS Look for **lactic acidosis** (high anion gap) with a "**rash,**" and "**alopecia,**" as well as **neurological** signs ranging from ataxia to coma.

TREATMENT It is treated with *biotin supplementation.*

BIO:

> **B**ald
> **I**tchy rash
> **O**ut cold = coma, ataxia, neurological signs

Maple Syrup Urine Disease

Besides the dead giveaway of "maple syrup-smelling urine," they will describe an infant with tachypnea, with a shallow breathing pattern and profound lethargy. They also can present with **hypertonicity**. The classic onset is during the **first week of life**.

To help remember which amino acids have elevated plasma levels[4] in Maple Syrup Urine Disease, think of the word **VIAL** (picture **maple syrup in a vial**):

> **V**aline
> **I**soleucine
> **A**lloisoleucine (never found in normal infants)
> **L**eucine

> **CASE STUDY**
>
> **You are presented with an infant with hypoglycemia and a variety of other symptoms such as seizures, hepatomegaly, or failure to thrive. What is the MOST helpful measurement to determine the etiology?**
>
> **THE DIVERSION**
>
> There may be choices there specific to the additional findings, in addition to hypoglycemia. For example, cortisol and growth hormone (if the infant is macrosomic), or they may include insulin level measurement. These are all diversionary choices.
>
> **ANSWER REVEALED**
>
> The most important measurement to determine the etiology of hypoglycemia in infants would be **urine measurement of *ketones* and *reducing substances***.

---

[4] It is the inability to break down these amino acids that causes the disorder. More details can be found in the 30-pound biochemistry text of your choice.

Amino Acid Metabolic Disorders

Alcaptonuria

Alcaptonuria results in **homogentisic acid in the urine**, which results in a **dark diaper.** Typically these patients will be described as being asymptomatic throughout most of childhood, except for the following unusual findings.

If you change "alcaptonuria" to "night captonuria" to associate the "dark" features of the disease, it will be impossible to forget.

Over time, the eye sclerae and ear cartilage develop dark pigmentation. Sweat and cerumen become dark.

Urine, if left standing, also turns black; thus the possible description of a "dark diaper."

As adults, they are at risk for developing early-onset arthritis and heart disease.

Intelligence is normal.

Tyrosine is not degraded well, resulting in increased tyrosine levels. *It is treated with a diet low in phenylalanine* and *tyrosine.*

Homocystinuria

Homocystinuria is due to cystathionine synthase deficiency, which results in **elevated methionine levels.**

There are 2 subtypes. Pyridoxine (B6) responsive and pyridoxine (B6) resistant. The IQ is typically higher in individuals with the responsive subtype when treated, which is why it is important to distinguish.

These patients present with **dislocated lens(es)**, **skeletal abnormalities**, and often **cognitive deficits**. They could describe an unpleasant odor. They will very likely describe the patient as having lighter-colored skin, hair, and eyes than other family members. The skeletal abnormalities are similar to those seen in Marfan syndrome. Homocystinuria is diagnosed by confirming homocysteine in the urine.

It is treated with **pyridoxine**; if this doesn't work, a ***diet high in cystine*** and ***low in methionine is the treatment.***

Marfan Syndrome can also present with dislocated lens(es) and skeletal abnormalities. Both Marfan syndome and homocystinuria patients may present as tall and thin with pectus excavatum. However, one *would not see any cognitive deficits with Marfan syndrome.*

Homocystinuria is due to an error in methionine metabolism.

Typical presentation is a child with thin body habitus, scoliosis, posteriorly dislocated lens, as well as cognitive impairment. They are at risk for thrombi and emboli, so watch for a presenting history consistent with a **pulmonary embolus**.

Most importantly, half of the cases have some residual enzyme activity, and these patients *respond to* **pyridoxine treatment.**

Marfan syndrome is very phenotypically similar to homocystinuria.

Marfan syndrome presents with **anterior lens displacement.**

Homocystinuria presents with **posterior lens displacement.**

MArfan syndrome is associated with Anterior lens dislocation and Aortic problems.

Oculocutaneous tyrosinemia

This will often be described with, you guessed it, the ocular findings. Due to tyrosine accumulation, patients develop *corneal ulcerations, plaques, and eventually corneal clouding. Skin thickening on the soles of the feet and palms of the hand* (areas that bear pressure) will also be described.

Treatment consists of a *low tyrosine* and *phenylalanine diet.*

PKU

Clinical Presentation of PKU

This is due to the deficiency of the enzyme that converts phenylalanine to tyrosine, thus the accumulation of phenylalanine.

Even though symptomatic PKU is not typically seen in the real world due to mandatory newborn screening, it can present on the boards. You need to be familiar with some of the important features.

These patients will be **asymptomatic** for a few months (with blond hair and blue eyes). If they are not treated, they will ultimately present with severe vomiting, irritability, **eczema**, or a musty or *mousy odor*[5] of the urine.

Later signs of untreated PKU could include **microcephaly, congenital heart disease**, and **low birthweight**.

It ultimately leads to **profound intellectual disability** and other neurological impairments.

PKU screening is only valid after a **"protein" feeding**, which is why it is typically done at 48-72 hours.

PKU and Pregnancy

Any mother with PKU who is contemplating pregnancy should be treated *before conception.* Otherwise, there is an increased risk for **miscarriage, SGA, microcephaly, cardiac defects**, and **intellectual disability**.

Treating PKU

 It is treated with a **low phenylalanine formula (Lofenalac®)**.

---

[5] I am not sure I know what exactly a mouse smells like, but if you see it described then consider PKU.

Benign Hyperphenylalaninemia

Here the levels are elevated but subclinical. In case they want numbers, **the clinical manifestations are evident with phenylalanine levels above 20.**

PERIL WARNING **Over-treatment** is a potential problem. A child *diagnosed with* PKU who presents with increased **lethargy, rash, and perhaps diarrhea** is being over-treated.

Because phenylalanine is not synthesized in the body, overzealous treatment, especially in rapidly growing infants, can result in phenylalanine deficiency.

HOT TIP In addition, it is important to note that tyrosine becomes an essential amino acid in this disorder, and its adequate intake must be ensured.

Mucopolysaccharidoses

With these, you must know the slight differences between similar disorders: all of them present with coarse facies (or faces for those unfamiliar with Latin). The differences start with the presence or absence of corneal clouding and intellectual disability. Modes of inheritance differ as well. Here goes:

Hurler's syndrome (MPS Type I)

Hurler syndrome presents before age 2. In addition to progressive facial coarsening, they will likely note *hirsutism, hepatosplenomegaly,* and *corneal clouding.*

They could also note lab findings significant for reduced **alpha-L-iduronidase** activity in WBCs.

Hunter's syndrome (MPS Type II)

BUZZ WORDS Coarse facial features are just the start. Watch for additional characteristics, including **organomegaly, joint contractures, and skin that appears "pebbly," especially over the upper back.**

They could also describe reduced **iduronate sulfatase enzyme** activity in WBCs.

Most hunters are male, so that tells you that it is "X-linked," and if that doesn't work, picture somebody hunting with a bow and arrow, and the points of the arrow are all "X's" instead of arrowheads.

You also need to see in order to hunt, and therefore you cannot have corneal clouding.

Sanfilippo Syndrome (MPS Type III)

Compared with other disorders in this category, Sanfilippo presents with minimal facial coarsening.

It also will not be described with *organomegaly*, which will likely be noted if they are describing the other mucopolysaccharidoses.

Sanfilippo **is** associated with *cognitive deficit*.

Sanfilippo syndrome is inherited as an **autosomal recessive** trait; therefore, it occurs in both males and females equally.

 Sanfilippo manifests during the first year of life. Urine may have increased heparan sulfate. There is no corneal clouding.

Morquio Syndrome (MPS Type IV)

It is my understanding that the sidekick on *Fantasy Island,* Tattoo, had this condition.[6] I cannot remember his name though—how's that for someone touting the importance of using a memory system? Kids with this disorder have **skeletal involvement** and **corneal clouding,** but **normal intelligence.**

Morquio-Boney abnormalities are the feature, but *no* **M**ental retardation (the only one that has an **M** in it), and there *is* corneal clouding. (You can hear the plane but you don't have to actually "see" the plane).

I-cell disease

I-cell disease is also called "Leroy" I-cell disease or mucolipidosis II.

They could present you with a neonate with coarse facial features, with *clubfeet* and *hernias*, as well as *hip dislocation.*

It is associated with severe intellectual disability and joint contractures. Children with the disease often do not live beyond age 10.

Purine and Pyrimidine Disorders

ADA[7] deficiency and *Lesch-Nyhan syndrome* are examples of Purine and Pyrimidine Disorders.

Watch for a family history and presentation of recurrent infections, developmental delay and failure to thrive.

---

[6] I could be badly aging myself here if you have no idea what I am talking about.

[7] Adenosine deaminase deficiency, which is an autosomal recessive disorder.

Glycogen Storage Diseases

Glycogen Storage Disease Type 1 (Von Gierke Disease)

In addition to non–specific findings such as *hypoglycemia* and a *distended abdomen,* watch for the description of a **doll–like** or **cherubic face. Consanguinity** is also a common feature in the history.

Additional features to remember are **poor growth, a large liver, seizures secondary to hypoglycemia**, and **elevated triglycerides and cholesterol**. Hypoglycemia and lactic acidosis with fasting is classic.

Important lab findings to remember include **elevated lactic acid** and **uric acid levels.**

In case it comes up, this is due to a deficiency of hepatic glucose-6-phosphatase. This is the *final step in the liver to produce glucose.* Glycogen storage diseases often present when an infant begins sleeping through the night, which results in "prolonged fasting."

Treatment is with **frequent snacks and meals, and sometimes continuous tube feedings.**

Treatment is the **infusion of glucose continuously, especially at night** *until the age of 2.* After the age of 2, **cornstarch** is often used, since it releases glucose slowly.

It is only the continuous feeding of glucose that is helpful. Choices that include the feeding of *formula high in fructose or galactose will not be useful. Glucagon injections are not useful.* They might present you with *liver transplant,* which might be appropriate down the road in the event of liver failure, but it will *not be the appropriate* <u>initial</u> treatment of course.

The keys to the treatment are avoidance of fasting, as well as frequent administration of carbohydrates, which is accomplished by feeding starchy food.

Pompe Disease (GSD II)

For those with the scorecard, this is a deficiency in lysosomal breakdown of glycogen.

They will describe this in an infant who is **one month of age or younger**, and normal at birth, who becomes **floppy**, **fails to thrive**, and develops a large liver with **macroglossia**. Eventually death is due to **respiratory failure**. They also present with cardiomegaly and the odd combination of hypotonia with muscles that are "hard" on examination.

To remember this, change it to **"Pope" disease**. One of the features is "**cardiomegaly**"—and the Pope has a "big heart"— along with **left axis** deviation on EKG, since the Pope sways away from Left Wing Politics. He is also not afraid to speak out when necessary, so he has a large tongue = **macroglossia**.

Hypoglycemia and acidosis are not part of Pompe disease.

Nonketotic hyperglycinemia

Yes this is spelled correctly, hyperglycinemia

This will typically be described in a newborn, presenting after being fed protein containing formula for the first time.

They then become lethargic and eventually comatose. If they survive it, they often will have spastic cerebral palsy.

Lipoprotein Disorders

Familial Hypercholesterolemia

Familial hypercholesterolemia is an *autosomal dominant disorder* due to the deficiency of LDL receptors.

There is a 50% chance of one parent passing along the gene. Xanthomas typically don't present until after age 10.

> **Watch the Spelling:**
>
> **Zellweger Syndrome** results in elevated very long chain fatty acids. They will describe facial features similar to Down syndrome and perhaps some MRI abnormalities.

Familial hypercholesterolemia is **not associated with obesity.**

Congenital Lipodystrophy

Here you have adipose tissue that is not on speaking terms with insulin, so you have fat tissue resistant to insulin. The result is a newborn that is *thin AND long*.

Farber's Disease

The **primary features are skin nodules and painful joints** that are noted in the **first week of life**. These patients also have a **cherry red spot** in the retina (see Tay-Sachs and Niemann-Pick for the other cherry red spots).

 I change this to "**Farmers Disease:**" farmers work hard "**picking cherries**" (cherry red spot), and their **joints ache**. They have **nodules on their skin** from getting down in the dirt so often.

Wolman Disease

Wolman Disease is due to defective lipoprotein metabolism, which results in **triglyceride** and **cholesterol esters in body tissue**. This is characterized by failure to thrive and a large liver and spleen. They may show you a **calcified adrenal gland**, which would be the clincher.

 Think of these "**fatty deposits**" as **white wool made up of fat**.

 Plasma triglycerides and cholesterol levels are normal. *Deposits are in body tissue only.*

They might describe some non-specific findings in the first few weeks of life (e.g., vomiting, malabsorption, failure to thrive, hepatomegaly) but the "different feature" will be the **calcified and enlarged adrenal glands**.

Menkes Kinky Hair Syndrome

Menkes Kinky Hair Syndrome is due to both **low serum copper** and **low serum ceruloplasmin, just as in Wilson's disease;** however, the **tissue copper level is high**. It is also recessive. They may show twisted hairs (pili torti).

Picture a "kinky" person in the "recesses" of society, to remember that it is a recessive trait.

Wilson's Disease

They will describe "liver deterioration" (i.e. **jaundice, large liver**) along with acute signs of **neurological deterioration**.

This is because of **deposition of copper in the liver and brain**. Also affected are the eyes (the classic Kayser Fleischer rings) and the kidney. **Visual deficits do NOT occur.**

It is diagnosed by liver biopsy. **Ceruloplasmin levels are low, but not diagnostic;** *liver biopsy is diagnostic.*

Lysosomal Lipid Storage Diseases (Sphingolipidoses)

Gaucher Disease

Gaucher disease should be considered in any child presenting with *organomegaly, bone pain, and easy bruisability. Short stature* is another important feature.

HOT TIP

These symptoms are due in large part to **thrombocytopenia. Osteosclerosis** and **lytic lesions** on x-ray may also be present.

Gaucher Disease

This comes in two flavors: "infantile" or "chronic juvenile."

Infantile Gaucher Disease

DEFINITION

It is due to decreased beta glucosidase activity. This results in a child in the first or second year of life who has progressive hepatosplenomegaly and CNS deterioration.

Chronic Juvenile Gaucher Disease

DEFINITION

This form isn't as severe and, usually, there isn't any CNS involvement. However, there is *splenomegaly* with chronic problems, including *thrombocytopenia* or *pancytopenia*.

Picture a "Gaucho Cowboy" falling off his horse resulting in bone pain, nose bleeds, and lots of bruises to lock this association into long term memory.

Fabry, Krabbe, and Tay Sach diseases are also sphingolipidoses with similar presentations; however, they are slightly different. Recognizing these slight differences will be the difference between passing and failing.

Fabry Disease

Fabry disease will present with **orange-colored skin lesions, opacities of the eye, and vascular disease of the kidney, heart, and brain.**

Krabbe Disease

Krabbe disease is a demyelination disorder with progressive neurological degeneration, resulting in death by age 2.[8]

Tay Sachs Disease

Tay Sachs Disease also presents with progressive neurologic degeneration over the first year of life, with death occurring by age 4 or 5.

Tay Sachs disease is a result of a deficiency of activity in the *hexosaminidase A* enzyme, which is a lysosomal enzyme. It is inherited in an autosomal recessive pattern.

The typical presentation of Tay Sachs is **normal development through the first 9 months.** At that point non-specific signs appear, including *lethargy* and *hypotonia*. Important signs specific to Tay Sachs include **exaggerated startle reflex, cherry red spot on the retina,** and **macrocephaly.**

This leads to continued deterioration, including *blindness* and *seizures,* with death occurring by the age of 5.

---

[8] Krabbe disease is technically a leukodystrophy, not a storage disorder.

While it is widely known to occur in Ashkenazi Jews, it can occur in other groups, including French Canadians. Due to widespread screening among Ashkenazi Jews, most infants born today with Tay Sachs disease are from couples where only one member is Jewish. *Therefore, screening is recommended even when only one parent is an Ashkenazi Jew.*

Niemann-Pick Disease

This also presents with a cherry red spot and CNS deterioration, **but there IS also hepatosplenomegaly**.

Both Niemann-Pick and Tay-Sachs have cherry red spots, but only Niemann-Pick disease has hepatosplenomegaly. Infantile Gaucher disease would also present with a cherry red spot and hepato-splenomegaly; however, you will more than likely be called upon to distinguish Tay-Sachs from Niemann-Pick disease.

I picture a "Pick Axe" attacking the liver and spleen, causing inflammation.

Prenatal screening

Prenatal screening is available through amniocentesis or CVS sampling.

The parents' carrier status does not need to be known. This may seem obvious, but they have been known to ask questions where several choices are based on the parents' carrier status. Taking a family history of premature deaths due to metabolic disorders, ethnic background, and geographical origin of the family are all important factors for screening disorders that are not part of *routine* screening. In this case, ethnic and racial profiling would be appropriate and helpful.

Class of Disorders	Age, Characteristics, Lab Findings
Inborn Errors of Metabolism	Infant with *sudden onset of lethargy, vomiting, tachypnea, apnea, irritability, or seizures*
Storage Disease	Late infancy or early childhood, with slowly progressive symptoms
Glycogen Storage Disease	When meals are more spread out, i.e., the infant is sleeping more
Fatty Acid Oxidation Disorders	When meals are more spread out, i.e., the infant is sleeping more Illness or stress increase metabolic demands, leading to hypoglycemia, metabolic acidosis, and hyperammonemia **Nonketotic**
Organic Acidemias (methylmalonic acidemia, propionic acidemia, and isovaleric acidemia)	Metabolic acidosis, increased anion gap, hyperammonemia, **Hypoglycemia** Neutropenia and thrombocytopenia can be a part of the picture with organic acidemias
Urea Cycle Defects	Hyperammonemia **without acidosis, Respiratory Alkalosis**
Mitochondrial Disorders	Elevated lactate and pyruvate
Maple Syrup Urine Disease	Acidosis and **hypoglycemia**
Non-ketotic Hyperglycinemia	Acute encephalopathy, **no metabolic acidosis, no hyperammonemia**

Vitamin Therapy that Works

Vitamin therapy is effective with a select group of metabolic disorders and you will be expected to recognize when this treatment applies.

BH4 you Pick PKU

The presence of elevated serum phenylalanine levels on PKU screening might not be garden variety PKU disease. In fact, 1-3% of the cases of positive screens are actually deficient in the co-enzyme tetrahydrobiopterin (BH4). Of course, the incidence is much higher on the boards.

In addition, it is important to note that elevated phenylalanine levels can be **transient,** which is why the test must be repeated before a definitive diagnosis is made.

CASE STUDY

You are presented with a toddler diagnosed in infancy with PKU who has been treated with an appropriate low phenylalanine diet. Despite this, neurological degeneration develops. You will then be asked to determine what deficiency can explain this.

THE DIVERSION

You could be presented with all sorts of diversionary choices to pick from, including the enzyme responsible for PKU, phenylalanine hydroxylase. If you pick the PKU enzyme, you have picked your way closer to a failing score.

ANSWER REVEALED

If you are presented with a child who presumably has garden variety PKU, and who has been treated appropriately and remains symptomatic, the diagnosis is probably off. Therefore, the correct answer regarding the deficiency responsible for this scenario would be BH4 (or its full name, to add more confusion, which is **tetrahydrobiopterin**).

Chapter 16

Is That an Orchidometer in Your Pocket?: Endocrinology

Sexual Differentiation

Normal Sexual Development and Differentiation

In order to better understand the breakdown in sexual differentiation, it is worthwhile to first review normal sexual development and differentiation, in order to clarify any potentially confusing concepts now rather than later.

This is important, as there are many questions on the exam covering this subject

· The **presence of androgens** is responsible for the **formation of male external genitals** in genetic males (XY)
· The **presence of müllerian inhibiting factor** results in the regression of female internal duct structure in genetic males.

HOT TIP

Therefore, the default pattern of differentiation of the genital system is toward phenotypical "femaleness," unless the system is dominated by the influence of testosterone and müllerian inhibiting factor.

XY

Precocious Puberty

DEFINITION

Precocious puberty in boys is defined as the appearance of secondary sexual characteristics before 9 years of age.

Precocious puberty in girls is defined as the appearance of secondary sexual characteristics before 7 years of age. This can appear as pubic hair development (adrenarche) alone, breast development (thelarche) alone, or a combination of both.

Premature Adrenarche

DEFINITION

If pubic hair is the only manifestation (without other secondary sexual characteristics), it is termed premature adrenarche. This may also include acne and body odor.

This would correlate with *elevated serum dehydroepiandrosterone (DHEA) and dehydroepiandrosterone-sulfate (DHEA-S) levels*. It would also correlate with low concentrations of testosterone. This does not usually require treatment unless bone age is advanced more than one year beyond chronological age.

In males or females, adrenarche can be caused by exogenous androgen or an endogenous androgen-secreting tumor. It can also be caused by late-onset congenital adrenal hyperplasia.

HOT TIP

In boys, androgen-secreting tumors may result in penile enlargement and pubic hair growth. Testes may be increased in volume (as in the case of increased androgen being produced by the testes). Tumors producing HCG can cause pubertal change in boys, but not in girls. Girls require LH and FSH to stimulate ovarian estrogen production.

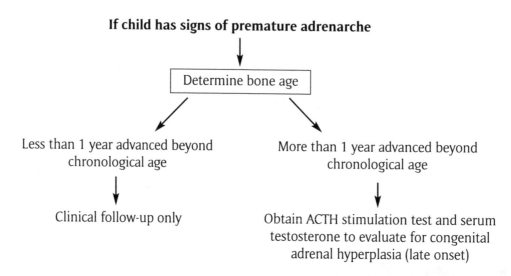

If child has signs of premature adrenarche

Determine bone age

Less than 1 year advanced beyond chronological age → Clinical follow-up only

More than 1 year advanced beyond chronological age → Obtain ACTH stimulation test and serum testosterone to evaluate for congenital adrenal hyperplasia (late onset)

* If measured, DHEA-S is somewhat elevated in children with premature adrenarche, and testosterone concentrations are typically low

* Insulin resistance is thought to be a primary factor in the increased incidence of premature adrenarche in overweight children.

* Premature adrenarche could be an early sign of polycystic ovary syndrome in adolescent girls.

Premature Thelarche

Premature thelarche is breast development in the absence of other sexual characteristics. Premature thelarche alone could be due to exogenous estrogen or a tumor producing estrogen endogenously. It can also be caused by the premature activation of the hypothalamic-pituitary axis.

Sources of *exogenous sex steroids* could be hinted at in the question, including *skin preparations, oral contraceptive medication exposure, weight lifting steroids,* and *plant-based phytoestrogens.*

Central Precocious Puberty

In central precocious puberty, the pubertal development would be sequential but premature. In boys, the first sign of true puberty or central precocious puberty would be testicular enlargement.

Please note that central precocious puberty can be due to *ovarian* or *adrenal tumors.*

> ### Benign Premature Thelarche and Adrenarche
>
> Benign premature thelarche, as the name implies, is a relatively benign finding, usually seen before age 4. It can present with unilateral or bilateral breast development in the absence of other symptoms. In 10% of the cases, true central precocious puberty will develop later on. In girls there is an increased risk for developing ovarian hyperandrogenism.
>
> In benign premature adrenarche, the presentation is consistent with adrenal sex hormone production, including pubic hair and acne.

Ambiguous Genitalia (What's in an Organ?)

A **micropenis** can look like **ambiguous genitalia**.

- With **micropenis**, they will have to show or describe a normally-formed penis with the **meatus in the right place** and **testes present** within the scrotal sacs.

- With **ambiguous genitalia**, you might not have testes present or the meatus in the proper place.

Male Pseudohermaphroditism

Male pseudohermaphrodites are genetic males with female phenotypical features or ambiguous genitalia.

Maternal exposure to androgens or progestins can result in virilized[1] female infants.

---

[1] No, that does not mean genitalia infected with virus but male features such as hypertrophied clitoris.

BUZZ WORDS A typical presentation would be an XY infant with "clitoromegaly" and *palpable masses in the labial folds.*

True Hermaphroditism

PERIL WARNING True hermaphroditism (both ovarian and testicular tissue) is extremely rare, even on the Boards, and thus it is unlikely to be the correct answer.

HOT TIP Often these children are raised as females who are ultimately infertile. Therefore, watch for a history of "aunts who are infertile."

PERIL WARNING 5-alpha-reductase deficiency (can't reduce testosterone to DHT) and 17-ketosteroid-reductase deficiency (impaired conversion of androstenedione to testosterone) must be ruled out in these patients as well.

Persistent Müllerian Duct Syndrome

The müllerian (paramesonephric) ducts are destined to become the *uterus, cervix, upper vagina,* and *fallopian tubes.* Since the fetal testes produce *müllerian inhibiting substance,* this process is interrupted unless there are genetic disorders resulting in:

A) müllerian inhibiting substance not being formed

B) lack of receptors for müllerian inhibiting substance

This results in the formation of *uterus, upper vagina,* and *fallopian tubes* or parts thereof in otherwise normal XY males (cryptorchidism may be present as well).

EITHER OR CHOICES Patients with **Klinefelter syndrome** genetically will be **XXY,** and might present with smaller testicles and phallus, but will not present with müllerian remnants.

BUZZ WORDS On routine procedures (eg., inguinal hernia repair or cryptorchidism management) or imaging studies, a male child may be noted to have *fallopian tubes* or a *rudimentary uterus,* along with *normal testicular tissue* and *normal testicular* and *phallus size.*

Testicular Feminization/Androgen Insensitivity

DEFINITION These are genetic males with end organ insensitivity to androgens, resulting in 1) the inability to develop male external genitalia and in 2) a blind-ending vagina and no uterus. [2]

---

[2] Testicular feminization is not a preferred term anymore.

At least from the outside, there is nothing ambiguous about the genitalia.

Here are the important features to remember:

❏ They are "genetically" male (XY)
❏ Peripheral receptors are resistant to the effects of testosterone.

Therefore, there is a normal looking vagina. However, testes will often be found in the inguinal canal.

HOT TIP Consider this as a diagnosis when presented with a patient with primary amenorrhea with no uterus or ovaries. This is an X-linked disorder! See scenario below.

HOT TIP Müllerian inhibiting factor IS produced; therefore, no uterus or ovaries develop, which is the reason for the vagina ending in a blind pouch. This is why it is important to have a basic understanding of embryological development.

Panhypopituitarism

DEFINITION Panhypopituitarism is a deficit in all hormones produced by the pituitary gland.

BUZZ WORDS It can also present as **micropenis**, and when it does, **hypoglycemia** will also be included in the description.

HOT TIP You want to also check thyroid function. TSH can be decreased when GH is decreased.

HOT TIP Panhypopit can be part of the following syndromes: Prader-Willi (slick Willy), Kallmann (poor sense of smell), or septo-optic dysplasia. Evaluating renal function should also be part of the workup.

CASE STUDY **You may be presented with a child who is phenotypically female. They may hint that the child is genetically male. Then the majority of the question will describe an x-linked disorder and ask for a diagnosis.**

THE DIVERSION By emphasizing the phenotypical identification of gender, i.e., a female, those who realize that females do not have these diseases may mistakenly rule out x-linked disorders.

ANSWER REVEALED If you watch for signs that you are dealing with a genetic male and watch for the description of a classic x-linked disorder, you will turn a difficult question into a slam dunk.

Congenital Adrenal Hyperplasia (CAH)

Congenital Adrenal Hyperplasia will often[3] present in the **newborn period** with a **shocky/septic picture**.

- With **males**, there will be **no ambiguous genitalia,** but there could be *excessive scrotal pigmentation*, so look for this in the question.
- With **females, ambiguous genitalia will probably be present**.

They will not come right out and hit you over the head with a hammer and say "ambiguous genitalia." Instead they will note "ruggated labia," "clitoral hypertrophy," and a wardrobe closely approximating 80s rock star Boy George.

The male features are due to increased androgen levels.

Not for Newborns Only

> **You are presented with a patient with growth delay. They point out that the patient "has received no medical care to date." They casually point out a recent history of hirsutism and amenorrhea. They ask for the most likely underlying condition.**
>
> The diversion here is their noting that the child has received no medical care to date. This will set you away from what is usually seen as a congenital condition causing growth delay.
>
> The correct answer will be CAH. This is an autosomal recessive (AR) disease. Remember that CAH can present beyond the newborn period. Therefore, do not rule this out just because they note that the child has required no medical intervention to date. There is also a *late-onset form of CAH* that should be considered as a possible cause of growth delay.

---

[3] But not always.

Another Traffic Report

CAH can be due to cortisol production being blocked along the endocrine highway. Like any highway with a bottleneck blockage, traffic builds up along the inroad that feeds it. The endocrine highway is no different. *21-Hydroxylase* is needed to produce both *aldosterone* and *cortisol.* When blocked, production of steroids *leading up to the block* is increased, just like cars behind a traffic jam stack up.

HOT TIP

This is the reason for the increased levels of testosterone resulting in virilization.

BUZZ WORDS

Watch for their mentioning a history of other family members taking prescribed testosterone gels for hypogonadism. If precautions are not taken, this can be absorbed by other close contacts, resulting in virilization in both males and females.

CASE STUDY

You are presented with labs that will imply other "salt-wasting disorders," and the question may mention a family history of early death. Buried in the description will be the implication of ambiguous genitalia.

THE DIVERSION

The implication and diversion is a diagnosis of cystic fibrosis, because CF has an increased amount of sodium present in sweat, resulting in decreased serum sodium, and therefore, in "salt wasting."

ANSWER REVEALED

Yes, cystic fibrosis is another salt waster. However, CF does not have anything to do with ambiguous genitalia, which all but rules out CF for the purpose of the exam.

Labs

While there are different varieties and flavors, the most common cause of CAH is **21-hydroxylase deficiency**. In addition, the "salt wasting" variety will present with **hyperkalemia** and **hyponatremia,** as well as an **elevated 17-hydroxyprogesterone**.[4]

Remember, with 21-hydroxylase deficiency, 17-hydroxyprogesterone levels are high.

> Accumulation of androgens will not be as alarming in a male, which is why they are often not picked up early or as easily.

---

4 The precursor just before the deficient enzyme.

Screening for CAH

 Screening for CAH is done via the 17-hydroxy progesterone assay.

If elevated, repeating the test is the next step.

If the repeat is positive, then measurement of serum electrolytes and urinary sodium/potassium excretion would be the next step.

Prenatal screening is also available via *molecular genetic testing of fetal cells.*

Measurement of 17-hydroxyprogesterone in amniotic fluid would not be the correct answer. This is *not* how prenatal screening is done anymore.

Treating CAH

Pharmacological treatment of congenital CAH is with glucocorticoid, usually administered as *hydrocortisone.* If given in high enough doses, it will have a mineralocorticoid effect in addition to a glucocorticoid effect.

Adrenal Disorders

The adrenals can simply stop functioning on their own (primary), or shut down if they are not receiving the signal from the pituitary gland (secondary) [5].

Primary Adrenal Deficiency (Addison Disease)

The adrenals stop working for a variety of reasons, ranging from *autoimmune disease* to *infection* to the always popular *idiopathic.*[6]

When the adrenals stop functioning – and cortisol is not produced, regardless of the reason – the message to the brain is "pour out ACTH by the bucketful."

The increased ACTH levels explain the **hyperpigmentation**.[7] When aldosterone isn't produced, salt wasting is the result and **hyperkalemia** and **hyponatremia** are seen. Fatigue and weight loss are other signs.

---

[5] The signal coming from the pituitary is ACTH.
[6] Latin for "we really don't know".
[7] Increased melanin.

Addison disease is usually an autoimmune disorder. Patients with Addison disease are also at risk for other endocrine disorders, including diabetes, ovarian failure, and hypothyroidism.

Secondary Adrenal Deficiency

With secondary adrenal deficiency, there is *no problem with the adrenal gland* itself. The problem is with the organ it takes orders from, the pituitary, which is "asleep at the wheel."

The pituitary makes ACTH. As they say, "No squirt, no ACTH, no cortisol service," or something like that. In this case, ACTH levels are low. With primary adrenal deficiency, ACTH levels are high.

In secondary aldosterone deficiency, which is really a central deficiency, ACTH levels **are low.** Since there is no aldosterone deficiency, there is *no hyperkalemia, hyponatremia, or salt wasting in secondary (central) adrenal deficiency.* There is also no hyperpigmentation.

Remember, CRH stimulates the pituitary to release ACTH. CRH can be used to distinguish pituitary disorders from hypothalamic failure in secondary adrenal deficiency. The cosyntropin[8] stimulation test (ACTH stimulation test) is used to test the adrenals, and results in no rise in cortisol levels in primary adrenal deficiency. If you have secondary disease, then the adrenals usually have normal cortisol stores, and cortisol will be released during the cosyntropin test.

Look for clues in the question of "midline defects," such as cleft lip and/or palate. This will be their way of telling you the problem is probably in the pituitary and, therefore, secondary adrenal deficiency.

Adrenal Insufficiency due to Medication Withdrawal

Patients who abruptly stop taking adrenocorticoid or glucocorticoid medications can present with signs of adrenal insufficiency, including muscle weakness, as well as decreased cardiac function (with increased pulse and decreased blood pressure).

Electrolyte imbalance would not be seen in this case.

---

[8] Synthetic corticotropin (ACTH 1-24)

Cushing Syndrome

Is characterized by core obesity as a result of glucocorticoid excess. Other typical findings include moon facies, hirsutism, easy bruising, as well as a buffalo hump.

In mild cases lab values could be normal

Short Stature

Rate of Growth

- ❏ **Prior to Puberty**: 5-6 cm/year.

- ❏ **During Puberty/Girls**: There will be a gradual increase in growth rate. Peak growth velocity is 9-10 cm/year.

PERIL WARNING They may not give you this information in centimeters. They may give it to you in inches so have those handy PDAs handy. (Or, if you are really smart, you can multiply by 2.5 to get cm from inches!)

Aging Your Bones and Looking at Bone Age

You will not be required to actually recognize a bone age by looking at it. That is what they have radiologists in dark rooms with flashlights, hot lights, dictaphones and disco balls for. However, they will tell you what the bone age is, usually in comparison to height and chronological age.

Peak Growth

HOT TIP In girls, peak growth velocity occurs ~1.5 years before menarche. Therefore, once females have reached menarche, they are within 1-2 inches of their adult height.

Better Late than Early

Maturing earlier usually means a shorter adult height. For boys, that may mean being the bigger, tougher kid in class, only to be shorter than average later in life. For girls, it will mean being taller than even most of the boys at first.

Let's look at some of the specific causes of short stature.

Growth Hormone Deficiency (GHD)

PERIL WARNING Intuitively, growth hormone deficiency is the easiest cause to think of, but it is rarely the cause of short stature on the Boards. Often it will be the wrong answer.

HOT TIP One exception would be that a child with headaches and growth attenuation could be due to a space-occupying lesion, resulting in GHD being responsible for short stature.

When you are presented with short stature, look for clues for other causes (including hypothyroidism, syndromes,[9] chronic illness, genetic short stature, or constitutional short stature).

---

[9] Examples would be Hurlers, Hunters, Morquio, or Turner syndrome.

The growth rate decline of children who have GHD can manifest as early as their first year.

These children often are chubby, and boys may have small genitalia. GHD is associated with a significant delay in bone age, as compared to chronological age (similar to constitutional short stature, which manifests later). Insulin-like growth factor -1 (IGF-1 for short), as well as IGF binding protein 3 (IGF-BP3) are appropriate screening studies for growth hormone deficiency (serum levels of both may be low).

Watch for:

· Sharp decline in the height percentile
· Weight may be normal for age but high for the height, with decreased muscle mass
· Delayed bone age by as much as 2 years

Congenital growth hormone deficiency usually presents during infancy (typically around 6 months of age), with slowed growth. Hypoglycemia could be one of the presenting signs.

In the context of hypopituitarism, associated findings could include hyperbilirubinemia and microphallus.[10]

Nutrition Deficiency

In addition to being proportionate, children with nutrition deficiency may also have a bone age that is equal to the chronological age. Of course the *height age will usually be below normal.*

CASE STUDY — **You are presented with a child with growth delay who is otherwise asymptomatic. You are then asked for the most likely cause or the next step to establish a diagnosis.**

THE DIVERSION — Among the choices you will be presented with will be Crohn's disease. However, since you have been told that the child is asymptomatic, you may be diverted into crossing out Crohn's disease among the choices.

ANSWER REVEALED — Crohn's disease can result in growth delay, which can precede the GI symptoms. Therefore, *ordering an ESR could be the correct answer.* Similarly, an elevated ESR in the lab values could be your clue in the question, and the correct answer will be Crohn's disease.

---

[10] In boys of course.

Constitutional Delay (Late Bloomers)

This is the classic "late bloomer." It is **more common in males**.

Typically they will describe a family history of a similar growth pattern in the father and brother.

· The **growth curve** may show a **decrease in growth rate**, usually in **early teen years**. **Delayed onset of puberty** and **bone age below chronological age** is the rule.

· There is a later onset of increased growth velocity. The growth rate may accelerate at around age 16 years.

Bone age is below (younger than) chronological age (think of the gap as the "bud" for the later bloomer to blossom in the spring). In addition to height, sexual development also lags behind.

If they ask for the best way to assess for growth delay, the answer is to compare bone age to chronological age. A look at family history is also important. Remember, the least invasive and less exotic the answer, the more likely it is to be correct.

Growth velocity may be blunted in early adolescence. However, when this is preceded by poor weight gain, it is abnormal, and a workup may be warranted. Celiac disease is an example of a cause which may be distinguished from constitutional growth delay through lab studies. Assuming normal serum IgA levels, the best way to screen for celiac disease would be to test for elevated levels of IgA antibodies against tissue transglutaminase (anti-tTG). Testing for IgA antibodies to endomysium is also used sometimes.

Low total serum IgA levels would invalidate the screening study.

SMR –
sexual maturity Rating

> **CASE STUDY**
>
> **You are presented with a 15-year-old boy who is short for his age, with a low SMR. His growth velocity is normal. The family notes that the father had the same "problem" and received "shots." You are asked to pick the most appropriate intervention at this time.**
>
> **THE DIVERSION**
>
> The father receiving IM shots is the diversion.
>
> **ANSWER REVEALED**
>
> The correct answer would be to reassure and wait, since the correct diagnosis would be constitutional growth delay. The fact that the father received IM shots tells you nothing, especially if it's in quotes.
>
> If they note a history of maternal delayed onset of menarche, this too is associated with constitutional growth delay in both boys and girls.

Familial Short Stature (Just Plain Short/Genetic Short Stature)

BUZZ WORDS

Sometimes short kids are just kids who are from "short stock," and will grow up to be short adults. They will be around or below the 5th percentile for height, with a bone age equal to chronological age. Growth velocity will be normal. They may even mention that the parents are short as well.[11]

> **CASE STUDY**
>
> **You are presented with a patient whose parents want to know his potential height. They will present you with the parents' heights, but buried in the question will be an implication that one or both of the parents were malnourished growing up.**
>
> **THE DIVERSION**
>
> The diversion here is their providing you with the parents' height. You will be diverted away from factoring in the parents' failure to reach their genetic potential due to malnourishment.
>
> **ANSWER REVEALED**
>
> The correct answer will be that the child will likely be taller than the parents, assuming the child is receiving adequate nutrition.

---

[11] More than likely, they will simply tell you the parents' height and let you figure out that they are short.

Here, the **bone age will equal the chronological age**, which would distinguish it from constitutional growth delay.

Syndromes that Make You Short

Turner syndrome

Turner syndrome is an example of a syndrome that might not become evident until puberty.

If they drop hints like "pedal edema" or "scant breast tissue," consider a karyotype as part of the workup to rule out Turner syndrome.

Turner syndrome patients are often **treated with** growth hormone.

Consider Turner syndrome in any short female.

Achondroplasia

Achondroplasia is an example of a syndrome that presents with short stature, among other things, but the short stature is *not proportionate*.

Congenital Adrenal Hyperplasia

Late onset congenital adrenal hyperplasia could result in short adult stature. The increased androgens result in premature closure of the growth plate.

This has a pattern of early *puberty followed by accelerated growth* that ends early with *short adult height*.

Turning on the Lab Lite

In addition to a karyotype, the following lab studies would be appropriate in a patient suspected of having Turner syndrome.

LSH and *FSH* would be expected to be elevated due to ovarian failure.

Although estradiol levels would be low in Turner syndrome, *estradiol assays may not provide an accurate picture in early puberty*. Therefore, this would not be a useful measure in girls in this age group with suspected Turner syndrome. In this case, it is better to "fish" for Turner with FSH and LH than turn the dial of estradiol.

TSH levels are warranted, since Turner is associated with a higher risk of hypothyroidism (and TSH would be elevated in primary hypothyroidism).

Hypothyroidism

 With hypothyroidism, they will be short AND overweight, but it won't be described that way.

 Children will have delayed bone age, so they could describe an 11-year-old with height consistent with a 9-year-old, and a bone age of a 7-year-old.

They may even drop in some hidden clues consistent with hypothyroidism, such as "cold intolerance," "constipation," "dry skin," or "myxedema."[12]

Bone age would be delayed in hypothyroidism.

Tall Stature

Don't forget the **genetic causes of tall stature**. Here we will review some of the endocrine components of syndromes associated with short stature.

If you are presented with a child who is "tall" for age, and are asked for the most important determinant for ultimate adult height, the answer will be sexual maturity rating. A bone age x-ray could be used to predict her adult height. This will help determine how much additional growth is left.

SMR

Klinefelter Syndrome

While these kids will appear **physically normal at birth**, eventually they will be tall. In addition to tall stature, they could have *learning disabilities* and/or *small testicles*. Gynecomastia may be seen in Klinefelter syndrome. If you are presented with male teenager with gynecomastia *and* other features of Klinefelter, then it cannot be simply passed off as a normal variant.

 Intelligence is often normal.

---

[12] Relatively "hard edema" of the subcutaneous tissue.

Marfan Syndrome

 One of the main features is a cardiac defect, including *aortic aneurysm*. These individuals are at risk for sudden death; therefore, the description of sudden death with tall stature is your clue. Patients with Marfan syndrome have disproportionately long legs and arms in comparison to trunk.

Soto's Syndrome

Soto's syndrome is a congenital cause of tall stature. They will likely also decribe a larger than normal head circumference as well as cognitive deficits. This would most likely be presented in the context of parents who are not tall.

High Caloric Intake

 Here they will be *tall*, often *overweight* and have *advanced bone age*.[13]

- Children with **exogenous obesity** tend to be **tall**.

- Children with **endogenous obesity** secondary to endocrine disorders, on the other hand, tend to be **short**.

Thyroid Disorders

Congenital Hypothyroidism

Patients with congenital hypothyroidism were previously known as "cretins." Neonatal screening thyroid tests are now performed routinely, making untreated hypothyroidism a rare disorder in real life, except on the Boards.

 In addition to the non-specific findings like *poor feeding* and *jaundice*, they will describe more specifics such as "*constipation*," "*hypotonia*," "*hoarse cry*," *large tongue (also known as macroglossia)*, *umbilical hernia*, and "*enlarged anterior fontanelle*."

---

[13] In other words they are big and fat.

Delayed treatment can have long-term consequences, including learning disabilities, cognitive deficits, as well as clumsiness and diminished fine motor skills. T4 and TSH levels should be looked at one month after treatment is started. Initial screening should take place within 24 hours of delivery.

Secondary Hypothyroidism

Hypothyroidism can be caused by hypothalamic or pituitary disease. In this case, TSH levels may be low or normal. Free (unbound) T4 is low in this case.

Hashimoto Thyroiditis

This is also known as **chronic lymphocytic thyroiditis**. Hashimoto's disease is an autoimmune disease characterized by antibodies to thyroid tissue and lymphocytic infiltration. Hashimoto thyroiditis is the most common cause of goiter in adolescents.

Patients are clinically euthyroid or hypothyroid. Most are **asymptomatic** and are discovered by the presence of a goiter. In such cases, TSH should be checked regularly.

In some cases, however, patients can develop thyrotoxicosis known as Hashitoxicosis. Therefore, watch for clues for Hashimoto disease in a patient who is also hyperthyroid.[14]

Hashimoto can also be a part of polyendocrine autoimmune syndromes such as Schmidt syndrome (adrenal involvement, APS or PGA Type II, typically in adults), or can occur with Type I diabetes.

TSH is the key, since T4 can be normal in compensated hypothyroidism. In addition, thyroid antibodies can be present; therefore, look for the presence of *anti-thyroglobulin* and *anti-thyroid peroxidase*. Thyroid ultrasound can be helpful if the antibody levels are not present.

Hashimoto has two "O's" to remind you that hypothyroidism is the more typical presentation. It has an "I" to remind you that it can present with transiently high thyroid hormone.

The Shake on TSH

If you are presented with a teenager on levothyroxine whose free thyroxine (fT4) and TSH levels are both elevated, the most likely explanation would be poor compliance.

In general, if you are presented with a teenager with lab results inconsistent with treatment, *poor compliance* will likely be the correct explanation.

If you are asked which lab results are important before changing the dose of thyroxine, the correct answer would be both fT4 and TSH levels.

---

[14] We included this under hypothyroidism since it is the more typical presentation.

Hyperthyroidism in Childhood

Graves Disease

It is caused by an IgG antibody, known as "thyroid-stimulating immunoglobulin."[15]

With Graves disease, they may describe "bulging eyes" (infiltrative ophthalmopathy). Since children with Graves disease tend to be "revved up," they will emphasize the **emotional lability** (trying to trick you into a psychiatric diagnosis), weight loss, sleep disturbance, and/or heat intolerance. They may even describe "lid lag."

Some of the findings can be more subtle, especially in more mild disease. Subtle findings could include increased appetite with weight loss or decreased muscle strength or endurance. Decreased school performance and hyperactivity are other subtle findings.

Additional signs could include itching, tremors, sweating, or increased urination at night. Females might present with decreased menstrual flow and/or decreased frequency of menses.

There are other causes of hyperthyroidism, but Graves will almost certainly appear on the test, so this is one to know well.

Radioactive iodine uptake would be important in distinguishing Graves disease from subacute thyroiditis. In Graves disease, there would be high uptake, and in subacute thyroiditis, there would be low uptake. Antithyroid therapy would be appropriate with Graves disease, but would be inappropriate with subacute thyroiditis (which is usually transitory and requires only monitoring).

Graves Disease (Neonatal Style)

Neonatal Thyrotoxicosis

Neonatal thyrotoxicosis will present as "irritability, tremors and tachycardia with SVT in the immediate newborn period." This is precisely how this would be differentiated from *any inborn errors*, which *usually do not manifest in the immediate newborn period.* **Symptoms in utero can include increased heart rate and a high output state.**

Failure to thrive, feeding problems, and hyperbilirubinemia are other associated findings.

---

[15] Previously known as LATS during the early 80's.

Because of the risk of cardiac arrhythmias, an immediate thyroid level is indicated. Neonatal Graves disease is caused by a thyroid stimulating antibody in the mother that crossed the placenta. Breakdown of these antibodies is slow.

CASE STUDY

You may be presented with a patient with emotional lability and hyperactivity, with information hinting at a diagnosis of Graves Disease buried in the question.

THE DIVERSION

The diversion is to draw you away from a diagnosis of Graves and towards a diagnosis of bipolar disease or ADHD by emphasizing the emotional lability or disorganization.

ANSWER REVEALED

Remember to consider a diagnosis of Graves disease in emotionally labile and disorganized children, especially if they provide physical and other findings consistent with Graves disease.

TREATMENT

Treatment of hyperthyroidism includes antithyroid meds (including methimazole and/or propylthiouracil), radioactive iodine (felt not to be the carcinogenic risk it once was), or thyroidectomy.

Thyroid Nodules

A solitary thyroid nodule can be a sign of thyroid cancer. There is a greater chance of a nodule being malignant in an adolescent than in an adult. Therefore, watchful waiting is not an option, even though it is an accepted practice in adults. Fine needle aspiration (FNA) is the diagnostic test of choice. FNA can identify virtually all thyroid malignancies.

HOT TIP

Past history of exposure to "ionizing radiation" is a risk factor for malignancy; exposure to "ultraviolet radiation" is not.

Hyperthyroid in Graves and Hashimoto: Telling the Difference

HOT TIP

Since Hashimoto and Graves can both present with hyperthyroid symptoms, how can you tell the difference? Glad you asked. Do the "eyes" have it? No. The presence of bulging eyes may tip you off that it is Graves, but the absence doesn't rule it out, especially on the Boards. Can you measure the human thyroid stimulating immunoglobulin? You can, but not everywhere. The answer will be radioactive iodine uptake. It is elevated in Graves and normal or low in Hashimoto.

If you are presented with a patient who has a thyroid mass, the most informative test would be to do a **fine needle aspiration biopsy**.

131-iodine thyroid scan, once in vogue to distinguish hot from cold nodules, is no longer felt to be useful and will now be the wrong answer on the exam.

Thyroid binding globulin (TBG) Deficiency

This can be a very confusing issue. Therefore, it is ripe for testing on the boards.

The following concepts are keys to understanding how TBG deficiency might present.

- T4 and T3 are reversibly bound to thyroid binding globulin.
- However, it is the **free unbound hormone which is metabolically active**.

A deficiency in TBG is suspected with the following findings:

- Abnormally low serum total T4 concentrations
- Normal free T4
- Clinically euthyroid patient
- Normal TSH

A key point to remember is that thyroid replacement therapy isn't necessary. Normal free T4 concentrations are maintained and the patients remain euthyroid.

Diabetes Mellitus

Since these are the Pediatric Boards and not the Endocrine Boards, a few good facts and concepts should set you up to be prepared.

Diabetes is diagnosed with

2 random glucose values > 200

Or

1 random glucose value > 200 with symptoms

Or

fasting glucose > 126

Or

2 hour post glucose tolerance serum glucose > 200.

Type 1 Diabetes

DEFINITION

Type 1 diabetes is due to islet cell destruction resulting in the inability to produce insulin. This is also known as *insulin dependent diabetes.*

BUZZ WORDS

Type 1 diabetes presents with the classic *polyuria, polydipsia, increased appetite, and weight loss.*

TREATMENT

Treatment would consist of *short and long acting SQ insulin.* Insulin pumps are also used with a baseline rate and manual override for bolus doses for meals. Health maintenance in children older than 10 would include an eye exam. *Lipid levels are monitored starting at age 12.*

Family education regarding disease management is a *crucial component of effective treatment.*

HOT TIP

Patients with *type 1 diabetes are at increased risk for other autoimmune diseases.* For example, there is an increased risk of celiac disease in patients who have type 1 disease, especially in those who have onset of diabetes before age 10.

> ### Honeymoon
>
> Soon after diagnosis of type 1 diabetes mellitus (DM), there will be a gradual reduction in the amount of insulin needed.
>
> This is because the last drops are being squeezed from the islet cells.
>
> **PERIL / WARNING** This does not mean the diagnosis is incorrect. Not remembering this on the exam can come back to haunt you.

Diabetic Ketoacidosis (DKA)

MNEMONIC

Here are a few principles to guide you on the exam.

HOT TIP

DKA is seen in Type 1 diabetes. *Always* consider poor compliance as a contributing factor.

Fluid Replacement

TREATMENT

The first step is rapid volume expansion with 20 cc/kg of NS boluses in the first hour. This is followed by additional replacement as needed. One-half the deficit should be replaced over the first 16 hours.

> *The K levels* will fall for a variety of reasons, mainly having to do with correction of acidosis. Less K comes out of the IC fluid into the EC fluid, plus more K is lost in the urine with correction.

> ### Reality Compliance Check
>
> The best way to check long term compliance in a diabetic is the glycosylated hemoglobin test (Hemoglobin A1C). This is frequently asked.

Watch the Bouncing Na

DKA is a sodium deficit at first. When the serum Na is high, then you have severe dehydration. If the serum sodium falls with rehydration, consider SIADH (or poor management) as the answer they are looking for.

Putting the K in DKA

In DKA there is a K deficit, regardless of the initial value they give you. Up to 60 mEq K/Liter can be given when the serum potassium is low at presentation, provided urine output is established.

Sugar and Spice

You begin to add glucose in the IV fluids when the serum glucose drops below 300. Insulin should be given IV until the patient is stable.[16]

Watch that Sign

When rehydration is too rapid, one thing to watch out for is cerebral edema. The treatment will be the same for any case of increased ICP, so this could be the last part of a series of questions.

Bicarb in DKA

Bicarbonate has very limited use in DKA and in most clinical scenarios you might be presented with, so be careful when choosing it as an answer.

Bicarb should only be used when the pH is below 7.1, and only to bring it up to a pH of 7.2. It should not be used if the patient is hypokalemic, unless potassium supplementation has been started.

The reason for this is as follows:

- Bicarb leads to increased CO_2, which is more permeable to the blood brain barrier, resulting in increased CO_2 levels in the CSF
- It can lead to metabolic alkalosis
- It can lead to hypokalemia, already a problem in patients in DKA with a low total body potassium level.

---

[16] This means a blood sugar no more than 300, pH greater than 7.3, and bicarb greater than 15.

Treatment with bicarb may increase the chance of cerebral edema in children. The treatment for ketoacidosis in DKA is insulin, not bicarb.

Type 2 Diabetes

Type 2 diabetes is primarily due to insulin resistance.

The typical presentation is an obese child. Physical findings, in addition to obesity, could include **acanthosis nigricans,** which will be described as *dark, thickened, velvety patches of skin.*

Initial treatment of Type 2 diabetes is non-pharmacological. This means improved nutrition, less sitting, and more exercise. If this does not work, then **metformin**, an oral hypoglycemic agent, is used.

Type 1 and Type 2 diabetes can be distinguished from each other by measuring **autoantibodies against pancreatic beta cells, which should only be present in type 1 diabetes**.

CASE STUDY

You are evaluating a child who presents with findings consistent with *acanthosis nigricans*. The child is obese. You are asked to pick the most likely laboratory finding.

THE DIVERSION

Right there waiting for you to pick up an easy answer would be elevated fasting blood glucose.

ANSWER REVEALED

Acanthosis nigricans is correlated with insulin resistance, not necessarily type 2 diabetes. It is more common to see an insulin-resistant and obese child who compensates with increased insulin and remains euglycemic. In this case, the expected laboratory finding would be **low HDL cholesterol**.

from sitting around

Hyperosmolar Diabetic Coma

Type 2 diabetics who are insulin resistant with high glucose may present with non-ketotic hyperosmolar diabetic coma.

The presentation will include elevated serum osmolality and serum glucose.

The goal of treatment is the same as DKA, which is to make the patient euvolemic and euglycemic without throwing the patient into cerebral edema. Fluid replacement should take place over 36-48 hours (similar to managing hypernatremic dehydration, for those of you who like to make connections).

Metabolic Syndrome

Metabolic syndrome is a series of clinical and laboratory findings as outlined below, which you are expected to be familiar with.

1. Elevated serum triglycerides
2. Low HDL
3. Hypertension
4. Hyperglycemia, typically a fasting glucose greater than 100
5. Truncal obesity

There is some controversy regarding the exact definition, **and a consensus definition may be newly available. Researchers have so far tended to use modified adult criteria.**

Acanthosis nigricans is **not** one of the criteria for metabolic syndrome.

Calcium Metabolism

I always found this a bit difficult to follow. It involves way too many organs and levels to measure and keep straight. However, it is well worth the time invested to study. So let's go to the blackboard.

Hypercalcemia = serum calcium greater than 11 mg/dL.

Hypercalcemia: The Causes

Prolonged Immobilization

If they present a patient with prolonged immobilization, then hypercalcemia may be a lab finding.

A wishbone is made of calcium, so think of the word **WISH** to remember the causes of hypercalcemia:

Williams Syndrome
Ingestion (Vitamin D and A Intoxication, Thiazide Diuretics)
Skeletal Disorders (Dysplasias and Immobilization/Body Casts)
Hyperparathyroidism

Treating Hypercalcemia

If a child has hypercalcemia secondary to being immobilized, and shows no specific signs like vomiting and irritability, the best treatment is with high volume fluid, furosemide (Lasix®), and EKG monitoring. In rare cases *calcitonin* is used.

Hypocalcemia: The Causes

Hypocalcemia = Ionized calcium lower than 4.5 mg/dL (1.0 mmol/L), and a total calcium lower than 8.5 mg/dL.

A classic presentation of hypocalcemia could include the following:

- **· Painful muscle spasms**
- **· Generalized seizures**
- **· Vomiting**
- **· Prolonged QT interval on EKG**

HOT TIP In particular, watch for a seizure that is resistant to diazepam. Also look for the classic **Chvostek** and **Trousseau signs. Watch out for hypomagnesemia as well.**

DEFINITION **Chvostek sign** is elicited by tapping just anterior to the ear lobe below the cheek bone. Contraction of the distal muscles is a positive finding.

DEFINITION **Trousseau sign** is much easier, it is elicited by inflating the blood pressure cuff above systolic pressure and leaving it there for 2 minutes (ouch! Don't forget to come back to the patient!) A positive finding would be carpal muscle spasm on that side.

MNEMONIC Remember the causes of hypocalcemia by picturing somebody getting drained of all the calcium (which is colored white = milk). Well, if you were drained of all of your pigmentation, you would look quite **PINK**.

Pseudohypoparathyroidism[18]

Intake (nutritional deficiency), **I**mmune Deficiency (DiGeorge syndrome)

Nephrotic Syndrome *(with a lowered albumin level, there is a lower calcium level)*

Kidney *(renal insufficiency results in higher phosphate, lower calcium, and a secondary hyperparathyroidism)*

Seizures can occur in the face of hypocalcemia.

EITHER OR CHOICES A combination of *hypocalcemia* and *hyper-phosphatemia* correlates with *hypoparathyroidism*.

Hypocalcemia and *hypo-phosphatemia* correlate with vitamin D deficiency.

Pseudohypoparathyroidism would present with high PTH *AND* **hypocalcemia,** because of end organ resistance to the hormone. They can be described as being developmentally delayed, short, and obese with moon facies and calcification of the basal ganglia.

HOT TIP If you are presented with a neonate who is LGA and hypoglycemic with hypocalcemia, there is a strong probability that you are being presented with an infant of a diabetic mother, even if this is not stated outright.

---

[18] Peripheral tissue is resistant to the effects of the parathyroid hormone; they are just not listening so PTH levels are high.

Hypoparathyroidism

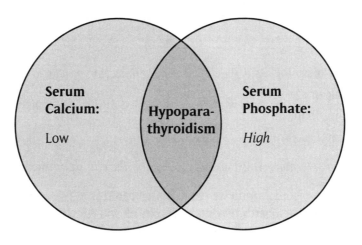

Vitamin D Deficiency

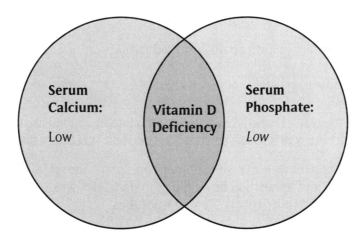

Rickety Rickets

Navigating the bridge of Rickets can get quite "rickety" indeed. However, if you take our hand and don't look down, we can navigate this bridge together and get across unscathed.

First what is **Rickets**? *Rickets is the deficient mineralization of bone.* This can be due to:

· Low Calcium

· Low Phosphate

· Both Low Calcium and Low Phosphate

You will be expected to determine which one it is, based on the clinical presentation and the lab findings.

Many, many, many, many disorders (and we mean many) can result in low calcium and/or low phosphate and subsequently, rickets. The boards may make you think you need a degree in metabolism, fluids, and lytes, but, rest assured that if you use the testing tips, and think through the question, you'll be A-OK.

There are a number of risk factors to watch out for in the presenting history that should point you toward a diagnosis of rickets:

1. Breast feeding without vitamin D supplementation

2. Poor exposure to natural sunlight (pay attention if they note the baby is dark skinned)

3. Low birth weight, prematurity, or both

In addition, children on certain **anticonvulsant medications** are at risk for developing rickets. Watch for this in the history.

Regardless of the type of rickets (which we'll jump into in a moment), there are classic characteristics in the history that should lead you to conclude rickets as a diagnosis.

Children with rickets present with a combination of **bone pain, anorexia, decreased growth rate, widening of the wrist and knees,** and **bowed legs**. In particular, look for the enlarged costochondral junctions, known as the **"rachitic rosary,"** and **craniotabes**.

Dental complications, including *delayed eruption of teeth,* could also be a part of the presenting history.

Serum alkaline phosphatase levels will be elevated in all forms of rickets.

Vitamin D Deficient (Nutritional) Rickets

Vitamin D deficient (nutritional) rickets occurs in infants who have inadequate **intake of vitamin D** and/or **poor exposure to sunlight**. This can be due to:

> · **Inadequate intake** – This would occur in the infant being breast-fed by a mother who is **vegetarian,** or a *mother who is not being supplemented with vitamin D or getting enough sunlight.*

> · **Malabsorption** – Any child suffering from a disorder leading to malabsorption would also be at risk for developing nutritional rickets.

African American babies are at particular risk, because of lower absorption of UV light. A typical presentation would be an African American infant, born in the fall or early winter, who is being breastfed without vitamin D supplementation.

Watch for children who are lactose intolerant since, by stating such in the history, they will expect you to realize that the patient (by avoiding dairy products) is vulnerable to vitamin-deficient rickets.

An *elevated PTH level*, decreased serum calcium and phosphate, along with a decreased 25-hydroxy vitamin D level, confirm vitamin D deficient rickets. Among the classic types we are describing, **this will be the only one where a 25-hydroxy vitamin D level will be low**.

Treatment is with vitamin D and calcium supplementation.

Do not get tricked into getting a 1,25-dihydroxy vitamin D level. You might think, "well, it must be a better test because it is the more active metabolite," but, unless there is a renal problem (see below), the 1,25- dihydroxy vitamin D level can actually be normal.

Vitamin D Dependent Rickets Type 1

Vitamin D dependent rickets (autosomal recessive) is due to *inadequate renal production of 1,25 dihydroxy vitamin D.*

This is treated with, you guessed right, 1,25-dihydroxy vitamin D.

This topic is confusing enough as a stationary target. But it is even more difficult when the nomenclature is a moving target.

This used to be called pseudo-Vitamin D-resistant rickets. What can possibly be more frustrating than studying and not even knowing if you are reading about the same disorder with two different names?

 Clinically, the presentation is the same as vitamin D deficient rickets. However, **there will be no clinical improvement with vitamin D replacement therapy**. In addition to low serum calcium and phosphate levels, the important lab finding of vitamin D dependent rickets type 1 is a **very low 1,25-dihydroxy vitamin D level**.

The 25-hydroxy vitamin D level will be normal.

Treatment is with **Vitamin D$_2$ and 1,25-dihydroxy vitamin D.**

Vitamin D Dependent Rickets Type 2

Vitamin D dependent rickets Type 2 (also autosomal recessive) is due to **end organ resistance to vitamin D.**

The primary difference between Type One and Type Two is that in Type One, 1,25-dihydroxy vitamin D is decreased due to poor or absent production, while in Type Two, 1,25-dihydroxy vitamin D is elevated due to end organ resistance.

This is the true "resistant" type, and it is starting to be called just that, "Hereditary Vitamin D Resistant Rickets." This might make more sense than calling it a Vitamin D "Dependant" type, as treatment is very difficult.

Vitamin D Resistant Rickets

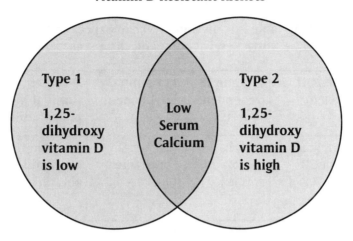

X-Linked Hypophosphatemic Rickets

At this point, you probably think that you can't get any crazier, and your eyes are rolling upside down in their sockets.

X-Linked Hypophosphatemic Rickets was also known as Vitamin D resistant rickets! How not fair is that?

In X-linked hypophosphatemic rickets, the problem is due to *excessive phosphate loss through the kidneys*. This is known as *X-linked familial hypophosphatemia*.

It's one of those rare **X-linked dominant diseases,** and it's the most common cause of rickets in industrialized countries.

X-linked hypophosphatemic rickets is also characterized by decreased conversion of 25-hydroxy vitamin D to 1,25-dihydroxy vitamin D. The two processes (phosphate loss from kidneys and lack of activation) are thought to result from the same gene mutation.[19] This is why it used to be called vitamin D **resistant rickets**, since Vitamin D won't help - but 1,25-dihydroxy vitamin D will.

Treatment of vitamin D resistant rickets is with phosphate supplementation. In addition, 1,25-dihydroxy vitamin D is needed.

---

[19] PHEX, for those of you who actually care about such things!

Crossing the Rickety Rickets Bridge

A variation on the following table is something you can expect to see on the exam. Knowing this information cold will be worth several points on the exam.

	Vitamin D deficient	Vitamin D Dependent Type 1	Vitamin D Dependent Type 2	X-Linked Familial hypo-phosphatemic	Renal Disease
THE UNDERLYING CAUSE	Nutritional Deficit OR Poor UV Light Exposure	1- alpha hydroxylase deficiency	End Organ resistance	Defect in tubular reabsorption of phosphate	Defect in phophate excretion
Phosphate	Low	Low	Low	Low	High
Calcium	Low	Low	Low	Normal	Decrease
Alkaline Phos	High	High	High	Elevated	High
PTH	High	High	High	Normal	High
1,25 Vitamin D	Normal	Low	High	Normal	Decrease

OK – so do you have all that, now?

Vitamin D deficient is just that, Vitamin D is missing or not absorbed.

Vitamin D dependent has two types –

> **Type I** just doesn't make 1,25-dihydroxy vitamin D well (or at all)
>
> **Type II** makes plenty, but is resistant to vitamin D
>
> **X-linked hypophosphatemic** has a conversion component and a hypophosphatemic component.

As we mentioned in the beginning of this section, they may throw other types at you. For example, there is a hereditary hypophosphatemic type that results (probably) from inability to resorb phosphate. This type has hypercalciuria, and would not need calcitriol (1,25-dihydroxy vitamin D) supplementation.

Our advice: know what you know, and if it looks like something you don't know, reason it out based on the clinical/lab findings that they give you.

Vitamin D *resistant* rickets can be distinguished from vitamin D *deficient* rickets by the serum parathyroid hormone level (PTH).

- **Vitamin D resistant rickets** (familial hypophosphatemia) has a **normal** serum PTH level
- **Vitamin D deficient rickets** has an elevated serum PTH level

 Renal tubular acidosis can also result in rickets.

Rickets of Prematurity

Rickets of prematurity bears mentioning here.

Vitamin D supplementation is inadequate treatment. Calcium and phosphorus supplementation are also needed.

The *most specific* risk factor for vitamin D deficient rickets is *very low birthweight.*

Chapter 17

GI: What to Know!

This is the section where you literally have to know everything from soups to nuts. Which soups, which nuts, and where can you find them floating around—that is the trick to passing.

First we'll look at the symptoms having to do with the GI tract and then we'll cover salient nutrition points.

GI

Acute Abdominal Pain

Acute abdominal pain isn't very cute at all, especially if you encounter it on the Boards. You need to take into account the age and gender of the child, as well as all the different bits of information they throw at you in the question. The following are common causes of abdominal pain and how they will be described.

CASE STUDY

A 6 year old with periumbilical pain yesterday now presents with RUQ tenderness and guarding, but no rebound tenderness. What is the best diagnostic test to determine if surgery is necessary?

THE DIVERSION

By noting that there is no rebound tenderness, they are hoping that you'll be fooled into believing that appendicitis is not in the differential, and therefore will choose a study that will rule out something else in the differential, i.e. *Yersinia* infection, mesenteric adenitis, or Crohn's disease.

ANSWER REVEALED

The correct answer is CT with contrast, because *the best way to determine if surgery is necessary is via CT with contrast.*

not UTZ!

Appendicitis

Appendicitis should be considered in a child *older than* 2 presenting with an acute abdomen. The diagnostic spot for pain is known as McBurney's[1] point.

The pain will be described in the right lower quadrant, periumbilical region, or midepigastric area, along with nausea, vomiting, anorexia, and low-grade fever. On physical examination, they might describe the "psoas sign" (pain on straightening out the leg).

X-ray findings include the "sentinel loop" and the *absence of air in the right lower quadrant*. A fecalith, which is a hardened mass (usually of stool), would be an important clinical sign that the patient has appendicitis. More often than not, the x-ray with appendicitis is negative. DO NOT let that dissuade you from considering this as a correct choice.

A child who wishes to eat does not have appendicitis. The absence of an elevated white blood cell count does not rule out the diagnosis.

Acute mesenteric lymphadenitis could present with an acute abdomen, but the child will be less toxic appearing. Don't forget to consider **lower lobe pneumonia** in a child described with abdominal pain.

CASE STUDY

A patient with JIA presents with epigastric pain. **What is the most likely mechanism for the GI distress?**

THE DIVERSION

You might be inclined to ignore their mentioning that the patient has JIA, thinking that it may be a diversion. Alternatively, you might get totally confused or try to over-analyze the question, thinking perhaps that the arthritic condition is associated with Crohn's Disease. However, it is a lot simpler than that. They may not mention that the patient is taking an NSAID medication, but *whenever they note an underlying chronic illness, you should consider medications the patient might be taking.*

ANSWER REVEALED

The correct answer will be **inhibition of prostaglandin synthesis**, the mechanism of action of NSAID dyspepsia.

---

[1] Apparently McBurney staked his flag about 1/3 of the way between the anterior-superior iliac crest and the umbilicus. Therefore, if you want a location on the abdomen with your name on it, you will have to move to another location.

NSAID-induced dyspepsia

NSAID-induced dyspepsia, and ultimately peptic ulcer disease, occurs by inhibiting cyclooxygenase, an enzyme that is essential for prostaglandin synthesis. Prostaglandins protect the gastric lining.

Pain from Gastroenteritis (Viral or Bacterial)

Vomiting and diarrhea will be followed by pain, not the other way around.

Pain from Pneumonia

This is a classic **presentation of acute abdominal pain** on the Boards and in clinical practice as well. A history of coughing and other respiratory signs is your clue. CXR is the answer to "what test do you use to diagnose the problem?"

Post Op Intestinal Obstruction

If you are faced with a post-op patient with acute abdominal pain, you must consider obstruction as the cause. X-ray findings would include the obstructive gas pattern.

TREATMENT If you are asked for the next step in managing this problem, the correct answer will be bowel decompression before anything else.

The Cute Players of Acute Pain

Remember the other causes of acute abdominal pain as follows:

MNEMONIC If you attended a summer camp known as "**CAMP HIT**" your abdomen would hurt for sure. Remember the causes of acute abdominal pain as follows:

Constipation (Cyst-Ovarian)   Hepatitis
Adenitis (Mesenteric)   Infection (UTI)
Mono   Trauma
Pancreatitis

Recurrent or Chronic Abdominal Pain

Recurrent or chronic abdominal pain includes all children who have abdominal pain for which a specific cause cannot be identified. **Recurrent abdominal pain** is basically the same thing **as chronic abdominal pain**, and synonymous with **functional abdominal pain**

Basically, recurrent or chronic abdominal pain is reserved for patients for whom an organic cause is not found.

However, just when you thought this would be easy, think again. There are actually subsets they expect you to know.

Before you succumb to recurrent abdominal pain as a result of this confusion, we offer you the following relief for your GI distress.

Functional Dyspepsia

The slippery heels of Helicobacter pylori

Even if the test for *H. pylori* is positive in the context of recurrent abdominal pain, it does not mean there is a causal relationship.

So why order the test? Good question! That is why routine testing for *H. pylori* in a question involving a patient with functional dyspepsia will likely be the wrong choice.

HOT TIP

Having said that, *H. pylori* is associated with low socioeconomic status, especially in those living in crowded housing. It is also more common in people immigrating from developing countries. Therefore, routine testing is not indicated, but it could be necessary if presented with a patient from these settings.

All of the following must be present at least once per week for at least 2 months before diagnosis:

Recurrent pain in the upper abdomen or periumbical pain. The pain cannot be relieved with defecation or changes in stool pattern. There must also be no organic cause or explanation for the symptoms.

If they describe the above clinical scenario in a child with a recent history of acute viral gastroenteritis, this is not functional dyspepsia. It is gastroparesis. Remember, this will be described after the viral illness has resolved.

If there are additional findings described, such as pain radiating to the back, bilious vomiting, bloody emesis, difficulty swallowing, or melena, they are pointing you in another direction. Systemic findings, including weight loss, fever, night sweats, or anemia are also signs you should steer clear of functional dyspepsia.

If you are sure that functional dyspepsia is what they are describing, then it is treated by eliminating items that can exacerbate symptoms, including NSAIDs and soda (especially sodas containing caffeine). Smaller more frequent meals could also be one of the correct choices.

If you are presented with medications, histamine-2 receptor antagonists or gastric proton pump inhibitors would be correct choices.

Although not proven in children, low dose antidepressants could be the correct answer, since they work in adults.

Irritable Bowel Syndrome

If each of the following is present once a week for at least 2 months in the clinical history, they are describing irritable bowel syndrome.

Abdominal discomfort improved with defecation, change in stool frequency, or change in form of stool. There also has to be no organic explanation for the symptoms.

A clinical history consistent with irritable bowel syndrome could be increased or decreased stool frequency, or loose or more formed stools. They could also describe straining or bowel urgency, with feeling of incomplete evacuation. Passage of mucous, bloating, and abdominal distention are also consistent with the diagnosis.

If the clinical description includes any of the following, you are not dealing with irritable bowel syndrome: pain limited to the nighttime, unexplained weight loss, oral ulcers, rash, pallor, or bloody stools.

Inflammatory bowel disease is the more likely diagnosis if they describe more systemic signs, such as anemia, fever, arthritis, delayed puberty, short stature, or a family history of inflammatory bowel disease.

Dietary changes and addressing psychological issues are all appropriate answers if asked about management and treatment. Dietary changes could include reducing intake of sorbitol (contained in sugar-free candies), fructose, and gas-forming foods. You know what they are, don't you? Brussel sprouts, broccoli, beans, and the winner of them all-Korean kim chee. There is some evidence that tricyclic antidepressants might work, although it remains controversial as of this publishing.

> ### Lactose Intolerance and Evidence Lacking
>
> Even if a patient responds well to a lactose free diet and experiences decreased bloating and diarrhea, it does not establish lactose intolerance as the cause. Lactose intolerance and recurrent abdominal pain are separate entities.

Childhood Functional Abdominal Pain

As always, they must describe the following as having been present at least once a week for the past 2 months.

Episodic or continuous abdominal pain that does not meet the diagnostic criteria for other GI disorders. In addition, there must be some evidence of loss of daily activity and presence of additional symptoms, including headache, limb pain, or sleep disruption.

Abdominal Migraines

The typical clinical presentation of abdominal migraines would be acute, incapacitating, periumbilical abdominal pain that lasts for more than 1 hour. Additional findings would include pallor, anorexia, nausea, vomiting, headache, or photophobia. There must also be symptom-free periods, lasting weeks to months in between episodes. A family history of migraine headaches could be included.

Treatment of abdominal migraines includes removing triggers such as caffeine or nitrate-containing foods (like smoked meats), and reducing psychological stress. Pharmacological treatment could include prophylactic use of propranolol, cyproheptadine, or sumatriptan.

Without any of signs of organic disease, if you are presented with a patient with signs of any of the above categories of functional abdominal pain, ordering lab and imaging studies would be incorrect choices. Watch for signs or indications of psychological stressors.

Anti-Anticholinergic Policy

Anticholinergic Meds

Watch out for a patient with recurrent abdominal pain presenting with

- Urinary retention
- Tachycardia
- Blurred vision
- Dry mouth

A patient presenting with these symptoms along with a history of recurrent pain may have been *inappropriately* prescribed anticholinergic medications to treat the recurrent abdominal pain.

Anticholinergics should <u>not</u> be administered to children who have either acute or chronic diarrhea.

Fecal overflow incontinence /Encopresis

The pain will be described in the **left lower quadrant** with a palpable "mass" on PE. Don't expect an obvious tip-off like a history of constipation or encopresis.

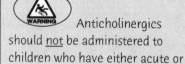

Typical presentation is a school aged child with **abdominal pain** and **soiled pants** who does <u>not</u> have diarrhea, weight loss, fever or other systemic manifestations.

Treatment

 Treatment is in 3 phases

1) Education – family must know that episodes are out of the child's control and not a purposeful behavior. Punishment and blame should be avoided.

2) Emptying the colon – Clean out with enema, and then mostly oral cathartics and stool softeners.

Enemas and suppositories may traumatize the child, and are not recommended unless there is encopresis.

3) Maintenance program – adjusting doses of medications until colon regains tone and one soft stool a day is obtained.

Parasites

Giardia lamblia

Giardia lamblia is a classic parasite that causes abdominal pain.

Typically the presentation includes several weeks of intermittent watery diarrhea, abdominal distension, anorexia, and no fever. A history of drinking bad water on a camping trip, or a child attending daycare, would also be suggestive of *Giardia lamblia*. Ultimately, a persistent malabsorptive diarrhea results.

The current best diagnostic test for *Giardia* is antigen-based, with a sensitivity of approximately 90% from a single stool sample.

Treatment (in *symptomatic* patients) is with metronidazole or nitazoxanide. Treatment seems to change frequently, and the correct answer could also include tinidazole. We suggest you check the latest Red Book® to verify the most up to date treatment for *Giardia.*

If asymptomatic carriers in the family are noted in the history, then the family pack would be indicated.

Diarrhea

Chronic Diarrhea and Malabsorption: This finding is common on the Boards and they ask a lot of questions about it too! We divide diarrhea into Acute and Chronic. When it is chronic, it may cause chronic abdominal pain. See chronic diarrhea later in this chapter.

Antidiarrheal medications are not to be used in children.

- If the question asks for treatment of diarrhea, antidiarrheal medications will be the incorrect choice
- If you are presented with a patient with GI distress who has been given antidiarrheal medications, then these medications will be the cause of the symptoms

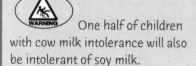

Cow Milk Protein Intolerance

The typical presentation is a child who, when given cow's milk for the first time, develops bloody stools and/or diarrhea. It is a **temporary problem**, but the immediate treatment is to revert to breast milk or give a non-cow's milk-based formula.

One half of children with cow milk intolerance will also be intolerant of soy milk.

Watery Diarrhea

Watery diarrhea derives from the small intestine and will be described as being high volume but not bloody.

No specific tests are needed when presented with a patient with *watery* diarrhea. The exceptions to the rule would be suspicion of *Clostridium difficile* or diarrhea due to *cholera*.

Picture watery diarrhea complicated by the presence of a "C" (sea) of diarrhea to remind you that in this case specific studies would be indicated for diarrhea due to **C**lostridium difficile or **c**holera.

Inflammatory Diarrhea

Inflammatory diarrhea is small and frequently contains blood, mucous, and white blood cells. In addition, a more toxic picture will be described.

Diarrhea and Feeding

Many pediatricians tell parents to limit the diet of children with diarrhea, even in the absence of dehydration. This is not the policy of the AAP;[2] according to them, children who have diarrhea and are not dehydrated should continue to be fed **age-appropriate diets**. If dehydrated, rehydrating fluids like Pedialyte® should be used.

The optimal mixture of oral rehydration solution should be **2% glucose and 90 mEq NaCl**. The AAP does agree that it is best to avoid fatty foods and foods high in simple sugars, such as sweetened tea, juices, and soft drinks.

The AAP states that the **BRAT** diet, which we all recite like a "**Pediatric mantra,**" contains well-tolerated foods, but it is too limited and does not supply optimal nutrition. In fact, "bowel rest" is considered to be "unnecessary starvation." Anything that reduces intestinal motility is also dangerous, since it results in pooling of fluids, with dehydration going unnoticed. In addition, it is important to note that *oral rehydration fluids do not reduce ongoing stool losses.*

By the way — tea is not part of the BRAT diet.

Acute Infectious Diarrhea

Neutrophils in the stool are more indicative of a diarrhea secondary to bacteria than occult blood. **You use methylene blue to find white blood cells.**

Virus

Viral diarrhea such as **rotavirus** will present with *low grade fever, vomiting,* and *large loose watery stools.*

Rotavirus is the leading cause of diarrhea in **infants worldwide;** the 2nd leading cause is adenovirus.

---

2 Guess whose policy dictates the correct answers on the exam.

Bacterial Diarrhea

 Bacterial diarrhea often presents with high fever, small frequent stools, and mucous or blood.

E. coli Diarrhea

Enteropathogenic E. coli

 Enteropathogenic *E. coli* results in acute and chronic diarrhea in neonates and younger children. It is more common in areas where there is poor sanitation.

Stools are non-bloody, but fever and vomiting are commonly seen.

Enterotoxigenic Diarrhea

 Presents with severe diarrhea and cramping and is self-limited. This is known as traveler's diarrhea (as in travelers to Mexico).

Prophylaxis against traveler's diarrhea is not typically indicated in otherwise healthy children. If you were asked to choose something for this purpose, bismuth subsalicylate or an antibiotic, such as trimethoprim-sulfamethoxazole, would be appropriate.

Entero-**TACO**-genic (Enterotoxigenic) *E. coli* causes traveler's diarrhea.

If there is no improvement after several days of supportive treatment, then antibiotics may be indicated.

However, assays for Shiga toxin must first be confirmed as negative. If diarrhea does not improve after several days of supportive care and assays for Shiga toxin are negative, antimicrobial therapy can be considered.

Treatment can include trimethoprim-sulfamethoxazole, azithromycin, or ciprofloxacin, depending on the age of the patient they present.

O157:H7 serotype

This type of *E. coli* has changed its name several times like Prince, to the point that it has now been assigned an impossible to remember number instead. O157:H7 serotype is a Shiga toxin-producing *E. coli* (STEC), the artist **formerly** known as enterohemorrhagic *E. coli* (EHEC) or verotoxin-producing *E. coli*.

The most important point to remember here in addition to the O157:H7 serotype ID card is the fact that it is a "Shiga toxin" -producing bacteria, and all the problems occur when the Shiga hits the fan.

It can initially present with watery progressing to bloody stools. General signs include cramping abdominal pain, nausea, and vomiting, followed by fever.

It can result in **hemolytic uremic syndrome** (HUS).

HUS is characterized by

- Renal failure
- Thrombocytopenia
- Hemolytic anemia

Antibiotics are contraindicated in enterohemorrhagic *E. coli* diarrhea. This is because it can result in the release of *shiga toxins*. It can also increase the risk of hemolytic uremic syndrome in children.

Enteroinvasive Diarrhea

Enteroinvasive diarrhea presents with a clinical picture similar to dysentery, i.e. *Shigella*. Stools are blood- and mucous-tinged, and tenesmus can be present.

Salmonella

The typical presentation will be 2 days after a picnic. "Green," "malodorous"[3] stools will be described. Note that *Salmonella* can present in the newborn, whereas *Shigella* rarely if ever does. If they present a child with bloody stools, *Salmonella* will not be the diagnosis.

Typhoid Fever

Typhoid fever is the more invasive form of the disease. *Salmonella typhi* invades the epithelial cells and gets hung up in the mesenteric nodes, but eventually invades the blood stream.

---

[3] As if there is any other kind of stool.

Treatment is with ceftriaxone and cefotaxime, especially in areas where resistance to trimethoprim-sulfamethoxazole is known.

Children with typhoid fever present with fever (of course!), headache, abdominal pain, muscle aches, and the classic finding of **rose spots.**

Remember, *Salmonella* can cause osteomyelitis in children with sickle cell disease.

Shigella (Shake-ella)

The onset of illness is several days after ingestion. The initial presentation is of watery diarrhea and fever. The characteristic bloody diarrhea appears after the fever subsides. There is also an increased number of bands on the CBC, *regardless of the actual white blood cell count.*

If they describe a child with bloody diarrhea who is also having a seizure, then the diagnosis is *Shigella.* They might describe the seizure without mentioning the diarrhea, but they will provide some "hint" somewhere that it is *Shigella.* That hint might be WBCs or RBCs in the stool with a left shift on CBC. Since resistance is high, trimethoprim-sulfamethoxazole is the treatment of choice.

"**Shake – ella**". Get it? "Shake" as in tonic clonic seizure.

Shigella and **Salmonella** — Which "Ella" Is It?

Shigella	Salmonella
❑ Person to person transmission	❑ Contaminated food
❑ Symptomatic when present	❑ Can be found in asymptomatic carriers
❑ Trimethoprim-sulfa is used for treatment	❑ Since they do not shorten the clinical course and can extend the carrier state, antibiotics are not recommended.[4]

Campylobacter can also present with a picture similar to *Shigella.* .

---

[4] Treatment would be indicated in children less than one year and for those at risk for systemic illness, including those with colitis or those who are immunosuppressed.

Campylobacter Diarrhea

Diarrhea due to *Campylobacter jejuni* typically sets sail 2 to 4 days after exposure. They will first dull your brain with non specific findings, including fever, malaise, abdominal pain, and diarrhea. Specific signs would include crampy periumbilical pain that is relieved by defecation.

They could describe it as localized right lower quadrant pain.

Treatment of *Campylobacter* is with erythromycin or azithromycin

Pseudomembranous Colitis

This manifests as diarrhea—often bloody—along with abdominal pain and vomiting. The diarrhea is caused by the ***Clostridium difficile* toxin** and is diagnosed by identifying the toxin. To distinguish it from other causes of bloody diarrhea, they will give you a history of recent use of antibiotics. Treatment is with Flagyl® (metronidazole) orally. Vancomycin would be indicated if there were no response to metronidazole.

C. difficile in infants –

Infants can be asymptomatic carriers of *C. diff* and rarely become symptomatic, even when toxin is present in the stool. Therefore, treatment for *C. diff* is not indicated in children younger than 6 months of age, unless they are symptomatic.

Yersinia

Infection with *Yersinia* can present with a clinical picture similar to appendicitis. However, when it is limited to the GI tract it is considered to be a benign self-limited disease, which *does not require treatment.*

Chronic Diarrhea

The causes vary with the age of the child. **Newborns** will have anatomical causes such as short gut syndrome; for **infants**, think of viral infection and protein intolerance; in **toddlers** (see Toddler's diarrhea) and in **older kids**, think of lactose intolerance.

	Passing through the Screen: Screening Tests for Malabsorption	
Malabsorbed Substance	**Test**	**Comments**
Sugars	Clinitest® (Quick Screen)	Tests for reducing substances, which are all dietary sugars except for sucrose. The presence of these reducing substances in stool would correlate with sugar malabsorption.
Sugars	Hydrogen Breath Test	A positive hydrogen breath test would correlate with sugar malabsorption. This is because the normal gut flora "ferments" the sugar, resulting in hydrogen production, which is absorbed in the blood and excreted in the lungs.
Fat	Fecal Fat Measurement	*PERIL WARNING* A single stool specimen for fat is not a valid verification. A 3-day fecal fat determination is necessary.
Fat	Serum Carotene and Prothrombin Time	These are indirect tests since they correlate with vitamin A and vitamin K absorption.
Protein	Albumin level, total protein	Typically occurs along with fat malabsorption. When it occurs as an isolated clinical finding, edema and other clinical findings will be noted (see intestinal lymphangiectasia later in this chapter).

DEFINITION Chronic diarrhea is defined as diarrhea beyond 2 weeks that cannot be attributed to an acute gastroenteritis.

PERIL WARNING The description of loose stools does not necessarily suggest or confirm "chronic diarrhea." Keep in mind that a child with steatorrhea may only have a couple of large firm stools a day yet still be suffering from chronic malabsorption.

Neuroblastoma can produce **vasoactive intestinal peptides** that can cause diarrhea.

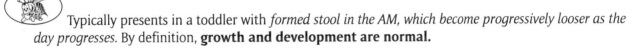
Oral Rehydration Fluid: The optimal mixture is **2% glucose and 90mEq NaCl**. This allows for the maximal absorption of sodium.

Transient Lactase Deficiency

This typically occurs after an acute gastroenteritis, and can take up to 3-6 months to return to normal.

Cryptosporidium

Cryptosporidium can cause a **chronic diarrhea even in a child with no immunological problems,** and especially in a child attending day care outside the home. In severe cases, it can result in malabsorption.

Toddler's Diarrhea (Chronic Non-Specific Diarrhea)

This is often due to fruit juices and excessive water intake. It can also be a result of severe viral gastroenteritis with mucosal damage. This is the so-called "Toddler's Diarrhea." **This is the most common cause of chronic diarrhea in children up to age 3.**

Typically presents in a toddler with *formed stool in the AM, which become progressively looser as the day progresses.* By definition, **growth and development are normal.**

Sorbitol, fruit juices, and even excessive water intake can cause chronic non-specific diarrhea.

Poor growth, fever, and melena are *not seen* with chronic nonspecific diarrhea.

Treatment consists of limiting carbohydrates in the diet, increasing fat intake, and increasing intake of high fiber foods such as fruits and vegetables. *Cold foods and liquids that stimulate colonic activity should be removed from the diet.*

Malnutrition

Malnutrition can be a significant cause of chronic diarrhea in children. Here the problem will be triggered by an acute gastroenteritis treated with high osmolar solutions (also known as fruit juices and other junk), leading to more diarrhea.

This leads to the erroneous conclusion that the acute episode is still ongoing, so the sugar water continues and things snowball in the wrong direction.

 The frequent passing of loose green stools would go along with this diagnosis. These are known as starvation stools.

Cow Milk Intolerance

While the incidence may be higher on the exam, confirmed cow milk protein intolerance is only present in 1% of the population. This is usually resolved by age 2.

 They will typically also present with other symptoms such as eczema and perhaps asthma.

Milk Protein Intolerance

There are two types of milk protein intolerance

Milk Protein Allergy – is IgE mediated and can cause anaphylaxis and trigger eczema.

Food Sensitivity (*"non-IgE mediated milk protein allergy"*) – This is commonly known as "Food Protein Enterocolitis Syndrome" or FPIES. This is more common than the IgE mediated form of enterocolitis. Symptoms include vomiting and bloody diarrhea. <u>Cow and soy milk are frequent culprits.</u> Elimination of the foods is the treatment.

 These children should avoid milk products for 1-2 years.

Colitis in a breast-fed infant can be a manifestation of food allergy to an allergen in the mother's diet.

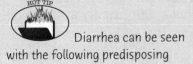

Protracted Diarrhea

Diarrhea can be seen with the following predisposing factors:

- Malnutrition
- Chronic infection
- Systemic Disease
- Immunodeficiency

Abetalipoproteinemia

Abetalipoproteinemia presents as steatorrhea and acanthocytosis;[5] it can result in retinal damage as well as neurological sequelae.

Intestinal Lymphangiectasia

Intestinal lymphangiectasia is a protein losing enteropathy that results in hypoproteinemia, hypogammaglobulinemia, steatorrhea, lymphedema, and lymphopenia.

Additional Causes

Additional causes of chronic diarrhea in children would be:

- *Giardia lamblia* infection
- Specific food allergies
- Cystic Fibrosis
- Shwachman Diamond syndrome

 Diets limited by food allergies can result in significant malnutrition.

Vomiting

Vomiting also occurs for different reasons in different age groups. Again, the presenting symptoms and facts included in the question, coupled with the age, should make these easy pickings.

Neonatal Vomiting

Since vomiting in the newborn period can be confusing, it will be tested on the exam. Therefore, we have decided to devote a specific section to this age group.

---

[5] Red blood cells with spiney projections- sort of what an erythrocyte would look like if it were a porcupine.

Antral Web

An antral web can cause non-bilious vomiting. This is similar to pyloric stenosis, except the outlet obstruction is before the pylorus. **It will manifest later than pyloric stenosis, but usually within the first six months of life.**

They usually mention *polyhydramnios and low birthweight.* It is diagnosed by ultrasound and resected surgically.

Antral web will present with polyhydramnios and non-bilious vomiting. Pyloric stenosis develops postnatally, therefore polyhydramnios will not be mentioned

In imaging studies, antral web will reveal a radiolucent filling defect in the prepyloric region, rather than a hypertrophied pylorus.

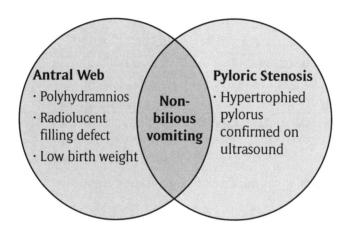

Pyloric Stenosis

Pyloric stenosis occurs in **males more than females**. However, a **maternal history of PS increases the risk more than paternal history.**

It is diagnosed with ultrasound and treated surgically **after electrolyte imbalance is corrected**.

"Progressive non-bilious vomiting" is the description. They will not provide projectile vomiting with palpable olive.[6] It typically occurs during the second month of life, but they may throw a curve ball by describing it in a child from 2-5 months of age.

Shine a Lyte: Pyloric stenosis presents with **"hypochloremic metabolic alkalosis"** with severe **hypokalemia**. The alkalosis would make sense because they are vomiting acid. And they will be low on Cl as well because they are throwing up HCl.

↓K
↓Cl ↑pH

---

[6] With or without the pimento.

Preterm infants present later, but the equivalent postnatal age.

Every year they give a patient with PS and then ask you to choose which value is not consistent. Therefore, know this well.

Elevated indirect Bili can occur in pyloric stenosis in up to 2.5% of cases, so don't let that throw you if it is included in the question of an otherwise classic description of PS. This is not a trick, just extra information.

Ultrasound Findings – Pyloric stenosis is diagnosed via ultrasound. In case they expect you to know the mind numbing ultrasound diagnostic criteria for pyloric stenosis it is:

A pyloric length greater than 14 mm

or

Pyloric muscle thickness greater than 4 mm

Inborn Errors of Metabolism

These are common causes of vomiting in early infancy. The description is similar to that of a septic infant.

When you are given an infant with a septic picture AND labs, **look for metabolic acidosis (with an elevated anion gap)**, hypoglycemia, **hyperammonemia,** and no fever as your clues pointing to inborn errors.

Duodenal Atresia

The key point to remember is that this presents as **bilious vomiting during the first day of life.** The classic double bubble sign on x-ray may not be presented to you. Because of diminished enterohepatic circulation, these infants are frequently **icteric.** The **double bubble sign** is seen on plain abdominal film x-ray.

Kidney and Pyloric Stenosis

Because of volume depletion, the **kidney** is called into action to **retain sodium**, but then it has to **toss potassium overboard**. This is a good way to distinguish pyloric stenosis from congenital adrenal hyperplasia, which has an elevated serum K. When the clinical picture further deteriorates, the serum K levels drop, and then the kidney really gets desperate. It starts tossing H overboard in exchange for Na (however, this results in worsening alkalosis). **Therefore, acidic urine is a bad sign**.

Pyloric stenosis presents with hypochloremic alkalosis and a low sodium and potassium; this is due in part to contraction alkalosis. **Adrenal insufficiency** will present with a high potassium AND a low (acidic) pH.

Be on the lookout: they both can present with vomiting and lethargy in the neonatal period and first few months of life.

There will be no air distal to the site of atresia if there is complete atresia.

CASE STUDY A 2 month old infant with Down syndrome presents with projectile non-bilious vomiting with hypochloremic metabolic alkalosis (or they might just present the lab findings themselves). What imaging study results are most likely?

THE DIVERSION The diversion is their telling you that the infant has Down Syndrome. Among the choices will be the double bubble sign. This, however, is just a diversionary choice, and if you are not careful the double bubble will be double trouble for you.

ANSWER REVEALED The correct answer will be "pyloric muscle measures over 6 mm in thickness" and the "pyloric channel 18 mm in length;" or, if they are actually fair and realize that this is not the pediatric radiology boards, "thickening and elongation of the pyloric muscle." They note that the infant is 2 months old, the time when a patient is likely to present with pyloric stenosis. Duodenal atresia will present in the first day of life, not at 2 months.

Malrotation   *Volvulus*

This is a **surgical emergency** that requires immediate intervention and is always on the Boards. It is caused by the **cecum's failure to descend while being handcuffed to the posterior right abdominal wall**. Therefore, it compresses the duodenum, causing duodenal obstruction.

BUZZ WORDS Malrotation will typically be presented as "bilious vomiting and abdominal tenderness, with **abdominal distension.**" The patient could also have crampy abdominal pain and could be passing blood via the rectum.

> ### Bile Stained Vomiting in the Newborn
>
> You will want to **order an abdominal film for any newborn presenting with bilious vomiting**. Keep in mind the diagnosis can be BENIGN idiopathic bilious vomiting.

EITHER OR CHOICES NEC presents in a similar fashion, but they will likely describe NEC in a preemie (**even though NEC can occur in a full-term infant**).

Volvulus

Presents in infancy as bilious vomiting and right-sided abdominal distension. It is associated with Ladd Bands, which constrict the large and small bowel. X-ray findings will be described as gastric and duodenal dilatation, as well as **decreased intestinal air** and **corkscrew appearance** of the duodenum — whatever that is. This is an example where knowing the association is the key.

Annular Pancreas

This can be a common cause of vomiting on the Boards,[7] because the pancreas literally forms a ring around the intestine, causing significant obstruction. One clue would be a **history of polyhydramnios,** because fluid was not swallowed effectively in utero.

> **CASE STUDY**
> If you are presented with an infant with one episode of bilious vomiting who is otherwise healthy, what is the MOST appropriate next step?
>
> **THE DIVERSION**
> You need to know that one episode of vomiting does not make a pathological cause! They will probably not underline this on the exam, but take note of every word. This is what it means to "read the question."
>
> **ANSWER REVEALED**
> The correct answer is to observe the patient, since this may be an isolated incident. This follows the "least invasive" rule and the "often no intervention and/or reassurance is the correct answer" rule.

GE Reflux in Infants

It manifests as regurgitation (or "spitting up" if you will), particularly when infants are lying down.

Gastroesophageal reflux can present with severe emesis and possibly abdominal pain, failure to thrive, or apnea in the newborn period. It doesn't usually present until 2 months of age.

---

[7] In the question, not you.

Many infants have daily episodes of spitting up at 4 months of age and it is normal, on the boards at least.

The upright position that is touted has not been shown to be helpful. Some have argued that it results in increased intraabdominal pressure.

Evidence of esophagitis (posturing), failure to thrive, or apnea would require further workup and/or treatment.

In older children, upper endoscopy and biopsy is the most valuable test, since it measures the chronic effects on the esophagus.

You will be expected to be familiar with the diagnostic tests indicated in evaluating an infant with GERD.

Evaluation and esophageal sphincter pressure	
Upper GI Series	To assess for malrotation and hiatal hernia
pH probe study (or esophageal impedance)	Measures the extent and duration of reflux over a 24 hour period
Gastric emptying scan	Tests for gastroparesis
Esophageal motility evaluation	Measures peristalsis and esophageal sphincter pressure

Sandifer Syndrome

They will describe unusual **dystonic movements** of the head and neck along with **GER**. Remember this by picturing a "sandpiper" blowing sand out of the pipe, as a reminder of reflux and the "twisted pipes" as a reminder of the twisting movements.

It is important to remember that regurgitation is often a normal finding in infants. Reassurance is often the correct answer. It can also be a sign of "overfeeding;" therefore, if they specifically mention the amount the baby is being fed, along with signs of reflux, then reducing the amount in the feedings will be the correct answer.

The baby will not be described as being sick in any other way. The vomiting will be described as *effortless*. However, if there is a repeated history of vomiting in infancy *with growth retardation* and no physiological explanation, consider emotional factors. In that case, intervention would be needed.

Remember, GE reflux can manifest as respiratory difficulties, including apnea.

Prognosis for Infants with GERD

Infants who simply have physiologic reflux will outgrow it by 1 year of age without any consequences.

However, if you are presented with the following in the history, they probably expect you to realize that there are higher risks for complications. These would include prematurity, underlying neurological impairment, or a family history of severe GERD.

Treating Reflux

Treatment of reflux, again, is limited to those with symptomatic disease and/or those with a neurological impairment.

Medications include antacids, which *can interfere with nutrition*, and H_2 blockers (ranitidine and cimetidine).

> **Anti serotonin antiemetic**
>
> Zofran®, which is also known as ondansetron, is an important antemetic. They might just ask you its mechanism of action; if they do, you will know that it is a serotonin receptor antagonist.

Cisapride, which was also known as **Propulsid®,** functioned to tighten the esophageal sphincter while relaxing the pylorus. However, due to potential cardiac side effects, resulting in the tightening of another sphincter in the lawyers representing the manufacturer, it was taken off the market and will, therefore, not be the correct answer.

Proton pump inhibitors[8] such as omeprazole, lansoprazole, and pantoprazole are frequently used to treat GERD.

Surgery for GERD

Surgery is only indicated where medication has failed. Duh!

Complications are highest in those with neurological impairment, those with underlying esophageal atresia, and those with chronic lung disease.

---

[8] Do you really want to know what that is? It inhibits the H/K adenosine triphosphatase enzyme, the last enzyme in gastrin formation. Now get back to real studying.

Non-Bilious, Infectious Causes of Vomiting

Antral web and inborn errors in metabolism (discussed under neonatal vomiting previously) are classic examples of non-bilious vomiting. Acute gastroenteritis (AGE) is the most common cause of vomiting in children. It presents with infectious diarrhea and abdominal pain, often due to rotavirus or other viruses.

 UTIs and **pneumonia** can also cause vomiting in children.

DKA

Don't forget this as a cause of vomiting. The lab findings would be suggestive of the diagnosis (see Endocrinology chapter).

Cyclic Vomiting

This entity may have **emotional overtones** with a precipitating event. Children with cyclic vomiting are also at risk for **migraines and irritable bowel syndrome**. The typical patient is early school age, and the episodes are separated by asymptomatic periods. It is a diagnosis of exclusion, so they will also need to tell you what has been ruled out.

If the diagnosis is cyclic vomiting, they will present a patient with intense periods of vomiting that last up to 48 hours. The patient will be described as feeling well between episodes.

You also need to know that conditions other than migraine variant can present with severe episodic vomiting, including pancreatitis and metabolic defects. Therefore, a workup that includes metabolic studies and imaging might be the answer they are looking for, depending on the context.

In addition to IV hydration, treatment could include antiemetics such ondansetron, and/or anxiolytics such as lorazepam.

A 5 year old is experiencing vomiting episodes that typically last 48 hours, and end suddenly after a long nap followed by an episode of *Sponge Bob Square Pants*. The mother has a history of severe headaches, and his uncle Billy, who accompanied them, has gone to the bathroom twice during this office visit. What is the most appropriate treatment at this time?

By noting the symptoms of the mother and Uncle Billy, they are letting you know that there is a family history of migraine headaches and irritable bowel syndrome. Both are associated with cyclic vomiting, which typically lasts 48 hours. Although long-term pharmacological treatment is similar to migraine treatment, i.e. *cyproheptadine, propranolol, or tricyclic antidepressants,* they asked for the best treatment *at this time.*

The correct answer therefore is *IV hydration.*

They will often note a family history of irritable bowel syndrome or migraines.

Münchausen Syndrome by Proxy (MSBP)

Watch out for Münchausen syndrome by proxy. Often, they will give hints of "hospital shopping" (going from hospital to hospital)[9] and no vomiting under observation.

Rumination

Rumination is the frequent regurgitation of ingested food into the mouth that is then re-chewed and swallowed or spit out. They will appear calm during episodes.

Rumination may be seen in **infants** of **severely disturbed caregivers**, and in older kids who are themselves disturbed or developmentally delayed.

---

[9] And, if wealthy enough, actually buying a few hospitals.

These children may **induce vomiting to seek attention** in environments where there is a failure in reciprocal interaction between the infant and caregiver.

Resolving the emotional trigger is the treatment of choice.

Some other disorders with a presentation similar to rumination are as follows. Please note that rumination is not associated with forceful emesis.

· **Achalasia** - is associated with forceful vomiting, weight loss, dysphagia, and failure to thrive

· **Gastric outlet obstruction** – presents with some of the same symptoms as achalasia, but also presents with abdominal pain and distension

· **Sandifer Syndrome** – also presents with abnormal movement and "unusual posturing"

· Infants with **GERD** present with nothing other than emesis. However, it often results in irritability rather than a calming effect, as seen in children with rumination

Going From Top to Bottom

Let's travel from the mouth to the other side of the GI tunnel.

Chew on This: The Mouth

If they describe a cyst on the floor of the mouth as a "mucocele," think **ranula**. However, a "midline mass" could be **ectopic thyroid**, which should not be removed.

Treatment of **ranula is excision. Take out your atlas and take a good look at what these both look like.**

Parotitis

They love to show parotitis and lead you down the false path to mumps. Remember, most cases of parotitis are idiopathic and require no treatment.

Another cause is **Mikulicz's disease.** Here, in addition to swelling of the parotid gland, there is **dry mouth and poor tear production**.

 Think of it as **milk** disease, and picture bottles of milk replacing the tear ducts and parotid glands.

Parotitis can also be caused by **Staph aureus,** in which case there will be more **marked tenderness and high fever** than with mumps.

Too Few Teeth

Ectodermal Hypoplasia

This can present with underdeveloped or absent teeth.

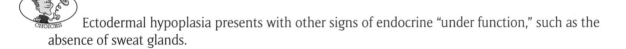 Change ectodermal to **"empty dental,"** and the image is clear and linked to the diagnosis. It is **diagnosed by skin biopsy, which shows lack of sweat pores.** It is also **X-linked**: in place of teeth, picture small X's sitting on the gums.

Hallermann Streiff Syndrome

This presents with underdeveloped small teeth.

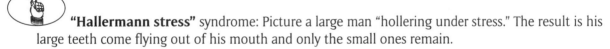 Ectodermal hypoplasia presents with other signs of endocrine "under function," such as the absence of sweat glands.

 "Hallermann stress" syndrome: Picture a large man "hollering under stress." The result is his large teeth come flying out of his mouth and only the small ones remain.

They can show this and give physical abuse as one of the choices, but it is the wrong choice.

Too Many Teeth (Supernumerary)

Gardner's Syndrome

Discussed later in the chapter.

Esophagus

Esophageal Varices

> ### Esophageal Burns
>
> **PERIL / WARNING** There can be serious esophageal burns from swallowing corrosive materials, **without any signs of burns on the lips or in the mouth**. Therefore, have a low index for choosing endoscopy as the answer in this situation.

BUZZ WORDS Liver disease leads to portal hypertension. If this is described in connection with "bright red, bloody stools," hematemesis, or tarry stools, "esophageal varices" is the correct answer. **Remember esophageal varices CAN cause tarry stools.**

PERIL / WARNING A child can have significant corrosive burns despite the absence of any burns in the mouth.

Foreign Body

BUZZ WORDS A child that swallowed a foreign body, which is stuck in the esophagus, will be "coughing" and "prefer liquids to solid foods."

Tracheo-Esophageal Fistula

HOT TIP The TE fistula with an upper esophageal pouch is the most common type. They present as coughing with feeding in the newborn period. They often show you a film with a feeding tube coiled up in the blind-ending esophagus.

TREATMENT It is managed by making the child NPO and draining the blind-ending esophagus prior to surgical correction.

BUZZ WORDS "Copious oral secretions," "polyhydramnios," "coughing and cyanosis with initial feeding," and "inability to pass a feeding tube" are all descriptions associated with TE fistula.

> ### NSAID SO Sad
>
> 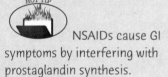 NSAIDs cause GI symptoms by interfering with prostaglandin synthesis.
>
> **Gastric ulcers are not treated with diet**. NSAID-induced ulcers respond well to H2 antagonists.
>
> Remember, there is no correlation between dyspeptic symptoms and the extent of the ulcer.

Stomach Disorders

Peptic Ulcer Disease

(BUZZ WORDS) This will be described in its classic form, which is vomiting after eating[10] and **epigastric pain severe enough to wake the child up at night**. They could throw in guaiac positive stools, which would be the clincher.

(PERIL WARNING) **A plain KUB** would be an important **first study** when evaluating the child with abdominal pain, **but not when PUD is strongly suspected,** or once other disorders have been ruled out.

The best diagnostic study is an **upper gastrointestinal endoscopy,** so that, looking at the histology and a culture for *Helicobacter pylori,* a biopsy can be done. Mild esophagitis can also be ruled out by endoscopy.

(MNEMONIC) Picture a helicopter swirling around the stomach causing ulcers.

(HOT TIP) If *Helicobacter* **is suspected** or confirmed, **"triple" therapy is also needed.** A PPI plus two antibiotics would be appropriate treatment.

(TAKE HOME MESSAGE) Uncomplicated dyspepsia due to NSAIDs can be managed with antacids and food.

(PERIL WARNING) Lower socioeconomic status is a risk factor for *H. pylori* disease.

Treatment of Peptic Ulcer Disease: How It Works!

There are 4 primary meds used to treat PUD in children: H2 blockers, sucralfate, prostaglandins, and PPIs.

1. The **H2 Blockers block** gastric acid secretion.

2. **Sucralfate** "coats" damaged gastric mucosa, protecting it from further damage.

3. The **prostaglandin analogues** enhance bicarb production, and to some extent decrease gastric acid production as well.

4. **Proton pump inhibitors (PPIs)** inhibit the gastric acid pump.

(PERIL WARNING) **Misoprostol** is an example of a prostaglandin that is used but **shouldn't be used in pregnant teens**; you can remember this by telling patients not to kiss under the "mistletoe" – misoprostol.

---

[10] Postprandial emesis for those who prefer Latin terms.

CASE STUDY A 12 year old with chronic periumbilical pain is positive for *H. pylori* on serological testing. What is the best next step?

THE DIVERSION They want you to believe that the positive serology is sufficient to make the diagnosis; however, this is only a screen door to more specific testing. Serologic testing for *H. pylori* IgG has a high sensitivity, but lots of false positives.

Therefore, a positive serology would not be reason enough to treat – one would want to do another study if this *screen* is positive.

ANSWER REVEALED The correct answer would be another study, such as fecal antigen or urea breath tests. But remember, even if you prove that H. pylori is present, that does not prove that it's causing the chronic abdominal pain, so read the question carefully.

PERIL WARNING Even though endoscopic biopsy is the gold standard, it violates the "least invasive choice" rule, and therefore, would not be the correct choice.

Treatment of *H. Pylori*

· Proton pump inhibitor (e.g., omeprazole, lansoprazole)
· 2 antibiotics (clarithromycin and amoxicillin OR clarithromycin and metronidazole)
· 7 day course is acceptable, but 14 day course has higher eradication rate

Zollinger-Ellison Syndrome

This is due to a gastrin-secreting tumor. They will present with symptoms related to peptic ulcer disease. It is diagnosed by obtaining **fasting gastrin levels**.

Intestinal Fortitude to Learn Intestinal Disorders

Celiac Disease

Children with celiac disease will present with **"bulky, pale, frothy, and foul smelling stools."** They will also describe **"proximal muscle wasting"** and abdominal distention.

Gluten is found in foods that contain **wheat or rye,** and must be avoided. **Oatmeal is fine in some patients,** and therefore, can be tested initially. Vitamin supplementations are needed. It is diagnosed by biopsy once it is suspected clinically.

Assuming normal serum IgA levels, the best way to screen for celiac disease would be to test for elevated levels of IgA antibodies against tissue transglutaminase (anti-tTG) or IgA antibodies to endomysium. However, **diagnosis is confirmed by biopsy.**

Irritable Bowel Syndrome

This has a high emotional component with hints in the question to indicate that. The clues could be **"worse diarrhea in the morning"** and no association of the pain with any particular foods.

The best treatment is a **high fiber diet** and close **attention to the emotional factors** that are contributing to the problem.

Cystic Fibrosis (GI Manifestations)

Malabsorption as a manifestation of poor exocrine function would be one sign of cystic fibrosis. **Hyponatremia would be another sign of CF.** Another cause of malabsorption is **short gut syndrome**, where they will note or imply previous GI surgery. **Shwachman-Diamond syndrome** can also cause malabsorption; however, it has other associations such as bone abnormalities and bone marrow involvement to distinguish it from CF. The main causes of malabsorption in children are **cystic fibrosis, celiac sprue,** and **cow milk** and **soy allergies**. In the latter two, exocrine function will be normal.

Intrinsic Factor and the Terminal Ileum

If they describe **small bowel resection** (for example, in an infant with NEC), and include a CBC in the lab profile, this is your clue that **B12 deficiency could be the answer**. Therefore, check and highlight findings, such as a macrocytic anemia in the CBC. Remember B12 is absorbed at the terminal ileum (with the help of intrinsic factor), and resection of this portion of the bowel results in B12 deficiency = Pernicious Anemia.

They might also describe other obstacles to B12 absorption like **parasites** or **inflammatory bowel disease**.

Rectal Prolapse

Cystic fibrosis is known to be associated with rectal prolapse. Other causes of rectal prolapse are anything that results in increased intra-abdominal pressure, such as **pertussis** and **tenesmus**, as well as chronic constipation. Rare causes include **meningo-myelocele** and **parasites** (especially if they tell you the child recently traveled or is a new immigrant from a place where parasites are endemic).

Look for a history of "**chronic diarrhea**," "**steatorrhea**," AND "**low sodium**" (lost through sweat). Also, malabsorption (as previously described), including poor absorption of fat-soluble vitamins. This poor absorption leads to the manifestations of fat-soluble vitamin deficiency. Therefore, any signs of fat-soluble vitamin deficiency could be a tip-off that the diagnosis is cystic fibrosis.

Meconium Plug Syndrome

In an infant presenting with meconium plug syndrome, you will have to rule out cystic fibrosis. However, only 10% of cases of CF present with a meconium plug. It appears as "ground glass" on x-ray.

Alone in the Colon/ Diseases Affecting the Colon

Gardner's Syndrome

This syndrome is associated with **extra teeth** and **polyps (pre-malignant) in the large and small intestines. Osteomas** are also part of the picture, and it is inherited in an autosomal dominant fashion.

Treatment is surgical.

Picture a gardener working his garden, but instead of the usual leaves, he has a garden made out of **bones** and **colonic polyps** (that's right — we have another delightfully grim and morbid image for you here). The polyps are indeed **pre-malignant,** and eventually win out by dominating the bones (to remind you that it is an **autosomal dominant** trait). However, along comes a power lawnmower driven by a surgeon to remind you that surgery is the answer. The lawn mower is made of supernumerary (extra) teeth that will pull out the bones and polyps.

Peutz-Jeghers Syndrome

"Mucosal pigmentation of lips and gums."

Treatment consists of removing any polyps.

Inflammatory Bowel Disease

Ulcerative Colitis vs. Crohn's: There will be several questions on Crohn's and ulcerative colitis and you will have to know the similarities and differences.

Ulcerative Colitis

Ulcerative colitis (UC) typically presents in a **teenager** with a history of **chronic crampy lower abdominal** pain, **with or without a history of bloody stools**.

Severe colitis can present with *fevers and hypoalbuminemia, as well as anemia.* So look for this in the labs and write the words in the margins when they appear.

Ashkenazi (European) Jews are at particular risk for this. ***Both Crohn's and UC* are associated with HLA B27 antigen and ankylosing spondylitis.**

Treatment

In the past sulfasalazine (Azulfidine®) was used to treat ulcerative colitis.[12] The treatment today is only with one of the components, which is known as 5-ASA, or 5-aminosalicylate (if they write the whole thing out).[13] Other medical options include corticosteroids and immunomodulators. **Drug therapy does help prevent relapses.**

Severe cases require initial hospitalization for rehydration and/or blood transfusion. When the disease is actually a medical emergency, fluids, blood transfusions, and steroids are required, and when infection is suspected, metronidazole is the treatment of choice.

The **first line of medical treatment is 5-ASA;** however, if this were not successful, the **second line of treatment would be:**

- Corticosteroids
- 6-mercaptopurine or azathioprine or methotrexate
- Cyclosporine or tacrolimus

A surgical consult is also needed because of the risk for perforation. **A barium enema is never the right answer with acute UC, because of the risk of perforation.** If possible, pain meds should be avoided, since the masking of pain makes it difficult to track the clinical status.

> ### Colectomy
>
> Colectomy will eliminate the risk for cancer in children with ulcerative colitis. This is not a small consideration given that the cancer rate is 20% per decade after the first 10 years of disease.
>
> The "extracolonic" manifestations of ulcerative colitis include arthritis, mucocutaneous lesions, and liver disease.
>
> Colectomy does not stop the progression of ankylosing spondylitis.

---

[12] If you really must know, sulfasalazine had 2 components, which were sulfapyridine and 5-aminosalicylate (5-ASA). It turns out that the sulfapyridine was not the important component, thus 5-ASA is now used alone.

[13] This is similar to ASA but not the same.

Crohn's Disease (Regional Enteritis)

HOT TIP

Crohn's can present as weight loss even before overt GI symptoms present. *The elevated ESR may be the only clue they give you.* Obtaining an ESR may be the correct answer in a child presenting with short stature.

BUZZ WORDS

"Skip lesions" on x-ray, "cobblestone" appearance on endoscopy, and "transmural lesions," as well as "noncaseating granulomas," are all typical descriptors of Crohn's disease.

TAKE HOME MESSAGE

Tuberculosis can be mistaken for Crohn's disease, because it can result in nodularity and mucosal thickening of the terminal ileum.

TREATMENT

Treatment - The medical management includes the use of corticosteroids, aminosalicylates, immunomodulators, and antibiotics (metronidazole [Flagyl®]) in addition to nutritional support.

Just as in ulcerative colitis, 5-ASA is now used instead of Azulfidine® (sulfapyridine) (see entry under ulcerative colitis).

Extraintestinal Sightings and Crohn's Disease

They can give you a case with no GI symptoms, and only the extraintestinal manifestations of Crohn's disease, as well as:

❑ Pyoderma gangrenosum of the foot
❑ Erythema nodosum (red tender nodules over the shin)
❑ Ankylosing spondylitis/ sacroiliitis
❑ Arthritis
❑ (Eyes) Uveitis
❑ Liver Disease
❑ Renal Stones

MNEMONIC

Think of it as "Cone" disease, since cone sounds like Crohn. The cone affects where you sit (sacroiliitis), where your shoe **fits** (pyoderma gangrenosum), where you get **kicked** (erythema nodosum), and where you can see **IT** (eyes – uveitis), and turns your liver into a useless **mitt** (liver disease).

	Ulcerative Colitis	Crohn's Disease
Lesions are continuous – no skipped lesions	YES	NO
Surgical excision is curative	YES	NO
Toxic megacolon can occur	YES	YES
Growth retardation and pubertal delay	YES	YES more common than with UC

Crohn's can present initially as an **acute abdomen,** mimicking appendicitis. Oral **aphthous** ulcers and **perianal fistulae** can also be presenting signs of Crohn's.

Treatment: Meds do not change the long-term course of CD; they just decrease morbidity. Those with mild symptoms are treated as outpatients, and those with more severe symptoms (e.g., massive weight loss, significant systemic symptoms) are hospitalized.

Steroids induce remissions in 70% of patients with small bowel involvement. There is a **high relapse rate after steroids are weaned.** Sometimes, 6-mercaptopurine or azathioprine and aminosalicylates can help. In addition, antibiotics (metronidazole and ciprofloxacin) are needed, for example in perianal disease.

Intussusception (You Don't Want This on a Spelling Bee)

"Sudden onset of severe paroxysmal and colicky pain in a previously healthy child, along with **intermittent asymptomatic** episodes." It typically presents between the ages of 3 months to 6 years.

Typical description – an infant with "**intermittent severe abdominal pain,**" who is "**drawing up his legs and vomiting.**" The pain may be relieved with the passing of a stool. However, the child ultimately becomes lethargic.

They probably won't describe the typical "currant jelly" stool. They might mention bloody stool and **palpation of a "sausage-like mass."**[14]

In the later stages, intussusception might be described as "bilious vomiting" with shock-like symptoms, so don't miss the diagnosis if you see **green** (bile) and **no red** (currant jelly stools) in the question.

Camp town Races

Chronic cramp and abdominal pain in a **febrile** child, that isn't quite as severe as the pain found in intussusception, could be *Campylobacter jejuni* diarrhea. Crampy severe *periumbilical pain* could also be **Yersinia** if it is one of the choices.

---

[14] I never knew what "currant jelly" was prior to medical school, but since training in pediatrics, I have never been tempted to try it, for obvious reasons.

They sometimes portray this as a child around age 2 who is **afebrile,** with **symptoms mimicking sepsis,** but with no GI symptoms. Think of intussusception when you see that. This should be high on your list in an **afebrile** child that looks toxic.

Treatment facts: "Air enema" resulting in hydrostatic reduction will diagnose and "cure" in most cases.

Most Popular Palpable Popping Mass in Infants

Multicystic dysplastic kidneys is the most common cause of palpable abdominal mass in infants.

Lymphosarcoma should **be ruled out** when a child **older than 6 gets intussusception.** The lymphosarcoma could be the "lead point" causing the intussusception.

A 20 month old presents with colicky abdominal pain and a right lower quadrant mass. He is intermittently in severe pain and lethargic between episodes. What would be the BEST diagnostic study to order?

If you are well prepared for the exam, there really isn't a diversion here. You should realize by now that they will not deliver a fast ball down the middle by noting that there are "currant jelly stools." There are sufficient code words, like *lethargic* and *severe pain*, here to let you know that this patient has intussusception. However, you could be thrown by their mentioning the abdominal mass, and think the correct diagnostic study is CT.

If they provide you with 2 correct choices, remember they want the best choice. Ultrasound may be correct, but it is not the best choice.

The correct choice is *air contrast enema*, since this may be both diagnostic and therapeutic.

Constipation

Hirschsprung's Disease

It presents early as constipation, or as intermittent loose stools, and rectal biopsy is diagnostic.

Treatment consists of surgical excision of the aganglionic segment, followed by colostomy and ultimately end-to-end anastomosis.

Think of Hirschsprung's disease for any significant defecation problem in a newborn, especially a male.

In addition to constipation or failure to pass first stool in the hospital, infants with Hirschsprung's disease can also present with: bilious vomiting, poor PO intake, and abdominal distension.

You may be called upon to distinguish just plain old constipation from Hirschsprung's. Keep the following in mind:

	Functional Constipation	Hirschsprung's
Delayed passage of meconium in the newborn period	RARELY	YES
Signs of obstruction	RARELY	YES
Soiling	YES	RARELY
Failure to thrive	NO	YES
Present after age 2	YES	NO[15]
Difficulty with toilet training	YES	NO
Stool in the rectal ampulla on PE	YES	NO

Different causes of constipation in infancy must be distinguished from each other.

---

[15] It is usually treated before age 2, which is why it won't present after age 2.

> **Cool Stool Facts**
>
> Ninety-nine percent of healthy newborns will deliver their first stool within their first 24 hours and the other 1% will within 48 hours, Hirschsprung's disease and cystic fibrosis should be your first considerations when there is no stool production in the first 48 hours.

Hirschsprung's disease Differential Diagnosis

Anal Stenosis - infants strain to pass small liquid stools, and there is a tight band narrowing on the anus. This is self limited and remits by age 1.

Functional Constipation - typically presents in infants fed cereal at an early age. Delayed passing of meconium will not be described in the vignette.

Congenital Hypothyroidism – in addition to constipation, the patient will present with poor growth, a hoarse cry, umbilical hernia, and delayed closure of the anterior fontanelle.

GI Bleeding

 Nasogastric lavage is the "first thing" you should do to distinguish upper from lower GI bleeding. When you are presented with a GI bleed, the first consideration is the age of the patient. In doing so, you will automatically narrow down the possible correct choices.

Lower GI Bleed (LGB)/Newborn Period

An apt test determines if the blood is the mother's or the infant's.

The important disorders to keep in mind with a LGB in the newborn are:

Hirschsprung's disease,[16] which can present as lower GI bleeding when there is an **associated colitis**.

Malrotation with an associated volvulus, which typically presents with bilious vomiting and sometimes **melena**.

NEC, especially if they describe a preemie.

Lower GI Bleed (LGB)/One To Two Years of Age

Anal fissures are the most common cause of a lower GI bleed in this age group, and they are quite benign. They are usually secondary to **constipation**.

---

[16] 5% of children with Down syndrome have Hirschsprung's disease. This is an association worth keeping in mind.

Intussusception typically presents in a child 9 months of age or older.

Hematochezia	Melena[18]
Described either as **"blood on toilet paper"**[17] (and is consistent with "distal bleeding," i.e. anal fissure) or a juvenile polyp.	The words "dark tarry stools" will be described. It is usually due to an upper GI bleed. Melena can also be **associated with Meckel's diverticulum**, so consider this diagnosis when melena is described instead of the classic painless bleeding.

LGB / Preschool (2 to 5 Years of Age)

A juvenile polyp is typically described as painless rectal bleeding in an otherwise healthy preschool child. **Juvenile polyps are not associated with an increased risk for malignancy**.

Entamoeba histolytica can cause bloody diarrhea. This is often described in a child **from Native American reservations or other rural areas** in the south, central, and southwestern United States.

Remember that 90% of those patients with amebic colitis have positive serology, and this would be the test to order if they ask you to "confirm the diagnosis." It is treated with metronidazole (Flagyl®) for colitis and liver abscess, and iodoquinol for asymptomatic disease.

Meckel diverticulum

Meckel diverticulum (MD) is a very common cause of lower GI bleeding. It is present in 2-3% of newborns. It manifests during the first 2 years of life (let's say age 2) and is **diagnosed by technetium 99m pertechnetate scintigraphic study.**[19]

I remember it because **pertechnetate is close enough to the word "petechiae."** MD consists of ectopic gastric mucosa, which takes up the material and lights up.

Treatment is surgical.

"Painless rectal bleeding."

---

[17] In which case you should write hematochezia in the margin, since this will be the word that will jog your memory.

[18] They won't use the word melena; they will instead describe tarry stools (hopefully not just before the lunch break).

[19] Whatever the heck that is.

Rule of 2 – It typically presents around the **age of 2,** with **2 types of tissue** (gastric and intestinal). In addition, it is usually found **2 feet from the ileocecal valve**, it is **2 inches in length**, and it occurs in **2% of the population**.

Think of it as Meckel's **diverTWOculum** to help associate it with **the rule of two's.**

Juvenile polyposis can also present as painless rectal bleeding, but they will likely describe it in a child that is older. This too presents with painless rectal bleeding.

Lower GI Bleed (LGB)/School Age Children

The school-aged child has a similar differential as the preschool child; however, you should also **consider Crohn's and ulcerative colitis**.

A Liver Runs Through It/Liver Diseases

> **Alagille syndrome** is a result of intrahepatic biliary atresia. Picture a liver filled with fish "Gilles" which disrupt the transport of bile.

Cholestatic Jaundice

This presents with elevated direct bilirubin, and is caused by **liver/parenchymal** disease or **anatomical/obstructive** disease. Intervention is required to prevent severe liver disease.

Hepatobiliary scintigraphy is a good first step to establish the diagnosis. With liver disease, the isotope is taken up and it makes its way to the biliary system. With obstruction, there will be uptake in the liver but no excretion down the biliary tree.

"Increased **Direct Bili**," "pale stools," and "hepatomegaly."

Neonatal hepatitis will present later (months after birth), whereas **obstructive disease** can present at birth **or** within weeks, *not* months, later.

Biliary Atresia

They will describe an *elevated direct bilirubin* in a child over **one month of age**. The *Kasai* procedure, which essentially joins the liver to the intestine, can be done if the infant is **younger than 2 months**.

When biliary atresia is suspected, the first test should be an *ultrasound,* followed by a HIDA scan and ultimately a biopsy.

The most common cause of cholestatic jaundice in a newborn is TPN (especially if they tell you it is a preemie).

If you need to distinguish **cholestatic jaundice** from **hepatocellular-caused jaundice,** remember: cholestatic disease has a very high alkaline phosphatase, and hepatocellular has a very high SGPT/SGPOT.

Gilbert Syndrome

Gilbert syndrome is due to **glucuronyl transferase deficiency,** and this results in an **intermittently** elevated serum Bili, particularly with illness or other stressors.[20] They will also likely drop a hint of a **similar history in other family members.** That will be your clue to pick Gilbert syndrome as your answer.

"Gil- bili" syndrome. Picture a "hill Bili" unable to transfer his yellow bananas because he lacks a truck (transferase), and his whole family is involved due to all that inbreeding.

Reye's Syndrome

This should be an easy one to figure out on the exam, since they will have to drop hints all over the place. They will likely mention a **recent URI,** during which **aspirin** was given. The child typically presents in the **ICU**, perhaps comatose with **elevated LFT's** and **serum ammonia levels**.

If they tell you this is the **second such episode**, Reye's syndrome is not the correct answer, although it will definitely be one of the choices given. In this case, *consider an inborn error of metabolism.*

---

[20] Like what you are experiencing right now.

Wilson's Disease

This is due to a **lot of copper floating around** and getting deposited, like unwanted pennies at a Michael Bloomberg[21] yachting extravaganza. They get deposited in the eyes (Kayser Fleisher rings), the liver, the brain, and the kidney (renal tubular acidosis is the result).

 Treatment is with D-penicillamine.

 Remember Copper ➔ Penny ➔ Cillamine. **Penicillamine can result in aplastic anemia**, so picture a fistful of pennies clogging up the bone marrow.

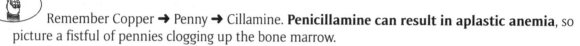 Excess copper can also be seen in **chronic active hepatitis**.

Pancreas

Shwachman Diamond Syndrome – See the "Heme Onc" chapter.

Acute Pancreatitis

 This is characterized by mid-epigastric pain radiating to the back with guarding and rebound, coupled with diminished bowel sounds and vomiting. In more severe cases, they could also describe signs of volume depletion, including decreased urine output and even pulmonary edema and pulmonary effusions. They could describe a child more comfortable lying on his side, with his knees to his chest. They might describe the absence of any family GI history.

Remember that **P**ancreatitis can be associated with **P**ulmonary edema and **P**leural effusion.

It is **diagnosed with abdominal ultrasound. Abdominal ultrasound**, not serum amylase, **is the most specific test in diagnosing pancreatitis**. ERCP (endoscopic retrograde cholangiopancreatography) is used to follow recurrent pancreatitis, not to diagnose acute pancreatitis.

A normal amylase does not rule out pancreatitis—a favorite Board trick. **Lipase** is a more specific test for pancreatic disease. Additional lab findings could include *hyperglycemia, hypocalcemia, elevated BUN/ Creatinine, and anemia, as well as evidence of coagulopathy.*

---

[21] Millionaire (or is it billionaire) mayor of New York City known for his extravagant vacations.

Recurrent / Chronic Pancreatitis

Familial dyslipidemia is an important cause for recurrent pancreatitis in children. They could hint at this by noting a family member had died of premature atherosclerosis. You might be fooled into believing the cause of the abdominal pain is cardiac.

If you are asked which test to order to reveal the underlying cause of the abdominal pain, the answer will be serum lipid levels, not the myriad of imaging or cardiac studies you will be offered.

HOT TIP Hypercalcemia is another known cause of acute or recurrent pancreatitis. Keep this in mind if presented with a child with hyperparathyroidism who is presenting with acute or recurrent abdominal pain.

You may be presented with a child with recurrent pancreatitis. However, because there is no obvious cause or explanation, you might rule it out as a cause. Don't be fooled by this. Often there will be no history of the typical causes of recurrent pancreatitis, such as medications, vasculitis, gallstones, or trauma.

Acute Sporadic vs Recurrent Chronic

EITHER OR CHOICES In case you are tested on it, there **is** a difference between *acute, sporadic pancreatitis and recurrent, chronic pancreatitis.*

Acute sporadic is more common and usually due to blunt abdominal trauma or just plain "we don't know," or idiopathic.

Chronic, relapsing pancreatitis is usually caused by infection, autoimmune disease, inherited conditions, or medications. The most common cause of recurrent pancreatitis is hereditary pancreatitis.

Bad Gall Bladder

Cholecystitis

BUZZ WORDS **Although it is not a cardinal sign in adults, jaundice is a presenting sign in over one fourth of children with cholecystitis.** Therefore, if they describe a child who is jaundiced with fatty food intolerance and has fever, pain radiating to the right scapula, and a palpable mass in the right upper quadrant, think of cholecystitis.

Referred Visceral Pain

Abdominal pain that radiates to the shoulder is likely to be gallbladder pain, which is a result of diaphragm irritation. The diaphragm and shoulder share common pain pathways.

Rolling for Stones

Risk Factors for Gallstones

- Cystic Fibrosis
- Ileal resection
- Treatment with ceftriaxone
- TPN

Cholecystitis can also present with fever and palpable mass in the RUQ.

There are several conditions that leave children predisposed to cholecystitis, and would be important clues included in the question. Examples include **hemolytic disease**, prolonged **use of total parenteral nutrition**, **small intestinal disease,** and even **obesity** or pregnancy.

CASE STUDY

A 15 year old icteric female presents with abdominal pain and hepatosplenomegaly.

What is the best diagnostic test? What is the diagnosis?

THE DIVERSION

You might be tricked into believing that this patient has hepatitis when the cause of the problem is quite galling, since it derives from the gallbladder.

ANSWER REVEALED

The diagnosis is **cholelithiasis** (the official title of gallstones), which is best diagnosed via **abdominal ultrasound**.

CASE STUDY

A 15 year old boy presents with right shoulder pain, nausea, vomiting, and lethargy.

What is the most likely diagnosis?

How would you make the diagnosis?

What is the best treatment?

THE DIVERSION

By noting vomiting along with right shoulder pain, they are hoping you will read this fast and climb the cardiac tree. However, the correct answer will be found in the gall bladder tree.

 Here are your answers:

- Cholecystitis
- Abdominal ultrasound
- Surgery

430

Notice the similar presentations of cholelithiasis and cholecystitis. Both are diagnosed by ultrasound, but the presentations are slightly different.

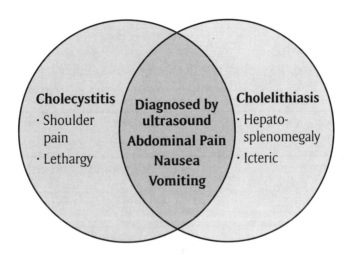

The Alphabet Soup of Hepatitis

Somewhere in the exam you will be called upon to decipher hepatitis A from hepatitis B, HBe antigen vs. core antigen vs. Auntie Jean from Ellie May vs. Non A, "**non-B, Non C and sometimes D**" and "tomorrow something else but today Non A." **Well, here is the ABC of Hepatitis for today's Board candidate**.

Hepatitis A

It is transmitted via the fecal-oral route. **IgM-specific antibody is the best way to diagnose this. Remember, IgG levels persist for life and tell you nothing about recent disease**. It is prevalent where there is poor hygiene and poor sanitation. It is contracted from household contacts and daycare centers.

The presentations will be "flu-like symptoms," along with elevated liver function tests on the lab findings. Also included in the history might be a recent trip to a place where hepatitis A is endemic.

90% of children younger than 5 years have asymptomatic infection and will not be jaundiced. Keep in mind that most children with hepatitis A infection will be asymptomatic. Hepatitis A is prevalent among Native Americans and Alaskan Natives,[22] whereas **hepatitis A is not commonly seen in Asians.**

---

[22] The old politically incorrect term that may still appear on the exam is "Eskimo".

Diagnosis of acute infection is via serum **IgM** for hepatitis A. IgM levels can remain elevated for 6 months. Elevated **IgG** confirms previous infection and immunity against the disease.

Hepatitis B

With hepatitis B, you need to keep track of the antigens and antibodies—and be familiar with their rise and fall.[23] Sort of like being a **hepatitis historian on a serological archaeological dig**.

Phase	Serological Test	Meaning[24]
Acute/ Positive	HB_sAg	Hepatitis surface antigen
	IgM anti-HB_C	IgM antibody to Hepatitis Core Antigen
	HB_eAg	Indicates "high viral load," infectivity, and replication
	HBV-DNA	A sensitive marker indicating "viral replication"
Recovery	**Disappearance of HBV-DNA and HB_sAg**	This occurs around 6 months after its appearance
	Appearance of anti-HBS, anti-HB_c,[25] and anti-HB_e	Antibodies to Hepatitis B surface antigen, core antigen and HBe
Window period	It would be difficult to determine if infection is present during the window period after the appearance of surface antigen and before the appearance of the surface antibody.	This is noted by the *presence of antibody to core antigen (anti-HB_c)* *Core stands for cavalry, and the anti -core cavalry stands in until the antibody to surface antigen comes in, which confers the real immunity.*
Chronic infection	The persistence of surface antigen HB_sAg beyond 6 months indicates chronic infection	It is detected in the serum lifelong in those with chronic infection.

---

[23] Insert your own rise and fall of the Roman Empire joke.

[24] Or added confusion depending on how many times you read it and the state of mind you are in while reading it.

[25] Anti-core antigen is an IgG antibody whereas IgM anti-HBc is, well, IgM.

HBsAg (Hepatitis B Surface Antigen)

It is present during active infection but does not differentiate between **acute** and **chronic** infection.

HBsAb (Antibody to Surface Antigen)

This is consistent with **previous infection** or **positive response to immunization**.

HBeAg (Hepatitis B e Antigen)

It correlates with a high rate of replication, and its presence correlates with **a high rate of infectivity**.

Think **E** as in **E**vil, or very infectious. You can also think of the "**E**" antigen as "**E**xcess" because it can spread to **E**veryone.

Anti-HBcAg (Antibody to Core Antigen)

Antibody to Core Antigen — Just tells you there was a previous infection.

IgM Class Antibody to Core Antigen would indicate a *recent* infection. IgM levels can remain elevated **up to 6 months post infection**.

It is spread by blood and through sex. Perinatal transmission is another major route of hepatitis B infection.

When HBeAg is positive, the mother is highly infectious. Almost ALL kids born to mothers with HBeAg positivity will develop chronic hepatitis B. The earlier the age of infection, the higher the incidence of chronic HBV (90% for infants, 10% for adults). Fulminant hepatic failure and hepatocellular cancer are the most feared complications of chronic HBV infection.

Hepatitis C Virus (HCV)

During my third year of medical school, this was called "*non-A, non-B*." During my residency it was known as "Clifford the Clip-haired Cutie." Now it is just known as **Hepatitis C**. It can result in liver disease and cirrhosis, and is associated with an increased incidence of hepatocellular carcinoma.

It is the most common bloodborne infection in the United States. Hepatitis C is the most common cause of chronic viral hepatitis. It is transmitted by the same route as Hepatitis B. Most infections in children are asymptomatic. Now that adequate blood screening steps are in place, in most cases the source of the infection is unknown.

Hepatitis **C** is associated with Liver **C**ancer and **C**irrhosis. The clinical presentation is quite similar to that of chronic HBV infections.

Hepatitis D Virus (HDV) (or Delta Agent)

If they mention "**Delta Agent,**" they are either referring to hepatitis D or Gene Hackman in *Mississippi Burning*. Remember, this is a virus that cannot replicate by itself. **It requires the presence of HBsAg to provide its outer coat**.

 D represents **D**ependent or **D**eficient. It cannot replicate by itself.

You can be infected with hepatitis D virus **after** hepatitis B infection or **at the same time**. Infection with HDV infection can be associated with chronic hepatitis and cirrhosis.

While chronic infection is rare after coinfection with both B and D, a severe acute hepatitis may result in the development of *cirrhosis*.

Hepatitis E

Hepatitis E is transmitted via the fecal-oral route and is most common in parts of Asia, Africa, and Mexico and is associated with exposure to contaminated water.

It does not lead to chronic hepatitis.

The Rest of the Alphabet

Apparently the professors of hepatitis alphabetology are now working on other letters in the growing list of hepatitis soup. These include hepatitis G and F. However, this is beyond the call of duty for the pediatric boards for the moment, and quite frankly way too boring to describe.

Chapter 18

Catching Your Breath: Pulmonary

Just as in clinical practice, asthma is commonly encountered on the boards. This is where we begin our breathtaking journey through the world of pulmonary disorders.

Asthma

Just the Facts

❑ **The mortality of asthma is on the increase**, which is something that they might want you to know.

❑ Asthma is more common in boys up until puberty, after which it is equally common.

❑ HFAs can be just as effective as nebulizers in older children who know how to use them, especially with the use of spacers.

❑ With **mild asthma**, 60% will outgrow symptoms by adulthood. With **severe asthma**, the rate is 30%.

❑ Routine pulmonary function testing is indicated for children with persistent asthma

Asthma Triggers

The following triggers will often be noted in the history to tip you off to a correct diagnosis of asthma:

· Weather changes

· Aspirin

· Beta Blockers

· Viral URI

- Preparing for and taking the boards

Classification of asthma by severity

Classification	Clinical Description
Mild Intermittent	· General symptoms less than twice weekly · Night symptoms less than twice monthly · No pulmonary function abnormalities · Exacerbations that can last hours to days
Mild persistent	Normal baseline pulmonary function tests General symptoms more than twice a week Night symptoms more than twice a month TREATMENT **Low dose inhaled steroids** **2nd line treatment – leukotriene inhibitor** (Plus bronchodilator prn)
Moderate persistent	A child who requires bronchodilators more than once or twice a week should be classified and treated as having persistent asthma TREATMENT Low-medium dose inhaler / Long-acting bronchodilator
Mild exacerbation of asthma	Mild exacerbation of asthma is defined as a decrease in pulmonary function that is still more than 50% of predicted TREATMENT Mild exacerbation of asthma can be managed with short-acting bronchodilators HOT TIP For some patients who have a history of repeated severe exacerbations, it may be appropriate to maintain a supply of oral steroids at home with instructions to initiate treatment early and call the clinician for further instructions.

Classification	Clinical Description
Mild exacerbation of asthma *(cont'd)*	Physicians tend to prescribe antibiotics for children who have a history of asthma and develop fever and cough. Viral infections are implicated much more commonly than are bacterial infections as triggers in children who have asthma. Bacterial infection will be incorrect on the exam. **Atelectasis in asthma is not a sign of pneumonia!** Steroids clearly improve pulmonary function, compared with use of bronchodilators alone in acutely ill children who have asthma.
Moderate and Severe acute Exacerbations	Pulmonary function tests less than 50% of predicted is consistent with severe obstruction. Levalbuterol has no hard data to support its superiority over albuterol. It would only be indicated in patients who have demonstrated tachycardia, tremor, and/or irritability. There is no role for inhaled mucolytics or chest physical therapy as part of routine care for asthma exacerbations.
Severe Persistent	Continual and frequent exacerbations. Treated with high dose inhaled steroids, long-acting bronchodilators, and oral steroids.

Regardless of the baseline asthma severity, patients can experience severe exacerbations. In general, if you are presented with a patient who is having an acute exacerbation of asthma which is not responding to beta adrenergic agonists, systemic steroids are the next step. *Steroids* only inhibit the late phase reaction of asthma, not the early phase. On the other hand, *leukotriene inhibitors* primarily block the early phase reaction.

Side effects of beta adrenergic agonists include *tremors, tachycardia, hypokalemia,* and in some cases *hyperglycemia* and *hypomagnesemia.*

Hypercapnia and Asthma

A low PCO_2 in the setting of acute asthma would reflect tachypnea.

However, an increasing PCO_2 would reflect CO_2 retention and fatigue.

A normal CO_2 following a period of tachypnea and low CO_2 could mean the patient is heading from a low to a high CO_2 secondary to respiratory fatigue, which would be an ominous sign.

Signs of *hypercapnia* would include *agitation, flushing, mental status change* (including disorientation), *headache,* or *tachycardia.*

Cough Variant Asthma

Reactive airway disease[1] will typically be described as a **"chronic nighttime cough"** which is not alleviated by over-the-counter medications.

The nighttime cough **can** be "productive," so that alone should not throw you off the reactive airway trail.

A **nighttime cough** could also be associated with sinusitis or **gastroesophageal reflux**. However, if this is the diagnosis they are looking for, they will be obligated to provide you with additional signs and symptoms.

Asthma in Pre-Schoolers

Special consideration must be given to preschool children with asthma.

CXR may help identify hyperinflation and increased peribronchial markings.

History from parents and caregivers must be relied upon.

Physical findings include tachypnea, nasal flaring, and/or poor air exchange.

In the acute phase, the child may not be moving enough air to elicit a wheeze.

---

[1] Or hyperresponsive airway disease, which is how it is described at pulmonary wine and cheese parties to justify 3 years of fellowship training.

Infants

All that wheezes, again, is not asthma, especially in an infant. For other causes of wheezing, consider **aspiration**, **bronchopulmonary dysplasia**, **foreign body**, and **vascular rings.** To put it another way:

❏ Aspirated **Drinks**
❏ Babies with **Kinks**
❏ Swallowed **Thinks** (=Things)[2]
❏ Vascular **Rinks** (=Rings)

Also consider **bronchiolitis**.

Allergies

Where there is allergic smoke, for example allergic rhinitis and/or atopic dermatitis, there is asthmatic fire.

80% of asthmatic children have positive immediate-type allergy skin tests.

Therefore, any description of allergic signs and symptoms should make you think of asthma.

Exercise Induced Asthma (EIA)

EIA is coughing and wheezing 5 minutes after exercising, with gradual improvement with 15 minutes of rest.

Cold, dry air is the worst; warm, moist air is the best. Therefore, jogging in the nude on an ice skating rink that hasn't been Zamboni'd in a while is the worst exercise for children at risk for EIA.

It is important to keep in mind that children with asthma should be encouraged to remain active. Severe EIA exacerbations may be considered a result of poor control or management.

> ## Foreign Body vs. Asthma
>
> **"Respiratory infection that is not clearing,"** a **"wheeze that is localized and fixed,"** "reduced breath sounds over one lung," a "mediastinal shift" that is seen on CXR, or a "very sudden onset" suggests foreign body as the cause of wheezing. If the foreign body is not removed, recurrent pneumonia, atelectasis, or bronchiectasis could result.

---

[2] Aspirated things (foreign bodies) are more likely in older children who are mobile, but it is still a consideration in an infant.

However, not all children experiencing shortness of breath are experiencing EIA. The following are other causes, and once again, they will be obligated to provide hints at the correct diagnosis in the presenting history.

To remember other causes of poor exercise tolerance, consider a child who is hanging around **CAMP**, drinking and smoking, while everyone else is playing kickball:

> **C**ardiac Disease
> **A**nemia
> **M**uscle Weakness
> **P**sychological Factors and **P**oor Shape (sometimes due to depression or distraction)

Long acting beta agonists (such as formoterol or salmeterol) may be needed for activities that last longer than a few hours. However, this is controversial, and since it is still being debated it may not appear on the exam.

Leukotriene inhibitors, such as *montelukast*, can help with exercise-induced asthma, but this varies from person to person.

Anticholinergic agents, including *ipratropium*, are not used for managing exercise-induced asthma.

Increased Risk for ICU Admission

The following are important risk factors for ICU hospitalization for asthma:

- · Chronic steroid use
- · Hospitalization within the past year
- · Low socioeconomic status/low educational level
- · Previous life threatening episode

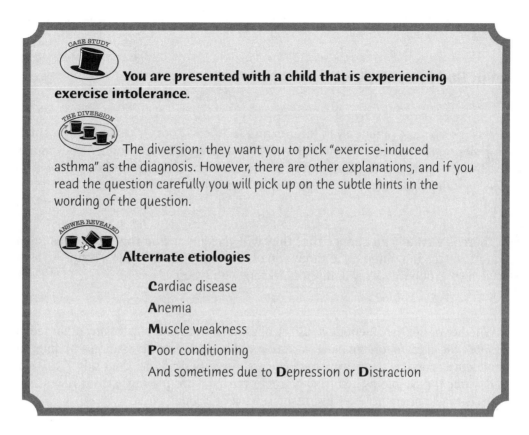

You are presented with a child that is experiencing exercise intolerance.

The diversion: they want you to pick "exercise-induced asthma" as the diagnosis. However, there are other explanations, and if you read the question carefully you will pick up on the subtle hints in the wording of the question.

Alternate etiologies

Cardiac disease

Anemia

Muscle weakness

Poor conditioning

And sometimes due to **D**epression or **D**istraction

Asthma Prognosis

Risk factors for persistent asthma – Rule of **E**'s and **3**'s (mirror images of each other):

- ❑ **3** years of age (onset before age 3)
- ❑ Ig**E** **E**levation
- ❑ **M**aternal history of asthma (think of the M as an E on its side)
- ❑ **E**osinophilia

· 60% of children with mild asthma will outgrow the symptoms by adulthood

· 50% of infants with severe RSV bronchiolitis will develop recurrent wheezing

Controlling Persistent Asthma

An inhaled corticosteroid is the best method because it not only decreases bronchial inflammation, but also reduces **bronchial hyperresponsiveness**.

The risk of oral candidiasis can be lessened by mouth rinsing after inhaling a dose.

Wheezing

Foreign Body Aspiration

This is seen most commonly in **infants and toddlers**. Another possibility is **a child with a developmental disability, or any child with CNS depression**. Most foreign body aspirations manifest within 24 hours. The classic **triad** is *cough, wheeze,* and *decreased breath sounds*. Infants and toddlers typically aspirate food, and older children typically aspirate objects.

There is virtually no chance that they will give you a clue that there was an object aspirated. In fact, they often try to throw you off the trail by mentioning a history of asthma and/or giving signs of croup with x-ray findings consistent with croup.

Whether or not they mention a history of asthma, signs of croup, or any other red herrings for that matter, the clues to foreign body aspiration will be "unlabored breathing with intermittent nonproductive cough" with an "expiratory wheeze" heard best on the "right side." They may, if you are lucky, describe the symptoms occurring just after the child was playing with a toy, but that hint would be a gift. They will often include a history of a cough of "sudden onset."

In nearly 50% of cases, **there is no recollection of an actual aspiration.** However, do look for it on the picture section;[3] if the object is radiolucent, inspiratory and expiratory radiographs showing the I/O discrepancy on one side will be obvious. Radiographs will need to be confirmed with bronchoscopy, which is how the FB will be retrieved anyway.

The "expiratory wheeze" can also be due to other problems that can cause obstruction to inspiration, such as a *vascular ring, bronchogenic cyst, or tracheal stenosis.* There will need to be other hints in the question pointing you to one of these diagnoses.

Another entity which can be confused with asthma is **vocal cord paralysis**. Vocal cord paralysis would present with difficulty during inspiration rather than expiration. In addition, you will be presented with a patient who has a normal pulse oximeter reading, clear lungs, and no response to beta agonists.

A blunted inspiratory loop on spirometry correlates with vocal cord paralysis, rather than asthma. Other associations with vocal cord paralysis include: recent viral *upper respiratory tract infection, exposure to chemicals, fumes,* or *cold air,* and *gastroesophageal reflux disease (GERD).*

---

[3] You may need to squint until you are cross-eyed.

Recurrent Wheezing

If you are presented with an infant with recurrent coughing associated with wheezing, the underlying problem might be a swallowing dysfunction. This would be confirmed by a swallow study with fluoroscopic guidance.

Treatment of swallowing dysfunction consists of thickened formula and/or human milk, with the infant placed in the upright position for feeding.

CASE STUDY

You could be presented with yet another long-winded description of a one-year-old child with acute onset of coughing coupled with a right-sided expiratory wheeze. Then, just as you pat yourself on the back for making the correct diagnosis, they provide you with the suspected diagnosis and then simply ask you to pick the best test to confirm your suspicions.

THE DIVERSION

Plain chest x-ray will be one of the choices. However, this won't be helpful since at this age, since a radiolucent food particle is what was most likely inhaled. Then, sitting right there for the taking is what you believe to be the juicy correct answer: "inspiratory/expiratory films" — right out of the textbook that is your brain. This will be incorrect, since it is impossible to have a child this age cooperate with such a test.

ANSWER REVEALED

Oddly enough, the correct answer will be **airway fluoroscopy**. This is the safest and most effective way to confirm foreign body aspiration in this age group.

Respiratory Failure

DEFINITION

Respiratory failure is present when a patient is incapable of compensating for the effects of respiratory compromise.

Tachypnea is the earliest sign of respiratory failure. Therefore, the evaluation of "**respiratory effort**" is more important than any lab value. Signs of respiratory failure include **tachypnea**, **retractions**, and **pulsus paradoxus.**

Late signs of respiratory distress and indications for intubation would include hypoxemia, grunting, and signs of fatigue. If you are presented with a patient with an underlying neurological disorder who is in respiratory distress, elective intubation would likely be the correct choice regarding management.

Let's go Clubbing

If you are presented with a patient with clubbing of the fingers or the toes, depending on other information presented, consider a diagnosis of *cyanotic heart disease, chronic lung disease,* or *cirrhosis of the liver.* It can also be a familial trait, in the absence of any other disorders.

Oh and by the way, the official term for digital clubbing is *hypertrophic pulmonary osteoarthropathy,* just in case they throw that term at you.

With pulsus paradoxus, the difference in blood pressure during inspiration and expiration should not be greater than 10 mmHg; more than 20 mmHg suggests pulmonary or cardiac problems.

The first thing to do in deciding whether to intubate is to **assess respiratory effort**.

Obtaining an ABG, or any other time-consuming lab, is **not the "first thing" to do** and would not be the correct choice in assessing a child in respiratory distress. You can almost never be wrong in choosing "assess airway" - the "A" in the ABC of managing acute situations.

They could present you with a child in respiratory distress and ask you the best way to assess and confirm this.

Assessing respiratory distress can be tricky. The diversionary answer will be to assess the respiratory rate. This is frequently the incorrect answer in ruling out respiratory failure since the "normal" respiratory rate may only be a transition from tachypnea to apnea.

When asked for the best way to assess for severity of respiratory distress, the correct answer will often be to watch for signs of anxiety (sweating and/or fast heart rate).

Chronic Hypoxemia

DEFINITION

Any disorder that compromises the ability to oxygenate blood results in chronic hypoxemia. Disorders resulting in **pulmonary hypertension** like cor pulmonale are an example.

PERIL WARNING

Any underlying disorder that results in chronic hypoxemia will have several consequences. They won't come right out and hit you over the head with a hammer and tell you the patient has chronic hypoxemia; it will be hinted at in the history.

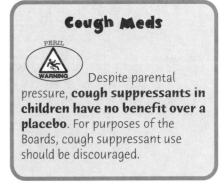

When a Cough is Not Effective

Cerebral palsy, muscle weakness, vocal cord dysfunction, CNS disease, thoracic deformities, and pain **all impair the effectiveness of coughing.**

MNEMONIC

TNT: **T**horaco **N**euro (Cerebral Palsy/ CNS Disease) **T**ied up with weakness and pain. It takes TNT to clear lungs when coughing isn't effective.

The Physiological Scoop

There is no memorization here, just cool explanation of the physiological facts.

The kidneys draw their own conclusion when they see hypoxemia. They assume all is okay with the lungs upstairs. The kidneys then respond by producing erythropoietin (the only thing they can do); red cells get produced, and the HCT goes up. A HCT of 65 is fine, but greater than that results in **headaches, joint pain, clots** (leading to **pulmonary emboli**), and "hemoptysis." Any of the above can be clues that chronic hypoxemia is the underlying problem.

For some reason, the platelet shelf life goes down, so there is also an **increased risk of bleeding**.

In addition, the respiratory drive of patients with chronic lung disease is often driven by hypoxemia, rather than acidosis and hypercapnia. You are expected to know that correction of hypoxia (by administration of oxygen) in a patient suffering from chronic lung disease may put the patient at risk for respiratory arrest. Therefore, oxygen supplementation should be provided at the lowest concentration needed to maintain an oxygen saturation of 90%. CO_2 measurements via ABG should be followed as well.

Calling All Coughs (Chronic)

Coughs present early without a lot of other clues, and you need to pick out the etiologies. Here is your roadmap.

Working Up a Chronic Cough

The initial screen should include **sweat chloride testing, TB skin testing,** and routine **CXR**. If findings from these tests are normal,

Cough Meds

PERIL WARNING

Despite parental pressure, **cough suppressants in children have no benefit over a placebo.** For purposes of the Boards, cough suppressant use should be discouraged.

spirometry can be performed in children who can cooperate (usually 6 years of age or older) to rule out asthma.

Psychogenic Cough

"Loud, brassy barking and/or honking that can be **produced on command.**" If they note that it disappears during sleep, you have your answer.

More Serious Considerations

TB and fungal infections can produce harsh, dry coughs. If they include the combination of fever, weight loss, and night sweats along with a chronic cough, skin testing is indicated.

Cystic Fibrosis

Signs and symptoms consistent with CF include *failure to thrive, steatorrhea, low serum albumin, low sodium,* and *pseudomonas infections.*

The Sweat Test: 60 mEq or greater is diagnostic. This number is critical in case they throw in a normal value, implying it is abnormal simply by including it in the description.

Genetics of CF

The gene is inherited in an autosomal recessive pattern. **Carriers show no signs, so any physical findings they tell you about are red herrings.**

In the past they have asked, "If a sibling of someone with CF marries someone from the general population, what are the odds of them having a kid with CF?"[4] Using the formula that oddsmakers in Las Vegas use, you can easily answer this question.

---

[4] They should tell you they are both Caucasian; otherwise, the risk is too low to bother with.

In the general Caucasian population, the carrier rate is **1 in 25 (1/25).** Memorize this.

· If 2 carriers are married, the risk (autosomal recessive) is 1/4.

· Therefore, the answer to the typical question they ask above is:

· (2/3)[chance of a sibling carrier] × (1/25)[chance in Caucasian population] × (1/4)[chance of child being double recessive] = 1 in 150.

Another very simple question they could ask is, "What are the odds of a **healthy sibling** of someone with **CF being a carrier**?" The answer is **2/3**.

They can present you with a child suspected of having cystic fibrosis, and ask for the most effective way to confirm the diagnosis.

The diversion will be DNA analysis or genetic testing. You will be tempted to take the bait, believing that modern methods must trump the old.

Sometimes an oldie but a goodie is better than new technology. This is the case in confirming a diagnosis of cystic fibrosis. DNA analysis *has not replaced sweat testing* as the gold standard. *False negatives are rare on the sweat test.* When it occurs, it is usually due to an *inadequate sample or technique.*

CF in Infancy

If they describe an infant with **hypoproteinemia**, **anemia**, **steatorrhea**, and recurrent pulmonary symptoms, think CF. Remember, **hypochloremic alkalosis** can be another sign of CF in infants. *During infancy, GI symptoms are more prevalent than respiratory symptoms.*

$\downarrow Cl, \uparrow pH$

GI Manifestations of CF

Vitamin E deficiency is a major problem with CF. **Vitamin E supplementation should be started before age 5**.

 The **E**'s of CF: **E**yes (Ptosis), **E**arth (Proprioception, Truncal Ataxia, and Muscle Sense), and Vitamin **E** deficiency.

Vitamin K malabsorption may lead to a prolonged prothrombin time.

GI manifestations of CF in the neonatal period could be **meconium ileus, meconium peritonitis, and/or unconjugated hyperbilirubinemia**.

Meconium ileus may present with a history of polyhydramnios. Abdominal films would show a "ground glass" appearance due to decreased bowel gas. **Meconium peritonitis** might present as a "pseudocyst" (which is calcified meconium) on x-ray.

Treatment of Acute Exacerbations of CF

Treatment of acute exacerbations of CF is with an **aminoglycoside** and a **penicillin** derivative such as **piperacillin** that attacks *pseudomonas.*

Staph infections are seen more often early in life. Later, *pseudomonas* is the main problem.

 Infections are controlled with antibiotics, but *never completely eradicated.*

Cor Pulmonale

"Lower body edema, hepatomegaly, gallop rhythm, and clubbing" are all signs of cor pulmonale.

Since cor pulmonale in most cases is caused by pulmonary hypertension, it is not reversible. However, when severe upper airway obstruction is the cause, it is surgically correctable and reversible.

In addition to cor pulmonale, life threatening manifestations of cystic fibrosis may also include development of pneumothoraces and/or hemoptysis.

Empyema

Empyema is the collection of pus in the pleural space.

If pneumonia is not improving despite treatment with appropriate antibiotics, think of **empyema**. This is especially true if there is some initial clinical improvement after treatment.

Hypercarbia vs. Hypoxia

Hypoxia will be described as "cyanosis" with "depressed sensorium."

Hypercarbia is often described as "flushing and agitation" and "headaches" because of elevated CO_2 leading to cerebral vasodilation.

Newborn Pulmonary Disorders

Central Apnea

When there is no respiratory effort because there is no signal from the CNS, this is central apnea.

Apnea of prematurity is a subset of central apnea. Apnea of prematurity cannot be diagnosed before other causes are ruled out, since it is a diagnosis of exclusion.

If there is another cause of the apnea, they will have to provide you with a hint of that cause. This may include *sepsis, medications, profound anemia,* or an *electrolyte abnormality.*

Apnea of prematurity is treated with *caffeine*, much the way the apnea of boredom is treated in those reading this book preparing for the boards.

Narcotic Overdose

Here we will see respiratory acidosis due to CO_2 retention with good PO_2 i.e., in the 60's, despite respiratory depression.

Apnea and Anemia in the premature arena

There is an association between anemia and apnea in premature infants. While more premature infants are anemic and do not experience apnea, anemia should be considered as a potential factor when both are present.

Hypoxia should be suspected in any premature infant experiencing tachycardia and tachypnea at rest who is not gaining weight. In such instances, transfusion with packed red cells should be considered.

Obstructive Apnea

Obstructive Sleep Apnea

Obstructive sleep apnea is often due to *adenoid hypertrophy*. Beware that the standard examination of the oropharynx might be negative, since the adenoids are not typically visible on routine exam. There may not be associated tonsillar hypertrophy.

You may distinguish adenoid hypertrophy from other entities as follows when presented with a patient with nasal congestion. *Adenoid hypertrophy* would typically be seen in a child between ages 2 and 5 years, where allergic rhinitis would typically be seen between ages 5-10 years. If they describe a patient that gets better on nasal steroids or other allergy medication, allergic rhinitis is more likely. If the patient responds to antibiotics, then sinusitis is the most likely diagnosis.

DEFINITION

When airflow ceases because the upper airway is occluded, this is obstructive apnea.

TREATMENT

If the obstructive apnea is complete (e.g., complete laryngeal atresia, severe web), treatment consists of *tracheotomy*. Some cases, such as severe subglottic stenosis and complete vocal cord paralysis, will require the more permanent tracheostomy.

EITHER OR CHOICES

You will be expected to distinguish between apnea and periodic breathing. **Apnea** would, by definition, last more than 20 seconds, or would be associated with bradycardia or cyanosis if less than 20 seconds. **Periodic breathing**, by definition, is a pattern of recurrent brief pauses in breathing, lasting less than 20 seconds. There may be a brief drop in heart rate or desaturation, but no "bradycardia" or cyanosis.

CASE STUDY

You are presented with a patient who is post-op from adenoidectomy and tonsillectomy, and is experiencing respiratory distress. They note a history of severe obstructive apnea. You will be asked for the most likely explanation of the acute respiratory distress.

THE DIVERSION

You might be tempted to pick pulmonary hemorrhage or hemothorax. Other diversionary choices could include tension pneumothorax, since this would likely be post extubation.

ANSWER REVEALED

The correct answer in this setting would be pulmonary edema, which is a postoperative complication in patients with severe obstructive apnea.

Plowing through Pleural Fluids

You will have to decipher different pleural fluids and their countries of origin based on the clothes they wear (color) and what they say (contents). Here is your travel guide.

Transudate/Pleural Fluid

I remember this as "transitional," as in "the source of the problem lies elsewhere." This is often due to one of the following:

- Cirrhosis

- Nephrotic syndrome

- Congestive heart failure

In a **transudate**, the *triglyceride level is low (less than 50)*.

Exudate is seen with inflammation. This can be expected when you are presented with a pleural effusion in the context of pneumonia, cancer, trauma, or inflammatory disease. With an exudate, the *lacate dehydrogenase concentrations are 2-3 times the concentrations* in serum, and *protein value will be greater than 3 grams/dL.*

Chylothorax

In a chylothorax, electrolyte **concentrations** are **close to those found in serum**. Besides history, the lab clues they will give are the triglyceride and protein levels in the fluid. Triglyceride **greater than 110, elevated lymphocyte count,** and **protein greater than 3 are consistent with chylothorax**. Typically they will describe it in a **post-op** patient, especially after cardiac surgery.

Pneumothorax (PTX)

You should suspect a pneumothorax if you are presented with a patient with *tachypnea, tachycardia,* and *unilateral decreased breath sounds.* If there is a *tracheal shift* with decreased blood pressure, you should suspect a tension pneumothorax. This is a medical emergency requiring needle and/or chest tube insertion. A pneumothorax can be seen in patients with asthma. It can also be seen in the context of intubation and ventilation.

Remember, small spontaneous PTX can occur with marijuana smoking in tall, thin adolescents, and this may be a clue they are handing you that drug use is an issue.

For a small pneumothorax, **watchful observation with oxygen administration is the first thing to do**. For a small PTX, needle aspiration may be the correct choice instead of chest tube placement.

PERIL WARNING The degree of pain does not correlate directly with the extent of the pneumothorax. Intubation is rarely the answer they want with a pneumothorax.

TREATMENT **If it is a small spontaneous** pneumothorax, **the first thing to do is "give oxygen."** If it is a **large "tension"** pneumothorax, it is a life-threatening condition; it should be evacuated STAT.

Sudden Infant Death Syndrome (SIDS)

This is a section in which when to reassure and when to be concerned will be tested in several questions. Here is what you need to know.

Risk factors for SIDS

Risk factors for SIDS are the following:

- Sleeping on Tummy, especially with soft bedding
- Sleeping with Mummy (co-sleeping)
- Living in the Slummy (low income)
- Smoking
- Cold Weather
- Young Parents

Apparent Life-Threatening Event (ALTE)

 An ALTE is an episode in which an infant:

❑ Ceases to breathe,
❑ Develops cyanosis or pallor, and
❑ Becomes unresponsive,
❑ But is resuscitated successfully.

A 2-month-old boy suddenly becomes **limp, cyanotic, and apneic**. He is revived with mouth-to-mouth resuscitation. When he is seen in the emergency room, findings on **physical examination are normal**.

The *most appropriate* next step in the management of this patient is to **admit to the hospital for evaluation**.

While the physical exam can be normal on presentation, it is the **history that is alarming and requires hospitalization, observation, and workup**. Diagnostic considerations are reviewed below. **Hospitalization is the answer they want**.

Discharge from the hospital after an ALTE would be appropriate if it was the first episode, the episode was brief and self- resolving, there is a non progressive explanation such as nasal congestion or even reflux, and there is no previous significant history of medical illness.

When you are faced with an infant with ALTE. Recall **NALS**:

> **N**euro (CNS anomaly, seizure)
> **A**buse/Trauma
> **L**ung Infection (RSV or other infections, sepsis, meningitis, etc.) /
> Lung Problems (aspiration, apnea, and GERD)
> **S**ugar is low (metabolic disorders, hypoglycemia)

> ## Pacifying An*iety
>
> Pacifiers may be protective, and the AAP actually now recommends "considering" them at naptime in the first year of life (after the first month for breast-feeders, so as not to interfere with successful breastfeeding).

> The most common **extra-pulmonary** causes of **cyanosis** are right-to-left shunting of blood and methemoglobinemia.

Risk for SIDS

Don't be misled into choosing an answer that states that apnea preceded or predicts SIDS. There is no evidence that apnea monitors are useful in reducing the risk of SIDS.

The only indication for a home apnea monitor is for an infant with bonafide apnea of prematurity that responds to stimulation when experiencing apnea.

Pulse Oximetry / What It Can and Can't Do

We have all become reliant on pulse oximetry without knowing its limitations. You will have to know these limitations. The easy part is to make sure the **pulse is correlating,** and that there are **no mechanical or artifactual problems**. That is for the real world; now for the Board world.

Watch out for the following conditions:

Carboxyhemoglobin

Carboxyhemoglobin is elevated in the face of carbon monoxide poisoning. Here, the pulse oximetries will *overestimate the level of oxyhemoglobin and, therefore, oxygenation.*

Methemoglobin

This will result in inconsistent and, therefore, unreliable values. Remember, this is one of the *non-cardiac causes of cyanosis.* Blood may be described as "chocolate" colored.

Impaired Perfusion

Anytime there are "shock-like" conditions resulting in impaired peripheral perfusion, consider the O_2 values to be unreliable. Watch for clues of shock in the question (e.g., heart failure, hypovolemia, septic shock).

Spirometry does not measure total lung capacity or residual volume.

Spirometry does not provide TLC or a ride home with an RV.

Best Gas

If you are asked for the best measure of pulmonary function in a newborn, the correct answer will be arterial blood gas measurement (ABG). Likewise, cyanosis in and of itself doesn't tell you much about the degree of hypoxemia. This too is best measured via ABG.

The least reliable test would be capillary blood gas. Pulse oximetry needs to be correlated with the ABG and therefore, would not be the correct answer.

If you are presented with an infant with "noisy breathing," the initial step is to obtain a thorough birth history and observe the breathing patterns in different positions.

Spying on Spirometry

Some important points regarding spirometry that you should be aware of:

Spirometry measures inspiratory and expiratory respiratory effort. It requires expiration for more than 6 seconds. Good luck getting a child younger than age 6 to do this. Therefore, if you are presented with a spirometry result in a child younger than 6, it is unreliable.

Apple Stridor

If you are presented with a patient with stridor, just noting the age should help narrow down the correct answer if you are asked for a diagnosis.

In a *neonate*, you are likely dealing with choanal atresia, laryngeal web /stenosis, vascular ring, or vocal cord paralysis

Envision the wind howling through an open CAVE, Choanal Atresia, Vascular ring, Vocal cord paralysis. You can picture a spider web covering the opening of the cave to remember laryngeal web/stenosis.

From *4 to 6 weeks* - laryngomalacia or tracheomalacia

1 to 4 years - croup, epiglottitis, foreign body aspiration

Older than 5 years - vocal cord dysfunction, peritonsillar abscess, or anaphylaxis

---

Viral croup is synonymous with laryngotracheobronchitis. It will be described as a harsh, nonproductive, "barking" cough, with inspiratory stridor preceded by a low grade fever and URI symptoms.

Spasmodic croup can also be described as a "barking" and nonproductive cough. It may be due to allergies or psychological factors. However, there will be no URI or low grade fever described, and this is your clue.

The Scoop on Croup

Etiology: **R**SV, **I**nfluenza, or **P**ara influenza (**RIP**).

They will either describe **an "inspiratory" stridor** or a **"biphasic"** (inspiratory and expiratory) stridor.

Bronchiolitis

❑ It most frequently occurs in children between 2-7 months, but can occur in those up to 2 years of age.

❑ It is obstruction of the small airways brought on by a viral infection, usually RSV.

❑ **RSV** is the most common cause of bronchiolitis (in case you are speed reading and missed it at the end of the last line).

❑ **Parainfluenza virus** is the second most common cause of bronchiolitis.

❑ Poor feeding and respiratory distress (characterized by tachypnea, nasal flaring, and hypoxemia) may be indicators of increased severity.

❑ O_2 saturation of less than 95%, PO_2 less than 65, PCO_2 greater than 40, atelectasis on CXR, and RR greater than 70 are all signs of severe bronchiolitis.

❑ Severe bronchiolitis is associated with the development of asthma later in life.

In addition to bilateral wheezing and crackles, they will also describe acute onset of rhinorrhea, low-grade fever, and shortness of breath.

CXR findings would include hyperinflation and patchy infiltrates. Focal findings would rule out bronchiolitis.

Bronchiolitis can be distinguished from chlamydia, which typically presents at 1-3 weeks of age with a staccato cough *without fever*. Wheezing is not part of the presentation.

Managing Bronchiolitis

CASE STUDY

You might be presented with a long-winded history, and in the end you are given a diagnosis of RSV. Besides realizing you wasted time reading the history, you then realize you are being asked how to prevent spread to other patients.

THE DIVERSION

Since bronchiolitis manifests as wheezing, you are tempted to pick "wear a mask" as the key to preventing spread of disease. This is the diversionary answer waiting for you.

ANSWER REVEALED

The correct answer is "hand washing," which is almost always the correct answer any time it appears.

Most cases can be managed without hospitalization and without albuterol. **The decision whether to hospitalize is based on the following factors**:

- ❏ Reliability of parents (compliance and follow-up)
- ❏ Duration of symptoms
- ❏ Underlying conditions (heart or lung disease)
- ❏ Condition on presentation (younger than 3 months of age, low O_2 sats, poor feeding, and dehydration are poor signs).

TREATMENT

Treatment is symptomatic and includes cool mist. If warranted, treatment consists of albuterol aerosols. Steroids can also be used (even though not conclusively proven to be effective).

Bronchiectasis

This is basically **permanent dilation of a small segment of airway, along with inflammation**. The most common cause is cystic fibrosis.

Watch for repeated *lower* **respiratory tract infections**, with a specific area of atelectasis on CXR (e.g., they might say R middle lobe atelectasis). In addition, the **coughing symptoms are made worse with changes in position (e.g., after lying down)**. If they are presenting you with a child with bronchiectasis associated with cystic fibrosis, they will likely present with GI symptoms and failure to thrive.

Diagnosis

The MOST helpful diagnostic test is **CT of the chest**.

Think bronchie**CT**asis.

The causes of bronchiectasis in addition to CF can be remembered with the following mnemonic

- **D**yskinesia (primary ciliary dyskinesia)
- **I**mmunodeficiency and **I**nfection
- **L**obar pneumonia, right middle **L**obe syndrome, enlarged **L**ymph nodes causing compression
- **A**spergillosis and disorders typically prevented by **A** vaccine, such as measles or pertussis
- **T**B
- **E**xtinsic compression caused by enlarged lymph nodes

Kartagener syndrome

Kartagener syndrome is due to ciliary dysfunction. If you ever wondered how important cilia were to your life, cilia dysfunction leads to chronic sinusitis and bronchiectasis in this syndrome. Cilia are also responsible for the heart moving to the left side of the chest during fetal development. Therefore, one sign of Kartegener syndrome is situs inversus. Cilia dysfunction may also result in male infertility.

If you are presented with a patient where they note the heart sounds are on the right side of the chest, consider Kartagener syndrome.

Vascular Rings and other Things causing vascular compression

Vascular rings and other entities such as a double aortic arch, which can cause external tracheal or esophageal compression, should be suspected in an infant with recurrent wheezing that increases with feeding and neck flexion. In addition to wheezing, the infant can also present with stridor and/or dyspnea during feeding.

Diagnosis is best confirmed with a barium swallow

Congenital Malformations of the Lung

Pulmonary Sequestrations - With pulmonary sequestration, you have lung tissue that is supplied by systemic rather than pulmonary arterial supply. **Intrapulmonary sequestration** usually presents in teenagers and young adults as a cough and fever, with a history of recurrent pneumonia. Dullness to percussion can be noted on physical exam. **Extrapulmonary sequestration** usually presents in infants, often with other congenital problems such as vertebral or GI anomalies.

Bronchogenic cysts can present with symptoms consistent with airway compression, or may be discovered incidentally on x-ray.

Congenital cystic adenomatoid malformation, which is dysplastic lung tissue, may present as recurrent pneumonia in early childhood.

Congenital lobar emphysema, which is the hyperinflation of one or more lobes of the lung, presents as respiratory distress and/or airway obstruction in newborns.

Managing Tuberculosis

You will need to know the proper management of TB exposures (and their workups), as well as cases of **active TB**.

Dealing with the Faces and Phases of TB

Most children with TB are **asymptomatic**, and the primary pulmonary focus (which is also known by its *nom de Guerre* "**the Ghon Complex**") **is not always visible on CXR**. Therefore, the PPD is the "eyes and ears" in the field looking for this guerilla warrior, the Ghon Complex.

Treatment of Latent Tuberculosis

Positive Skin/Negative CXR

Isoniazid monotherapy is for positive skin tests with negative CXR. Once again, this is given for a full gestational period = **9 months**.

Rifampin is given for 9 months if it is an INH-resistant strain.

Treatment of Active Pulmonary Disease

Typical buzzwords for a child they identify as "at risk" for TB or having active TB are: "**low-grade fever and cough for a month**" or perhaps longer. On physical exam they can describe "**rales usually at the bases.**" If they are kind enough to describe it, the CXR finding will be "hilar adenopathy."

There are a few options for such active pulmonary TB:

- ❏ 2 months of **RIP** (**R**ifampin, **I**NH, and **P**yrazinamide) and then you
- ❏ **P**ass on to **4** months of INH and Rifampin or
- ❏ **P**ass **P**yrazinamide altogether and go directly to 9 months of isoniazid and rifampin.

Extrapulmonary Tuberculosis

Pulmonary is a guerilla warrior, but extrapulmonary fights fair and is diagnosed after symptoms or signs have presented themselves. It's all out in the open; therefore, they are easily **MAPD:**

> **M**eningitis
> **A**denitis
> **P**leuritis
> **D**isseminated (Miliary disease)

 Treatment is virtually the same as that for pulmonary disease. It is more tailored to clinical response since there are more signs to monitor.

The one exception is meningitis. In this case you use **RIP** (see above) for 2 months **AND streptomycin**. Afterward, RI is fine for another 10 months and you can stop the streptomycin after isolating the strain and confirming sensitivity to INH.

Steroids are **used with TB meningitis**.

Primary TB can **present with a localized pleural effusion**. However, if they describe it in a preschool child, it will be a clinically significant finding in its own right. They will describe symptoms similar to bacterial pneumonia, but it will be in the context of TB exposure or other clues.

Managing Chest Wall Trauma

With respiratory symptoms following blunt trauma to the chest, they want you to know that the **MOST important procedure to perform initially**[5] **to determine management of this child is *physical examination* of the chest.** Physical examination is almost always going to be the correct answer to any question if it is one of the choices.

You will want to examine the chest even if[6] there are signs of respiratory distress and tachycardia.

Physical evaluation is implemented even in the absence of any respiratory distress.

If the chest wall trauma has resulted in flail chest, intubation and pain management are the correct initial steps.

---

[5] Once airway and breathing have been confirmed.
[6] Make that "especially if".

Acute Respiratory Distress Syndrome

Acute respiratory distress syndrome (ARDS) used to go by the name "adult respiratory distress syndrome" until it was discovered that it can also occur in children and on the pediatric board exam. ARDS may occur with sepsis, lung contusion secondary to trauma, smoke inhalation, and near downing episodes.

The prognosis is better if it occurs in the context of trauma.

The initial presentation may include hypoxemia, atelectasis, and pulmonary edema. This could progess to decreased lung compliance and the development of a pneumothorax, and eventually multiorgan failure.

While steroids are not indicted for acute near-drowning episodes, steroids would be indicated if you are presented with a patient with ARDS who is not improving on supportive measures.

The cause of <u>death</u> in ARDS is <u>multiorgan failure</u> rather than respiratory failure.

You could be presented with a patient who is relatively asymptomatic following the initial triggering insult. Don't be fooled. It can take several days for symptoms of ARDS to present.

> ### Acute Respiratory Distress Syndrome
>
> In near-drowning episodes, this starts out as pulmonary edema, which is a result of increased permeability of the alveolar capillary membranes. It is a result of some insult, in this case the submersion episode. The x-ray findings will be described as "<u>fine reticular infiltrate</u>," and <u>8 hours</u> later things get <u>worse</u>.
>
> The lungs are only the opening act. The headliners include liver, kidney, brain, and bone marrow dysfunction. It is this multi-organ involvement that poses the greatest risk to survival. And is what you want to avoid.

Drowning

Hypothermia

Hypothermia is a common complication with near drowning and, therefore, rewarming is important.

External rewarming by placement in a warm bath will <u>not be</u> the correct choice. This is in part because monitoring will be impossible. The correct answer will be <u>external rewarming of the head and neck</u>.

Homeward Bound?

If they have been submerged for **less than 1 minute** with no loss of consciousness and required no resuscitation in the field, the patient can usually be observed at home.

Hospital Bound?

Children rescued from near-drowning episodes can **look** quite **stable** upon **arrival to the emergency department**, and **then go downhill and require advanced life support.**

Duration of asphyxia is the key to prognosis. **The duration of time from submersion to when adequate respiration is restored determines the extent of the damage**.

Any one of the following *predicts risk for future deterioration* and *warrants continued medical supervision:*

❏ A history of **apnea and CPR in the field.**

❏ Neurological concerns (seizure or disorientation) or respiratory failure from aspiration.

❏ Arterial desaturation and/or tachypnea.

Hemoptysis

The most likely causes of hemoptysis in children are:

1. Infection
2. Cystic fibrosis (bronchiectasis)
3. Foreign body aspiration
4. Hemosiderosis

If you are presented with a patient with acute hemoptysis and are asked for the best next step, the answer will be any choice which is diagnostic, since the most important task when faced with a patient experiencing hemoptysis would be to identify the source of the bleeding.

Correct choices would include pH of the emesis to determine if it is acidic (stomach content) or alkaline (from the lungs), CBC, and coagulation studies.

Pneumonia

Pneumonia by Age

You are expected to understand pneumonia broken down by age.

Neonatal Pneumonia

The common causes of pneumonia from 3 weeks to 3 months would be

 Chlamydia transmitted during delivery. They will be afebrile, with interstitial infiltrates on CXR.

 RSV presenting as bronchiolitis with wheezing (typically late fall)

 Parainfluenza bronchiolitis, typically fall through spring

 Pertussis, with paroxysmal cough and no fever. This may also lead to aspiration pneumonia

Pre-school

The common causes of pneumonia from age 3 months to 4 years would be

 Viral, including RSV, parainfluenza, human metapneumovirus, influenza, and rhinovirus

 S. pneumoniae, which is the most common treatable form of pneumonia in preschool children

 Mycoplasma pneumoniae would likely be presented in a child that is close to entering school

School age through Teen Years

 Mycoplasma pneumoniae is the most treatable form of pneumonia in this age group

> ### No New Labs for Pneumonia
>
> Unltess there is something compelling in the presented history, lab studies would not be necessary in establishing a diagnosis of pneumonia. Chest x-rays in general would not be indicated if the pneumonia is minor enough for outpatient management.

 ***Chlamydophila pneumoniae* presents similarly to mycoplasma pneumonia**

 S. pneumoniae in this age group can lead to complications, including empyema

 Mycobacterium tuberculosis, if they present a child among the high risk pool. Higher risk in pregnant teens.

Pneumonia By Etiology

S. pneumoniae

 S. pneumoniae or pneumococcus typically presents with abrupt onset of productive cough and fever, with a somewhat toxic picture preceded by URI symptoms. Abdominal pain with vomiting can be part of the picture, possibly even mimicking an acute abdomen.

Mycoplasma pneumonia

Characterized by low grade fever with a more insidious onset. CXR will have diffuse non-focal infiltrates.

Viral Pneumonia

The primary symptoms will be upper respiratory, including nasal congestion and rhinorrhea. The patient will either be afebrile or present with a very low grade fever.

Complications of Pneumonia

Necrotizing pneumonia

Necrotizing pneumonia occurs as a result of toxins produced by bacteria, leading to necrosis and liquification of lung tissue. It is diagnosed on x-ray.

 Treatment is with vancomycin or clindamycin

Lung Abscess

This will typically be described in a child at risk for aspiration, including a child with a seizure or a neurological disorder.

Effusions

Sterile effusions require no specific interventions. Purulent effusions can lead to empyema. Watch for specific findings, such as dullness on chest percussion and decreased air movement, planted in a sea of general findings (including ill appearance, tachypnea, and chest discomfort). Simple aspiration pneumonia without effusion is treated with amoxicillin or amoxicillin clavulanate.

Surgical drainage of effusions is controversial, and therefore will not likely be the correct answer regarding management.

The Undercurrent of Recurrent Pneumonia

Recurrent pneumonia might be placed in quotes on the exam. This is your hint that the diagnosis is not necessarily correct. Unless they describe a patient with more than one confirmed positive x-ray in a year or more than 3 episodes of pneumonia in a lifetime (with no symptoms in between episodes), you are not dealing with recurrent pneumonia.

Without this history, you may be dealing with recurrent asthma, with the atelectasis on x-ray being mischaracterized as pneumonia.

Preventing Pneumonia

Children over 2 years old who are at high risk for pneumococcal disease should receive the 23-valent pneumococcal vaccine. High risk children include those with chronic heart or pulmonary disease, sickle cell disease, diabetes, or HIV infection.

CASE STUDY You are presented with a patient with a diagnosis of pneumonia confirmed on x-ray. You are asked to pick the best diagnostic study to confirm the diagnosis.

THE DIVERSION You will be provided with several diversionary choices that might seem correct, such as sputum or nasopharyngeal culture. None of these will be correct.

ANSWER REVEALED The correct answer would be blood culture, which is very helpful, if positive. Pleural fluid or culture of lung tissue would also be definitive, but would not likely be among the choices, and would be a bit too invasive anyway.

Musculoskeletal Impact (or lack thereof) on Pulmonary Function

Scoliosis

Childhood-onset scoliosis can impair pulmonary function. Therefore, treatment will be indicated to minimize the impact on pulmonary function. *Adolescent-onset scoliosis does not necessarily carry the same concerns.*

Pectus Excavatum

Pectus excavatum does not typically result in any pulmonary issues. It is primarily a cosmetic concern, although I've been told by a friend with this condition that this is offset by the fact that it serves as a nice spot for guacamole dip when lying on the beach.

Chapter 19

Don't Go Breaking My Heart: Cardiology

Cardiology, although it can often be a difficult subject, is only a small part of the exam. What you need to know is limited to a set of core areas, which, if mastered, should earn you easy points on the exam. There is some overlap, and some cardiology topics are covered in other chapters. This chapter will focus on specific core topics in cardiology.

Congestive Heart Failure

 Congestive heart failure will present differently in infants than in older children.

CHF in Older Children – CHF in older children will present with *fatigue*, especially with *exertion or exercise*. This would include activities they enjoy, not just chores (for those of us who have asked our kids to take out the garbage, only to be told they are too tired). Subtle signs could include poor *appetite* and *coughing*. This presentation could include shortness of breath and/or diaphoresis.

On physical exam, they could describe a *gallop rhythm*, distended jugular veins, or peripheral edema.

CHF in Infancy – CHF in infancy would present as *difficulty feeding, weight loss* or *failure to gain weight, tachypnea, tachycardia*, as well as *hepatomegaly*.

If the congestive heart failure is due to left to right shunting, the goal of treatment is to reduce volume overload. Diuretics such as furosemide would be indicated.

Beware that certain medications would not be indicated in children, and would be the incorrect choices in this setting.

Hydralazine, which is a vasodilator, would not always be appropriate, since it can lead to sinus tachycardia, thus worsening congestive heart failure.

> ### Systemic AV Malformation and CHF in Newborns
>
> Systemic arteriovenous shunting of blood (as might be seen in the case of an AV malformation in the brain or liver) results in left to right extracardiac shunting, and ultimately leads to right-sided congestion. This is because the blood can move directly from the higher pressure arterial side to the lower pressure venous side. The end result is volume overload to the right side of the heart, leading to jugular vein distension and hepatomegaly in cases of significant congestion.

Verapamil, a calcium channel blocker, is contraindicated in infants younger than 1 year of age.

Congenital Heart Disease

Coarctation of the Aorta

The classic findings of coarctation of the aorta are "*decreased perfusion/pulses in lower extremities.*" If severe enough, coarctation of the aorta could also be associated with decreased pulses in the *upper* extremities.

They are unlikely to present you with the classic description of differential blood pressures or brachial/femoral pulse differences. They might just present you with classic signs of congestive heart failure and nothing else. This would include signs of shock and *acidosis*, in addition to an infant who is *lethargic* and *not feeding well*. Physical findings could also include a *non-specific gallop, nasal flaring,* and *sweating while feeding.*

The goal of treatment is to maintain a PDA[1] with a prostaglandin drip, thereby increasing blood flow to the descending aorta. Coarctation of the aorta is ultimately treated surgically. However, recurrence can still occur. In addition there is a higher risk for the development of **hypertension, even after surgical correction**.

Presenting Signs for Newborns

Cardiogenic shock may be the only presenting sign of congenital heart disease.

Congenital Heart Disease, Cyanotic

If you are presented with a newborn in respiratory distress whose oxygen saturation does not improve with 100% oxygen, you are likely dealing with cardiac rather than pulmonary disease.

This is an important piece of information they will present in the question.

---

[1] Patent Ductus Arteriosus.

Different Strokes

You also should keep in mind that infants with *cyanotic heart disease* and *polycythemia* are at high risk for cerebrovascular accidents.

Another risk factor would be *iron deficiency anemia*, which increases viscosity and risk for cerebral strokes.

Cyanotic Heart Disease and Anemia

You will be expected to determine the presence or absence of cyanotic heart disease when provided with a hematocrit value.

If an infant is anemic, he may not show signs of cyanosis on physical exam, even with O_2 sats around 88%. Infants have high fetal Hgb levels, so cyanosis may not be clinically apparent until O_2 sats are quite low.

Cyanosis Without Heart Disease

Methemoglobinemia

Be on the lookout for methemoglobinemia, a condition in which the iron in the hemoglobin molecule is defective, making it unable to effectively carry oxygen to the tissues. In this case, Hgb is not transporting oxygen (think of it as a trucker's strike). This can be congenital or acquired. **This results in cyanosis in the absence of cyanotic heart disease.**

They could describe the child as having his formula mixed with **well water**.

Without proper treatment, it can lead to *acidosis, tachycardia,* and *signs of shock*.

Treatment consists of eliminating the triggering agent and/or methylene blue.

Remember, cyanosis in the absence of respiratory distress is a tip that the likely diagnosis is methemoglobinemia.

The Tease of the 5 T's

Here are the 5 Ts of cyanotic congenital heart disease:

> Truncus Arteriosus
>
> Transposition of the Great Arteries
>
> Tricuspid Atresia
>
> Tetrology of Fallot
>
> Total Anomalous Pulmonary Venous Return

However, these are not always described with the T prominent in the description, i.e. total anomalous venous return might be described as anomalous venous return.

Transposition of the great vessels is the only cyanotic heart disease which presents in the first few hours of life.

Isn't it a PDA?

In the presence of a PDA, you can have high O_2 sats, even with a low PO_2. They might describe the classic to-and-fro "machinery type" continuous murmur associated with a PDA.

Therefore, O_2 sats in the 90's with an "oxygen challenge" does not rule out cyanotic heart disease.

CASE STUDY

A frantic mom presents in your office with her 6 month old infant, whose hands and feet are blue and have been this way on and off since birth. Five minutes later, the grandmother comes in carrying 14 pounds of blankets because of the draft she detects from the open window in the office 140 feet down the hall. The baby is otherwise normal. They both note that, when the hands and feet are not blue, they are mottled. You try to hide your own mottled and cyanotic appearance and figure out what's going on.

THE DIVERSION

You might be diverted into doing a workup for methemoglobinemia, obtaining an EKG, or something simple like an oxygen saturation reading.

ANSWER REVEALED

This is nothing more than *episodic acrocyanosis*, which requires no workup at all other than reassurance to all involved (including you).

Total Anomalous Pulmonary Venous Return (TAPVR)

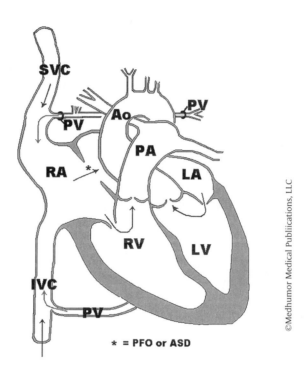

* = PFO or ASD

©Medhumor Medical Publiications, LLC

With Total Anomalous Pulmonary Venous Return, none of the four veins that drain blood from the lungs to the heart is attached to the left atrium. *In TAPVR, oxygenated blood returns to the right atrium instead.* There must be a connection to the left side of the heart, or the condition is incompatible with life.

The severity of this condition depends on whether the pulmonary veins are obstructed. **There are two subtypes of TAPVR.**

- In one, the veins course into the abdomen, passing through the diaphragm. This squeezes the veins and narrows them, causing the blood to back up into the lungs. This type causes symptoms *early in life.*
- The second type of TAPVR has no obstruction; the veins do not course through the abdomen.

Tricuspid Atresia

Tricuspid atresia will result in cyanosis. They often focus on the details of the other causes of cyanosis discussed more extensively in this chapter.

Total Anomalous Pulmonary Venous Return will often present in a full term infant as **increased right ventricular activity**. They present with **cyanosis** and **pulmonary edema**. There will be a *fixed split S2* and a *short systolic murmur.*

With Total Anomalous Venous Return, you typically have an infant that is cyanotic with signs of *hypoxia, hypercarbia,* and a "**normal sized heart.**"

The **CXR** will be significant for findings consistent with **pulmonary congestion** (because of the increased venous return), along with a normal to small heart. The ABG will have an increased PCO$_2$.

TAPVR and RDS can present in similar ways; however, if they are describing **a full term baby, consider TAPVR first** even though RDS <u>can</u> occur in full term infants.

Ductal Dependent Lesions

They may describe an infant with good Apgars who was pink and well-perfused; some time during the first or second day of life, the infant became **cyanotic due to the closing PDA**, which resulted in diminished mixing at the ductal level. In addition, "**tachypnea**" might be described. They might also describe the **lack of increased vascular markings** on CXR, ruling out pulmonary disease.

Treatment

Treatment consists of **prostaglandin** to maintain a patent ductus arteriosus.

In the event of **pulmonary hypertension**, **nitric oxide** would be the answer.

Ni-Tric does the Tric for pulmonary hypertension.

Tetralogy of Fallot (TOF)

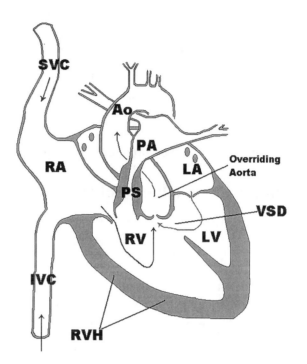

Tetralogy of Fallot (TOF)

©Medhumor Medical Publications, LLC

You might be asked to pick out the 4 components of TOF from among a list of 5:

1. Pulmonary Stenosis
2. Overriding Aorta
3. Insatiable desire to sing 50's R and B songs with lyrics containing the word Fallot, as in "I Will Fallot You", or Judy Garland Show tunes: "Fallot the Yellow Brick Road"
4. VSD
5. Right Ventricular Hypertrophy

In most instances choice 3 will be incorrect.

Common Blues

TOF is the most common cyanotic heart condition overall. However, in newborns, transposition of the great arteries is the most common cyanotic lesion seen.

Children with Tetralogy of Fallot present with a palpable right ventricular impulse and a **single 2nd heart** sound (the pulmonary component is absent). The EKG shows **right ventricular hypertrophy** and the CXR shows a **"boot-shaped"** heart with decreased pulmonary vascularity.

Remember, this is **often asymptomatic in early infancy**, especially on the Boards. The typical presentation is in an infant of 3-5 months of age.

After surgical repair there is a chance for *arrhythmias* and *episodes of syncope*.

The Tet Offensive Redux: Under a "Tet Spell"

Recognizing a Tet spell is worth a point or two. These are basically **hypercyanotic hypoxic episodes**, similar to a prima donna athlete being denied his big contract. In this case, the triggering agent is often **"anemia."** It is a result of **increased R to L shunting during an acute episode.**[2]

During a tet (hypercyanotic and hypoxic) episode, the infant will often be described as being agitated, with absence of a heart murmur, due to decreased pulmonary blood flow. The episode will often be described as following an episode of viral gastroenteritis, since dehydration can precipitate a tet spell. *The inability to hear a murmur is an important feature of a tet spell.*

Cognitive Effects of Cyanotic Heart Disease

This is a ripe topic for the exam. Factors that correlate with cognitive prognosis are:

- ❑ **Neurological baseline before surgery**
- ❑ **Seizures occurring after surgery** (especially early)
- ❑ **Coexistent problems** such as a chromosomal abnormality
- ❑ **Duration of intraoperative circulatory arrest** (e.g., greater than 75 minutes makes for a worse prognosis)

Correcting Your Tet Spelling

If they describe a classic spell in the question (**the acute onset is often the clue**), then the treatment consists of placing the child in a squatting position (to increase peripheral vascular resistance) just like a free agent baseball catcher. And if they are real little, don't pick them up and simulate a squat on the table or bed – just do a knee to chest move – but you knew that, right? In addition, **morphine**, **phenylephrine, IV propranolol**, and **volume expansion** are given.

The overall prognosis for infants undergoing surgical correction for TOF is 95% survival. However, all children who undergo cardiac bypass procedures are at increased risk for neurodevelopmental delay and/or other cognitive deficits.

---

2 Shunting deoxygenated blood through the VSD to the left side.

Hypoplastic Left Heart Syndrome

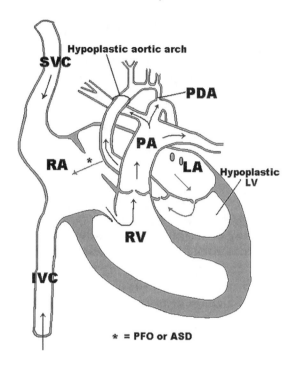

Hypoplastic Left Heart Syndrome

Hypoplastic left heart is due to a congenital cardiac disorder resulting from the underdevelopment of the left side of the heart (left ventricle, aortic valve, and aorta).

Infants with hypoplastic left heart syndrome have signs of **severe congestive heart failure** and marked **cardiomegaly** on chest radiography in the immediate newborn period. The trouble starts when the PDA starts to close - they often look like *normal healthy babies at birth.*

Additional findings include **precordial hyperactivity** and a **loud S2.**

CASE STUDY

A 10 day old newborn is brought to your office. You immediately notice that the infant is tachypneic, with thready peripheral pulses and an enlarged liver. You accompany the infant to the emergency room and obtain an ABG, which reveals marked metabolic acidosis and an EKG consistent with aortic stenosis. From a list of dobutamine, epinephrine, nitric oxide[3], prostaglandin, and IV fluids, you are asked which therapy should be used immediately.

THE DIVERSION

Since you are being presented with an infant with signs of *cardiogenic shock*, you might be tempted to pick IV fluids, or a pressor like dobutamine, or even epinephrine. The key to remember is that hypoplastic left heart syndrome presents after the immediate newborn period, and presents with a picture of cardiogenic shock.

ANSWER REVEALED

Since cardiogenic shock is the primary problem and started with the closing of the ductus arteriosus, keeping it opened is the most important step to ameliorate the cardiogenic shock. In other words, fix the pump, and the hoses and water will take care of themselves. Therefore, *prostaglandin E_1* would be the correct answer to this question.[4]

Genetic Echo

There is a strong association between chromosomal abnormalities and congenital heart disease.

Therefore, cardiac echo is routinely done in patients with Down syndrome and any other syndrome that is associated with congenital heart disease.

PERIL WARNING

There is no murmur associated with hypoplastic left heart syndrome, even though the ductus remains open. This is because pulmonary and aortic pressures are equal, resulting in no turbulence across the patent ductus.

HOT TIP

This is why an EKG and cardiac echo are important parts of a workup of a child presenting in cardiogenic shock.

---

[3] Not to be confused with nitrous oxide, AKA happy gas.

[4] Does anybody know what the E1 stands for and why E2 or D5 or Prostaglandin MP3 wouldn't work? Does anybody care?

Transposition of the Great Arteries

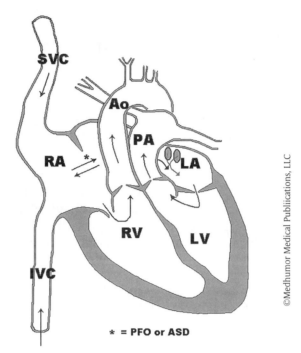

* = PFO or ASD

Transposition of the Great Arteries

©Medhumor Medical Publiications, LLC

Transposition of the great arteries is due to the connection of the aorta to the right ventricle and the pulmonary artery to the left ventricle. It is the most common congenital heart defect presenting with severe cyanosis in the **first week** of life. The result is two circulations in parallel.[5]

Blood mixing must occur either through the foramen ovale (at the atrial level) or through the PDA; thus, it is "ductal dependent."

Transposition of the great arteries should be your first thought when presented with any cyanotic newborn. They typically present with tachypnea and a **single 2nd heart sound.** On CXR there is an **egg-shaped heart** (which can be absent in the first week of life) and **increased pulmonary vascularity.**[6]

---

[5] Sort of like a couple not on speaking terms.

[6] Some now say that the egg shaped heart is a non-specific finding. However, on the exam it would be wise to still consider it to be an association with transposition of the great vessels.

Both *Tetralogy of Fallot* and *transposition of the great arteries* present with a *single 2nd heart sound*. However, transposition of the great arteries presents with increased pulmonary vascularity, while Tetralogy of Fallot does not.

Since this is a normal finding in the first week of life, the right ventricular hypertrophy noted on EKG is not helpful.

Treatment consists of IV **prostaglandin E₁** to maintain the PDA and, if this does not work, a **balloon septostomy** to maintain a patent ASD. Ultimately, surgical correction is needed (the specifics of which are not tested on the general pediatric board exam).

Superior Vena Cava Syndrome

Superior vena cava syndrome results when the flow to the superior vena cava is impeded.

Superior vena cava syndrome presents as **generalized facial swelling,** as well as **fatigue, weight loss, night sweats,** and a **dusky color.**

The dusky color is due to the venous stasis seen with impeded blood flow — **not arterial desaturation,** so do not expect to see low oxygen saturations peripherally.

Persistent Fetal Circulation

Persistent fetal circulation occurs when pulmonary vascular resistance exceeds systemic resistance. This results in right to left shunting of blood. It is common in pulmonary disease that increases pulmonary vascular resistance.

Cardiac — post-ductal higher

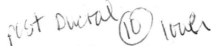

Typically, they will present to you an infant who develops respiratory distress shortly after delivery, with oxygen saturations in the lower extremities lower than that seen in the upper body. This is because of desaturated blood reaching the descending aorta and below. In addition, because of the *increased workload of the right ventricle, a precordial lift*, or at least a prominent precordial impulse, will be described.

Endocarditis, Myocarditis, Hiscarditis, Pericarditis and Theircarditis

Infective Endocarditis

This is self defined, basically an infection of the endocardial surface of the heart, usually involving the valves.

This may be characterized by "a one to two week history of lethargy, along with a low-grade fever," physical findings of "splenomegaly," "petechiae," "tender lesions on the pads of the fingers and toes,"[7] "a systolic ejection click (usually at the apex)," and/or a "diastolic murmur on the right side."

· **Osler Nodes** are the "tender nodules on the pads of fingers and toes."
· **Janeway Lesions** are the non-tender red nodules on the palms or soles.

Envision the Osler Nodes as gigantic O's on the toes causing pain.

JRA (now known as JIA) is usually associated with *carditis, not vascular heart disease. Rheumatic fever is the opposite.* This is one way of distinguishing them.

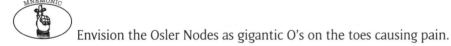

If they give you the classic description of endocarditis and ask what is the **BEST** study to **confirm the diagnosis**, the answer will be **blood culture**, not cardiac echo or the other decoys waiting for you. This is because the infection can only be identified by isolating the pathogen in the blood.

---

[7] Osler Nodes.

Acute Bacterial Endocarditis

Streptococcus viridans, Strep bovis, as well as *Staph aureus* are the most common causes of acute bacterial endocarditis in children. There is also a group of bacteria known as **HACEK bacteria** which have been known to cause infective endocarditis. This stands for *Haemophilus, Actinobacillus, Cardiobacterium, Eikenella, and Kingella,* in case you are asked.

Subacute Bacterial Endocarditis

Streptococcus viridans is the responsible organism in subacute bacterial endocarditis.

Dental Plan

Routine antibiotic prophylaxis is no longer recommended before dental procedures.

This is now reserved for patients with congenital heart disease in specific situations including:

- Incompletely repaired cyanotic heart disease, especially those with shunts and other hardware
- Heart disease surgically corrected with hardware and other devices within the previous 6 months
- Any residual defect near a prosthetic cardiac device

The main take home message is routine prophylaxis is no longer indicated. When prophylaxis is indicated, PO amoxicillin 30 -60 minutes prior to the procedure is appropriate.

Myocarditis

Myocarditis will typically follow a **viral illness**. If myocarditis is the correct answer, they will usually slip in something about a **recent URI** that precedes the current presentation. They will likely describe a new murmur, arrhythmia, and/or acute onset of heart failure described clinically. The clinical signs can be as subtle as fatigue and lethargy (similar to what you are experiencing while reading this material), to signs of shock.

In an infant, watch for tachypnea and tachycardia, as well as a *holosystolic murmur.*

Coxsackie group B virus is the most common cause of myocarditis.

Even though the star virus is **group B coxsackievirus**, other viruses can result in myocarditis, but don't let that stop you from picking viral myocarditis as the correct answer. It can have a benign or more fulminate course, ranging from tachycardia to CHF, pulmonary edema, and arrhythmias.

With **pulsus paradoxus** (drop in systolic pressure with inspiration), EKG typically reveals low voltage abnormal T waves, and ST depression.

Use of steroids to treat myocarditis is controversial and, therefore, very unlikely to be the correct answer.

Pericarditis and Pericardial Effusion

Pericarditis is the inflammation of the pericardial sac, typically involving the epicardium and pericardium. The more common causes are **viral** or **collagen vascular disease**, for example, JIA.

Pericardial effusion is the inflammation of the pericardial sac coupled with fluid effusion. If a definitive cause is needed, then it must be done by obtaining a sample via cardiocentesis. Viral serology and cultures are needed to document the etiology. When pericarditis is caused by bacteria, it is usually due to a preceding or concurrent bacterial infection elsewhere, i.e., pneumonia. *Staph aureus* is the most common *bacterial* cause of pericarditis.

Children with pericarditis tend to lean forward. ECG would demonstrate *ST segment* **elevation**. Additional findings could include nonspecific chest and epigastric pain. The fact that the pain is positional could lead you to believe it is musculoskeletal, but the *EKG findings and muffled heart sounds* would tell you that pericarditis is the most likely cause. If the patient has an underlying rheumatological disorder, this is further information pointing to pericarditis.

Typical phrases you will see that tip you off to pericarditis are "**muffled heart** sounds" and "**pericardial friction rub**" (due to pericardial fluid). A "**low grade fever**" could be thrown in for good measure, as well as "**jugular venous distention.**" And finally there is left sided chest pain that is worse while lying down (supine) and better when sitting up. It will occur following a URI of viral origin.

Pulsus paradoxus is a finding in pericardial effusion, which is the diminished peripheral pulses with inspiration. This is due to impeded venous return of blood by the pericardial effusion.

Study results will **include enlarged heart on CXR** with **no heart failure clinically**, and **confirmation** of pericardial fluid on echocardiography.

Penny Carditis. Envision a penny on the chest causing pain. When you sit up, the penny falls off and the pain is gone.

The most important study to order when pericarditis or effusion is suspected is a **CXR.**

Purulent Pericarditis

A pericardial friction rub will be described. In this case, there will be no change in sound with change in position. Therefore, it is not a "positional lesion."

CASE STUDY

10 days after having corrective open heart surgery, a 6 year old is noted to have anorexia, fatigue, nausea, and vomiting. The patient appears pale with barely palpable peripheral pulses, especially when the child takes a breath. The heart rate on direct auscultation is within normal range, but peripherally, when it is palpated, it is much slower. What is the most important next step? You could be provided choices that include surgical intervention, as well as medical interventions such as digoxin, steroids, NSAIDs, and more dramatic interventions like cardioversion.

THE DIVERSION

The key to not being diverted to the wrong choice in this question is to follow the logic of what they are telling you. First, the patient had cardiac surgery. Here they didn't tell you the specifics of the indication for surgery, but even if they did, it would be a red herring designed to throw you off. Second, you know there was surgery and you need to consider *postpericardiotomy syndrome*, which is a post-op complication that results in pericarditis and pericardial effusion. Therefore, it will be very tempting to pick the least invasive and dramatic management such as steroids or NSAIDs. However, since there was more going on than simple pericarditis and effusion that would not be correct.

ANSWER REVEALED

The clinical vignette described a child with signs of *pericardial tamponade*, as well as *pulsus paradoxus*. Therefore, the correct intervention is *pericardiocentesis* to relieve the tamponade.

I say Murmur, you say Mummur

Evaluating and Distinguishing Innocent Murmurs

Evaluating and distinguishing innocent murmurs is an important component of general practice, and one you will need to navigate with ease on the exam as well. Here are the guidelines to getting the answer correct on the exam.

Up to 90% of children will have a murmur at some point in their lives; more than that if they are appearing on the Board exam. *Less than 5% of these will actually represent pathology.*

Here are some of the typical descriptions of innocent murmurs:

"Vibratory," "Venous hum," and "Carotid bruits."

V's: **V**ery good, **V**enous hum, **V**ibratory, and "**V**ascular – Carotid" bruit.

Any description of associated physiological problems suggests a pathological murmur. If they mention any of the following in the question, you are **not** dealing with an innocent murmur: **exercise intolerance, feeding difficulties, dyspnea, cyanosis, syncope, or wheezing and hacking like a diesel engine when seeing what pictures of you were posted on Facebook**.

In infants, watch for signs of tachypnea. Watch for any family history of cardiac disease if they describe any — and I mean *any* — associated physical findings; that could be your clue that the murmur is not innocent and is probably part of a syndrome.

Often the mother of a child with complete (3rd degree) heart block is diagnosed with SLE retrospectively.

VSD Murmur

The murmur associated with a VSD is best heard at the **left lower sternal border,** and is typically **pansystolic**.

Suddenly, at your 2 mo WCC, this murmur is clearly audible and you wonder how you possibly could have missed it at all your previous visits. The answer: you didn't miss it. The right and left ventricular pressures were roughly equal, so there was no interventricular flow to create a murmur previously.

With a **large VSD, there might be no murmur**. However, the clue is that **the 2nd heart sound won't be split or will be loud**. They may also describe a **hyperdynamic precordium**. All of this could be your only clue to a VSD in an infant with no mention of a murmur.

Maternal Meds on Board

Have your highlighter ready for any mention of maternal use of meds or drugs during pregnancy. The following are your associations and memory aides:

Medication	Cardiac Defect	Mnemonic
Lithium	Epstein Anomaly	Picture a Manic Guy named **Upstein**
Alcohol	(Fetal Alcohol Syndrome) VSD/ASD	Picture a Shot Glass in the VSD and ASD

Cranial Bruits

Cranial bruits are typically associated with a "**bounding carotid pulse**" and perhaps "**decreased peripheral pulses.**" This can signify an AV malformation of the brain, and can lead to congestive heart failure.

Carotid bruits, **not cranial bruits,** are usually associated with innocent murmurs in kids.

More than a Murmur/ Indications of Pathology

Continuous Murmur

Auscultating[8] the Murmur (Described in Plain English)

The nice thing about the exam (aside from the fact that it will eventually end) is that the little old lady from Pasadena (your proctor) *won't walk over and ask you to actually listen to[9] a murmur.* They will describe them for you. Since these descriptions are very specific for their associated disorders, anyone can memorize these descriptions and should get the answer correct.

You, on the other hand, might get the question wrong if you don't commit these descriptions to memory. Yet, in your career you may have detected more murmurs than Terrell Owens elicits at a nationally televised football game (even when he's not playing – which is a lot these days).

 Any murmur described as "harsh sounding" or "with intensity greater than 3/6" is abnormal.

The following are the different "stages" of the typical heart sound and their typical "pathological descriptions":

- ❏ **Systolic**: pansystolic or late systolic
- ❏ **Diastolic**: any diastolic murmur is abnormal
- ❏ **4th Sound**: a fourth heart sound is not normal, nor is an S4 gallop
- ❏ **Clicks**: ejection and/or mid systolic clicks are not normal

 If they describe a 3rd heart sound, check the position[10]. **If the child is lying down, it could be normal**. If it is a normal finding, when the child sits up the 3rd heart sound should disappear; if it does not, you could be dealing with an abnormal sound.

 Picture a number 3 lying down, murmuring, and stopping when it sits up, which is normal for a 3.

---

[8] Auscultating means "listening" to the rest of the non-medical world.

[9] Or auscultate.

[10] Of the child, not you.

Sounds for Musing

ASD Sounds

Patients with an ASD will present with specific auscultatory findings (also known as heart sounds). This would include a fixed and split 2nd heart sound. They might describe this in a patient with decreased exercise tolerance.

Pulmonary Stenosis

Pulmonary stenosis will often be described with a systolic click and normal splitting of S2.

Aortic Stenosis

Aortic stenosis could also be described with a systolic (ejection) click, regardless of position. There will also be a murmur best heard at the upper right sternal border and radiating into the neck.

Marfan Invaders

Since children with Marfan syndrome are at risk for aortic enlargement and/or aortic dissection, you need to know which physical restrictions are appropriate. They should *refrain from activities that involve muscle straining, such as weight lifting,* as well as contact sports.

Referral to a cardiologist would be appropriate for all first degree relatives of a patient with hypertrophic cardiomyopathy or certain other known heritable cardiac conditions, such as in Marfan syndrome.

EKG Findings and the Disorders that Love Them

Aortic Stenosis

Aortic stenosis leads to *left ventricular hypertrophy.* This makes sense because the left ventricle has to work harder against resistance.

PERIL / WARNING *Coarctation of the aorta in newborns presents with right ventricular hypertrophy* because, in a fetus, the RV is the dominant pumping chamber.

Tetralogy of Fallot

Tetralogy of Fallot results in *right ventricular hypertrophy.* This makes sense because it is pumping against the resistance of pulmonary stenosis. This results in right axis deviation on EKG.

AV Canal Defect

"Superior" QRS axis (e.g., 30°–90°)[11] occurs because the conduction system has to go around the large defect in the middle of the heart. It also has left axis deviation.[12]

 Right ventricular hypertrophy goes hand in hand with R axis deviation.

However, *disorders like hypertrophic cardiomyopathy that result in LVH* **DO NOT result in left axis deviation on EKG.** Left axis deviation will be seen with tricuspid atresia and AV canal defects because of its effect on the conducting system's orientation.

Arrhythmias

The following are some of the basic arrhythmias that frequently appear on the exam.

PAC's (Premature Atrial Contractions)

When we refer to a PAC, we are not referring to the folks who hang around the corridors of Congress, syphoning money to our poor and humble politicians, called "Political Action Committees."

 Remember that most of the time, PAC's are benign (much unlike their political counterparts).

Two exceptions to this rule are children on *digoxin* and *children less than 1 year old.* They are at risk of PACs progressing to atrial flutter.

Atrial Flutter/Fib

This is clearly more serious. Look in your Atlas for the classic pattern (**saw-tooth waves**).

---

[11] Note that this is associated with Down syndrome.
[12] Not to be confused with the axis of evil.

Sinus Arrhythmia

This is another name for a *normal variant.*

Wolff Parkinson White Syndrome (WPW)

Wolff Parkinson White Syndrome was named after Bernard Wolff Parkinson, an eccentric dog physiologist and part-time canine couple's therapist who did all his research in the Alaskan Tundra. His obsession with white snow earned him the moniker "White." He also discovered, and later designed, the first Parka coat. Rumor has it that Frank Zappa had him in mind when he wrote the lyrics, "Don't go where the huskies go, don't you eat that yellow snow."[13]

They will show or describe a *shortened PR* interval and/or a *delta wave*[14] that distorts the QRS upstroke.

Prolonged QT Syndrome (Prolonged Cutie Syndrome)

The QT interval is the time it takes the heart muscle to recover between beats.

When the QT interval takes too long, it can lead to arrhythmias.

They will typically describe a **family history of sudden death in young people**. In addition, they could describe a patient who was *previously asymptomatic who presents with syncope* brought on by vigorous exercise such as sports training. It could also be triggered by emotional stress. Unusual presentations could also include *syncope followed by a seizure.*

Prolonged "Cutie:" If someone dies young, he/she is forever young and "cute," and thus a "prolonged cutie."

---

[13] My editor says that this story is not factually accurate.

[14] The wave on the EKG – not the sleep stage you are in right now.

CASE STUDY You are presented with a patient who has recurrent episodes of syncope, usually while standing for prolonged periods of time. There is no family history of sudden death in anyone younger than 50 or other premature cardiac disease. What is the most likely diagnosis?

THE DIVERSION You might be fooled into picking prolonged QT syndrome. However, the clue here will be the absence of a family history of sudden death in anyone younger than 50 or other significant cardiac disease.

ANSWER REVEALED The correct diagnosis when presented with recurrent syncope, particularly with prolonged standing, would be **neurocardiogenic syncope**.

CASE STUDY You are taking care of a very athletic teenage boy. He has been playing varsity level basketball and is in great condition. In the past 6 weeks he has passed out twice during practice, despite maintaining adequate hydration. His drug screen is negative. There is no known family history of any cardiac arrhythmias and no known history of sudden death in anyone younger than 50. What would be the most appropriate management at this time?

THE DIVERSION The diversion here is the lack of "known" history of sudden premature death. Read the question carefully. Even in the absence of a known history, long QT syndrome could exist in the family. The key here is the history of syncope during exercise, as opposed to occurring with prolonged standing.

ANSWER REVEALED The correct answer here would be to obtain a cardiology consultation. In addition, the patient should not be allowed to return to sports until cleared by a cardiologist.

By the way, had they asked for the most important additional history, the answer would have been to uncover the true family history.

SVT (Supraventricular Tachycardia)

SVT is the most common rapid rhythm in children. For most children, in the absence of any other cardiac defects, it is a benign finding and all that is needed is reassurance.

 If they ask what is the **"first thing to do"** in a *stable* patient in SVT (HR greater than 220), **the correct answer is a "12 Lead EKG."**

Of course, if they describe hemodynamic instability and tachycardia, then cardioversion would be the answer. However, you would first need to take other measures while getting ready. These measures would include vasovagal maneuvers, such as brief facial stimulation (cold, wet cloth or ice bag); this maneuver induces the "diving reflex."

Adenosine is the drug of choice to slow the heart down, and in some cases **atrial overdrive pacing** would be appropriate.

If you are presented with a patient in SVT who is demonstrating signs of cardiac failure, vasovagal maneuvers would not be the correct choice. In this case, adenosine would be appropriate immediately. If no IV and adenosine are available immediately, cardiovert.

Digoxin is sometimes used in the long-term management of children with SVT.

Digoxin is contraindicated in children with Wolff-Parkinson White syndrome.

Verapamil is not indicated for SVT in children, especially those younger than one year, because it can cause cardiac arrest. And that's bad.

AV Block

 The important thing to remember is that an *AV block with a widened QRS complex* is more ominous than a narrow one. With the widened complex, blood flow to the brain can be compromised, resulting in risk for *seizure* and *syncope* (the double S).

Picture a double S falling through a wide QRS.

AV block can be associated with **viral myocarditis**.

Sinus Tachycardia

If you are presented with an anxious patient with tachycardia which has been noted on more than one occasion, the most likely diagnosis is sinus tachycardia.

In this case you need to consider non-cardiac etiologies, including pheochromocytoma, hyperthyroidism, infection, or dehydration.

Chest Pain

If you are presented with one of the less than 1% of cases of chest pain that is cardiac in origin, it will be described as pain that **radiates to the neck, back, shoulders,** or **left arm**. Additional findings that tip you off to a cardiac origin include pain that is *constant/frequent*, **dull,** and **pressure-like**.

Pain that is *infrequent, brief,* and *sharp* that increases with a deep breath would be consistent with **musculoskeletal** or **pulmonary-related pain**.

Chest pain in children, especially on the boards, will rarely be due to a myocardial infarction or anything cardiac. There is only a 1% chance that chest pain in a child is cardiac in origin.

They could include a history of a family member older than 50 suffering from heart disease. This is often nothing but a diversion that you should simply discount, especially if the pain is inconsistent with cardiac disease as outlined above.

On the other hand, if they present a history of a patient with chest pain consistent with cardiac disease as outlined above, along with a history of a relative **younger than 50 with cardiac disease who is taking lipid lowering medications,** then the chest pain is very likely due to cardiac disease, and referral to a cardiologist would be appropriate.

You will be expected to be familiar with the common cardiac causes of chest pain in children, which include:

- Pericarditis
- Aortic stenosis
- Aortic regurgitation
- Anomalous origin of coronary arteries
- Cardiomyopathy
- Mitral valve prolapse
- Sequelae of Kawasaki disease

Chapter 20

Heme Onc

This chapter will deal with diseases of the blood and neoplastic disorders, otherwise known as "heme-onc." Basically, the focus is on the ABCs of RBCs and WBCs, and of course, oncologies...

Oncology

General Considerations

A febrile child who is neutropenic and on chemotherapy needs to be worked up immediately. Treatment is (**after** blood cultures!!) broad-spectrum antibiotics as quickly as possible. If the patient has an ANC<500 or looks ill, they should be admitted to the hospital.

Fragile Chromosomes

Remember, many chromosomal fragility syndromes are associated with leukemia. Examples include Down syndrome, Bloom syndrome, and Fanconi's anemia.

Bone Tumors

The two types of bone tumors they will ask you about are **Ewing** and **osteogenic sarcoma**. Each has its own very distinct characteristics, and they love to focus on these for a few questions. This is a typical favorite for the match section, so invest in some of the easy-to-remember details below and you will be rewarded with a few slam-dunk lay-ups.

Ewing Sarcoma vs. Osteogenic Sarcoma (OS)

Ewing Sarcoma	Osteogenic Sarcoma	Both
· Soft tissue component · Ewing Sarcoma is not usually seen in African Americans	· OS is more common in blacks than whites · **Teenager, usually going through a growth spurt, who presents with pain** · Common sites for OS are the **proximal and distal long bones (femur and humerus)**	· Both will involve bones · Both Ewing sarcoma and OS can occur in long bones · **Treatment for both is chemotherapy, radiation, and surgery** · **Both can metastasize to the lungs, but this is the main site of OS mets**

They could present a patient with unilateral pain in a long bone (i.e., the leg), emphasizing that it is an adolescent going through a growth spurt.

The distracter will be "growth spurt," which will lead you to the incorrect "growing pains" as the answer.

However, growing pains are usually bilateral and usually occur at night only.

Osteogenic Sarcoma

Treatment is **amputation** or **limb salvage,** with **chemo to prevent spread**.

Mets go to the lungs.

Picture a teen with an **amputated leg trying to run**. Well, he will be **out of breath** pretty fast, which should remind you that mets go to the **lungs**.

They will often try to throw you off by including a history of trauma, followed by bone pain or swelling. Don't go for this distracter if there are other signs of a possible tumor, such as preceding *recurrent persistent* pain. They are describing osteogenic sarcoma despite the mention of trauma.

Osteoid Osteoma

Osteoid Osteoma: this is a Board favorite and very easy to get correct because the history is as unique as are the x-ray findings. For a typical picture, look at your favorite Atlas. They will describe **"tibia pain"** or **"femur pain,"** worse at night, **"relieved by ibuprofen."**[1]

The picture will have a central radiolucent (white area) surrounded by thick sclerotic bone.

---

[1] In past years this was described as pain relieved by aspirin. However it seems that finally this has been updated to reflect that the use of aspirin in children has been phased out with 1970's rotary phones.

Brain Tumors

Brain Tumors (taken as a whole) are the most common type of **solid** tumors.

If they describe headaches that are worse in the morning and get better with standing and/or vomiting, the correct diagnosis is likely to be a "brain tumor." Additional findings could include deteriorating school performance and/or ataxia.

Leukemia

Acute Lymphocytic Leukemia (ALL)

ALL is by far the most common pediatric malignancy.

The following are poor prognostic signs:
- Younger than age 2 years at time of diagnosis
- WBC > 50
- T Cell

Pre-B cell type is a good prognostic sign.

T Cell is Terrible.

Boys were once thought to have a worse prognosis than girls, but this is no longer accepted dogma (though it may be so on the Boards). In general, the cure rate for ALL is very high.

They could present you with a child with **"bone pain"** and/or **"joint pain or swelling."** There will often be fevers. Labs may show pancytopenia, though the WBC count may also be normal or elevated.

To be fair, they will have to include something in the history to differentiate ALL from aplastic anemia, such as an enlarged liver or spleen. Leukemia should not be diagnosed without a bone marrow examination.

ALL vs. AML - You should not be required to make this distinction on a blood smear. AML tends to present in older kids. The prognosis is worse; however, even with AML the cure rate is now close to 50%.

> ### Acute Myelogenous Leukemia
>
> Whereas one would see a more homogenous pattern in the bone marrow with ALL, there is a more varied picture seen with AML. The clinical picture is similar and the focus of the exam is usually not on differentiating the two types of leukemias.

Treatment goals of leukemia

The treatment goal in kids with ALL is to induce remission with one course of chemotherapy.

Even after treatment, children who have had ALL and AML are at risk of relapse. In ALL, the CNS and testes are sanctuary sites of ALL which is more resistant to therapy. These are common sites of relapse. Early relapse has a worse prognosis.

Infection in leukemia

Infection is a major cause of death in kids with leukemia. Indwelling catheters and neutropenia combine to increase the risk for infection. **Therefore, children receive broad-spectrum parenteral antibiotics.**

Lymphoma

Lymphoma can be confusing. Basically, there is Hodgkin's lymphoma (Hodgkin's disease) and "everything else" (non-Hodgkin's lymphoma).

A chest x-ray would be the correct choice if you are presented with a patient with unexplained lymphadenopathy, especially if there are symptoms suggesting chest pathology (including cough, chest pain, or shortness of breath).

Hodgkin's Lymphoma

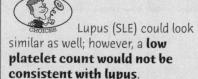

Atypical Limps and Lymphs

They might even throw in the term "atypical lymphs" to throw you off the trail, with some choices consistent with mono. In the context of a clinical picture of ALL, the **"atypical lymphs" are actually "lymphoblasts,"** incorrectly reported in the CBC as atypical lymphs.

Lupus (SLE) could look similar as well; however, a **low platelet count would not be consistent with lupus**. Distinguishing leukemia from infectious mono can be difficult. Both can present with cytopenias and atypical lymphocytes on peripheral blood smear, in addition to joint pain and splenomegaly. The degree of cytopenia in leukemia should be worse than in mono. Leukemia may have circulating blasts. Finally, although other symptoms can guide you, if there is doubt and urgency for a diagnosis, a bone marrow examination will give you the answer quickly (though not painlessly!) A marrow specimen with greater than 25% blast forms is leukemia.

 Hodgkin's lymphoma typically presents in **teens as non-tender enlarged cervical lymph nodes**. Patients often have weight loss, fevers and night sweats. It is a slow-growing malignancy.

They will typically describe a teen with *a **non-tender** cervical node* or a **supraclavicular node** and then mention, describe, or show a **Reed Sternberg** cell on the biopsy. The white count will be high with a **relatively low lymphocyte** count.

Atypical mycobacteria may present with a cervical node, but there will be other signs, i.e., a positive PPD less than 10 mm, and there will be *no supraclavicular nodes*.

Sepsis and Splenectomy

If you are presented with a patient with Hodgkin lymphoma who has undergone a splenectomy (or any patient who has undergone a splenectomy, for that matter), know that he/she is at high risk for sepsis.

If they present you with such a patient with a high fever, know that a sepsis workup is indicated.

Non-Hodgkin Lymphoma

Non-Hodgkin lymphoma is more likely if they present you with a **small child rather than a teen**. It usually involves the **head and neck region**. It can also present in the **abdomen as a non-tender mass**. Keep this in mind in addition to *Wilms and neuroblastoma.*

N-H Lymphoma, **N**eck **H**ead **L**ymphoma: Usually a younger child presenting with a non-tender abdominal mass. It is fast growing. **NHL** hockey is a fast sport.

Subtypes of NHL

Non-Hodgkin Lymphoma is divided into two subtypes.
- One is *lymphoblastic,* which is "T Cell" in origin.
- The other is *nonlymphoblastic,* which is B cell in origin (Burkitt lymphoma is an example of this subtype).

Children with the lymphoblastic subtype will present with mediastinal masses and sometimes with pleural effusions.

NHL vs. Leukemia

Both leukemia and NHL involve an abnormal clone of a B or T cell. So what's the difference? It is all semantics. The presence of more than 25% blasts in the bone marrow is leukemia – no matter how many or how big the nodes and masses are. If there are less than 25% blasts in the marrow along with a mass, it is lymphoma.

Other Tissues

Langerhans Cell Histiocytosis (Long Hands Hysterical X)

Langerhans cell histiocytosis (LCH, formerly Histiocytosis X) has several typical features that will be included in the presenting history. Once these features are committed to memory, the answer will jump out while you are reading the question.

Patients may present with a solitary focal bone lesion, often in the skull. Other typical features include:

❑ Seborrheic rash

❑ Ear discharge

❑ Lytic lesions in the skull

❑ Diabetes insipidus

❑ Excessive urination[2]

LCH is diagnosed by **skin biopsy** and **electron microscopy**.

 Treatment is with surgery (to remove a single lesion), steroids, or chemotherapy. Let's come up with a visual to memorize this by linking it to "Long Hands Hysterical X."

Let's start with **_Long Hands and X_**. (Picture _Edward Scissor Hands_[3])

❑ You are in a room full of people who have 8-foot-long hands with a sharp X at the end.

❑ In reaching across the room they keep hitting your head, which puts holes in your scalp (**Lytic Lesions**).

❑ This eventually penetrates deep enough to cut into your _posterior pituitary_, resulting in **Diabetes Insipidus**.

❑ In addition, they punch a hole in the eardrum, resulting in **Ear Drainage**.

❑ This results in a "Rash" on your cheek (**Seborrheic Rash**).

❑ You can only stop this by using a Giant Electronic Light and Cutter (Electron Microscope and Biopsy) to clip off the Sharp X's.

Neuroblastoma

With the exception of brain tumors, this is the most common **solid tumor** in childhood.[4]
It presents initially in the adrenal glands in 50% of cases. **When neuroblastoma occurs before 12 months of age, the survival rate is 95%.** In fact, neuroblastoma is the only known tumor to spontaneously regress.

---

[2] Both from diabetes insipidus and from pituitary involvement.

[3] From the motion picture a few years back.

[4] Leukemia is not a solid tumor.

Typical presentations of Neuroblastoma include:

- ❏ Non-tender abdominal mass
- ❏ Weight loss, anorexia
- ❏ UTI from obstructing abdominal mass
- ❏ Raccoon eyes *(due to metastases)*
- ❏ Horner syndrome (*due to a mediastinal tumor compressing the recurrent laryngeal nerve*[5])
- ❏ Irritability, hypertension, and diarrhea all due to catecholamine production

If given hypertension as a symptom, choose renal artery compression as the reason over excess catecholamine production if you're given both choices.

Diagnosis of neuroblastoma is made either by:

(1) Biopsy of tumor
(2) Elevated urine VMA and HMA along with a tumor found in bone marrow

CT with contrast will locate the tumor. Other lab abnormalities common at diagnosis are **pancytopenia** (from bone marrow involvement), **elevated ferritin**, and **elevated LDH.**

Neuroblastoma Prognosis

The most important *prognostic feature is age.*
· If younger than 1 year, the prognosis is excellent
· If older than 1, the prognosis is poor

You **are** expected to know the following relatively arcane fact.

Surgical staging, once all the rage in the late 80's, is now no longer in vogue, just like other late 80's icons like MC Hammer. If surgical staging makes its way onto the exam, it is wrong, and MC equals wrong answer squared.

---

[5] Which would affect speech.

Retinoblastoma

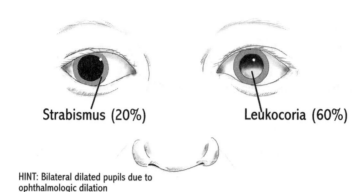

Strabismus (20%)　　　Leukocoria (60%)

HINT: Bilateral dilated pupils due to ophthalmologic dilation

Genetics of Retinoblastoma

There is a heavy genetic component to this, and they like to harp on this point. Remember, if a parent had it in **2** eyes there is a 1/2 **(50%)** chance of any child having it.

However, if a parent had only **1** eye affected, then there is only a **1/20 (5%)** chance of a child having it. The same odds apply if one sib has unilateral disease.

In the typical presentation they will show or describe "leukocoria" (white pupil).

BUZZ WORDS A typical presentation would be a mom who brings in a picture showing the normal red light reflex in only one eye.

PERIL WARNING Despite the genetic association of retinoblastoma, only 5% will have a family history. The mainstays of treatment are surgical excision, chemotherapy, and radiation.

HOT TIP Retinoblastoma also places a child at risk for **osteosarcoma later in life**.

You are presented with a child just under 1 year old who is vomiting, but not experiencing diarrhea. Among the physical findings (which will be consistent with dehydration, including dry oral mucosa and decreased urine output), they note a full anterior fontanelle. He is provided with two normal saline boluses, and then postures by fully extending his arms and legs. You are asked what would be the best next step.

If you do not read the key words carefully[6] you might mistakenly read "full fontanelle" as "flat fontanelle." This is the key to the question. If you read it as flat fontanelle, you might pick the diversionary choice of continued boluses and IV fluids. If you misinterpreted this as a seizure, you would have picked fosphenytoin or other anticonvulsants incorrectly.

The history is consistent with a space occupying lesion, most likely a brain tumor. The full fontanelle is what gives this away. The arm and leg extension and posturing is secondary to increased intracranial pressure, *not a seizure*. Therefore, IV dexamethasone and other steps to reduce increased intracranial pressure would be the correct response.

Rhabdomyosarcoma

Rhabdomyosarcoma is the most common soft tissue sarcoma in children and is a Board favorite.

They could describe a child with constipation. On rectal exam a mass is **visible or palpated**. This description should tip you off to the diagnosis.

Young patients (2-6) tend to have head and neck rhabdo, while older patients (teenagers) are more likely to have truncal or extremity tumors. Diagnosis is made by biopsy. Treatment is with chemotherapy, surgery, and radiation.

When rhabdomyosarcoma occurs in an extremity, they **often describe a history of trauma to throw you off**. Don't be fooled, and don't go for the distractor. What will tip you off is that the area of **trauma is getting worse after a couple of weeks**. This is a typical presentation of rhabdomyosarcoma, as is "atypical" pain following routine trauma.

---

6 Again, sounds like a cliché, but it is important to read the key words carefully.

They may show a grape-like mass protruding from the vagina. This is classic rhabdomyosarcoma.

Change it to "grape-domyosarcoma" and you won't forget that image if they present it to you on the exam.

Two disorders that can get worse after trauma injury are rhabdomyosarcoma and osteogenic sarcoma. Don't be deceived by the mention of the trauma.

Wilms Tumor (Nephroblastoma)

Wilms tumor is the most common pediatric abdominal malignancy. The median age for diagnosis is 3 1/2 years.

The most common presentation is an asymptomatic abdominal mass. Sometimes it causes hypertension and/or gross hematuria. Diagnosis is made by histology.

Following nephrectomy, the patient receives chemotherapy and radiation according to the stage of their disease. Today, close to 90% of children with Wilms tumor may be cured.

Aniridia is one of the characteristics of Wilms tumor. *Abdominal mass* and *hemihypertrophy* are other important findings.

Think of Wilma from the Flintstones, who had no iris.[7]

Wilms does not calcify. Remember this since Wilma Flintstone lived in the Stone Age, not the Calcium Age.

 Both **Wilms tumor** and **Beckwith Wiedemann syndrome** are associated with hemihypertrophy. In addition, children with Beckwith Wiedemann syndrome are at risk for developing Wilms tumor.

---

[7] If you do not know who this is, check it out on the Internet, but don't get carried away unless you have met your study quota for the day.

They most likely will not use the word "hemihypertrophy." Instead, they will likely describe "half the body being larger than the other."

Think of Beckwith-Wiedemann, as a "Wide Man," as in Fred Flintstone, and Wilms as Wilma: **Fred and Wilma Flintstone, sharing "half a body."**

Oncologic Emergencies

Tumor Lysis Syndrome

> ### Very Bad Varicella
>
> Patients on chemo have a lot to fear regarding varicella. You are expected to know that varicella-zoster immunoglobulin is indicated for any patient on chemo who is exposed to varicella.

Tumor Lysis Syndrome occurs with the rapid breakdown of a large number of tumor cells. It is most common at the **initiation of chemotherapy** for **large tumors or leukemia**. The classic tumor is *Burkitt's lymphoma*, but it can occur with any malignancy. Children need to be monitored for hyper**P**hosphatemia, hyper**K**alemia, and hyper**U**ricemia (PKU if you will).

 It is treated with hydration, **A**lkalinization, and **A**llopurinol.

If you end up with tumor lysis, you go to the PICU- **PKU** to help remember elevated **P**hosphate (potassium) and **U**ric acid.

Cord Compression

Any tumor in or around the spine can cause cord compression, which often presents with **neurologic symptoms or bowel/bladder dysfunction**.

 This emergency is usually *treated with steroids and/or radiation.*

Anterior Mediastinal Mass

Symptoms are respiratory distress, especially when supine.

Treatment is to make the diagnosis and treat the underlying condition. In an emergency, radiation can be used.

Intubation is NOT the answer because the airway compression is BELOW the vocal cords, and once the patient is anesthetized, there will be no way to maintain oxygenation and ventilation.

Any of the four **T**'s can result in the symptoms associated with anterior mediastinal masses: **T**hymoma, **T**eratoma, **T**hyroid, and **T**errible (**T**-cell lymphoma). Any of these can cause *airway compromise;* however, lymphoma *most commonly* results in airway compromise.

Superior Vena Cava Syndrome

Superior Vena Cava Syndrome is usually due to extrinsic **compression of the SVC**[8] **by an anterior mediastinal tumor**, most commonly **Hodgkin's disease or T-cell lymphoma**.

Superior Vena Cava Syndrome typically presents with red face *(plethora), facial swelling, upper extremity edema, distended neck veins, and, if bad enough, neurologic symptoms.*

Treatment is aimed at the underlying disorder, but if emergent, *steroids and/or radiation* can be used.

Think about a big heavy Donald Trump type at Christmas after a few drinks – big red swollen face. That is plethora.

If an anterior mediastinal mass is suspected, the choice to anesthetize the patient should NEVER be chosen.

Side Effects of Chemotherapeutic Agents

This is an excellent topic for the matching section. Having these at your fingertips will provide you with a few easy lay-ups if you need them.

---

[8] Superior Vena Cava.

Cyclophosphamide: Hemorrhagic Cystitis

Cyclophosphamide and **Cy**stitis both begin with **Cy**. Or you can picture somebody riding a cycle in your bladder, causing bleeding. Management includes serial U/A's to monitor for cystitis as well as bleeding. Management is through hydration to increase urine output.

Bleomycin: Pulmonary Fibrosis

"Blow My Icing:" When you take this medication, your **lungs are so bad**, you **"blow icing"** instead of air.

Anthracycline (Doxorubicin, Daunomycin) - Cardiac Toxicity

One way to remember this is to picture the **Doc exchanging your heart for a giant ruby**, which is **not very functional**. Or picture **"anthrax cycling in your heart,"** causing toxicity.

Vincristine/Vinblastine

Neurotoxicity and **SIADH** are the side effects here. Picture a guy named Vin whose head is blasting (Blastine) and is replaced by a giant crystal ball (Cristine).

Asparaginase - Pancreatitis

Envision, instead of a **pancreas, a very long, green asparagus bunch**.

Procarbazine: CNS Problems

"Pro Car BAM Scene:" Picture a **"Pro Car"** going **"Bam"** into **a giant head** at an accident scene.

Cranial Irradiation and Growth Attenuation

Cranial irradiation can impact pituitary hormone secretion, including growth hormone secretion

It is important to monitor for growth hormone deficiency in children receiving cranial irradiation therapy. This could be worth a point on the exam.

Methotrexate: Oral and GI Ulcers

 "**Moutho Tray X:**" Picture a mouth **filled with trays of sharp X's** resulting in oral and GI ulcers.

Disorders of Red Cells

Anemia Mania

Anemia of the newborn

A physiological drop in the HCT is to be expected by the 2nd or 3rd month of life (8-10 weeks of age) in term infants.

If they describe garden-variety **physiologic anemia of infancy**, the correct answer will likely be "**no further laboratory evaluation is necessary**." The only time further intervention is needed is if cardiovascular compromise exists, or possibly if the patient is a premature neonate.

But don't be fooled – even in a premature neonate; the likely cause of a drop in hematocrit at 2-3 months is still the physiologic nadir.

Should they ask for the "etiology" of physiological anemia in newborns, the answer is "**low erythropoietin production**."

Sizing It All Up

The best approach to questions concerning anemias is to break them up into size order. Note the MCV, and write in the margin whether it is micro-, macro-, or normocytic. It shouldn't be subtle. Remember that the normal MCV for babies and toddlers is 70-90, as opposed to 80-100 for adults. Since these are not the Heme-Onc Boards, there are only a limited number of anemias you need to know, and a limited number of ways they can present them. So here goes:

Microcytic Anemia

The primary disorders are iron deficiency, thalassemia, anemia of chronic illness, and lead poisoning. The MCV will be less than 70.

In a kid with a microcytic anemia (MCV<70) and normal iron studies, consider thalassemia and lead as the most likely causes.

Beta Thalassemia

Thalassemia Minor or Thalassemia Trait

Thalassemia Minor or **Thalassemia Trait** is caused by a *defect in one of the beta globin gene alleles*. These patients are *asymptomatic*, though their *mild anemia* may be found on routine laboratory examination and be *mistaken for iron deficiency anemia*. It is also sometimes diagnosed in a parent when two supposedly healthy persons have a child with thalassemia major.

Thalassemia Major or Cooley's anemia

Thalassemia Major, or **Cooley's anemia**, results from severe deficiency of **beta** globin due to a mutation in both beta globin gene alleles. It is also known as **beta thalassemia.** These patients present in the first year of life with profound microcytic, hypochromic anemia. Hepatosplenomegaly will also be present. Patients require regular blood transfusions and frequent monitoring, and need to be under the care of a hematologist.

Beta thalassemia can be diagnosed on hemoglobin electrophoresis. There will be very **low levels of hemoglobin A1** and **increased levels of hemoglobin A2** (alpha-delta). **Hemoglobin F will also be elevated**, though this is not specific for beta thalassemia.

In beta thalassemia, the beta is missing or low, so the alpha is lonely. Since it can't form hemoglobin A1, it resorts to pairing up with other forms of hemoglobin like delta (making A2) and gamma (making F).

With **thalassemia major,** they will typically describe a small-for-age Greek child with anemia and an **enlarged liver or spleen**. They may even give you a hemoglobin electrophoresis that shows **increased hemoglobin A2 and F**. They could also describe or show an x-ray that has **thickened bone**. The skull x-ray will often have the classic **"hair-on-end" appearance**, as one would see in hair exposed to static electricity (this is secondary to extramedullary hematopoiesis).

The mainstay of treatment is *chronic transfusion therapy*.

The two **long-term complications** seen in these kids are

1. Cholelithiasis[9]
2. Hemosiderosis (iron deposition in the heart, liver, and pancreas).

Sickle cell anemia and **beta thalassemia** can be distinguished on **hemoglobin electrophoresis** as follows:

· sickle cell anemia ➜ high hemoglobin F and high hemoglobin S
· beta thalassemia ➜ low hemoglobin A1, high hemoglobin A2, high hemoglobin F

CASE STUDY

You are presented with a 10 week old infant of Mediterranean descent with a hematocrit of 12.4 and an MCV of 89. What is the most likely explanation for the anemia?

THE DIVERSION

The diversion here is the child of Mediterranean descent. If your eyes were drawn to this word and you ignored the numbers and picked thalassemia, you would be adrift in the Mediterranean.

ANSWER REVEALED

This is an example where "putting numbers into words" would be helpful. You would have noted that this is a normocytic anemia, and given the age of the infant, the most likely cause of the anemia is *physiologic anemia of infancy.*

Alpha Thalassemia

There are two alpha globin genes on chromosome 16 (thus 4 alleles = aa/aa), and alpha thalassemia results from mutations in one to all four of these alleles.

Other than a mild microcytic anemia, you will most likely not be asked to recognize a diagnosis of Alpha thalassemia.

---

[9] Known as gallstones to the rest of humanity.

Iron Deficiency Anemia

Infants

The risk for iron deficiency anemia in infants begins after 6 months, *particularly in breast fed infants.*

Iron deficiency anemia is treated with ferrous sulfate until 2 months after hemoglobin levels are normalized. This is to replenish iron stores. Think of it as paying off all your bad debts first (resolving the anemia) and then putting some savings away in the bank (building up iron stores).

> **Watch That Iron** – Any patient who undergoes **regular transfusion therapy** (thalassemia, sickle cell, aplastic anemia, vampires) will eventually have **iron overload**. These patients must begin chelation therapy to remove excess iron, or they will have toxic buildup in their livers (hemosiderosis) and hearts. This is a significant cause of morbidity and mortality in chronically transfused patients.

How now Bad Cow

Because of the low amount of iron absorbed, **infants** given cow's milk (versus formula or breast milk) before 12 months of age are also at increased risk for **iron deficiency anemia**. Microscopic GI bleeding can lead to iron deficiency anemia, but the most common cause (in real life and the Boards) is nutritional.

Look for this common scenario – An 18 month-old kiddo with pallor and tachycardia. The **hemoglobin** will be very **low** (<6) and the MCV will also be low (<60). The tip-off for iron deficiency anemia in this child will be a history of drinking lots and lots and lots of cows milk and probably still on the bottle, to the exclusion of anything else containing iron.

A response to iron is not diagnostic. For example, if the hematocrit was low due to an infection—any infection, including viral—the hematocrit will rise after iron therapy. It would respond after Earl Gray Tea Therapy. Basically, the hematocrit comes back up with resolution of the illness. Watch for this trick question.

Parenteral iron administration will never be the right answer, unless 1) the kid cannot take oral iron, or 2) in very extreme social circumstances.

RDW, the Road to Passing: You can be presented with a grid with at least five forms of anemia, along with their associated lab findings. At one point, you will narrow down the choices to two microcytic anemias: one with a high RDW and one with a low RDW.

Without knowing the reason, even your accountant can get this one correct. Iron deficiency has an "**I**" and no "L" therefore, the RDW is **high**. Thalassemia has an "**L**" early on; therefore, the RDW is Low.[10] Slam Dunk!

Anemia of Chronic Disease

The size of the cells can be variable, but are *usually normocytic or microcytic.*[11] However, there are certain features in the history and/or the labs that will clue you in that you are dealing with a chronic disorder.

The anemia of chronic illness can present as a microcytic anemia.

With anemia of **chronic disease**, *total iron binding capacity* **is low.**[12]

Think of the iron binding capacity as "vehicles to carry iron." In the absence of iron, there are plenty of empty vehicles around and the TIBC is high. With chronic illness, there is no energy for the vehicles to come by and pick up the iron. Therefore, the supply builds up (see next entry), and the TIBC is low.

Serum ferritin[13] is high in **chronic illness**. "The reserves were there before the illness," is one way to remember this. In addition, there are no TIBC vehicles to carry the iron away; therefore TIBC is **low** in anemia secondary to chronic illness.[14]

Anemia	Ferritin	TIBC
Chronic Illness	High	Low
Iron Deficiency	Low	High

---

[10] Or possibly normaL, but definitely not high.

[11] Since it can be microcytic we included it in this section.

[12] In iron deficiency, it is high.

[13] Iron stores, essentially. Remember, ferritin is low in iron deficiency.

[14] TIBC is high in iron deficiency.

CASE STUDY **You are presented with a child with a *microcytic anemia*. They will note that the child has sickle cell disease. You will be asked "What is the anemia due to?"**

THE DIVERSION The decoy, of course, is noting that the child has sickle cell disease. Clearly this will not be the answer; however, it will be among the choices for those willing to pick the most obvious incorrect answer.

ANSWER REVEALED Since it is a microcytic anemia, the correct answer will be *iron deficiency anemia* or *beta thalassemia*. You would have gotten this correct if you noted the cell size in the labs, and wrote "microcytic" in the margins, realizing iron deficiency anemia is microcytic.

HOT TIP With anemia of chronic illness, **treatment with iron is NOT necessary** since they have adequate stores, but not enough "carrier energy." Treatment of the underlying illness is curative. Treatment of children with chronic renal or chronic inflammatory disease includes erythropoietin.

HOT TIP With any illness or inflammatory process, ferritin goes up (it is an acute-phase reactant). This includes a minor URI. Therefore, anytime the sedimentation rate (ESR) is high, the ferritin level should be elevated as well.

HOT TIP The most important lab studies to diagnose iron deficiency are:

- Serum ferritin
- Serum iron binding capacity
- Total iron binding capacity

If you want to separate whether the ferritin level is due to acute phase reaction or true iron stores, order a CRP. If the CRP is normal, there is no acute illness, and the serum ferritin is a true measure of your iron stores.

Lead Poisoning

Lead poisoning is the most common environmental illness in kids. It acts by interfering with various enzyme systems; most notably it can affect the production of heme.

Look for a pale kid with vague symptoms (irritability, lethargy, sleeplessness, headaches, belly pain, or constipation). "Lead lines" on long bone radiographs are rare in kids (except on the Boards). Lead can affect any organ system, especially the developing brain.

It is important to remember that **iron deficiency usually coexists with lead poisoning** and this enhances lead absorption.

Measuring a whole blood lead level is the gold standard test.

Treatment is with chelation therapy (penicillamine, dimercaprol, or EDTA).

Lead Poisoning and FEP

FEP (free erythrocyte protoporphyrin) is elevated in both Pb poisoning and Fe deficiency. It is normal in thalassemia. Although not very common in clinical practice, it might creep up in a question.

A **ringed sideroblast** (immature red blood cell with iron-bloated mitochondria surrounding the nucleus) could be an important clue that lead poisoning is the diagnosis, though the much rarer sideroblastic anemia should also be considered.

Macrocytic Anemias

The MCV in macrocytic anemias will be >100, often around 110.

Vitamin B12 Deficiency / Folate Deficiency

Frequently this is due to poor absorption of B12, often as a result of a gastrointestinal disorder such as Crohn's disease.

B12 deficiency can also be due to:

- · Intrinsic factor deficiency[15]
- · Bacterial overgrowth
- · Following bowel resection.
- · Infants whose mothers are vegetarians

Often they will drop a hint as to the etiology of the deficiency in the question. Vitamin B12 deficiency will frequently be the underlying problem if a compromised gut is combined with a heme question.

MNEMONIC Remember the **B** Rule: **B**acterial overgrowth, **B**owel resection, **B**12 deficiency, HLA-**B**27 (Crohn's).

HOT TIP On the Boards, B12 will be known by its formal name: that's "Mr. Cobalamin." **The "Schilling" test is for B12 absorption.**

MNEMONIC "Cobra Ladder Min:" Cobalamin – Picture a cobra climbing a ladder to the 12th Floor. With B12 deficiency, they may also describe hypersegmented polys; just picture the same cobra, coiled up in the white cell. In addition, picture the cobra climbing the ladder and paying a "schilling" to **enter** the 12th floor to help remember that it is the schilling test that measures B12 **absorption**.

Pernicious Anemia

Pernicious anemia is caused by a *lack of intrinsic factor*, which leads to impaired B12 absorption. The *classic triad* is **weakness, paresthesias, and sore tongue**. Treatment with IM cobalamin[16] should provide some relief within 24 hours.

PERIL WARNING **Remember**: Administration of folate will correct the hematological abnormalities without addressing the underlying vitamin B12 deficiency, possibly leading to irreversible neurologic damage.

TREATMENT Before treatment with folate, the proper diagnosis MUST be made.

MNEMONIC Imagine a pernicious snake. It bites your legs, making you weak and causing paresthesias. It climbs down your mouth, giving you a sore tongue. When it reaches your stomach, it steals all your intrinsic factor.

Fanconi anemia and Blackfan anemia are both macrocytic anemias.

MNEMONIC Picture the large Red Cells as a giant electric fan, and you will remember that FANconi's and BlackFAN are both macrocytic anemias.

Got Goat Milk? – If you see the words "goat milk" in the question, it is macrocytic anemia. It is caused by folic acid deficiency. That points you to the treatment.

MNEMONIC Well, we know that goat's milk results in megaloblastic anemia, but this is due to **"folate"** deficiency. Remember, goats are "foolish animals;" therefore, drinking their milk results in **"foolate"** deficiency. Don't pick B12 deficiency, even though that trap will be waiting for you.

---

[15]See " Pernicious anemia" below.

[16] That's Mr. Cobalamin to you.

You are presented with a patient who they suggest or come right out and tell you has folate deficiency. You are then asked for the next most important step in diagnosing and/or treating the patient.

Among the choices for diagnosis will be serum folate levels, and for treatment, *immediate* replacement therapy with folic acid before diagnostic steps are taken.

Both of these diversionary choices are incorrect. **Erythrocyte folic acid concentration** would be preferred over serum folate levels. In addition, with a diagnosis of folic acid deficiency, vitamin B12 deficiency must first be ruled out. If B12 deficiency is present, then treatment with folic acid may delay the diagnosis.

Normocytic Anemias

When you see a normocytic anemia, consider (1) the patient is bleeding, (2) the patient has a chronic disease, or (3) there is a hemolytic process.

Hemolytic Anemias result in an **elevated reticulocyte count (normal is 1%).** One exception to this would be a parvovirus infection leading to an aplastic crisis.

Therefore, if you have a question that points to a hemolytic anemia, but there is **no elevated retic count, parvovirus** could be the correct answer regarding etiology.

Breaking up is Hard to Do: Hemolytic Anemias (G6PD deficiency, HS, PK deficiency, Sickle Cell)

There are a few types of hemolytic anemias, each with its own unique characteristics and descriptions. These should be easy-to-answer questions once you have them down straight. They each have different inheritance patterns, a subject ripe for the matching section. Follow the bouncing memory aides and you won't go wrong.

Consider the reasons that a red cell might be destroyed. There could be enzyme problems (G6PD, PK), structural problems (HS), or a weird shape that causes its removal from the circulation (sickle cell).

Contents Under Pressure

When hemolysis is occurring, the products of red cell breakdown have to go somewhere. You will find them in the **urine**, usually in the form of **hemosiderin** and **bilirubin.** In addition, **serum haptoglobin** will be low in hemolytic anemia. Finally, an important lab finding you will see is the **Coombs test**. The direct Coombs identifies antibodies on the surface of the red cell. This is extremely useful in determining whether a hemolytic process is immune-mediated.

G6PD Deficiency

 Glucose-6-phosphate dehydrogenase protects the red cell from oxidative stress, which can lead to hemolysis. There may be a reference to "**Heinz Bodies,**" which are small, purple granules in the red cell that form as a result of damage to the hemoglobin molecule.

They typically will describe a black or Mediterranean child (almost always a boy) with "**dark urine,**" who is also "**jaundiced**" and "**anemic.**" They may describe exposure to a causative agent (i.e., mothballs, antimalarials, nitrofurantoin) that triggered the "hemolytic crisis."

Watch for the *sudden onset* of pallor and anemia in an otherwise healthy child. Often they will describe an agent that might cause the oxidative stress, such as treatment with a sulfa-containing antibiotic.

To remember that this is X linked, remember G**X**pd deficiency. You can also picture the cells as "Heinz®" bottles of ketchup ready to explode (hemolyze).

G6PD deficiency is the most common sex-linked disorder in black males.

Shades of Gray

G6PD deficiency is classified according to the **degree of enzyme activity** (mild, moderate, or severe enzyme deficiency). Most patients are asymptomatic, but there may be a history of neonatal jaundice or transfusion.

There may be a history of **drug-induced hemolysis** (sulfonamides, ciprofloxacin, antimalarials, nitrofurantoin) or a crisis precipitated by ingestion of fava beans.

Type A G6PD deficiency

Type A G6PD deficiency (both A+ and A-) mainly affects African Americans, and the A- variant is usually episodic, with hemolysis occurring mainly after exposure to oxidants. This is because the G6PD activity decreases with the age of the red blood cell. This is why an oxidative stress is required.

African Americans often have Type **A.**

Type B G6PD deficiency

Type B G6PD deficiency is found mainly in Mediterranean populations and is characterized by *chronic hemolysis,* in addition to the acute episodes described for Type A. Low enzyme activity and Heinz bodies confirm the diagnosis.

When testing for G6PD deficiency, **testing right after or during an episode is not reliable,** because reticulocytes have a large amount of G6PD and can lead to a false negative test. Testing should be done several weeks after the episode. **Therefore, if the question includes a negative test right after an episode, G6PD deficiency has not necessarily been ruled out.**

Hereditary Spherocytosis (HS)

HS is due to *defects in the surface of red cells* resulting in loss of erythrocyte surface area. The most common form is moderate *autosomal dominant* **HS.**[17] These small fragile cells will have an **increased mean corpuscular hemoglobin concentration (MCHC)** because there will be more hemoglobin per volume (the cell is smaller with the same amount of hemoglobin). These cells will break open more easily when subjected to osmotic fragility testing, which is the diagnostic method of choice.

On the boards, the etiology of HS will be **spectrin deficiency** or spectrin mutation (they really have asked this in the past). Technically, ankyrin deficiency can also cause HS, but if they give you both choices (and they might), choose spectrin.

Think of **HS** as **H**ereditary **S**pectrin deficiency, and you won't forget this.

HS typically presents with mild or moderate anemia, *splenomegaly,* and *intermittent jaundice. Gallstones* are also common.

---

[17] The most common HS is autosomal dominant, but an autosomal recessive form can also occur.

Treatment

Treatment of Hereditary Spherocytosis is with **folic acid**, monitoring for growth, and transfusions if needed, particularly with a parvovirus infection (aplastic crisis). **Splenectomy** is sometimes done and is usually **curative**.

Parvovirus B19 is the most common cause of aplastic crisis in children with hereditary spherocytosis.

A description of a **hemolytic anemia** coupled with **hyperchromia or increased MCHC** tips you off to **spherocytosis**, which is usually **autosomal dominant**. They may also describe an "aplastic crisis," which would be noted by the inappropriately *low reticulocyte count*.

Sickle Cell Anemia (Sick as Hell Anemia)

Sickle cell disease is caused by a substitution at amino acid six of the beta globin chain. In the abnormal gene, a valine is substituted for a glutamic acid. Past Board exams have asked which diseases are results of an amino acid substitution.

Sickle cell anemia **does not usually present clinically until after 6 months of age**, but children are usually **diagnosed when their newborn screens come back** abnormal. Children are started on prophylactic penicillin early in infancy, and are given the **pneumococcal vaccine at 2 years of age (PPV)**. Any older child should be considered asplenic and treated as such (antibiotics and a septic workup for fevers). The spleen removes Howell-Jolly bodies from the red cells, so once asplenic, you will find these nuclear particles. Priapism may be seen in sickle cell disease, particularly on the boards.

Antibiotic prophylaxis with **penicillin** is recommended for all children with sickle cell disease (at least through age 5).

Defects of structure (e.g., membrane) are dominant traits. **Enzyme defects** are usually recessive.

Crisis with SCA

Vasoocclusive Crisis: This will present with acute pain secondary to ischemia and infarction. Rehydration and pain control are the staples of management. Infants can have dactylitis – pain and swelling of the hands and feet, also treated with aggressive pain control.

Sequestration Crisis: They will describe **signs of shock**. This is due to pooling of blood in the liver and spleen, often in response to an infection. This is a medical emergency and requires aggressive medical intervention, including hospitalization and transfusion.

Aplastic: Aplastic crises are typically due to parvovirus infection. A person with sickle cell(or HS for that matter) needs to keep a high reticulocyte count to keep up with increased red cell destruction. If this is turned off (say, by parvovirus), the person is in dire straits indeed, and their hemoglobin will plummet.

Hyperhemolytic Crisis: Usually they will describe an infection as well as a history of SCA. It can often precede an aplastic crisis or sequestration crisis.

Howell-Jolly bodies are associated with sickle cell disease and Heinz bodies with G6PD deficiency. Memorize Heinz body as "Hein6" body to keep this straight. Another way to remember this association is that **6** year olds like **Heinz**® ketchup on everything.

Most states screen newborns for sickle cell disease, so there are fewer and fewer diagnostic surprises. However, things always lag behind on the Boards, so it is still possible to have an infant of several months who has not been diagnosed yet.

Spleen Truth

By age 5, children with SCA have **functional asplenia**, and many will have a small, hard, non-palpable spleen. If they describe a child older than that with SCA and a **palpable spleen,** then they are telling you it is a variation on the theme, either hemoglobin-SC or sickle cell and thalassemia together (hemoglobin-S, beta-thal).

Children with SCA and thalassemia are resistant to **malaria**, which is thought to be how these abnormal genes have selectively remained in the gene pool.

Acute Chest Syndrome

Acute chest syndrome is defined as **chest pain**, **infiltrate on x-ray**, and **hypoxia**[18].

If they describe a sickle cell patient with these symptoms and signs, the next study to get would be an **ABG to confirm the hypoxia** —*the oxygen saturation, especially if borderline, is usually not good enough to make the diagnosis of ACS*. The treatment for ACS is **transfusion**. If the starting hematocrit is low, a simple transfusion may suffice. But if the hematocrit is relatively high to start with, the patient may require an exchange transfusion.

Chest pain in a child with SCA is difficult to distinguish between *"pneumonia"* and *"pulmonary infarct."* Therefore, "fever, cough and chest pain" should be treated for both.

Cerebrovascular accident (CVA):

If they were to describe an African American child with symptoms of a stroke, treatment would consist of transfusion first, followed by an MRI. You want to treat before you diagnose because you don't want the CVA to progress on the MRI table.

---

[18] As an intern, I once dictated this diagnosis and the transcriptionist typed it out as "A Cute Dress" Syndrome.

Call the doctor for Cholelithiasis

Cholelithiasis, or gallstones (as they are commonly called), is associated with sickle cell disease. Consider this diagnosis or obtaining an abdominal ultrasound in a child with sickle cell disease presenting with right upper quadrant tenderness.

CASE STUDY **You are presented with a child with sickle cell disease and symptoms of a stroke. However, the diagnosis is not given, and they ask how to diagnose the underlying disorder. They might mention that the child is new to the U.S., implying an undiagnosed chronic illness.**

THE DIVERSION Among the choices will be a head CT or MRI, but this will not be the correct answer. It is the decoy.

ANSWER REVEALED The correct answer is **hemoglobin electrophoresis** since sickle cell anemia is the underlying disorder and this is how it is best diagnosed.

PERIL WARNING If they had asked what would be the first thing to do, the answer would be an exchange transfusion (to replace sickled forms with normal red blood cells). If they asked how to "diagnose" the problem (not the underlying cause), the answer would be MRI. This is yet another example of the importance of reading the question.

Hypoplastic and Aplastic Anemias

In general these are anemias due to suppression of the red cell line in the bone marrow.

HOT TIP Whenever the bone marrow isn't functioning well, as is the case in aplastic anemia, the cells revert to fetal synthesis, and there is an **increase in fetal hemoglobin** and **macrocytosis**. So look for increased fetal hemoglobin levels noted in the lab findings.

The question will contain a description of labs consistent with marrow suppression across-the-board, along with associated physical findings such as **anemia (pallor), low WBC (mucosal ulcerations), and low platelet count (ecchymoses, bruises, petechiae).**

Aplastic anemia and acute leukemia can look very similar. They will have to give you something to help differentiate them. **Normal liver and no lymphadenopathy** would steer you towards aplastic anemia and away from leukemia. A high LDH or uric acid, as well as fevers and bone pain (and, of course, circulating blasts), make the diagnosis of leukemia more likely. Diagnosis for both must be made by bone marrow biopsy.

Just because **chloramphenicol** is rarely used in practice does not mean it will not make an appearance on Boards. It is still used in the Board's world, and can cause an **aplastic crisis**.

Neuroblastoma can metastasize to the marrow, resulting in **cytopenias**.

They would have to give you something in the history and physical to indicate that neuroblastoma is the primary problem.

Fanconi's Anemia (A Fan Made up of Ice Cream Cones)

In addition to Fanconi's Anemia being a form of *aplastic anemia*, there are chromosomal structural abnormalities, as well as distinct **physical characteristics,** associated with it. It presents later in childhood, usually **after age 3.**

It is a **macrocytic anemia** with **elevated fetal hemoglobin**.

The following **physical characteristics** are associated with Fanconi's Anemia:

- ❑ Abnormal skin pigmentation
- ❑ Growth retardation
- ❑ Renal abnormalities
- ❑ Absent thumb (or hypoplastic thumb) – orthopedic surgeons sometimes refer kids to the hematologist for this sign, often leading to a new diagnosis of FA

We already established that we would think of a **"fan made up of ice cream cones."**

❑ First, the fan chops off the thumbs, then the feet (elevated FEET-al-Hemoglobin), which results in short stature.

❑ Because the fan is made up of ice cream cones, picture the cones spraying odd-colored pigment all over the room, resulting in **abnormal skin pigment.**

❑ The pigment turns into hard plastic. You can't go to the bathroom covered in hard plastic. This results in **urinary retention** and a plastic kidney (**renal abnormalities**).

It is **re**cessive. Remember this by picturing the fan in the "**re**cess" of the ceiling. These patients are also at risk of transformation to AML or myelodysplastic syndrome.

Treatment

Patients invariably require transfusions of red cells and platelets. The only **cure for aplastic anemia is a bone marrow transplant**, although medical therapy with immunosuppressants or, less commonly, androgens, can lead to a prolonged remission (it takes a muscle builder on androgen to take down the fan). Even children in remission require periodic bone marrow examinations to monitor for transformation to AML or MDS.

Diamond-Blackfan Anemia (DBA) vs. Transient Erythroblastopenia of Childhood (TEC)

Both DBA and TEC are profound isolated red cell anemias that present in infancy/toddlerhood. Differentiating them can be tricky, but you will be given some important clues.

Diamond-Blackfan Anemia (DBA) is due to an *arrest in the maturation of red cells.*

Transient Erythroblastopenia of Childhood (TEC) is a consequence of a *suppression of erythroid production.*

In both TEC and DBA, the reticulocyte count and hemoglobin will be low at the start. Both may have gradual onset, though DBA often presents with anemia at birth. Both are likely to be relatively asymptomatic.

Both TEC and DBA **affect the red cell line exclusively**, and you will be expected to distinguish them. As noted, DBA affects infants, so if they describe a 2 or 3 year old they are NOT describing DBA. Also, DBA is chronic, while transient erythroblastopenia is, well, transient.

Features of DBA can be remembered as :

· **D**ysmorphic facies (unlike Fanconi's anemia)
· **B**abies (unlike TEC), with
· **A**nemia

	TEC	DBA
Median age of onset	18-26 months (**TEC=T**oddler)	2-3 months (**DBA=BA**by)
Spontaneous recovery	Almost always	Rarely
Dysmorphology	Uncommon	Common
Transfusions	Uncommon	Common
Steroids	Not indicated	Often helpful
Incidence	Common	Extremely rare

It is very important to look for clues suggestive of **DBA**. If you see mention of thumb abnormalities, urogenital defects, or craniofacial problems in a kid with severe anemia, they are probably talking about DBA.

MCV in TEC will usually be normal, unless the patient has already started to recover and there is a reticulocytosis, in which case it may be elevated.

You could be presented with a child with fairly severe anemia (hemoglobin 3-5), who has a reticulocytosis (retic count 5-10%). They may even give you the history of a recent viral illness. Unless there are other clues, this is probably someone who had TEC and is now in the recovery phase.

If there is no cardiovascular compromise, transfusion is usually not warranted.

Donations?

Blood donations are tested for Hep C and B and HIV. This actually rhymes.

Checking Blood = Hematology; they all begin with the letter H.

Also, Blackfan is **MACRO** (remember the big fan). **Steroids** are used with DBA and *not in TEC*.

Remember to watch for signs of hemolysis. **If they describe dark urine or a positive Coombs test (DAT), you should put DBA and TEC aside and think about hemolytic processes.**

Transfusion would be indicated for children with transient erythroblastopenia with hemodynamic or other instability.

Transfusion Confusion

To avoid confusion regarding the ill effects of transfusion reactions, keep the following in mind.

Febrile nonhemolytic transfusion reactions present as fever and chills. Risk is reduced by using leukocyte-filtered blood.

Pre-medicating with antipyretics does not help prevent this reaction.

Hemolytic reaction

This occurs when blood is not properly cross- matched.

Allergic reaction

This typically presents with urticaria. Cessation of transfusion and administration of an antihistamine is the correct response. If the urticaria resolves rapidly, the transfusion may resume.

Abnormal White Cells

Try to keep these straight – they may be tested on the exam several times.

Chediak-Higashi Syndrome (CHS)

This should be a slam-dunk if memorized properly.

The characteristics are all related to abnormal white cells and platelets. The WBCs contain **lysosomal granules** and have **abnormal chemotaxis**.

Apart from frequent infections, the other symptoms to keep in mind are easy bruisability and oculocutaneous albinism.

Remember: Infections in CHS mostly occur in the lungs and skin, and the most common pathogens are *Staph aureus*, *Strep pyogenes*, and pneumococcus. They may ask you this in one form or another.

"**Cadillac Hibachi:**" If you sat on a hibachi (grill) instead of a Cadillac and tried to drive, you wouldn't go far (**poor chemotaxis**) and your butt would have some serious granules (**lysosomal granules**). A Cadillac is a receding "auto," which should help you remember that CHS is AUTOsomal recessive. The Hibachi would burn your skin and the smoke would make you cough (infections of the skin and respiratory tract).

Think of a very fair-skinned, blonde, blue-eyed kid with frequent bad skin infections and you won't forget Chediak-Higashi.

The diagnosis is made on blood smear with giant granules in the neutrophils. Without bone marrow transplant, most kids die before age 10.

Chronic Granulomatous Disease

CGD is a disorder of phagocytes – they cannot kill the bugs they ingest. Think of your "chronic granny" who eats but has trouble digesting her food.

There is no abnormality in the neutrophil count or in chemotaxis.

These kids present with recurrent bacterial and fungal infections in organs that normally provide a barrier (skin, lungs, GI tract, liver, spleen). The granulomas of the skin are only a tissue response to antigenic stimuli. Watch out for "recurrent Staph" or "gram negative" infections.

Remember the test for CGD. The nitroblue tetrazolium test (NBT) measures the oxidative burst (think NITROglycerine and a BURST). The genetics of CGD is complicated – they should not ask you this.

Mainstays of treatment for CGD are infection prophylaxis and control, interferon, and BMT.

Leukocyte Adhesion Deficiency (LAD)

The name itself pretty much describes the problem. The WBCs do not adhere well. There will be a high white count, but the cells don't move or work.

 Think of a "lazy LAD in Scotland."

With LAD they might describe "**delayed separation of umbilical cord**," "**impaired wound healing**," or "**severe periodontal disease.**"

Look for a high WBC (over 20) in the absence of infection that increases to 40-100 with infection. Most patients with LAD present in the first few months of life and die younger than one year of age unless they undergo bone marrow transplantation.

Because movement is the underlying problem, **the umbilical cord won't move** and the ambulance doesn't arrive (**poor wound healing**). If your jaw doesn't move and your mouth doesn't open, and you can't brush your teeth and you will have "**severe periodontal disease.**"

Neutropenia Encyclopedia (Differentiating Neutropenias)

Neutropenia is defined as an *absolute neutrophil count* (ANC) of **less than 1000 during the first year** and an **ANC less than 1500 beyond that.**[19]

Neutropenia is further classified by severity with:

- **Mild** being an ANC between *1000-1500*
- **Moderate** being an ANC *between 500-1000*
- **Severe** being an ANC *less than 500*

Watch for signs of **gram negative infections** from organisms that ordinarily colonize *skin, mucosal linings,* or *the GI tract.*

If **mucosal ulcerations** are described in the history, you should immediately write the word **neutropenia** in the margin.

---

[19] That is to say, the first year of life and first year of residency training.

Antibiotic Neutropenic Panic Button

HOT TIP

A patient known to have neutropenia (from any cause) needs to have a blood culture and antibiotics when they have a fever. If they give you a kid with an ANC<500 and a fever, the treatment is IV antibiotics and admission to the hospital.

Congenital vs. Acquired

Think of neutropenias as being congenital or acquired.

The congenital ones you should know about are **cyclic** neutropenia, severe congenital neutropenia (**Kostmann syndrome**), benign neutropenia, and the ones where you look weird (**Shwachman-Diamond, Chediak-Higashi**).

The most common cause of **acquired neutropenia** is **infection**. Many, many, many **drugs** cause neutropenia, but the ones to know for the Boards are the **macrolides**.

Transient Neutropenia

Once again don't forget the ever-present "viral suppression" that usually follows a cold and lasts a couple of **days** (**not quite as long** as in cyclic neutropenia). **No treatment or monitoring is needed**.

CASE STUDY

You are presented with a previously well child with a febrile illness, with no hepatosplenomegaly or lymphadenopathy. They provide you with the results of a CBC, with the only significant result being a WBC of 3.5. You are asked for the next step in the management of this apparent neutropenia.

THE DIVERSION

The diversion here is the neutropenia and your call to manage it. You will be provided with several decoy choices including *antibiotics, bone marrow, referral to a hematologist-oncologist, a call to the man on the moon, whatever!*

ANSWER REVEALED

The correct answer will be to repeat the WBC in a few weeks (when it will of course be normal). This is *transient neutropenia due to a viral illness.*

Cyclic Neutropenia

Cyclic Neutropenia is inherited in an **Autosomal Dominant** pattern. Picture someone dominant whipping the white cells into submission in the marrow.

The low WBC count **lasts around a week** and **reappears every month or so**. Often they will describe oral lesions, and it will be in a child **younger than 10 years old**. The diagnosis can only be made with frequent CBCs (twice per week) in order to document the cycle.

They often ask how long the neutropenia lasts and how long the cycles are. It is easy to remember that it is similar to a **menstrual period**, since it lasts around **one week** and occurs on a **monthly cycle**.

Oral **lesions are common:** picture white blood cells sharp around the edges cycling around the mouth causing oral lesions. *Clostridia perfringens* is a typical cause of the infection.

Change the name to *Clostridia "perfume-gin"* and envision the oral lesions giving off an odor of perfumed gin.

Treatment is to manage infections and to use **G-CSF** only if the patient is symptomatic during the periods of neutropenia. The disease is often self-limited.

Chronic Benign Neutropenia

These children usually present because the pediatrician did a CBC at the one-year visit and *discovered it as an incidental finding*. These children rarely have oral ulcers or other signs of infection, but when they do, G-CSF may be helpful.

Distinguishing *Chronic Benign Neutropenia* from *cyclic neutropenia* can be done with very frequent CBCs, but this not often necessary, as the treatments are the same. Children **usually outgrow Chronic Benign Neutropenia by the age of 2.**

Kostmann Agranulocytosis

Kostmann Syndrome, or Kostmann Agranulocytosis, is also known as **Severe Congenital Neutropenia**, which should help you remember what it is. This autosomal recessive disorder results in an arrest in the development of neutrophils. The consequence of this neutropenia may be severe, and may lead to life-threatening infections.

It can be difficult to distinguish Kostmann syndrome from cyclic neutropenia (both in real life and on the Boards).

> · In babies with **cyclic neutropenia**, the *ANC will rise to normal as the cycle ends.*
> · In **Kostmann syndrome**, the *ANC will remain low.*

Be careful – in BOTH disorders, the ANC may rise in response to G-CSF.

Shwachman-Diamond Syndrome

In addition to **pancreatic exocrine insufficiency** (which leads to steatorrhea), these kids all have some degree of pancytopenia.

Patients usually present with short stature, diarrhea/steatorrhea, and recurrent infections, especially those of the upper respiratory tract and skin. They may also have skeletal abnormalities like *clinodactyly and syndactyly.*

Change the name to "**Squashman Diamond**" syndrome. Picture a hammer smashing the bone marrow and diamonds falling out and forming the shape of the pancreas. Squashed bones would remind you of the bone abnormalities.

You can also remember it by its initials **S**hwachman-**D**iamond **S**yndrome, which can stand for **S**ubstandard neutrophils, **D**umb pancreas, and **S**teatorrhea and **S**keletal abnormalities.

Since Cystic Fibrosis also has pancreatic insufficiency, you may have to distinguish between the two. Of course, **Shwachman-Diamond Syndrome is the one with the neutropenia**. Remember that Shwachman-Diamond Syndrome also has **normal electrolytes, no history of pulmonary problems,** and the **sweat test will be normal.**

In addition to neutropenia, other cell lines can be affected, so there can be pancytopenia as well as skeletal abnormalities with Shwachman-Diamond Syndrome.

The treatment of SDS is to control/prevent infections, give pancreatic enzyme supplementation, prevent orthopedic abnormalities, and to monitor for **leukemic transformation**.

Platelet Abnormalities

 Thrombocytopenia is defined as a platelet count lower than 150,000/cubic millimeter.

Thrombocytopenia is the most common hematologic abnormality in neonates admitted to the ICU. The most common cause of true neonatal thrombocytopenia is related to maternal factors such as allo- or autoantibodies. But the MOST COMMON reason for a low platelet count is clumping from improper collection.

Remember to write down the word "thrombocytopenia" if you note a low platelet count in the CBC. With thrombocytopenia, look for "**recent meds**" in the question and note it, since it may be the key to the question. Certain meds can lower platelet counts.

Also, aspirin and ibuprofen result in abnormal platelet function; however, the platelet count will be normal.

Thrombocytopenia in a newborn can be a sign of sepsis.

Thrombocytopenia or functional **platelet disorders** can cause bruising, petechiae, epistaxis, or gastrointestinal bleeding.

However, deep muscle or joint bleeding will likely be due to a **coagulopathy**, not a platelet problem. Remember, "dinner" plates (platelets) are too big to penetrate a joint or a muscle.

ITP – Idiopathic Thrombocytopenic Purpura

They will describe an otherwise healthy 3-year-old with a **recent viral illness** and a **low platelet count, ecchymoses,** and perhaps **petechiae**.

50% of cases will resolve within 3 months; 75% within 6 months. When to transfuse platelets is controversial, but 10-20K is a good guideline. The best therapy for ITP is probably IVIG, but it is expensive and inconvenient to administer. If the patient is Rh positive, an excellent treatment is WinRho® (Anti-Rh D). Splenectomy is a second-line therapy for ITP and not a good choice for very young patients or in ones where conventional therapies have not yet been tried.

If you are presented with a patient with ITP who has persistent or severe headaches, you are expected to realize that the patient may be experiencing an intracranial hemorrhage.

Prognosis is worse if it presents in an older kid, i.e., older than 10 years. In such cases it can become a chronic problem. *The younger the patient, the more likely it will be a single occurrence.*

The ABC's of treating ITP

ITP is not usually treated unless the platelet count is lower than 20,000 and/or there is bleeding. Intravenous immunoglobulin is a mainstay of treatment and will raise the platelet count more quickly than steroids or WinRho®.

A mother with ITP may have an infant with thrombocytopenia, and treatment is usually supportive. However, infants may require IVIG or platelet transfusion in cases of severe thrombocytopenia (< 20K) or bleeding. Platelet transfusions for these newborns is considered to be less effective than IVIG.

Anemia is a contraindication to WinRho® use (anemia is a side-effect of this treatment). With chronic ITP, splenectomy may be the only option, although it should be avoided in children younger than 5.

Steroids are an excellent treatment for ITP, but since ITP and leukemia can look similar, **it has been the practice to not use steroids as a first-line therapy for ITP**. Steroids for thrombocytopenia caused by leukemia would almost certainly induce a remission, but it would be short-lived, and the disease would be much more difficult to control once relapsed. **A bone marrow aspiration is no longer considered necessary by many institutions; however, on the exam you should only choose steroids if IVIG and WinRho® are not choices,** if they show you results of a bone marrow examination, or if it is obviously not leukemia (for instance, if the patient has chronic ITP).

Wiskott-Aldrich Syndrome (WAS)

Wiskott-Aldrich Syndrome (WAS) is an immunodeficiency seen ONLY in boys (X-linked). Look for a baby boy with really bad diaper rash, bruising, and ear infections or pneumonia. They may even give you a low platelet count with a low MPV (mean platelet volume) or "small platelets." Bone marrow transplantation is the treatment.

Children with *Wiskott-Aldrich syndrome* are at *risk* for developing *other malignancies* down the road.

Both ITP and WAS have low platelets and can be difficult to distinguish. Although few in number, **big platelets** on the smear are indicative of ITP whereas **small platelets** are seen more commonly in WAS.

· **W**BC problems
· **A** topic problems
· **S** mall platelets / bruising

Platelet Hall of Fame

Here are some more disorders that are easy to recognize:

Kasabach-Merritt Syndrome

Here you have a hemangioma that serves as a "sand trap" for platelets. Thrombocytopenia is caused by a localized consumptive coagulopathy. The bone marrow is normal. Patients are at risk for DIC.

Treatment is to control the hemangioma and support with transfusions.

If you had a "**sand castle on your back,**" your back would be black and blue and your platelets would be destroyed.

TAR Syndrome

The name says it all—**T**hrombocytopenia **A**bsent **R**adius. Often they just hand this to you either by describing it or showing you the x-ray. You won't miss the absent radius. In addition, the *WBC count is high.* **50% are symptomatic in the first week of life and 90% have symptoms by 4 months.**

 There is really no excuse for getting this wrong.

Thumbs Away! – You may have noticed that there are three disorders associated with upper limb abnormalities and low blood counts.

	Upper Limb Abnormalities	Thumb Abnormalities	Platelets	Hemoglobin	Presents in infancy
DBA	Yes	Yes	Normal	Low	Yes
Fanconi	Yes	Yes	Low	Low	Not usually
TAR	Yes	No	Low	Normal	Yes

Coagulopathies

Vitamin K Dependent Factors

Yes, they do ask this every year. The Vitamin K dependent factors are 2, 7, 9, and 10. Committing this to memory is worth at least one correct answer on the exam.

 The letter K looks like 2 Sevens (7) stuck to each other and turned around; 7 + 2 = 9 plus one "fact" = 10.

Deficiency in the vitamin K factors (i.e., hemorrhagic disease of the newborn) results in **elevated PT**.

Remember, "KEPT" – Vitamin **K**, **E**xtrinsic pathway, **PT**. Because of the vitamin K in formula, this occurs mostly in breast-fed infants.

Early Onset Vitamin K-dependent bleeding

In early onset vitamin K-dependent bleeding, consider maternal factors, such as medications that interfere with her vitamin K stores (anticonvulsants, warfarin, some antibiotics). Common sources of bleeding are at venipuncture sites, penis after circumcision, and mucous membranes and GI tract.

The classic Boards presentation for this disorder is a baby born **at home** who is **breast-fed**. The baby will present at a week or less with the bleeding described above.

Hemophilia

The main types of hemophilia to know are Hemophilia A (factor VIII deficiency) and Hemophilia B (factor IX deficiency, Christmas disease). They are both seX-linked recessive.

You will remember factors 8 and 9, so **just remember that they are in order (A=8, B=9).** Boys (ALWAYS boys) with hemophilia will often have a family history (**boys/ men on the <u>maternal</u> side**). They will always have a prolonged **PTT**. Diagnosis is made by measuring the activity of the specific clotting factors. In addition "A" and "8" sound alike. "B" and "9" both come right after "A" and "8".

> ### Circumcisions
>
> If they describe a child with excessive bleeding after circumcision, a workup for a congenital factor deficiency is the answer. Remember, **C**ircumcision and **C**oag both start with a "**C**."

Kids with hemophilia often present in the neonatal period with bruising, bleeding from their circumcision, or bleeding at the site of venipuncture. The PTT is found to be very prolonged, and the diagnosis is made by measuring factor 8 and 9 levels. Older kids are subject to deep joint bleeds. Mortality can occur from intracranial bleeding.

If you are presented with a patient with hemophilia who suffers severe head trauma, replacement therapy is indicated even in the absence of clinical signs.

Treatment is with factor supplementation.

Hereditary

With bleeding disorders, even if they **do not describe** or specifically mention the presence of a **family history** for bleeding disorders, **"hemophilia" cannot be ruled out**. Remember that hemophilia can present in the absence of family history.

In addition, if they specifically mention that the mother has a **family history** of a bleeding disorder, they are hinting at an X-linked recessive disease.

Male offspring (also known as boys) of a mother who is a carrier have a 50% chance of being born with the disease.

Von Willebrand's Disease – mucosal bleeds.

Hemophilia – bleeding into joints and muscles.

HOT TIP — If you are presented with a patient with hemophilia who has bleeding in the antecubital area following a blood draw, this is serious. It can lead to nerve compression and is considered to be a medical emergency.

Blood should not be drawn from the jugular or femoral veins of individuals with hemophilia who have not received replacement therapy. It could be fatal to your chances of passing the boards.

MNEMONIC — Santa Claus is a "benign" fellow; therefore, it is easy to associate "B9" with Christmas disease. Call it X-mas disease and you will remember it is X-linked recessive. Whoosh!

PERIL WARNING — If they give you a girl with bleeding, it is NOT hemophilia (but it may be von Willebrand's disease).

PERIL WARNING — One common trick on the Boards is to describe a child who develops a hematoma from the vitamin K shot. The reason the child got the hematoma may be hemophilia. They are trying to hypnotize you by mentioning vitamin K – don't let them!

Von Willebrand's Disease

DEFINITION — Von Willebrand's Disease (vWD) is due to an abnormal von Willebrand factor, which is required for normal Factor VIII function as well as normal platelet aggregation.

BUZZ WORDS — They will commonly present a child who has (1) excessive bleeding after a **dental procedure or tonsillectomy,** (2) **epistaxis,** or (3) **a girl with menorrhagia**. It is also commonly picked up from an abnormal PTT on preoperative screening. **The hallmark of vWD is a normal PT. PTT is often normal, but may be slightly prolonged in some cases.** Levels of von Willebrand factor activity should be low. If it is a girl, you are done – the diagnosis is most likely vWD. If it is a boy, you need to measure Factor VIII and IX levels to establish the diagnosis. **Bleeding time is prolonged**.

HOT TIP — Most of the time, no treatment is indicated. For minor bleeding, intranasal or intravenous DDAVP (desmopressin, Stimate®) can be used, as it causes an increase in plasma vWF and factor VIII. For major surgery or life-threatening bleeds, replacement with a factor VIII concentrate should be administered.

If given the choice, choose Factor VIII <u>concentrate</u> over cryoprecipitate administration. Amicar® (aminocaproic acid) helps with mucosal bleeding by inhibiting fibrinolysis, and is often used in vWD.

Consider changing it to Von Wi**TT**erbrand's disease to remember that the P**TT** may be prolonged and PT is often normal. Again when we say "may be" and "often is," this is especially the case on the boards. It is autosomal **dominant**, so picture a person being dominated by someone dressed in a German WWII outfit, bleeding for a prolonged period of time. **Their hat has 2 TT's on it.** The torture stops only after *you start crying* (cryoprecipitate). (Morbid thought, I know: remember to make up your own wild pictures if you don't like ours!)

Disseminated Intravascular Coagulopathy (DIC)

With disseminated intravascular coagulopathy, there will be a history of sepsis or other major illness such as malignancy or severe burns. The platelets will always be low. Other supporting labs are a low fibrinogen and elevated D-dimers. PT and PTT are unpredictable. Thrombin time will be prolonged.

Treatment of the underlying condition is the most important factor in management. Support with blood products as needed - platelets, fresh frozen plasma (if clotting factors are low), cryoprecipitate (if fibrinogen is low), and/or RBCs.

Chapter 21

Renal

Microscopic Hematuria

To paraphrase the Byrds, who paraphrased Ecclesiastes, "there is a time to reassure, a time to work up, and a time to follow-up." Here is "the way" to know which. First, some definitions:

 Microscopic hematuria is 3 or more red blood cells per high-powered field (hpf) *in 2 centrifuged samples of freshly voided urine.*

The urine is not discolored when there is microscopic hematuria.

Transient Hematuria

Transient hematuria may be caused by minor trauma, exercise, or fever. Free hemoglobin, myoglobin, and peroxidase-producing bacteria will be positive on urine strip tests. As the name suggests, there **is** hematuria.

 0-2 cells per high-power field (hpf) is not hematuria.

Family history is important in assessing hematuria. If other family members have a history of hematuria without complications, then benign familial hematuria is a strong possibility. Typically the hematuria is microscopic, so other than monitoring for hypertension and proteinuria, no further workup or intervention is necessary.

Heeding Hematuria

If you are only told that the urine dipstick is positive for blood, then the next step will be to obtain a urinalysis since a dipstick that is positive for blood could be positive for:

- Hemoglobin
- Myoglobin
- Porphyrins

Patients with hemoglobinuria will also be jaundiced and present with anemia. There will be no RBC in the urine, and, therefore, no hematuria.

If they present you with a patient who is a runner, or engages in other vigorous sports activities and has no hematuria, (i.e. 1-2 cells) and dark urine, then the most likely diagnosis is **myoglobulinuria**.

CASE STUDY

You could be presented with a child who engaged in vigorous activity and presents with "gross hematuria." He is otherwise asymptomatic, and they note 0-2 RBCs on microscopic urinalysis. What is the most likely diagnosis?

THE DIVERSION

Here the diversion is the description of "gross hematuria," which is really "gross blood." If you assume that hematuria is present, then you might pick transient hematuria or other disorders associated with hematuria, including renal stones, as the diagnosis.

ANSWER REVEALED

You need to remember that 0-2 RBCs per hpf is not hematuria. If you are given a patient who engaged in vigorous exercise, has grossly bloody urine and a U/A with 0-2 RBC per hpf, you are dealing with a patient with myoglobinuria.

Your Workup for Microscopic Hematuria

HOT TIP

When you are presented with a patient with hematuria you should immediately note if the following is also part of the presentation:

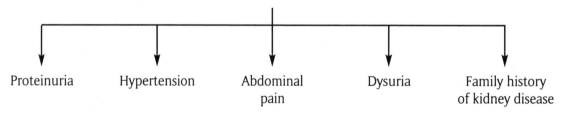

| Proteinuria | Hypertension | Abdominal pain | Dysuria | Family history of kidney disease |

If none of these are present, then all that is necessary is a repeat urinalysis in 2 weeks.

Normal Microscopic Hematuria

Remember, microscopic hematuria is seen normally in **2-3% of school-aged children**. At 6 months follow-up, only 1% remain positive. In the absence of any other clues, the correct answer will simply be to repeat the urinalysis.

Persistent hematuria

If you have persistent microscopic hematuria, then the next step after checking blood pressure would be to look closely at the urinalysis findings (which should be repeated several weeks apart) for proteinuria or other abnormalities. If there are "crystals" noted on the UA, hypercalciuria should be on the differential (this is the most common cause of crystals on a UA). If a hint of hypercalciuria is suggested in the history, you need to check a urine Ca/Cr ratio.

A calcium/creatinine ratio **greater than 0.25** would be consistent with hypercalciuria, which may result in hematuria.

These parameters would not be valid in an infant, because even 0.8 can be normal in an infant. In all fairness, they should not present you with a patient younger than 2, the age when a value greater than 0.25 is abnormal.

Hypercalciuria can result in microscopic hematuria or gross hematuria.

If a patient has persistent microscopic hematuria with no evidence of hypercalciuria or other obvious concerns on UA, the next step would be to obtain serum BUN, creatinine, and lytes. Based on other findings in the history, it may be necessary to order C3, C4, ANA, ASO titers, ANCA, as well as a renal/bladder ultrasound.

Watch for a patient with an underlying condition that has nothing to do with renal disease, such as an infant with bronchopulmonary dysplasia who happens to be on **furosemide**. If they ask what is the cause of the hematuria, the answer may be hypercalciuria, a side effect of furosemide therapy.

Hypercalciuria is a common cause of hematuria. It can present with abdominal pain and dysuria, even in the absence of kidney stones.

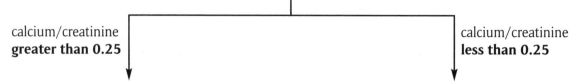

calcium/creatinine
greater than 0.25

calcium/creatinine
less than 0.25

24 hour collection

If the spot urine collection result is greater than 0.25, then a 24 hour total calcium excretion measurement is indicated. A value > **4.0 mg/day** would confirm hypercalciuria. At this point, a **renal ultrasound** should be done to rule out a *renal stone.*

Ureteropelvic junction (UPJ) obstruction

If the screen for hypercalciuria is negative, then an **ultrasound** would be indicated to rule out structural anomalies, especially UPJ obstruction.

UPJ Obstructions

One scenario could be a child presenting with *microscopic hematuria after an MVA or sports injury.* Another scenario could be a one day old with a *palpable flank mass* and confirmation of the *unilateral flank mass on ultrasound.*

UPJ obstruction would first be suspected because of *hydronephrosis* on **CT,** followed by confirmation on **renal scan** which would demonstrate *delayed excretion from the hydronephrotic kidney.*

An additional diagnosis to consider:

> · **Dysplastic Kidney**- CT would show abnormal parenchyma with a similar renal scan result.

VCUG should be done in the opposite kidney because of the increased risk of *vesicoureteral reflux.*

Sickle Cell Disease / Hematuria

In addition, keep in mind sickle cell disease as a cause of hematuria. Therefore, a **sickle cell screen** would be appropriate in any patient at risk. **Even a child with sickle cell <u>trait</u> (Hb AS) can develop hematuria.**

Cystoscopy would never be indicated in a pediatric patient, since bladder carcinoma will be unlikely and not worth the trauma of a cystoscopy.

Gross Hematuria=RBCs in a urine sample that is discolored.

The following can present with gross hematuria, depending on what else is included with the history they present to you:

- **Post strep glomerulonephritis**
- **Membranoproliferative glomerulonephritis**
- **Henoch-Schönlein purpura**
- **Immunoglobulin A (IgA) nephropathy**
- **Hereditary nephritis**
- **Alport syndrome**
- **Benign familial hematuria**

In addition, **sickle cell disease, uteropelvic junction obstruction, stones,** and **trauma** can result in gross hematuria.

 Remember this as follows:

H Henoch Schönlein Purpura and Hereditary nephritis

E Easy benign familial

M Membranoproliferative

A Alport and IgA

T Trauma

U Ureteropelvic junction obstruction

R Renal stones

I Post Infectious (i.e. strep)

A Abnormal blood cells (i.e. sickle cell)

>
> ### Shades of Red
>
> The color of the urine described can be a clue to the correct diagnosis.
>
> **Painless, tea or coke colored urine, without clots is typical of glomerulonephritis.**
>
> Bright red urine with clots is usually due to non-glomerular disease, ie lower urinary tract below the level of the kidneys. Often this is due to a structural anatomical abnormality, including kidney stones, Wilms tumor, or even cystic kidney disease.

Kidney Stones

In addition to hematuria, children with kidney stones will often be described with abdominal/flank pain, urinary frequency, dysuria, and possibly fever.

The initial diagnostic study would be plain x-ray and/or ultrasound. Increased fluid intake is an important component of treatment.

The most common cause of kidney stones in children is hypercalciuria.

Proteinuria

Working up Proteinuria

Orthostatic Proteinuria

This is a *normal variant* where the first morning urine is protein-free, and it becomes positive over the course of the day when the patient is upright and walking about.

In orthostatic proteinuria, proteinuria is higher with standing. It is usually benign, and can be documented by comparing the first AM urine (right after the patient was lying down) with mid-afternoon urine. **This accounts for 50% of benign proteinuria.**

In the absence of any urinary dysfunction and/or any anatomical defects, children with this diagnosis require no intervention other than followup.

Transient Proteinuria

Fever, exercise, and **dehydration** can all cause temporary proteinuria. So if they give you a patient who is doing gymnastics and is febrile, keep this diagnosis in mind.

Proteinuria, in the absence of hematuria or other clinical findings, is most likely benign or simply orthostatic proteinuria.

Orthostatic proteinuria is present during the daytime, but disappears when the patient has been lying down, which typically occurs when they are asleep. Therefore, a negative fresh urine sample upon waking up and a subsequent positive one would confirm this diagnosis.

By the way — Orthostatic proteinuria is a benign condition.

This is best confirmed by a **first void spot urine.**

· If the proteinuria disappears with the night's sleep, then a **serum creatinine** is checked. If the serum creatinine is normal, then a **3 month followup is fine.**

· If the proteinuria is confirmed, then the urine should be checked with a **protein/creatinine ratio, which, if greater than 0.2,** suggests **renal disease**

Proteinuria can be a benign finding in several scenarios, for example:

❑ Concentrated urine (high specific gravity)

❑ Alkaline urine

Picture the protein looking like "cigarette **ASH**":

Alkaline
Specific gravity
High $\Big\}$ = concentrated urine

Remember, proteinuria and a small amount of bacteria can be normal. When both are present, they want you to focus on the protein.

The following are important points in the history to keep in mind, since they will often be the key to the correct diagnosis. Note when they mention edema, history of a UTI, and/or possible exposure to toxins.

Repeating the test and obtaining a **protein/creatinine ratio** distinguishes clinically significant from clinically insignificant proteinuria.

A 24-hour urine collection is generally not used in children. Serial spot checks are the standard.

Hereditary Nephropathy

Alport Syndrome (Familial Nephritis)

Alport is inherited primarily as an x-linked dominant disorder. In addition to hematuria, important parts of the presentation include **bilateral sensorineural hearing loss, ocular defects** and ultimate **renal failure**. It occurs more frequently in **males.**

Males with Alport syndrome are more likely to develop end-stage renal disease than females.

Change the word Alport to Airport and picture a giant plane with the two wings replaced by kidneys landing on an eye. The loud noises cause everyone on the runway to become deaf. Remember, the larger and more illogical the image, the easier it will be to remember the associated features of a given disorder.

Despite this being an x-linked **dominant** disorder, most females are **asymptomatic carriers.** You want an explanation? Okay, but only if you can handle it — read the footnote![1]

---

[1] The variability in disease severity in females is due to the degree of random inactivation of the mutated X chromosome due to lyonization. Now, after you wake up, you can return to the main text!

Renal Dysplasia

Multicystic Dysplastic Kidney Disease (MCDKD or MCDK)

The most commonly palpated masses in infants are due to **hydronephrosis** and **cystic dysplastic kidneys (MCDK)**.

MCDK is an **enlarged kidney** with **non-communicating cysts,** along with **thin parenchyma** (if any) and, of course, dysplasia. The **kidney does not function** and there is no treatment.

A "unilateral flank mass" is a clue to renal dysplasia. The diagnosis (especially if bilateral) can be suspected prenatally with the presence of **oligohydramnios** and **minimal fluid in the bladder**.

It is usually **unilateral,** with other **urinary tract anomalies** occurring around **50%** of the time, including:

- · UPJ obstruction
- · Vesicoureteral reflux
- · Posterior urethral valves
- · Megaureter and duplication

If you are presented with a patient **with** MCDK, the next step is a **VCUG** to rule out these comorbid anomalies. However, if MCDK is suspected, and it hasn't already been done, **renal ultrasound** would be the best initial study to order. Read the question carefully to see if the diagnosis was confirmed with renal ultrasound.

Watch for a child **younger than 10** who presents with a **kidney mass in childhood** and signs of chronic portal hypertension, i.e., **hematemesis, palpable liver, thrombocytopenia** and/or **splenomegaly.**

Autosomal Recessive Polycystic Kidney Disease

PCKD and the Liver

Congenital hepatic fibrosis is seen in children with autosomal recessive polycystic kidney disease and can result in **portal hypertension**.

The typical presentation in infancy is bilateral flank masses at birth, along with a history of oligohydramnios.

Older children with ARPKD will be described as having bilateral kidney masses and signs of chronic portal hypertension, i.e., **hematemesis, palpable liver, thrombocytopenia** and/or **splenomegaly.**

Adult (Autosomal Dominant) Polycystic Kidney Disease

Even though this is primarily an adult disease, it could make its way onto the pediatric boards.

It is important to know the following:

- The workup for adult polycystic kidney disease should include a **renal ultrasound**

- Adult polycystic kidney disease is associated with **intracranial aneurysms**

- They will almost always include the **history of adults in the family** who died of renal disease and/or cerebral aneurysms

Juvenile-Onset Medullary Cystic Disease (Nephronophthisis)

Juvenile-onset medullary cystic disease is an **autosomal recessive disorder** that presents with **polyuria, enuresis, polydipsia, and hyposthenuria.** In addition to the renal manifestations, look for **short stature** and ophthalmological problems (including **retinitis pigmentosa),** and **anemia.** Juvenile-onset medullary cystic disease is also known as **nephronophthisis.**

It is important to remember that retinal disease is frequently associated with juvenile-onset medullary cystic kidney disease, and ophthalmologic follow-up is an important part of the management.

Collecting System Pathology

Ureteroceles

Ureteroceles are the most common cause of urinary retention in females, and can present as a mass protruding from the urethral meatus or a round filling defect on IVP. It can lead to urinary tract obstruction.

Ureterocele presents with symptoms that mimic **UTIs,** such as **dysuria, hematuria,** and/or **abdominal pain.**

Vesicoureteral Reflux

The **earlier** a UTI presents in life, **the more likely** that reflux is a contributing factor. The diagnosis is confirmed with **VCUG.** Management depends on the grade of reflux. **The goal of management is to** *avoid* **hypertension and renal insufficiency and/or ultimate failure**.

Grades 1 and 2	No treatment; periodic cultures
Grade 3	Prophylactic antibiotics with followup VCUG to see if it is resolving
Grade 4	Surgical intervention is often unnecessary
Grade 5	Surgical correction is needed to resolve the problem

Patients with vesicoureteral reflux need to be started on prophylactic antibiotics until the reflux is resolved.

Urethral Strictures

Urethral strictures in boys usually result from urethral trauma. Of course, this can be iatrogenic (as in the placement of catheters). Therefore, watch for a history of a recent surgical procedure that may be unrelated to the urinary tract.

Other causes of urethral strictures are infections, including GC.

 Insertion of a catheter is contraindicated in a patient who is experiencing gross urethral bleeding following trauma.

Posterior Urethral Valves

 Typical presentation in a newborn is a **palpable bladder** and a **weak urinary stream.** Watch for a **prenatal ultrasound** with **bilateral hydronephrosis and reduced renal parenchyma.**

If you are presented with an infant with a palpable bladder with no urine output, the most appropriate next step will be to pass a urine catheter.

> ### Narrow Urethra Go no Furtha
>
> If you are presented with a girl with a narrow urethra discovered as an incidental finding, no further treatment is necessary.

Immediate urological consult for surgical correction is indicated.

· If the other signs are present, a **strong urinary stream does not rule out posterior urethral valves** with flow not completely occluded.

· **Renal failure** can occur even **after surgical correction of posterior valves.** Therefore, long-term followup of bladder function is important.

· **Posterior urethral valves occurs exclusively in males.**

CASE STUDY

You are presented with an infant with posterior urethral valves and vesicoureteral reflux who received appropriate surgical treatment. In addition, they note that the serum electrolytes and urine output are normal. They will then ask you for the long-term prognosis.

THE DIVERSION

The diversions will range from "unlikely to reach end stage renal disease (ESRD)" to "start dialysis immediately." Clearly you should eliminate these two extreme choices. Now the tough part! Do they go on to ESRD in the teen years, adulthood, or within 5 years?

ANSWER REVEALED

In this case, if you chose the most moderate answer, "teen years" you would be wrong. Despite surgical intervention, patients who have posterior urethral valve repair still go on to ESRD within 5 years.

Infections (UTI)

DEFINITION

A UTI would be diagnosed by a culture result of greater than **100,000** colonies from a *reliable sample.*

However, you will need to know that it is possible for patients with symptomatic pyelonephritis to have urine with less than 100,000 organisms/mL.

PERIL / WARNING

Contaminated specimens typically contain **10,000** colonies or less. False negative results can occur with high urine volumes and/or low osmolalities and low pH.

Etiology

Remember, a UTI is not always due to a bacterial infection. It can be caused by **adenovirus**. However, most UTI's *are* caused by bacteria. **E. coli** is the most common organism associated with UTI. Other less common organisms are **klebsiella** and **enterococcus**. Remember that urinary tract infections may be seen more commonly in children with constipation.

Prune Belly (Eagle Barrett) Syndrome

Not many disorders present with a baby with an abdomen looking like a prune. These children are prone to chronic UTIs, dilated ureters, and large bladders.

Posterior urethral valves are the cause of the problems.

BUZZ WORDS

Typical presentation is a newborn with decreased urine output, soft abdominal musculature, bilateral undescended testicles, and a distended bladder.

Picture the bladder as a cave. You "**club**" *(klebsiella)* your way in, and **enter** (enterococcus), and then you hear a loud **echo** *(E. coli)* that repeats itself over and over (to remind you *E. coli* is the most common cause).

Children who have "**chronic**" pyelonephritis are often **asymptomatic**.

So how *DO* you workup a preschool age child after their first UTI? When is a renal U/S indicated? (See the reflux entry previously).

A **renal ultrasound to rule out urinary tract obstruction** is indicated in the following cases:

❑ Symptoms of pyelonephritis
❑ Newborns
❑ Males

> Recurrent UTI with anatomical pathology ruled out requires a trial of prophylactic antibiotics.

A **renal scan** and a **VCUG** are used to initially define the specific pathology. Renal ultrasound is a good way to follow any further changes when abnormalities are detected.

Positive leukocyte esterase is only suggestive of a UTI, but not diagnostic. Even though we often treat empirically, UA alone is not enough to diagnose a UTI; a positive urine culture is needed to make the diagnosis.

Calling in a specialist is rarely the answer on the Boards. Urology consult is indicated with evidence of severe urinary tract obstruction, valves, renal scarring, and difficulty voiding. **Asymptomatic bacteruria** can be something they present on *routine screening* and will require no further intervention.

Who Gets UTIs

The following information can come in handy on the exam:

During the first 3 months of life, boys are at higher risk than girls for UTIs (especially boys who are uncircumcised). After that time, UTIs are more common in girls.

In adolescence, UTIs are more common in sexually active females and homosexual males than in other demographic groups.

Appropriate antibiotics to use to treat acute pyelonephritis prior to culture results include trimethoprim-sulfamethoxazole or a 3rd generation cephalosporin (such as cefixime or cefdinir).

IV options for hospitalized patients being treated for pyelonephritis include cefotaxime, ceftriaxone, or ampicillin/gentamicin.

This is, of course, until sensitivities come back.

Nephrotic Syndrome

Nephrotic syndrome consists of the triad of:

1. Hypoproteinemia
2. Proteinuria
3. Edema

Most cases of nephrotic syndrome are due to **minimal change nephrotic syndrome (MCNS).** It occurs primarily between the ages of **2-8, primarily in males (2:1).** Important findings include **decreased urine output, abdominal pain, diarrhea,** and **weight gain.**

Renal function is normal.

The triad of hypoproteinemia, proteinuria and edema are related, and it flows logically: Low serum protein ➔ exerts oncotic pressure ➔ resulting in edema. Everything else is a consequence of this triad.

A Liver Flows Through It

The *low oncotic pressure* does not make the liver too happy, and it begins to act out in a variety of ways:

VLDL[2] production increases ➔ resulting in a *high* LDL/HDL Ratio.

Fibrinogen, Factor V and VII increases ➔ and combines with decreased volume ➔ and increased platelet count ➔ resulting in **hypercoagulability.**

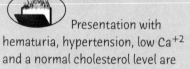

Poor Signs

Presentation with hematuria, hypertension, low Ca^{+2} and a normal cholesterol level are all poor prognostic signs.

Treatment is with prednisone, cyclophosphamide, and cyclosporine.

Kidney Runneth Over

Even though it started all the trouble, the kidney won't be undersold by its rival, the liver, and it too begins to act out.

Since protein is spilling out of the kidneys, **important proteins are lost,** including:

❑ **Immunoglobulins** ➔ Complement levels decrease as well ➔ **Immunodeficiency**

❑ **Albumin** ➔ low albumin decreases bound and available calcium, resulting in ➔ **Hypocalcemia**

❑ **Thyroxine Binding Globulin** ➔ resulting in *functional hypothyroidism*

---

[2] Very low density lipids.

Complications of Nephrotic Syndrome

3 Important complications of nephrotic syndrome are:

- Hyponatremia
- Vascular thrombosis
- Peritonitis

Vascular thrombosis should be suspected in a child with a diagnosis of minimal change disease who then develops **hematuria, decreased urine output,** and **acute abdominal pain.**

Prognosis in nephrotic syndrome is often based on response to treatment. **Most important is the response to steroid treatment.**

Treatment of nephrotic syndrome

The first episode requires hospitalization for education and initial treatment which includes **sodium restriction and prednisone.**

In the absence of severe edema, fluid restriction is unnecessary.

*If treatment with steroids fails, then a **renal biopsy** is indicated (and possibly treatment with **cyclophosphamide** or **cyclosporine**). 1-2 relapses per year are not uncommon and this usually ceases during adolescence.*

Specific Nephropathies/ Nephritides

When I was in medical school (back when dinosaurs and Ronald Regan still roamed the earth), I recall not so fondly poring over renal histopathology slides. Each one looked strangely familiar to the woody grain seen in cheap paneling, and I tried to distinguish them — only to discover they are all treated with steroids.

Here are a few salient points that will get you through this section of the Boards.

Glomerular disease is suggested by the presence of RBC *casts.*

ASO and C_3 levels, blood pressure, Lytes, BUN/Creatinine, and serum albumin are important values to note in the question.

The following words, values, or smoke signals in the question will tip you off as to the cause of hematuria: "positive family history," "recent trauma," "abdominal pain or mass," "recent strep infection," or "sickle cell disease."

Low Complement

Post-Strep GN, Membranoproliferative GN, and Systemic Lupus

MNEMONIC **PMS**: If you were having PMS, you would not be in the mood to "**compliment**" someone, so remember this as:

Post Strep
Membrano-
proliferative   } = Low complement
Systemic
Lupus

Normal Complement

Here, the causes are: Henoch Schönlein Purpura, Idiopathic Vasculitis, and Rapidly Progressive GN.

MNEMONIC This takes a bit of imagination, but it works and will be there on the exam ready for quick recall. Think of the word HIGH as in high complement:

HSP

Idiopathic Vasculitis

Glomerulonephritis (Rapidly Progressive)

H Ig H = IgA nephropathy

MNEMONIC We all remember what the glomerulus looks like all coiled up. Now picture a bad glomerulus where the coil is made up of "**rope,**" which would not work well. The word ROPE will help you remember the symptoms of glomerulonephritis.

Red urine (hematuria)
Oliguria
Proteinuria
Elevated BP and BUN (azotemia)

Kidney Punch: The Causes of Glomerulonephritis

These can be divided into 2 camps:

1) Those with low complement

2) Those with normal serum complement levels

PERIL / WARNING Remember, cystoscopy will rarely be the correct answer in the face of microscopic hematuria.

MCNS, FSGS, MPGN, MSNBC, CNN, ESPN

Once again, the different glomerulonephropathies are difficult enough to spell, let alone keep straight. The good news is there is a limit to what you need to know about each. Knowing the basics will allow you to score easy points on the exam.

Minimal Change Disease (MCNS)

MCNS **is successfully treated with prednisone; however, relapses are common**. The long-term prognosis is good, with most children going into remission by adolescence.

MCNS will typically present with generalized edema and decreased urine output.

Look for proteinuria, hypoalbuminemia, and edema.

 Minimal change is caused by a loss of "foot processes."

Focal and Segmental Glomerulosclerosis (FSGS)

FSGS is typically seen in teenagers. Remember, FSGS usually **leads to progressive renal failure**. You would expect to see low serum albumin and edema. In addition, look for normal C3 levels.

Membranoproliferative Glomerulonephritis (MPGN)

MPGN results in **low C$_3$** (you knew this because it is part of "**PMS**").

 Aggressive treatment is necessary to prevent renal failure.

Post Strep Glomerulonephritis

Post Strep Glomerulonephritis (PSGN) is a nonsuppurative sequelae of an infection with a nephritogenic strain of group A beta hemolytic strep. Both throat and skin infections can lead to PSGN. It is due to the deposition of immune complexes in the kidney. PSGN does not typically lead to renal failure.

They always describe the triad of **hypertension, edema,** and **hematuria**. They may not mention a recent strep infection, just a subtle hint that the patient was "recently ill." The edema will typically be described in the eyelids and/or the face, often noticed by the family rather than the physician.[3]

The hematuria will typically be described as tea- or cola-colored, rusty, or smoky.[4]

In case they get technical, the low serum albumin levels are due to hemodilution rather than proteinuria.

---

[3] Which is pretty scary.

[4] Not unlike the way single malt scotch is described.

A Time to Biopsy

A renal biopsy would be indicated for:

- ❑ Hematuria > 8 weeks
- ❑ Low serum complement levels
- ❑ Hypertension
- ❑ Proteinuria
- ❑ Abnormal renal function

C_3 levels are lowered for up to two months, but then go back to normal. Therefore, documentation of the C_3 returning to normal differentiates it from the two disorders that result in more sustained low C_3 levels. Lupus and membranoproliferative GMN are examples. (Remember, they are part of "PMS" - low complement).

Treatment of PSGN is largely supportive, including fluid restriction.

Hematuria with proteinuria indicates glomerulonephritis.[5]

Berger's Disease (IgA Nephropathy)

IgA Nephropathy is associated with elevated serum IgA and IgA deposits noted on renal biopsy; the same as Henoch Schönlein purpura (complement is normal).

IgA nephropathy will rarely occur in any child younger than 10. The typical presentation is **gross painless hematuria several days after an upper respiratory infection.** While the hematuria is usually painless, **mild abdominal pain can be part of the history.**

You are presented with a patient who you figure out has IgA nephropathy. However, the diagnosis is not what they are after. Instead, they present you with a variety of clinical findings, all consistent with the disease. You are asked to determine which one *correlates with worsening disease.*

Since you already figured out that this is IgA nephropathy, your eyes will zero in on the choice that includes IgA levels. They know this, so this decoy choice will be sitting there for you, drawing you away from "A" passing grade.

The correct answer would be **persistent proteinuria** which correlates with worsening or progressive disease.

---

[5] Or red-hot chili peppers.

Acute Renal Failure

Acute renal failure (ARF) can occur in the context of acute fluid loss, cardiac failure, or a variety of renal diseases.

In patients with prerenal causes of ARF, the urine sodium concentration and fractional excretion of sodium (FeNa) will be low. In those with renal causes of ARF, the FeNa will be high.

Patients with prerenal causes of acute renal failure typically need isotonic fluid replacement to maintain intravascular volume.

Regardless of cause, **hyperkalemia** is also a problem with acute renal failure. This may be treated with calcium gluconate, insulin and glucose, or sodium polystyrene sulfonate.

If **acidosis** is severe enough, sodium bicarb is indicated.

If you are presented with a patient in acute renal failure taking medications, the dosages have to be adjusted accordingly.

Dietary considerations in acute renal failure

· **Dietary changes with acute renal failure** would include giving infants formula that is low in phosphorus.

· Older children may receive formulas that contain high biological value proteins (which contain essential amino acids and come from animal sources of protein).

· More than 70% of calories should come from carbohydrates, and less than 20% from lipids.

Chronic Kidney Disease

They might tell you a child has chronic kidney disease, or they might work backwards by letting you know that a child has some of the common features of kidney disease listed below.

Failure to Thrive and Growth Failure

If they present you with a child with failure to thrive or with growth failure, chronic kidney disease should be in the differential. The cause of this is thought to consist of many factors, including acidosis, nutrition status, and problems with bone mineralization. Growth hormone is often used to treat growth failure.

Anemia

This is due to **decreased erythropoietin production by the kidney**.

Treatment with exogenous erythropoietin is indicated when the **Hgb level drops below 8**. The anemia will be *normocytic.*

However, the downside to erythropoietin therapy is that polycythemia may occur, and it is associated with hypertension and thrombosis.

Metabolic Acidosis

Metabolic acidosis is a result of bicarbonate loss, decreased production of bicarbonate by the renal tubules, and decreased acid excretion. This is a contributing factor to growth failure in chronic kidney disease.

Secondary Hyperparathyroidism

In chronic kidney disease, 1,25-dihydroxyvitamin D3 production decreases. This results in decreased calcium absorption (causing hypocalcemia), resulting in elevated PTH. Calcium levels are already low, and phosphate levels are already high due to kidney disease. The **serum calcium being lowered** can result in tetany. Phosphorus cannot be secreted by the kidneys in CKD, and PTH receptors are downregulated. This is best managed by restricting oral phosphorus intake, using phosphate binders (calcium carbonate), and, if severe, administering IV calcium.

Uremia

Elevated BUN is an important component of renal failure and obstructive uropathy.

Restricted protein intake is a key component of management.

Kidney Punch to the Memory Load

Life was simple when chronic renal failure was simply a patient with a GFR less than 75.

Now they are throwing the kidney punch, making it even more difficult to remember the new subcategories.

Stage 1: Kidney damage with a normal or increased GFR (>90)

Stage 2: Mild reduction in the GFR (60 to 89)

Stage 3: Moderate reduction in the GFR (30 - 59)

Stage 4: Severe reduction in the GFR (15- 29)

Stage 5: Kidney failure (<15 and/or on dialysis)

These values are only valid in children older than 2, since the normal GFR values are different in children younger than 2.

Hypertension

Hypertension in renal failure is due to salt and water retention, and sometimes increased renin levels.

Neurological abnormalities

Changes in mental status, seizures, and peripheral neuropathies can all be manifestations of kidney disease.

Hypocalcemia

Decreased production of calcitriol[6] results in decreased intestinal absorption of calcium, increased parathyroid hormone (PTH) levels, and calcium resorption from the bones.

Increased serum phosphorus levels are also a complicating factor, which further suppresses calcitriol production, resulting in additional calcium losses and increased PTH levels. The result is a snowball effect.

Dermatological abnormalities

Dry skin, pruritus, and easy bruisability can all be a part of kidney disease.

Immunizations in Chronic Kidney Disease

Maintaining the recommended immunization schedule in children with chronic kidney disease is important.

If they are not up to date on immunizations, children may not qualify for a kidney transplant. Live vaccines should be given prior to transplant, since these vaccines would be contraindicated once patients are on immunosuppressive therapy.

Children undergoing dialysis must have their hepatitis B titers checked regularly, since these antibodies may be removed by dialysis.

Hemolytic Uremic Syndrome

Questions on HUS will usually include the classic triad, making it one of the easier questions to answer. The triad is implied in the name:

- Hemolytic anemia
- Renal failure (elevated BUN)
- Thrombocytopenia

Anemia and pallor are the typical initial signs, followed by abdominal pain and decreased urine output. Purpura and ecchymoses will also be typically described. CNS signs can be part of the presentation, so consider HUS when seizures, lethargy, and even coma are part of the scenario they present. Hypertension can also be part of the clinical scenario of HUS.

---

[6] 1, 25 dihydroxycholecalciferol

HUS is typically caused by a strain of *E. coli*[7] transmitted through **bad meat and milk.** This information should be included in the question.

Serum complement levels are normal in HUS, and the Coombs test will be negative.

HyPertension

Hypertension is defined as BP **greater than the 95th percentile for age and sex, taken on 3 separate occasions**.

> **High BP Labs**
>
> The appropriate lab studies for a hypertension workup include **BUN** and **creatinine**.

With hypertension in childhood, particularly essential hypertension, the kidney is always the main suspect. Don't forget post strep glomerulonephritis.

Look for a hint in the question that the **wrong cuff size** has been used. This is often the answer they are looking for.

Pressure Elevators

In addition to pure renal etiologies, there are other causes, and often the clues in the question are obvious.

To remember the causes of hypertension in children, link it to the phrase "**Pound Hard,**" since high blood pressure "pounds hard."

Polycystic Kidney Disease
O (Zero) Enzyme (11 hydroxylase deficiency)
Urinary Reflux Nephropathy
Neonatal Problem (Bronchopulmonary Dysplasia), **N**eurofibromatosis
Deficiency (17 Hydroxylase Deficiency)

Heart = Coarctation of the Aorta, Renal Artery Stenosis
Adrenal = Pheochromocytoma
Reflux Nephropathy (in case you missed it the first time)
Difficult to fit in "Cushingoid" unless you spell it backwards

---

7 If they get that technical and/or you get your jollies off of such minutiae, the name of the strain is E. coli 0157:H7.

Historical Clues/Hypertension

Here, more than anywhere, the clues will be in the wording of the question.

If the question includes the following terms and buzzwords on the left side, then think of the etiology on the right side (see table on following page).

Children who are obese are more than three times more likely to develop hypertension than children who are not. A secondary cause (other than essential hypertension) is more likely in a pre-adolescent child.

Children placed in prolonged traction after orthopedic procedures are at increased risk for acute hypertension.

> **Drugs and Hypertension**
>
> If they describe a child with hypertension taking any of the following medications, these could be the cause.
>
> Medications that may cause HTN include albuterol, contraceptives, corticosteroids, and decongestants.
>
> If they describe a child with HTN and hint that he/she is using illicit drugs, this can also be the cause.

"Family history of hypertension"	**Renal or endocrine problems that run in families**
"Prematurity"	**Renal injury secondary to umbilical catheterization**
"Joint pain, swelling"	**Connective tissue disorder like lupus**
"Flushing," "palpitations," "fever," "weight loss"	**Either a teenager in love or pheochromocytoma**
"Muscle cramps, weakness"	**Hypokalemia secondary to hyperaldosteronism**
"Onset with sexual development"	**One of the enzyme deficiencies**

Physical Evidence/Hypertension

In addition to the history, the physical findings may also include clues pointing to the cause of the hypertension. If the physical findings include the descriptions on the left, then think of the diagnosis on the right:

"Pale color, edema"	Kidney disease (pallor is due to poor erythropoietin production)
"Pale color, increased sweating even at rest, flushing, abdominal mass"	Pheochromocytoma
"Wide spaced nipples, webbing of the neck"	Turner syndrome (coarctation of the aorta)
Elfin facies, high serum calcium, friendly personality	Williams syndrome; supravalvular aortic stenosis
"Decreased femoral pulse or low BP in legs vs. arms"	Coarctation of the aorta

Treatment of Hypertension

The most important non-pharmacological intervention is **weight reduction** if obesity is a problem.

Pharmacological treatment of hypertension may include the following:

- Calcium Channel Blockers: nifedipine or amlodipine
- Vasodilators: hydralazine or minoxidil
- ACE inhibitors: enalapril or lisinopril
- Angiotensin Receptor Blockers: losartan
- Beta Blockers- propranolol or atenolol
- Alpha 2 Agonists – clonidine
- Diuretics – thiazides, furosemide, or spironolactone

Pheochromocytoma

PERIL WARNING Before surgical resection, patients with pheochromocytoma must have their blood pressure under control via **alpha adrenergic blockade,** an example of which is **phenoxybenzamine.**

Even though tachycardia can be a problem, **initial treatment via beta blockers alone is contraindicated since it would lead to unopposed alpha effect and paradoxical increase in blood pressure.**

Cushing Syndrome

If presented with a short obese patient with hypertension, think of Cushing syndrome.

Renal Causes of Hypertension

When a renal cause of hypertension is suspected, the next step is a **renal arteriography with differential central venous renin determination.**

For example, when renal stenosis is the suspected cause, **renin** levels will be higher in the renal vein of the involved kidney. **Renal scars** can also cause hypertension.

Dysuria

Age of Dysuria

Pay close attention to the age of the patient presenting with dysuria:

Age	Possible causes of Dysuria (not comprehensive)
Pre-adolescent female	Pinworms Poor hygiene Trauma Vaginitis
Adolescent female who is not sexually active	Urinary tract infection
Adolescent female who is sexually active	Urinary tract infection Chlamydia or gonococcal infection
Adolescent male	Chlamydia or gonococcal infection

CASE STUDY **You are given the scenario of a teenage girl treated empirically for a urinary tract infection who is still experiencing dysuria. What is the most appropriate next step?**

THE DIVERSION Among the tempting diversions would be a change of antibiotics or addition of other medications.

ANSWER REVEALED In this setting, additional treatment would not be correct. Additional history, physical exam, or lab tests would be appropriate. If you were provided with any of these choices, including pelvic exam, these would be correct.

Urinary Frequency and Incontinence

You may be tested on causes of urinary incontinence other than UTI. This could include:

Ectopic urethral opening in females

BUZZ WORDS This would be presented as a girl who, despite a thorough negative work up, is always wetting her pants.

Unstable Bladder

BUZZ WORDS Children with unstable bladders will experience daytime urinary frequency, but usually a lack of symptoms at night. They could be described as engaging in leg crossing or squatting to compensate for their unstable bladders. This can lead to UTIs due to urine retention. Timed urination is one management strategy, and, if necessary, anticholinergic agents may be used.

Neonatal Renal Numbers

Some Definitions and Facts

Bladder Capacity: A rough estimate of capacity is the child's age plus 2.

Urine Output/Infants: The normal U/O in an infant is 1-2 cc/kg/day.

Premature infants have increased fractional excretion of sodium.

The glomerular filtration rate is significantly slower in the premature neonate compared with the older infant. (Due to an increase in glomerular capillary surface area).

Normal Values in a 2 Week Old

The normal values for a 2 week old infant can be quite different than those in other age ranges. **The following would be considered normal in a 2 week old infant:**

· **Serum Creatinine – 0.2-.04**

· **Serum Potassium -3.0-7.0 (relative hyperkalemia)**

· **Urine Specific Gravity – 1.002-1.030**

· **Urine pH 5-7**

· **Increased fractional excretion of sodium**

· **Serum Phosphate (higher)**

· **Decreased capacity to reabsorb bicarb (relative acidosis)**

Creating Creatinine

Serum creatinine levels correlate with muscle mass. Therefore, serum creatinine levels are higher with increasing pediatric age, since older patients generally have more muscle mass due to growth. After adolescence, males usually have higher creatinine levels than females.

On the other hand, creatinine is typically elevated in the newborn period, which is a reflection of maternal creatinine levels. It has also been shown that premature babies tend to have higher creatinine levels than full term babies.

Nephrotoxic Medications

Nephrotoxic medications include the aminoglycosides, cyclosporine, and tacrolimus, as well as specific chemotherapeutic agents (including cisplatin, carboplatin, and ifosfamide).

Chapter 22

Genital-Urinary

GU Conditions/ Infants

Inguinal Hernia

Inguinal hernias in infants will be described as a bulge through the external inguinal ring that increases in size with crying or straining.

Incarcerated Inguinal Hernia

In addition to the symptoms of a reducible inguinal hernia, an incarcerated inguinal hernia will present with irritability, tender abdomen, and vomiting. The mass will appear tense, and attempts to reduce it will be unsuccessful.

You will be expected to differentiate an incarcerated hernia from other causes of inguinal masses. A hydrocele can mimic an incarcerated hernia, since they both present as masses. The hydrocele will be **painless, will transilluminate,** and does not reach the inguinal ring. Another diagnostic possibility is **inguinal lymphadenitis**. This too will present as a tender mass; however, it will also present with the skin over the mass being **red** and **warm to touch**, and there will also be an infection distal to the node that they will need to include in the history.

Hydrocele

A hydrocele will typically be described in an infant with bilateral painless swelling of the scrotum. It transilluminates on exam.

Varicocele

A varicocele typically presents on the **left side**, and will be described as a **heavy sensation** or a **"bag of worms."** The swelling will decrease when the patient lies down and will be painless.

CASE STUDY

You are called in to the ER to evaluate a 2-year-old girl on peritoneal dialysis for progressive abdominal pain. The child has been afebrile, and her immunizations are up to date. On physical examination, you do not notice anything in the dialysis drainage that is abnormal. In addition to some crusted edges around the catheter site, you note a large mass in the left lower abdomen just lateral to the catheter, but no guarding or rebound tenderness.

What is the most likely cause of the patient's symptoms?

THE DIVERSION

You could be provided with several diversionary choices including bacterial peritonitis, cellulitis, incarcerated omentum, and incarcerated inguinal hernia. Noting that the child is on dialysis is not necessarily a diversionary tactic, although it could be if you automatically assume some of the worse case scenarios implicated in these choices. For example, picking incarcerated omentum will only impede your momentum en route to passing the exam.

ANSWER REVEALED

Clearly an afebrile child with a benign abdominal exam is unlikely to have any of the diagnoses noted. The only correct answer would be "hernia." This should be the logical choice without even knowing that children on peritoneal dialysis frequently develop abdominal hernias because of increased intraperitoneal pressure.

Maternal Estrogen Influence

Gynecomastia

Gynecomastia secondary to maternal estrogen influence is common, typically presenting at 2-3 days of life, up to the 3rd week of life.

Galactorrhea, known as witch's milk, is also not uncommon; if this is presented on the exam, then nothing more than reassurance is indicated.

Neonatal Vaginal Discharge

Pink vaginal discharge in an otherwise healthy newborn is most likely due to the influence of maternal estrogen withdrawal; no intervention is necessary in that case.

Vitamin K deficiency would not be the cause unless they describe other signs such as petechiae.

Vaginal Conditions

Labial Adhesions

Vaginal adhesions are commonly seen during infancy and in pre-school girls. They are similar to the adhesions seen in the foreskin in males, and usually resolve spontaneously if asymptomatic.

Symptoms would include dysuria or secondary bacterial infection - in these cases, treatment with **estrogen cream** would be indicated.

Imperforate Hymen

Imperforate hymen will present in a girl who has reached full sexual maturity in the absence of menarche. Additional findings will include **cyclical abdominal pain, midline abdominal mass, and/or bluish bulging hymen.**

Another condition to consider and differentiate from imperforate hymen is **tubo-ovarian abscess.** Tubo-ovarian abscess can also present with intermittent abdominal pain; however, the abscess is usually not palpable midline.

Hydrometrocolpos is the collection of fluid in the uterus, in this case due to imperforate hymen and retained menstrual fluids.

If they present you with a patient with signs and symptoms consistent with imperforate hymen and/or hydrometrocolpos, and ask for the *most appropriate* step in the patient's evaluation, the correct answer will be *physical examination of the external genitalia.*

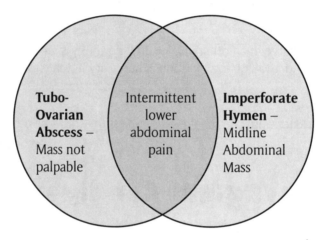

Vulvovaginitis

Vulvovaginitis presents as vaginal irritation, pain, and pruritus. It can also present as *dysuria.*

Non-sexually transmitted causes

Vulvovaginitis can be due to *non sexually transmitted diseases,* including:

· *Enterobius vermicularis* (pinworms)
· Group A beta hemolytic Strep
· *Staph*
· *Candida*

Sexually transmitted causes

 Sexually transmitted causes include:

- · Gonorrhea
- · Chlamydia
- · *Trichomonas Vaginalis*
- · Herpes Simplex

 Most vulvovaginitis that will present on the boards is not due to sexual activity in teens or sexual abuse in children. Usually it will be non-specific due to poor hygiene, chemical irritants such as bubble bath, or tight clothing.

- · Vaginitis can also be due to a **foreign body** (such as toilet paper), which may also include discharge and a **foul odor**.

- · **Candida infection** could be seen in a pre-pubescent girl if there is a history of recent antibiotic use.

- · **Neisseria gonorrhea** will typically include a description of *green discharge*. A *beta hemolytic strep infection* could present similarly.

Bartholin Gland Cysts

Bartholin gland cysts are usually soft masses which are non-erythematous and occur in the absence of vaginal discharge or bleeding.

A Bartholin gland cyst should be differentiated from sebaceous cysts, which are *flesh-colored bumps that arise from the skin.*

Male Conditions

Undescended Testicle

 Management of an undescended testicle

Orchiopexy by the age of 1 year is the appropriate treatment for an undescended testicle.

The following are some important tips and points to remember:

- The longer the testicle remains uptown, the lower the chances of having a baby downtown.
- Bringing the testicle downtown may improve fertility, but it does not lower the risk of malignancy.
- The descended testicle on the other side also has a higher malignancy risk, but not as high as the one stuck uptown.

Neither *human chorionic gonadotropin* nor *testosterone* are considered to be effective treatment, and will therefore be the incorrect choice.

> **CASE STUDY**
>
> **You are evaluating a 3-year-old boy who is new to your practice for a routine physical. You are having difficulty palpating the right testicle. You review his previous record, and bilateral descended testicles have been documented in the past. What is the most appropriate next step?**
>
> **THE DIVERSION**
>
> You could be presented will several diversionary choices consistent with an undescended testicle, such as testicular ultrasound, family history, pelvic ultrasound, and genetic studies.
>
> **ANSWER REVEALED**
>
> Well, all of these steps will be incorrect. If the previously documented bilateral descended testicles wasn't considered authentic, they would have placed it in quotes. Therefore, they are describing retractile testicles secondary to an overactive cremaster muscle. The correct answer would be related to re-examining the patient, usually in the "tailor position," which is the cross-legged position (knees out, ankles crossed). We are not sure why this is the tailor position, but this would be the correct answer.

Hypospadias

If you are presented with a newborn with hypospadias, surgical correction should be done during the first year of life, preferably at 6 months. Circumcision should not be done in a patient with hypospadias.

With a distal hypospadias, the incidence of renal anomalies is low and no intervention is needed. Hypospadias can be associated with some syndromes.

Because someone with hypospadias is likely to urinate all over the floor, he would be a **slob**. That is an easy way to remember the syndromes associated with hypospadias:

> **S**ilver Russell Syndrome (Russell Silver Syndrome)
> **L**aurence-Moon-Biedl Syndrome
> **O**pitz Syndrome
> **B**eckwith Wiedemann Syndrome

Congenital micropenis

If you are presented with boy with the following triad:

> *1. Micropenis*
> *2. Poor feeding*
> *3. Hypotonia*

You are most likely dealing with a boy with **Prader-Willi syndrome.**

In addition to Prader-Willi syndrome, micropenis is also associated with **Kallmann syndrome,** which is also associated with *hypoglycemia, septo-optic dysplasia,* and *anosmia (the absence of the sensation of smell).*

The mean penile length for a full term boy for the first 5 months is 3.9 cm. Therefore, if they present you with an infant whose penis length is greater than 2.5cm whose father projects his own inadequacies by expressing concern over his son's penis length, the answer is to reassure the father (well, at least reassure him that his son's penis length is normal).

With a penis length less than 2.5 cm (one inch), an endocrine and/or genetic workup **would be** indicated.

> ## Beware the Fat Pad
>
> Size may be important, but you have to make sure you are measuring what you believe you should be measuring.
>
> *If they hint at a large suprapubic fat pad, accurate measurement requires gentle stretching of the penis to its full length, measured from pubic symphysis.*

Epididymitis vs. Testicular Torsion

The typical presentation is unilateral pain, dysuria, and/or fever. Pertinent negatives will include no testicular masses or urethral discharge.

In sexually active males it is usually due to Chlamydia or *Neisseria gonorrhea*.

Epididymitis must be distinguished from other conditions with similar presentations. **Orchitis** can be similar in presentation, but they will *not describe dysuria*.

Epididymitis and **E**levation both have **E**'s in them. With torsion it already is high and elevated with no place to go, so the cremaster reflex is not maintained.

You are presented with a 16 year old patient from Panama, who is febrile and presents with a 2 day history of right testicular pain. The testicle is swollen and diffusely tender, with erythema of the overlying skin. There is no urethral discharge or history of dysuria. He is Tanner Stage 4 and he denies any sexual history. Testicular ultrasound is negative, with normal bilateral blood flow. The most appropriate next step would be to order a:

You might be tricked into picking non-specific lab studies such as an ESR, a CBC, or even a blood culture. Chlamydia cultures might be another you could be tricked into picking, since perhaps his denial of sexual activity is unreliable and he could be asymptomatic.

We rarely if ever see mumps anymore given widespread immunization in the United States. However, if you remembered to read the question carefully and noted that they mentioned his coming from abroad, you would have made a note to consider *1) diseases we immunize for here in the US* or *2) an undiagnosed chronic illness.*

In this case, the patient's symptoms are consistent with orchitis, which occurs in mumps 30% of the time. The appropriate next step would be **mumps serology.**

Epididymitis vs. Testicular Torsion

Epididymitis	Testicular Torsion
❑ The cremaster reflex is maintained. ❑ The testicle will be described as low lying. ❑ White cells will be noted in the urine. ❑ You need to treat for GC and Chlamydia with IM Ceftriaxone and PO Doxycycline.	❑ Elevation makes the pain worse. ❑ The cremaster reflex is not maintained. ❑ The testicle will be described as being "high" or retracted.

HOT TIP Testicular torsion can be bilateral. Testicular torsion is best diagnosed by ultrasonography with Doppler flow.

Phimosis

DEFINITION Phimosis is the inability to retract the foreskin. In order for this to be considered clinically significant, they should present this in a boy older than age 4 (since this can be a normal finding up to age 3). Treatment would consist of a topical steroid cream, along with periodic gentle retraction.

Paraphimosis

DEFINITION Paraphimosis is foreskin that, once retracted, cannot be brought to usual position, resulting in constriction. This is a **surgical emergency**.

HOT TIP The accumulation of tissue (smegma) under the prepuce in an uncircumcised child up until age 3 is a normal finding and requires no treatment. At age 3 the foreskin should be fully retractile in most uncircumcised boys.

Balanitis

 Inflammation of the glans penis is usually associated with phimosis.

For purposes of the boards, the foreskin is fully retractable after age 3. Foreskin which does not retract in a boy younger than 3 generally requires no intervention.

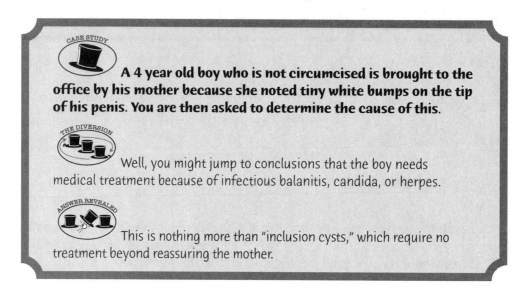

CASE STUDY

A 4 year old boy who is not circumcised is brought to the office by his mother because she noted tiny white bumps on the tip of his penis. You are then asked to determine the cause of this.

THE DIVERSION

Well, you might jump to conclusions that the boy needs medical treatment because of infectious balanitis, candida, or herpes.

ANSWER REVEALED

This is nothing more than "inclusion cysts," which require no treatment beyond reassuring the mother.

Urethritis

Gonococcal urethritis

Discharge that will reveal Gram-negative intracellular diplococci is characteristic of gonococcal urethritis.

Chlamydia urethritis

Chlamydia urethritis can present with a gram negative urethritis.

CASE STUDY

A 3rd year medical student presents a 15 year old boy who has recently had unprotected sex. He is complaining of dysuria and swelling of the foreskin. His urinalysis is positive for 3+WBC, and the Gram stain is negative. In addition, you also note conjunctivitis on physical exam. Additional physical findings would most likely include which of the following?

THE DIVERSION

The negative gram stain noted would point away from gonococcal urethritis. However, with conjunctivitis included in the description you might be tricked into thinking it is chlamydia, and that, therefore, pneumonia is probably the correct answer. After all, this occurs in infants exposed to chlamydia and this must be what they are alluding to.

ANSWER REVEALED

You would need to know that **Reiter syndrome** is felt at times to be due to an **autoimmune response** to chlamydia infections, which is very possible given the history of unprotected sexual activity. Since Reiter syndrome can be remembered as "It hurts where you see (conjunctivitis), where you pee (urethritis), and your knee (arthritis)," the correct answer for additional physical findings would be **arthritis**.

MNEMONIC

Another common mnemonic is:

Can't see, Can't pee, Can't climb a tree

Urethral Instrumentation

HOT TIP

Urethral instrumentation following a surgical procedure is a common cause of non-sexually transmitted urethritis. If a bladder infection is suspected, then a urinalysis and culture should be obtained.

Testicular Cancer

You are expected to be familiar with some important points regarding risk and diagnosis of testicular cancer. This includes:

- Testicular masses should be evaluated using bilateral ultrasound, even when the mass is unilateral
- Lab studies include lactate dehydrogenase, B-HCG, and alpha-fetoprotein.
- It is more common among Caucasians
- High risk factors include cryptorchidism, previous testicular cancer, family history, and Klinefelter syndrome

Dermatological GU Disorders

Condyloma acuminata (Venereal Warts)

Venereal Warts will be described as "flesh colored" verrucous lesions. They are caused by the *human papillomavirus.* The lesions are *non-tender,* but will *bleed with minor trauma.*

It is a risk factor for the development of cervical cancer.

The cause of condyloma acuminata is human papillomavirus. It appears as flat papular lesions, which are often pedunculated in the genital and/or anal mucosa. Transmission in adolescents and young adults is almost always via sexual contact.

There is no specific treatment for condyloma acuminata. However, vaccination would still be recommended if you are presented with a patient who has contracted genital warts. The vaccine would protect against strains other than the one contracted by the patient.

Condyloma acuminata vs. Other

 You will be expected to differentiate condyloma acuminata from similar genital lesions as follows:

Molluscum contagiosum differ in appearance, location, and size. Molluscum is much smaller, is rarely genital, and will be described as *smooth and flesh colored,* with *central umbilication.*

Bartholin cysts are large and tender; and may present as a fluctuant mass on vaginal wall.

Condyloma lata is part of secondary syphilis, and will be described as *whitish-gray papules that have coalesced* in the genital area. They are flatter than condyloma acuminata, and will also present with systemic symptoms, including fever.

The words condyloma *lata* and condyloma *acuminata* can look alike at first glance, and this is something that will definitely be taken advantage of on the exam. Even though they are clinically dissimilar, they will both appear among the choices in any given question since they both have condyloma as their first names.

Congenital condyloma acuminata

One mode of transmission of anogenital warts is through a contaminated birth canal.

While anogenital warts can be transmitted through the anogenital canal, this will usually manifest by age one. Some would argue that it can be attributed to perinatal transmission up to age 3. Therefore, if they present a child with new onset of condyloma genital warts *after age 3, it is due to child abuse.*

> **Vulvitis**
>
> You could be presented with a child with benign vulvitis, which presents simply with mild perianal and vaginal pruritus and dysuria. If they note the absence of sexual abuse, trauma, or signs of pinworms, then sitz baths and reassurance are all that is needed.

Herpes Simplex

The **primary lesion** (initial infection) will be painful, and usually they will describe tender inguinal nodes.

Genital herpes will be described as ulcerative lesions.

Treatment of primary HSV infection is acyclovir 400 mg TID for 7-10 days. Other correct treatment choices would include famciclovir and valacyclovir.

You are presented with a patient with a history of unprotected sexual intercourse several weeks ago who now has several vesicular lesions on the penis. What would be the best diagnostic test to do initially?

You very astutely recognize that this is a herpes lesion. One of the choices you are given is a Tzanck test, which you know is associated with diagnosing herpes, so you lock into this answer. If you do this, you have locked into the wrong answer, and you and the patient described in the vignette both should be more careful and less impulsive.

The correct answer is **viral culture for herpes simplex**. The *Tzanck test* does detect multinucleated giant cells, but its sensitivity is less than 50%. In addition, it does not differentiate herpes from varicella. Therefore, when it comes to herpes viruses, "Tzanck you but I don't know **HSV** from the next "**ella**."

Pediculosis Pubis

Pediculosis pubis, or as it is known in less lofty circles — "crabs" — will have a classic presentation described below.

Patients with pediculosis pubis will present with red, crusted suprapubic macules. They could also be described as "blue-gray dots," which are *maculae cerulea*.

Some important points regarding pediculosis pubis that you might be tested on include that they are slow moving and sluggish, which is why they spread primarily by close contact, especially sexual contact. They can last 1-2 days without a meal, which for them is blood. In addition to the pubic area, they can infest anal hairs as well as facial hair, including eyelashes.

Finding of pubic lice in any child should raise the suspicion of sexual abuse.

 If you are asked for the correct treatment for pediculosis pubis, the correct choices would include *permethrin 1% or 5%, pyrethrin with piperonyl butoxide*, and *malathion*. For the eyelashes, application of petroleum jelly several times a day for 10 days is sufficient.

Lindane is considered a 2nd line treatment, but *not in neonates or pregnant women.*

Abdominal Pain

CDC on PID

The CDC criteria for diagnosing PID is:

- Adnexal tenderness
- Cervical motion tenderness
- Lower abdominal pain

Additional criteria include:

- WBC in vaginal secretions
- Temp > 101F
- Elevated ESR or C-reactive protein
- Gram negative diplococci from endocervix
- Lab evidence of GC or chlamydia at cervix
- Abnormal cervical or vaginal mucopurulent discharge

CASE STUDY

You are presented with a female teenager with right upper quadrant pain along with nausea and vomiting. They will note that oral contraceptive pills are the only medications she is taking. You will be asked for the best initial step in making the correct diagnosis.

THE DIVERSION

Since you will be focusing on the right upper quadrant pain, you may ignore the fact that she is on oral contraceptives — you have been diverted away from thinking it is important, because they noted them as the "only" pills she is taking. Therefore, you will be tempted by all the diversionary choices, including serum amylase, lipase, abdominal ultrasound, plain abdominal film, and maybe even serum LFT levels.

ANSWER REVEALED

By falling for all the diversions, you probably would have dismissed the correct answer, which would be cervical cultures. Whenever they mention the "only medication" a patient is taking, you should read it as a "very important" medication that reveals a part of the history. Putting this together, you have a sexually active female with right upper quadrant pain, which would be consistent with Fitz Hugh Curtis, which is perihepatitis - a manifestation of gonococcal and chlamydial infections.

Ovarian Cyst

BUZZ WORDS

A typical presentation of an ovarian cyst would be a teenager with unilateral abdominal "discomfort," typically mid-cycle. They will probably throw in a positive ultrasound showing a fluid-filled cyst on the ovary.

The question will focus on management. Here, size is important.

- Cysts smaller than 6.0 cm will only require a followup ultrasound
- Cysts greater than 6.0 cm or those causing significant symptoms beyond discomfort would require laparoscopic cyst aspiration.

Ovarian Torsion

Ovarian torsion will present as **sudden lower abdominal pain which radiates to the back, side, or groin/leg on the same side,** with nausea and vomiting.

Diagnosis is confirmed with Doppler ultrasound, but this should not delay surgical consultation if ultrasound access is not immediately available.

Chapter 23

The Neuro Bureau: Neurology

With Neurology, you have to pay close attention to the details in the wording of the question. Many of the disorders are quite similar, with only fine differences that distinguish them. We will call attention to these fine differences, and by committing them to memory, you will be on the road to getting these potentially tricky questions correct each time.

Encephalitis

You will be expected to diagnose and understand the underlying causes for a child presenting with symptoms consistent with encephalitis. The time of year and other epidemiologic information in the history will be critical. The following are important considerations to keep in mind on the exam:

- **Arboviruses** - Typically occur in warm climates and are carried by insects, especially mosquitos. This would include St. Louis and West Nile Viruses.

- **Enteroviruses** - Present with generalized neurological findings, and are transmitted from human to human. Watch for non-specific findings preceding confusion and irritability.

- **Herpes encephalitis** - Often presents with non-specific findings, without a history of oral lesions. It is best diagnosed by DNA PCR.

- **Mumps encephalitis** – Present with or after parotitis. Watch for a child or teenager who is from another country, or other hints that the patient wasn't immunized. Late winter and early spring is when this will present.

CASE STUDY

You may be presented with a febrile toddler with a focal or generalized seizure. The toddler is lethargic one hour after the seizure. Additional information might include a CBC that is unremarkable, and results of a lumbar puncture may show a negative gram stain and a moderate amount of WBCs, consistent with viral meningitis. You will be presented with several treatment choices.

THE DIVERSION

This clinical vignette could be consistent with a typical febrile seizure. However, the fact that the child is lethargic one hour later suggests otherwise, as does the WBCs in the CSF. Therefore, reassurance would be the incorrect choice. Anticonvulsants such as phenobarbital would be incorrect, since the seizure is not ongoing.

ANSWER REVEALED

The correct answer would be acyclovir to cover for the possibility of HSV encephalitis. If they were to present IV antibiotics as one of the choices, this too could be correct, since you would want to cover for bacterial meningitis as well as HSV encephalitis. The key point is that HSV encephalitis can present with non-specific findings. Don't look for a history of HSV lesions either; that will never be part of the presentation of HSV CNS infections on the boards.

What a Headache

You will need to know how to distinguish different types of headaches and their etiologies — which shouldn't be hard, considering that you will have much real life experience with headaches while studying for the Boards. Just remember to keep in mind that answers can often be found in the questions.

Stress/Tension/Emotion

Stress headaches should be one of the easier ones to distinguish, because they will be describing what you are experiencing at the moment...

It is typically described in a teenager as a *frontal* headache or *band-like pressure* sensation.

Treatment consists of eliminating the stressor (in your case passing the Boards and getting on with your life).

If they describe *a headache in the absence of a history of trauma or signs of potential brain tumor or increased ICP... complicated studies are usually not indicated.*

Headaches **can be** caused by depression. Therefore, look for other signs of depression such as malaise, excessive sleeping, and/or declining school performance.

Migraine Headache

Migraine headaches are episodic, with no symptoms in between episodes. It will be described as frontal or temporal, lasting up to 48 hours. Nausea and vomiting will likely be described as well.

Hard neurological signs, including hemiparesis, eye movements, and/or temporary visual deficits may be clues telling you they are describing a migraine headache.

They will not likely describe an aura in the description of a migraine headache on the boards.

An important point to remember is that patients experience *photophobia.*

 Treatment most commonly consists of *ibuprofen, acetaminophen, fluids*, and *rest*. Other treatments include *ergotamines* and *sumatriptan (Imitrex®)*.

If *subcutaneous* sumatriptan is one of the choices for treating migraines in children, it will most likely be incorrect.

Depression can trigger migraine headaches. However, headaches due to depression will be described as chronic daily headaches, without the other signs associated with migraines.

While placebo alone can eliminate pain, this, in and of itself, does not rule out migraine headaches.

CASE STUDY

You are presented with a patient who has had a headache for several months. They note that the patient suffered a minor head injury with no loss of consciousness. He now presents with daily headaches that are not relieved despite frequent acetaminophen, ibuprofen, or naproxen. The headaches are frontotemporal. What is the most appropriate next step in managing this patient?

THE DIVERSION

If you are not careful, you will go down the path leading to a headache caused by picking the wrong answer. The answers will include "obtain a head CT." By noting that there was no loss of consciousness and that the patient "now" presents with headaches, they are implying that the patient was asymptomatic until this point. Therefore, a head CT would not be appropriate.

They might provide additional medications among the choices. However, the vignette is not consistent with a migraine headache.

ANSWER REVEALED

The key to the diagnosis: the medication is being used chronically and its effect is blunted. Rescue medications such as ibuprofen should not be used chronically. The correct step in this case would be to stop all medications.

Headaches Associated with Increased Intracranial Pressure

Progressive and intermittent visual disturbances are tip-offs to increased ICP and a space-occupying lesion. Of course, "**papilledema**" on physical exam is another confirmatory sign. Blurred vision occurring **only** before the headache is more typical of a migraine.

You need to order a CT when increased ICP is suspected.

BUZZ WORDS

Remember: red flags for headaches due to a space-occupying lesion are "headaches worse in the morning" or "headaches relieved by vomiting."

PERIL WARNING

Nausea and vomiting are non-specific findings. Negative Babinski sign is also bogus. They will throw these in to trick you.

California, Oregon, and Other Altered States of Consciousness

If you are presented with a patient with an "altered state of consciousness," pay particular attention to the **age** of the child, since this will help determine the etiology and should make these questions some of the easiest ones on the exam (leading to a euphoric state of consciousness in yourself). If the onset is abrupt, the cause is more likely to be trauma or a cerebrovascular accident. If they describe the onset as having occurred over several hours, along with specific physiological signs, then a toxic ingestion is more likely.

Older Kids

In older children, an important diagnosis will be **encephalopathy,** with a preceding history of *hepatic, renal, pulmonary,* or *cardiac pathology.*

HOT TIP

Another possibility is **toxic** ingestion. The hints in the history will often be subtle, such as a **family member with a condition that requires medication** (i.e., depression, seizures, or heart disease). It is also important to consider the possibility of head trauma causing the altered state of consciousness. Even if the question specifically states "no *history* of head trauma," you would be correct in choosing head CT as an initial study. This is because the head trauma might have been unwitnessed. What the question is really stating is, "no *known* history of head trauma."

CASE STUDY You could be presented with a child presenting in the ER with hypoglycemia that is resistant to glucose replacement.

THE DIVERSION You could be provided with options for all sorts of workups to find the reason for the hypoglycemia. This is the diversion.

ANSWER REVEALED The correct answer will be to ask the parents if anyone is taking any medication. They might even drop a hint that there is no significant family history, except for an aunt with diabetes who is visiting for the weekend. Ingestion of oral hypoglycemics could be the answer they are looking for.

Neonates

Neo Poetry Night

If they describe a non-responsive neonate, don't automatically jump on the Sepsis ship. They may want you to measure a serum ammonia and organic acid levels.

MNEMONIC Remember this with the following poem: "Neo Coma Order Organic Ammonia." (Read that at poetry open mike and check out the response).

Wilson's Disease

DEFINITION Wilson's disease is an autosomal recessive disease of copper metabolism. Because the *liver cannot get rid of copper*, it accumulates in the liver, kidneys, brain, and eyes (corneas).

BUZZ WORDS

· **Younger patients** mostly present with **symptoms of liver disease**.

· **Older patients** have more **neuro/psych symptoms**.

Common neurologic manifestations are **tremors, emotional problems, difficulty with handwriting, depression, and abnormal eye movements.**

When they describe evidence of **acute hepatic failure** coupled with **dystonia** and **mental status changes,** think of Wilson's disease.

By the time neurologic or psychiatric symptoms are present, there will almost always be ***Kaiser-Fleischer rings*** in the eyes (greenish-yellow rings seen at the edge of the cornea – seen best on slit-lamp exam and in close-up shots on the board exam).

Since **ceruloplasmin** is the "carrier vehicle," all vehicles are "taken," and are busy depositing copper into tissue. Therefore, **ceruloplasmin levels are low. Serum copper levels are low because most of the copper in the body is deposited into tissue.** There should be **increased copper in the urine**.

Patients with Wilson's disease may have **hemolytic anemia** and disorders of **calcium metabolism** as well.

Wilson's disease is **treated** with **chelation**, usually with **penicillamine**, along with a low copper diet. Wilson's disease is fatal if untreated. Occasionally, acute hepatic insufficiency will necessitate a liver transplant.

Think of yourself as "**rec**eiving" a copper penny, and you will remember that this is a **rec**essive disorder. If you remember the copper ***penny,*** it will be easy to remember that **penicillamine** is the treatment.

Ataxia Attackia

You need to distinguish different forms of **ataxia** from each other. A systematic approach that looks at the clues in the question will help you avoid getting "*tripped up.*"

Acute Ataxia

With an **acute** onset, your first thought should be a **post-viral** etiology. They may even mention a recent viral illness such as

---

Vein of Galen Malformation

If they include a cranial bruit in the description of a neonate, along with hydrocephalus and a history of congestive heart failure, the answer is likely Vein of Galen malformation.

Tin walk

To remember the possible causes of ataxia, remember the stilted walk of The **TIN** Man in *The Wizard of Oz.*

Toxic ingestion
(e.g., ethanol, pesticides)

Infection
(including Guillain Barré)

Neoplasm
(e.g., glioma, medulloblastoma)

Additional causes would include a cerebral hemorrhage and a variety of metabolic disorders.

chickenpox[1], Epstein-Barr, or mumps. The prognosis of acute cerebellar ataxia after infections or vaccinations is generally excellent. Additional causes of acute ataxia would include toxic ingestion, neoplasm, trauma, metabolic problems, and/or other infections.

Ataxia Telangiectasia

Ataxia Telangiectasia (AT) is an autosomal recessive disorder due to a defect in DNA processing and repair. The disease has CNS effects, skin and eye findings, and immunologic sequelae.

Ataxia Telangiectasia can be associated with hematologic malignancies. Think about this when presented with **abnormal hematologic** values, **ataxic gait**, and **oculocutaneous lesions**.

There is a high incidence of malignancy in AT, especially *Hodgkin lymphoma* and *leukemia*.

Telangiectasias are capillary dilatations, causing red blotches on the skin and conjunctiva.

When they are learning to walk, kids often display signs of cerebellar ataxia (*clumsiness, unsteady gait*). Over the next few years, they get *telangiectasias* of the conjunctiva as well as cheeks, ears, and other areas. Children with AT may have intellectual disability.

The immunologic effects of this disease lead to both decreased levels of immunoglobulin and T-cell dysfunction, manifesting as *frequent upper and lower respiratory tract infections*.

Once the ocular telangiectasia becomes advanced, it can simulate conjunctivitis. Patients are unable to voluntarily make rapid eye movements.

This should be a piece of cake because the question will likely include a description of the *pigmentation in the eye*. Otherwise, they may give information on the decreased *immunoglobulin levels* coupled with a description of ataxia.

Despite these eye findings, both acuity and pupillary reflexes are often normal.

---

[1] Always referred to by its formal title, varicella, or sometimes as nom de-Guerre chicken pops. While this is seen more and more rarely out there in the real world, it is another example of something that is still seen on the boards (much the way old Hollywood has-beens are seen in Las Vegas).

Friedreich Ataxia

 Friedreich ataxia is an autosomal recessive disorder accounting for about half of all cases of *inherited* ataxia.

 It typically presents in late childhood or early adolescence. Children tend to present initially with a *slow and clumsy gait*. This ataxia is due to both a cerebellar component, as well as a *loss of proprioception*. Watch for signs of spinal cord and peripheral nerve problems. This could be described as decreased strength in the feet, as well as decreased reflexes in the lower extremities.

The only good treatment for Friedreich ataxia is supportive.

Clinical features that distinguish Friedreich ataxia from other forms of ataxia are:

- **Elevated planter arch**
- **Absence of lower extremity deep tendon reflexes**
- **Diabetes**
- **Cardiomyopathy leading to CHF**

Friedreich ataxia presents later than ataxia telangiectasia.

Remember "*Fried Arch*" (= Friedreich) ataxia and picture the elevated arch. If you ate "fried" arches or any fried food for that matter, you would have "cardiac" problems too.

Strange Movements (in D Minor)

Chorea

The two main types of chorea to know for boards are **Sydenham chorea** and **Huntington chorea**.

Sydenham Chorea

CASE STUDY

You are presented with a child who is *fidgety* in class and has poor tone and "quick *random jerky movements*." She has difficulty paying attention because she easily becomes emotional. What is your next step?

THE DIVERSION

Here you are being led to believe that this is a child with ADHD, and you can easily be tricked into picking stimulant medication as the next move.

ANSWER REVEALED

However, the description is more consistent with a child with Sydenham chorea, rather than ADHD. Therefore, the correct next step would be obtaining *antistreptolysin-O levels*.

HOT TIP

If they note that the antistreptococcal antibody titers are normal, it does not rule out Sydenham chorea.

PERIL WARNING

If they note that the antistreptococcal antibody titers have returned to normal, it does not rule out Sydenham chorea.

Treating Chorea

You could be questioned on the appropriate treatment of chorea.

Dopamine-blocking agents in the antipsychotic category are used as treatment. Specifically, haloperidol is effective.

Sydenham chorea is essentially self limited. However, low dose haloperidol would be correct if listed among the choices.

Other medications that could be considered correct choices include fluphenazine, risperidone, or tetrabenazine.

Huntington Chorea

DEFINITION

Huntington chorea (Huntington disease) is an autosomal dominant disorder that involves chorea and dementia. This presents with the **triad** below, and is inherited in an *autosomal dominant* pattern.[2]

1) Chorea

2) Hypotonia

3) Emotional lability

---

[2] By the way, this is what Woody Guthrie died of. (He wrote *This Land is Your Land.*)

Most of the time, symptoms are not apparent until adulthood (after age 35), but about 10% will have juvenile Huntington chorea (which is more likely to present with rigidity), and this is important to keep in mind for the exam.

CASE STUDY

You are presented with a 2 year old who has a fixed upward gaze. Throughout the exam, he remains alert and appropriately frightened. His parents and the paramedics who brought him confirm that he has remained alert. His airway is patent and his vital signs are stable. A toxic ingestion is a possibility. You are asked to pick a pharmacological treatment until ingestion can be confirmed. Which would you use?

THE DIVERSION

You could be provided with choices such as rectal diazepam, which will lead you to believe this is a seizure, even though the wording of the question serves as a neon beacon that says "NO SEIZURE." NG tube, activated charcoal, and even syrup of ipecac can be among the choices, since ingestion is a possibility.

ANSWER REVEALED

If they tell you or strongly hint that there was no seizure, then treatment of a seizure is not the answer. If they specifically state that ingestion is suspected, then a simple answer like charcoal or NG tube placement will probably be incorrect, since everyone taking or even proctoring the exam will get it right. No, they want you to identify the specific toxin ingested and treat it specifically. That is what it takes to grab the brass ring of board certification. In this case, the upward gaze is a dystonic reaction, which is probably due to ingestion of promethazine or a related drug. Therefore, treatment with *diphenhydramine* would be most appropriate.

Tips on Tics

CASE STUDY You are presented with a 10 year old diagnosed with ADHD who has been on methylphenidate for the past 3 years. He briefly experienced eye blinking, which has since resolved with no intervention. Other than the diagnosis of ADHD, which has responded to medical and behavioral interventions, he has done well and has no other issues or medical problems. You will be asked for the most likely explanation for the eye blinking, and for appropriate intervention.

THE DIVERSION The combination of the eye blinking and a child with ADHD on methylphenidate (or other stimulant medication) may trigger you to consider a diagnosis of a tic disorder such as Tourette syndrome. This is exactly the diversion they want to lead you to.

ANSWER REVEALED However, in this patient the tic was limited and resolved spontaneously, despite the continuation of methylphenidate. Therefore, the correct explanation would be a *simple motor tic* and *no additional intervention*.

Simple Motor Tics

Simple motor tics typically present as *eye blinking* and *movements of the head, face, and/or shoulders.*

Although tics can be seen with anxiety disorders, they are *not caused by anxiety.*

Choreiform movements are *repetitive, jerking movements.* Although they may describe voluntary movements designed to stop the jerking movements, **choreiform movements cannot be suppressed.**

Tourette syndrome is part of a continuum of tic disorders that are **present for at least 1 year**. In the vignettes presented in the box above, the tics were short-lived, and therefore not consistent with a comorbid diagnosis of Tourette syndrome.

There is co occurence between Tourette syndrome and ADHD, however. Tourette syndrome also occurs frequently in children with *obsessive-compulsive disorder.*

In the past, the presentation of *tics* and *throat clearing* meant that stimulant medication for ADHD had to be discontinued. This is no longer the case. However, parents need to be made aware of the fact that stimulants may unmask an underlying tic disorder.

Meds that Move

You should be familiar with various medications that can cause movement disorders.

Ataxia can be caused by anticonvulsants, alcohol, and thallium.

That's easy to remember: ataxia, anticonvulsants, and alcohol all begin with the letter A.

You will just have to remember that thallium is also associated with ataxia.

Tremors can be caused by amphetamines, valproic acid, phenothiazines, and tricyclic antidepressants.

In addition, methylxanthines such as caffeine and theophylline may cause tremor.

Stimulant medications do not cause tics. However, they may unmask an underlying tic disorder in predisposed patients who are placed on stimulants.

Space Occupying CNS Lesions and Other Anatomical Problems

Posterior Fossa (Infratentorial) Tumors

BUZZ WORDS

   You will be expected to recognize the clinical presentation of a child with a posterior fossa tumor. Most likely you will need to know that when you are dealing with a suspected posterior fossa tumor, a CT or MRI is indicated.

Look for "ataxia, gait imbalance, incoordination, neck pain, and increased intracranial pressure" in the history. A posterior fossa lesion should be considered in any *afebrile* child with *ataxia* and a *headache*.

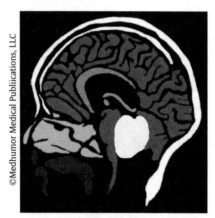

Contrast MRI scan showing midline, posterior-fossa medulloblastoma
- Contrast-enhancing 4th ventricle mass
- Hydrocephalus

Supratentorial Tumors

Craniopharyngioma

 Craniopharyngioma is a *common supratentorial brain tumor in kids.*

 Craniopharyngioma is usually present with pituitary and hypothalamic problems. Pressure on the optic tracts can lead to *visual deficits.* Look for a *chronic progressive visual field deficit*, along with a headache.

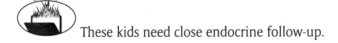 However, neck pain without fever should point you away from an infectious process necessitating an LP.

Surgery and possibly **radiation** are the treatments, and most patients do well.

These kids need close endocrine follow-up.

They could also describe growth delay and show or describe a skull film with *calcification in the sella turcica.* These classic descriptions should make it an easy question.

Optic nerve gliomas can lead to decreased vision (imagine that). They are mentioned here to remind you that they are associated 25% of the time with neurofibromatosis.

Increased Intracranial Pressure

The clinical signs for increased intracranial pressure in **infants** include: irritability, decreased PO intake, and failure to thrive, as well as macrocephaly with wide sutures and a bulging fontanel. Additional findings would include the "setting sun" sign: downward deviation of the eyes with hydrocephalus.

Signs of increased intracranial pressure in children include: hypertension, bradycardia, and abducens paresis.

If you are presented with these findings, then brain imaging studies are indicated.

If increased intracranial pressure is suspected, a head CT must be done before the LP is done.

Additional contraindications to performing an LP include focal neurological signs, history of a coagulopathy, and cardio-respiratory instability.

Remember that your ABC's come before an LP

Pseudotumor Cerebri

Pseudotumor cerebri is *increased intracranial pressure of unknown etiology*. It leads to *papilledema* and eventual *optic disc atrophy* and blindness if not treated. This is an important consideration and often shows up on the exam.

Pseudotumor cerebri will typically present with **double vision**, **papilledema**, and evidence of increased intracranial pressure (**headache**, **tinnitus**). There should be something in the question to suggest this. *Megadose vitamin intake*, particularly *vitamin A*, is a favorite cause.

Other **medications** *that may cause pseudotumor cerebri* include:

· Steroids
· Thyroxine
· Lithium
· Some antibiotics

Patients may be **treated** with **carbonic anhydrase inhibitors (acetazolamide).** Severe cases require steroids and possibly surgery to shunt CSF.

Yes, steroids can cause and be the treatment of pseudotumor cerebri, just like alcohol can be the cause of, and solution to, all of life's problems, in some cases.

Muscle Weakness and Hypotonia

The following table helps organize your approach when presented with a question involving a child with muscle weakness:

Type of Disorder	Presentation	Examples
Muscular Disorders (Acute Weakness)	Proximal weakness affecting hips and shoulders	· Polymyositis · Dermatomyositis · Electrolyte imbalance
Muscular Disorders (Chronic weakness)	Proximal Weakness	· Muscular Dystrophy · Mitochondrial myopathies · Congenital myopathies
Neuromuscular Junction	**Progressive onset**	· Myasthenia gravis
	Rapid onset, descending	Botulism
Acute Peripheral Nerve Processes	Loss of deep tendon reflexes	· Guillain Barré · Polio · Diphtheria · Tick paralysis · Lead Poisoning
Chronic Peripheral Nerve Processes	Loss of deep tendon reflexes	· Chronic demyelinating polyneuropathy · Hereditary neuropathies · Leukodystrophy
Spinal cord weakness	· Loss of motor and sensation function · Loss of bladder and bowel function · **Increased reflexes**	· Transverse myelitis · Anterior spinal artery infarction · Spinal Cord Compression (tumors) · Epidural abscess · Tethered cord · Trauma

HOT TIP

CNS causes of hypotonia may include hypotonic cerebral palsy, genetic disorders (e.g., Prader Willi, Angelman, and Down syndromes), or metabolic problems (e.g., leukodystrophies, peroxisomal disorders).

Peripheral Nerve and Muscle Disease

Guillain Barré Syndrome

With Guillain Barré Syndrome, there is *progressive motor weakness, as well as areflexia.*

Patients often present with *leg weakness and/or an unsteady gait,* as well as pain. The muscle weakness *starts in the lower extremities* and *progresses upward in a symmetric fashion* ("ascending paralysis"). It is often preceded by a **viral illness,** or perhaps another illness such as *Campylobacter jejuni,* which may be subtly noted in the question.

On physical exam, in addition to the leg weakness and unsteady gait, there will often be *cranial nerve findings* and dysautonomia (tachycardia, orthostatic hypotension, and/or dizziness).

Areflexia is always seen in GBS. If reflexes are present in the lower extremity, it is not GBS they are describing.

On lumbar puncture, one can also see **increased protein in the CSF,** along with a normal cell count. Remember that proximal muscle weakness is a classic sign.

They will rarely come right out and say "proximal muscle weakness." Instead, they will simply describe it. They might note a child who has *difficulty rising from a sitting position* or *cannot shrug his/her shoulders.* Sometimes they will present a child who becomes clumsy or starts falling.

The **biggest risk is respiratory failure** secondary to ascending **paralysis.** Therefore, they expect you to know that *lung function must be followed closely.*

Tick Bites and Paralysis

This is caused by a neurotoxin secreted by the tick. It is seen during the summer months. It can present exactly like GBS with ascending paralysis. This is opposite of the descending paralysis seen with botulism.

You need to measure pulmonary function tests; **oxygen saturations are inadequate** and will be the incorrect answer since they only decline once the patient is severely compromised. Correct parameters or studies to follow would include "vital capacity" or "negative inspiratory force" or "PFT" – never "oxygen saturation" (unless it is the only choice relating to pulmonary function).

GBS is treated with supportive measures (including intubation if needed) and also with **plasmapheresis** and **IVIG**. Most patients who survive have a full recovery, but there is permanent disability in about 10% of cases.

Steroids have no proven benefit in the treatment of Guillain Barré syndrome.

Neuromuscular Junction disease

Myasthenia Gravis

Myasthenia gravis is an autoimmune disorder in which the patient develops antibodies against the acetylcholine receptor in the neuromuscular junction. The cause of myasthenia gravis is unknown. In most cases, though, *penicillamine* is known to cause it. Other drugs, as well as illnesses, can exacerbate symptoms.

The weakness of myasthenia gets worse with activity and improves with rest. Patients will report feeling *good in the morning* but *tiring as the day goes on.*[3] **Ptosis** is a very common finding in myasthenia gravis. Many patients present when someone else notices their droopy eyes – look for this in the question.

Myasthenia gravis is associated with *thymoma.* A diagnosis of myasthenia gravis should prompt a search for a thymoma.

Tensilon it in

When suspected, myasthenia gravis can be confirmed by the "Tensilon test" which uses edrophonium, a short acting **acetylcholinesterase inhibitor**. In kids with myasthenia gravis, the symptoms will be temporarily alleviated with a small dose of Tensilon.

Tensilon (edrophonium) is NOT a treatment for myasthenia gravis – it is very short acting and is only used for testing.

The Tonic for Dystonic Reactions

If you are presented with a patient who presents with an acute dystonic reaction characterized by neck hyperextension and decreased extraocular movements, watch for certain medications, especially neuroleptics, which may have caused this reaction and can be reversed with diphenhydramine.

Metoclopramide, though not always thought of as a neuroleptic, in fact is one.

---

[3] Of course, this describes everyone with a job, family, kids, or anyone who is alive.

Testing for anti-acetylcholine receptor antibody further supports the diagnosis. **Anti-Smith antibodies** are also often present. *Electromyelogram (EMG)* is also used to support the diagnosis.

The mainstay of chronic therapy is **pyridostigmine (Mestinon®)**, which inhibits acetylcholinesterase, thus increasing the amount of acetylcholine available in the neuromuscular junction. *Plasmapheresis* and *plasma exchange* are also used. *Prednisone* and other immunomodulating agents are less commonly used. *Thymectomy* is often done, especially in kids, and can be curative.

Myasthenia Gravis in Infancy

There are two types of myasthenia gravis in infancy, and you will be expected to be able to distinguish them.

Congenital myasthenia gravis

Congenital myasthenia gravis is due to a genetic defect of the neuromuscular junction and, therefore, is a *lifelong disease*.

Transient myasthenia gravis

Transient myasthenia gravis is due to mother's antibodies that crossed the placenta. It will *resolve within 6 weeks*. **Most babies born to mothers who have myasthenia gravis do not get transient myasthenia gravis.**

Remember that both congenital myasthenia gravis and transient myasthenia gravis occur in newborns. **Transient myasthenia gravis does not involve the eyes; congenital does.** Both will respond to the Tensilon test.

To help you remember that *congenital* myasthenia gravis involves the eye and *transient* does not: **C**ongenital and **C**onjunctiva both start with a **C**.

Infantile Botulism

You may be presented with a case of infantile botulism – clues to look for are **"weak cry,"** **"constipation," "listlessness," "hypotonia",** and/or **"poor feeding."** In textbooks and on the boards, a lot of infantile botulism is caused by unpasteurized honey. In reality, most infant botulism results from intestinal colonization in an immature GI tract. But if given honey in the history or as a choice, choose it as the source of botulism toxin in infantile botulism.

Treatment is supportive, and most kids do fine if treated in a timely fashion, though most require ventilatory support.

The *paralysis* in **botulism** is _descending_, while that in **Guillain Barré syndrome** is _ascending_.

Infantile botulism can look similar to **myasthenia gravis**. Botulism has a rapid onset (as in hours). Myasthenia gravis is more progressive, occurring over the course of weeks.

The toxin blocks the release of acetylcholine from the neuromuscular junction.

Picture a giant "BOXER" (box-ulism) blocking acetylcholine from getting through. Now picture him beating up the the folks who write the board question. There, did that feel better?

Dermatomyositis

Dermatomyositis will present initially as proximal muscle weakness and is diagnosed by elevated CPK levels. They will also describe the butterfly malar rash on the face.[4]

---

4 See the Rheum chapter.

Muscular Dystrophy

There are three major types of muscular dystrophy. The primary focus is on **Duchenne muscular dystrophy**. However, **Becker muscular dystrophy** could show up as well. This is not as severe; this limited seriousness would be the tip-off that they are talking about Becker. The 3rd type is myotonic muscular dystrophy.

Duchenne muscular dystrophy

This is an X- linked recessive disorder (**only boys get it**). An absence of dystrophin (easy to remember) is the underlying cause. The diagnosis is made by muscle biopsy.

Children with Duchenne muscular dystrophy are not usually symptomatic at birth. In fact, they usually achieve their baby milestones at the right times. Poor head control may be the first sign in infancy, as well as weakness in the hip muscles. Toddlers have a lordotic posture to compensate for their gluteal weakness.

Look for a child with "**poor head control**" who, in order to stand, walks his hands up his legs for support. This is "**Gower's sign,**" which is associated with proximal muscle weakness. Look for "**hypertrophied calves**" or the term "pseudohypertrophy." It is not actual muscle hypertrophy; it is fat deposition and proliferation of collagen. Most kids with DMD have some degree of *intellectual disability*, but *it is mild in most.*

CPK is elevated at all times in kids with DMD, **even at birth. Therefore, CPK levels can be elevated before weakness appears.** Muscle biopsy is diagnostic. Genetic testing would be via **Xp21 gene testing**. Just remember that it is carried on the X chromosome to avoid being confused with other choices on the exam.

Most patients have some degree of cardiomyopathy, and heart failure is a frequent cause of death in these patients, often by the third decade which would be by the time the patient is in their 20's. Other common causes of death are respiratory failure and pneumonia.

An item that distinguishes this from other neuromuscular disorders is the *absence of tongue fasciculations and eye muscle involvement.*

Think of it as **DuXchenne** muscular dystrophy to remember that it is **X**-linked recessive.

Remember that there is a significant spontaneous mutation rate. They could try to trick you by providing a choice that states that the mother is *always* a carrier. In 1/3 of the cases, the mother is NOT a carrier.

Asymptomatic Carriers: The CPK level can be elevated in asymptomatic female carriers.

Myotonic Muscular Dystrophy

Myotonic muscular dystrophy affects **both striated and smooth muscle**, and thus impacts multiple systems in addition to skeletal muscle, including the *heart* and *GI tract*.

Myotonic muscular dystrophy typically presents at around 4-5 years of age with muscles that have **"slow relaxation after contraction,"** particularly those in the hand – this is called "*myotonia.*" Patients also have endocrine problems. Diagnosis is by muscle biopsy.

The muscle wasting in myotonic muscular dystrophy is distal, compared to proximal for most other neuromuscular disorders. As opposed to **Duchenne muscular dystrophy,** CPK may be normal in **myotonic muscular dystrophy**. Myotonic muscular dystrophy is inherited in an autosomal dominant fashion.

They might describe myotonic dystrophy and tell you the mother has it, so what are the chances of subsequent children getting it? They will say "mother" to trick you into believing it is X-linked recessive. However, if it were an X-Linked recessive disorder, Mom wouldn't have it. Myotonic muscular dystrophy is also known as *Steinert disease;* remember that it is inherited in **autosomal dominant fashion**.

Spinal Neurology

HOT TIP

If you are presented with a patient with symptoms consistent with a spinal cord lesion, then the study to order would be an *MRI* of the *spine.*

Epidural Abscess

BUZZ WORDS

An epidural abscess compresses the spinal cord and can cause *spinal pain, paresthesias,* **weakness** and/or *paralysis.* There can be *fevers,* and most people have *localized back pain as their initial symptom.* Other signs of localized spinal compression include *decreased anal tone, reduced sensation in the lower extremities,* and *increased* reflexes.

Infection can occur by direct extension from the paraspinal tissues or seeding from a distant infection (e.g., UTI, dental abscess, central venous catheter). *IV drug users* are particularly susceptible.

Urgent spinal imaging is mandatory. If *MRI* is not available, a *CT* should be performed.

TREATMENT

Treatment is with antibiotics that have good antistaphylococcal activity. In addition, emergency surgical decompression should be performed.

Brain Abscess

BUZZ WORDS

Remember that patients with **pulmonary, sinus, and cyanotic heart disease** are at increased risk for developing a brain abscess. Watch for a patient with evidence of a space-occupying CNS lesion presenting with seemingly irrelevant upper respiratory findings consistent with chronic sinusitis. They are most likely describing a patient with a brain abscess.

TREATMENT

There is a witch's brew of potential bacterial causes of brain abscess. Therefore, the initial treatment is a broad-spectrum combination of vancomycin, metronidazole, and ceftriaxone. This should be adjusted if necessary based on culture results.

Acute Transverse Myelitis

This is also known as **post-infectious myelitis. It is due to lymphocytic infiltration and demyelination of nerves/spinal cord secondary to inflammation.**

This is one of the many "serious" presentations triggered by a virus that they want you to know about. They present with fever and a sudden onset of paralysis. The CSF has increased polys and a negative gram stain. There is pain on palpation of the spinal canal, and the MRI shows cord swelling. Respiratory arrest or compromise is the main consequence of concern. In this way, it is similar to polio. Before an LP can be performed, an MRI with gadolinium should be performed first.

They may describe a child with an *abrupt onset* of weakness, hypotonia, and decreased reflexes. This is followed by the opposite: increased tone and hyperreflexia. Bowel and bladder dysfunction are common. Most cases have spontaneous recovery over a few months.

Extrinsic Spinal Cord Mass Lesion

If you are presented with a question dealing with a patient with extrinsic spinal cord mass lesion, the most immediate treatment should be high dose IV dexamethasone to reduce pain, edema, and the risk for ischemia.

Werdnig-Hoffmann Disease

Werdnig-Hoffmann is one of the spinal muscle atrophies (SMA type 1). This is due to the degeneration of anterior horn cells; therefore, only *motor function* is affected, and there are no sensory deficits.

Werdnig-Hoffmann typically presents in infancy as severe hypotonia and weakness. Diagnosis is made by muscle biopsy. There is no treatment, and most kids die by two years of age. **"Hypotonia," "poor suck," and "tongue fasciculations"** are key phrases to look for.

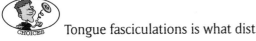

Tongue fasciculations is what distinguishes this from infantile botulism.

Myelomeningocele/Spina Bifida

A myelomeningocele is a protrusion of the spinal cord and surrounding membranes through a defect in the vertebral column. Affected children often have hydrocephalus as well, and frequently require surgery for shunt placement.

A key point you can be tested on: when it is suspected in the newborn period, early orthopedic and urological evaluation is important.

It is important to remember that children with spina bifida can do well during preschool years. However, in later years they may have difficulty with organization, memory, or other learning skills. Their IQ is typically low- average.

Shunt malfunction is always a concern in patients who have spina bifida and a shunt. If you are presented with a patient who presents with a *headache, nausea/vomiting, gaze disturbance, academic or behavior changes, or new onset seizures (or change in occurrence or type of seizure)*, consider shunt malfunction and/or worsening hydrocephalus as a possible cause.

Occult Spinal Dysraphism

You are expected to recognize some of the more subtle signs of occult spinal dysraphism.

Some of the more subtle findings they might mention in the history include a lipoma, patch of hair, hemangioma, discoloration, and of course a sacral dimple.

Later, not-so-subtle findings they could present you with include *discrepancy in leg strength, elevated arches*, and gait abnormalities.

More frightening signs are diminished sensation in the perineal area, urinary and/or stool incontinence, and urinary tract infections.

An MRI of the spine should be ordered if spinal dysraphism is suspected

Spinal Trauma

This will typically be described as focal pain along the spine following trauma. They may also describe weakness and/or sensory deficits. Bladder and bowel function can be lost as well.

If there is a high index of suspicion for spinal trauma, in addition to immobilizing the cervical and lower spine, **methylprednisolone 30 mg/kg** should be administered over an hour.

Dexamethasone would be indicated for spinal cord compression, but not spinal trauma. If mannitol is among the choices you are given in this setting, it would only be indicated with signs of increased intracranial pressure.

Hail Seizure

When you are presented with a question that seems to involved a patient having a seizure, make sure it is actually a seizure and not a "pseudoseizure" or other medical concern such as syncope or tics.

If you follow these guidelines, you are less likely to be, ahem, "shaken" off the trail to the correct answer.

Pseudoseizures will typically be described as occurring during the day, often with other people around. Most importantly will be the absence of the post-ictal state.

To differentiate tics from seizures, they will likely note the patient's ability to suppress the movement.

Seizures typically occur suddenly. At most, the patient might describe an "aura" that preceded the event. Syncopal episodes, on the other hand, are preceded by dizziness, loss of color, or blurred vision.

A seizure is an abnormal, sudden electrical discharge of nerve cells from the gray matter, which progresses to the white matter, having a measurable effect on the innervated organ.[5]

You need to distinguish different categories of seizures based on the history and physical findings. They will not simply just ask what kind of seizure it is. Instead they will ask you to pick the prognosis and treatment based on the associated features they describe.

---

[5] It is also defined as the illegal or forceful attainment of land or property (as in seizure of property), but this is the Board exam, not the Bar exam.

The myriad of different names for different types of seizures can be confusing, but most can be put into one of the following categories.

Seizing Seizure Nomenclature	
1. Neonatal seizures	These occur within the *first month of life* and have a variety of causes, ranging from birth defects to perinatal hypoxia to drug effects.
2. Febrile seizures	These are very common[6] (2-5% of all children) seizures that occur during a rapid rise or decrease in body temperature, usually in response to a common infection such as otitis or other URI.
3. Partial seizures	These are **focal** and only involve part of the brain. They come in two main flavors. **Simple partial seizures** have a *localized motor component* limited to one part of the body. The seizure can progress to other parts of the body. *Children remain awake* during a partial seizure (Jacksonian seizure). **Complex partial seizures** also involve motor activity, but the child is unaware of what he or she is doing, thus making it more "complicated."
4. Generalized seizures	This class of **non-focal seizure** has *several subgroups*. This can get confusing, but follow the bouncing strobe light and it will flow logically. **Absence seizures** (petit mal seizures) are short episodes in which the child *stares into space* with no awareness of their environment. **Infantile spasms** usually occur in children *under a year of age*. They are associated with *intellectual disability* and have a very poor prognosis. **Convulsive seizures** and **tonic/tonic-clonic seizures** are the common seizures your non-physician friends witness while watching *Grey's Anatomy* and munching on stale popcorn. These seizures typically last around 5 minutes and have a *post-ictal period* during which the patient is drowsy.
5. Status epilepticus	This is defined as seizure activity of *more than 30 minutes* in duration, or repeated seizures without a return to normal in between. This is a medical emergency.

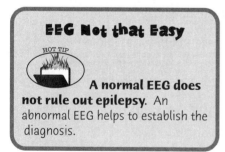

EEG Not that Easy

HOT TIP

A normal EEG does not rule out epilepsy. An abnormal EEG helps to establish the diagnosis.

Apparently the nomenclature was selected to maximize confusion and to increase the chances of actually experiencing a seizure while trying to memorize and remember the appropriate associations. Let's face it, using the term "partial seizure" to describe a focal seizure is quite bizarre.

---

[6] You guessed it, even more common on the Boards.

If **not dealing with neonatal or febrile seizures**, you can usually classify the seizure as being either focal (partial) or non-focal (generalized).

It might be easier to remember partial as being **local** and **focal**, or perhaps this is even more confusing.

We go into greater detail further down. First we go over some general principles.

EEGs

They will not show you EEG tracings. For most non-neurologists (and many neurologists, for that matter), EEG printouts are indistinguishable from the Richter scale printouts by the Geological Society. However, they **will** *describe* the EEG pattern. Becoming familiar with the EEG "descriptions" associated with different disorders will allow you to often recognize the diagnosis based on this alone.

If they describe a child who still has a seizure despite being on anticonvulsant medication, the initial step is to *obtain drug levels*, since poor medication compliance is the likely cause. In addition, weight gain resulting in a child outgrowing the dose and/or a factor interfering with absorption could be the cause behind this *breakthrough seizure*.

Todd's Paralysis

This is postictal motor weakness (focal).

If you are lucky, they might describe the preceding seizure. More often, though, they will describe a child with localized motor weakness in an extremity, and you will need to work backwards to figure out that this is postictal weakness.

> ### Metabolic Seizure
>
> Common causes of metabolic-related seizures, especially in the newborn period, include:
> - Pyridoxine deficiency
> - Hypoglycemia
> - Hyponatremia
> - Hypocalcemia
> - Urea cycle disorders

> ### First Things First Seizures
>
> You might be tricked into believing a variety of myths, both medical and non-medical, regarding first seizures.
>
> Medications are not indicated after a first unprovoked seizure.
>
> Other than a dextrose stick, routine labs and workup are not indicated.
>
> Parents are to be educated on safety, including wearing a helmet while biking and no bathing without supervision.
>
> The risk of swallowing the tongue during a seizure is a myth; therefore, sticking a spoon or other object in the mouth is incorrect.
>
> Seizures in and of themselves do not cause brain damage.
>
> EEG in the ED after a first unprovoked seizure is not indicated routinely.

Seizing the Pharm

A variety of medications are known to cause seizures.

These include chemotherapeutic agents such as:
- Cyclosporin
- Intrathecal methotrexate

Other medications known to cause seizures include:
- Isoniazid
- Insulin/ oral hypoglycemics
- Bupropion (and other psych meds)
- Theophylline

Although not a medication, you should know that cocaine is also known to cause seizures.

Treating Status Epilepticus

Remember your ABCD's. Attend first to the airway, breathing, and circulation (and check Dextrose). Ativan® (lorazepam) is shorter acting but has a rapid onset. If the seizure continues after lorazepam administration, then IV *fosphenytoin* should be administered. This "prodrug" (inactive precursor) is much less likely to produce the skin necrosis ("purple glove syndrome") seen with phenytoin. If IV access is not available, the patient can get rectal diazepam (Diastat®).

Generalized Seizures

Febrile Seizures

Febrile seizures are the most common type of seizure seen in children, occurring in around 3% of kids by their fifth birthday. Most febrile seizures are short (less than 15 minutes) and have no focal component. If there is focality to the seizure or if focal signs are present at the time of presentation, it is not a simple febrile seizure.

Complex Febrile Seizures

Patients experiencing a complex febrile seizure **first** (as opposed to a simple first febrile seizure) are at increased risk for developing epilepsy

A complex febrile seizure is defined as follows:
- Lasts longer than 15 minutes
- Recurs within 24 hours
- Focal

Recurrence of Febrile Seizures

About a third of kids will go on to have a second febrile seizure.

Risk factors for recurrence include:
- A low fever at time of first seizure
- Young age
- Family history of febrile seizures
- A short period of time between onset of fever and the seizure

Appropriate workup for a Febrile Seizure

Unless there are focal signs or other concerning aspects, an EEG, head CT, or LP are not indicated. The choice to do a workup for the second febrile seizure is somewhat controversial, and therefore it is something they should not ask you about.

A lumbar puncture should be considered in a child younger than 18 months presenting with any febrile seizure (strongly considered if less than 12 months).

Even though we tell parents that there is little or no risk for developing epilepsy after a single febrile seizure, this is not entirely true, particularly when it comes to the Boards. Children who have had a single febrile seizure have twice the rate of epilepsy as the general population (1% vs. 0.5%).[7] The risk is still very low, and it is appropriate to reassure parents; however, keep this fact in mind on the exam.

Okay, now let's look at the other types of generalized seizures you should consider, in addition to febrile seizures. Once again, these are:

- Absence
- Tonic Clonic
- Myoclonic
- Infantile Spasms

Absence Seizures

Absence seizures are brief staring spells. The child is not responsive during the episode, and there is no postictal period.

Key words include "spacing out" with "blinking." Afterwards, patients have no recollection of the event.[8] The EEG will be described as "**3 per second spike and wave**" – whatever that is – but if you see that phrase in the question they are talking about an absence seizure. Absence seizures are also called "potato chips" seizures because you can't stop with one (i.e., they come in clusters).

If all this sounds like a **complex partial seizure**, you are right. Absence seizures and complex partial seizure can be difficult to distinguish. Some differences:

---

[7] This is an example of how statistics can be manipulated. If one wanted to be an alarmist or a journalist looking for a story, one could correctly state that the risk for developing epilepsy "doubles."

[8] Reminds me of one of those cult leaders who ask for donations and subsequently direct deposit the money into their Cayman Islands account after rolling their eyes back and communicating with Satan's Secretary.

· A complex partial seizure may start as a simple partial seizure (with the child being aware of the seizure), while an absence seizure is abrupt in onset.

· In contrast to complex partial seizures, absence seizures are usually short (less than thirty seconds).

· Absence seizures end abruptly (like they began), while complex partial seizures end gradually, progressing into the postictal period.

"3 per second spike and wave." Picture a surfer spiking a wave 3 times and then "spacing out" into the horizon.

Hyperventilating can induce an absence seizure, and this maneuver is diagnostic.

Absence seizures are treated with **ethosuximide** (specific for absence seizures) or **valproic acid** (a more general anticonvulsant). The younger the child, the more likely that he/she will respond to therapy and remain free of seizures, even after discontinuation of therapy.

Tonic-Clonic Seizures or Generalized Tonic-Clonic Seizure (GTCS)

These patients can have an aura or prodrome minutes, hours, or even days before their seizure. A key component of a tonic-clonic seizure is the **loss of consciousness and possibly bladder control** with **full body tonic clonic movements**.

Generalized Tonic-Clonic Seizure (GTCS) occurs in three phases:

1. Tonic
2. Clonic
3. Postictal

Tonic Phase

The tonic phase is characterized by flexion of the trunk and extension of the back, arms, and legs, which typically lasts less than 30 seconds. There is no loss of bladder control during this phase.

Clonic Phase

The clonic stage is characterized by clonic convulsive movements, along with tremors. These clonic movements alternate with short periods of atonia, *during which the person may void.* The child is *apneic* during this phase of the seizure, which usually lasts for 1-2 minutes.

Postictal Phase

During the postictal phase, the patient is *initially unconscious* and then sleepy and confused, gradually awakening and becoming more oriented. The patient is unable to recall the events of the seizure. In essence, it is similar to somebody coming out of general anesthesia.

 Treatment of GTC seizures is with anti-epileptic drugs (imagine that!) The drug of choice is **valproic acid**. *Phenytoin* and *carbamazepine* are other options. Lamotrigine (Lamictal®) is another anti-epileptic drug that you may need to know. *Phenobarbital* is still widely used, but is falling out of favor.

 A potential side effect of lamotrigine (Lamictal®) is Stevens Johnson Syndrome.

Myoclonic Seizures

Myoclonic seizures are single or repetitive contractions of an isolated group of muscles.

The key description is "loss of muscle tone" and "sudden brief shock-like muscle twitches," with the child "falling" forward. *There is no impairment of consciousness or memory.*

Infantile Spasms (West Syndrome)

West syndrome is the **triad** of:

1. Infantile spasms
2. Hypsarrhythmia (on interictal[9] EEG)
3. Developmental delay

Infantile spasms represent only 2% of all epilepsy, but they account for 25% of epilepsy seen in the first year of life and maybe more than that on the exam.

---

[9] This would be "in between seizure episodes," for those who prefer English to Latin Medicalese.

Most kids present between 4 and 6 months. The spasms occur in clusters, sometimes 20 or 30 in a row. These spasms are sudden flexion or extension of the body, sort of like a Moro reflex in a child too old to be demonstrating the Moro reflex. *Almost all patients have developmental delay.*

"Repetitive flexing of the head, trunk, and extremities," with an EEG description that includes the word "**hypsarrhythmia.**" These were called Salaam movements in the past.[10]

Where the Tube Grows

It is important to remember that there is a definite **association between Tuberous Sclerosis and infantile spasms.** Remember that TS is an autosomal dominant disease that can present with various tumors (cardiac, kidney) and ash-leaf spots, in addition to seizures.

Recall that babies love their sweet "potatoes," and you can remember that infantile spasms are associated with "tuberous" sclerosis.

Treatment

First line treatment is with **ACTH**, and the prognosis is dependent on developmental status *prior* to the onset of the seizures. If there was a developmental delay present prior to the onset of seizures, then the prognosis is poor.

Other medications used include *steroids* and *benzodiazepines*, as well as other anti-epileptic drugs. In some cases, focal resection is indicated.[11]

Partial Seizures

Remember "**partial** seizures" are **focal** seizures.

Complex Partial Seizures

Complex means **alteration in consciousness**. The description will include facial movements. They can appear to be responding to auditory or visual hallucinations.

---

[10] These were called Salaam movements in the pre-politically correct days when ethnic and religious traits were attributed to children (e.g., kids with Down syndrome were called mongoloids). The term still helps with memorizing the movement and passing the Boards.

[11] Don't try that at home… or on the exam.

Consciousness may not be impaired completely – patients may respond to simple commands. Patients may also have automatisms, which are movements or vocalizations that accompany complex partial seizures (such as moaning or simple talking).

With complex partial seizures, they could describe weird movements like "lip smacking." Head MRI and EEG are part of the workup.

Anti-epileptic drugs are the treatment of choice. Surgery is only rarely used.

Once again, complex partial seizures can be similar to absence seizures, and this is a classic example where knowing the subtle differences between the two can win you points on the exam. With **absence seizures**, patients "just snap out of it" and resume normal activity, as if nothing had happened. With **complex partial seizures**, patients are "postictal" afterwards.

Simple Partial Seizures

"Simple" means **consciousness is maintained**.

They may describe *motor activity in the extremities (usually the arms) or the face*. They often occur as the patient falls asleep or just wakes up. The abnormal movement may "march" to other locations. In addition, simple partial seizures may occur as sensory seizures or autonomic seizures.

Remember: **"simple"** means **consciousness is maintained**. Therefore, if they note that *consciousness is maintained*, then a ***complex** partial* seizure is essentially ruled out.

Simple partial seizures are treated with carbamazepine. Many cases remit during adolescence, and *treatment is not always necessary.*

Partial Leading to ➜ Generalization

Consider this if they initially describe a *focal* seizure that *leads to a generalized seizure* by the time you are done reading the entire question.[12]

---

[12] The seizure would occur in the patient being described, not (necessarily) you, the person reading the question.

Benign Rolandic Seizures = Benign Epilepsy of Childhood

Benign Rolandic seizures are the most common form of epilepsy in childhood. These are self-limited seizures involving the **face**. In addition to the facial motor seizure, there is often *unilateral sensory involvement (commonly involving one side of the tongue).*

These often occur **at night while the child is asleep**. There is also a common association with migraine headaches.

Treatment may not be indicated, but when it is, carbamazepine is usually the first choice. They are a **dominant trait,** so look for mention of a family history.

Picture a child rolling (Rolandic) around in bed, making weird **facial movements**. Certainly anyone rolling around like that would dominate the bed.

Complex partial seizures can also involve weird facial movements; however, **complex partial seizures** occur during the day while the child is awake. Rolandic seizures occur while the child is asleep at night.[13]

Cyanotic Breath Holding Spells

While this is not a seizure, all choices will lead you to believe it is. They will describe a toddler having a temper tantrum, turning blue, passing out, and then coming to. It is a benign, although frightening, process. Parental reassurance is the answer they want.

There is NO postictal phase with breath-holding spells... at least not in the child. The parents, however, are often in a state of shock closely mimicking a postictal state.

Facts and Myths regarding patients with epilepsy

Patients with epilepsy can bathe or swim, but not alone. They must be monitored by an adult.

Teenagers can drive unaccompanied, even if they are on anticonvulsant medication. They must be seizure free for 3-12 months. The exact period varies from state to state, but on the boards the time period will be greater than 12 months.

Withdrawal from medication can be attempted if the patient has remained seizure-free for 2 years.

Withdrawal would not be appropriate with a diagnosis of **juvenile myoclonic epilepsy**, for which valproic acid is the treatment of choice. Likewise, it would not be indicated in the presence of complications, including:

· Onset of seizures after age 12

---

[13] Rolandic seizures can occur during both sleep and wakefulness, with only about 1/2 to 2/3 occurring exclusively during sleep. However, this rate is closer to 100% on the exam, which is why we state this as such.

· Neonatal seizures

· Multiple medications tried before control of seizures was obtained

Adrenoleukodystrophy

This may be confused with ADHD. With adrenoleukodystrophy, they will likely describe a child who, in addition to having difficulty paying attention and concentrating, is "clumsy." The most important descriptive component in the history will be abnormal motor function.

A key finding will be **adduction of the contralateral leg with stimulation of the patellar reflex.**

In this case, the correct steps would include neurology consultation and/or MRI imaging studies.

Cerebral Palsy

This is a topic that will show up in several questions.

CP is a static encephalopathy characterized by gross and fine motor abnormalities evident early in life. *There are dozens of proposed etiologies.* Contrary to popular belief, CP is not always caused by birth asphyxia, which is the documented cause in only about 10% of cases. In most cases, the etiology is unknown, though a variety of prenatal, perinatal, and postnatal factors have been *proposed.*

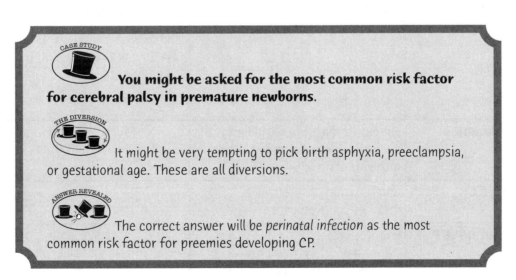

You might be asked for the most common risk factor for cerebral palsy in premature newborns.

It might be very tempting to pick birth asphyxia, preeclampsia, or gestational age. These are all diversions.

The correct answer will be *perinatal infection* as the most common risk factor for preemies developing CP.

Do not automatically pick "birth asphyxia" as the answer – consider the clinical scenario and look at the other etiologies that may have affected the developing brain. **A specific cause of CP is often not found**.

Another myth is that children with CP are always intellectually disabled. On the contrary, many children and adults with CP have normal (or above normal) intelligence. **Unless the question specifically states that the child is intellectually disabled, do not assume this is so because they have CP.**

Cerebral palsy can be broken down into several types as noted in the table below:

Subtype of Cerebral Palsy	Buzz Words	Associations
Spastic Diplegia	Bilateral spasticity of legs **Walking is delayed** **Tip-toe walking**	Excellent for normal cognitive function without seizures More likely to involve lower extremities
Spastic hemiplegia	Spasticity of half of the body, left or right, involving the arm, trunk, and leg. If it occurs prior to age 2, it is considered to be cerebral palsy.	1/4 are cognitively impaired May involve upper extremity more than lower
Spastic quadriplegia	Increased tone in all 4 extremities Lower > upper	Are *more likely* to be associated with: · Intellectual disability · Seizures · Feeding difficulties · Speech difficulties · Visual difficulties
Dyskinetic[14]	Similar to spastic quadriplegia; in addition, **dystonia and strange movements**	
Mixed CP	Combination of spastic and dyskinetic movements	
Hypotonic CP	Hypotonia seen in the trunk and extremities. They might also describe retention of primitive reflexes and/or hyperactive reflexes.	

[14] Also known as athetoid cerebral palsy

Cerebrovascular Accident

BUZZ WORDS

The typical presentation would be an afebrile child with a headache and neck pain who then develops focal paralysis.

HOT TIP

If you are presented with a patient with a CVA confirmed with CT, then cerebral angiography would be the next step to identifying a specific diagnosis.

CASE STUDY

You are presented with a child who comes in with acute unilateral hemiparesis; other than blunt trauma to the chest yesterday during football practice, his history is benign. Which diagnostic study would be most helpful in making the diagnosis?

THE DIVERSION

You might be tempted to pick a head CT, which will be conveniently listed among the choices for your diversionary pleasure. However, if you remember the "don't pick an answer so obvious that your next door neighbor, the hospital CFO, would pick it," you won't be diverted to the incorrect answer.

ANSWER REVEALED

The CVA or stroke in this case was caused by the blunt trauma to the chest, which resulted in carotid dissection, leading to an embolic stroke. This would be best diagnosed via carotid angiography.

HOT TIP

If you are presented with a clinical history consistent with a stroke and they note an **elevated lactate level** and **sensorineural deafness,** they are describing a patient with a **mitochondrial disorder**.

If they ask for the best diagnostic step to **establish the underlying diagnosis,** the answer will be *molecular analysis of mitochondrial DNA.* If you read the question carefully, you won't be tricked into picking head CT.

Vascular malformations, including arteriovenous and cavernous malformations, are the most common causes of hemorrhagic stroke in children. This can present initially as severe headache and/or mental status change.

Neurodiagnostic Testing

Please note some of the indications for Head CT and MRI in the table below.

Test	Acuity	Indications
MRI / Head	Non-urgent	Partial seizures Herpes encephalitis (confirmed with HSV polymerase)
CT/Head	Urgent	Hemorrhage Tumors Abscesses
Head Ultrasound	Non-urgent	Infants with accelerating head circumference across percentiles.

Vertigo

Benign Paroxysmal Vertigo

Consider a diagnosis of benign paroxysmal vertigo in a patient with an acute onset of self-limited vertigo in the *absence of vomiting or loss of consciousness*. The episode is brief, typically presenting in a toddler. In addition, nystagmus will be described, as well as pallor.

If the vertigo lasts hours or days, then benign paroxysmal vertigo is unlikely. If hearing loss is also part of the history, then labyrinthitis is the more likely diagnosis.

Chapter 24

Musculoskeletal

Much of this chapter includes orthopedic conditions. "Strong as an ox and twice as smart" is the old adage about our orthopedic colleagues.

They have to be strong in order to lift the words that describe the geography of bones in diagnosing musculoskeletal disorders. With words like varus, valgus, Las Valgus, and Las Vegas, it is easy for the uninitiated to get confused. Before embarking on the specifics of what you will need to know for the Boards, here is a glossary of terms from the orthopedic cabinet.

Defining Orthopedics

Physeal: Growth plate.

Metaphyseal: The end of the long bone, adjacent to the growth plate or physis.

Metaphysical: Having to do with the non-physical world.

Varus: When the distal part of the deformity points inward.

Valgus: When the distal part of the deformity points away from midline.

Picture a "gust of wind blowing things away." If you just think of a gust of wind blowing out the distal portion of the deformity, everything else will flow from there.

For example, you would know that **Genu Valgum** is "knock-kneed" since the distal part of the leg is pointed outward, and the proximal (knee) is inward. Or you can picture "gum" keeping the knees stuck together.

Heart: Pumps nafcillin to the bones. Also a 1970s band from Seattle.

Sprains, strains, and pains

Ankle Sprains

The *immediate treatment* of an ankle sprain would be the *application of ice.* This should continue for 20 minutes at a time over the first 36-48 hours.

If you are presented with a child who "recovers" from an ankle injury, returns to competitive sport, and then sustains another more severe injury in the same ankle, what is the most likely cause?

The diversion (and implication) is that the child has sustained a new injury, since they tell you he has "recovered" from the previous injury before returning. However, this is often in quotes, or should be in quotes, since the child probably never fully recovered from the initial injury.

The most likely answer will be *reinjury* because the child *returned to competitive play too soon.*

Pain over a bone *physis* in a pre-adolescent child should be assumed to be a Salter Harris I fracture, *even if the x-ray is normal.*

Spraining Degrees

You are expected to understand what defines different degrees of ligament sprain as follows:

Grade 1 Sprain – A grade I sprain only involves minor stretching of the ligament, with minimal discomfort or loss of function. This initial injury often does not come to medical attention or appear on the boards by itself.

Grade 2 Sprain – **In a grade 2 sprain, the ligaments are partially torn.** They will describe tenderness and swelling. Ecchymosis will also be consistent with a grade 2 sprain. There will be some loss of function.

Grade 3 Sprain – In a grade 3 sprain, the ligament is completely torn and there is significant pain, tenderness, swelling, and loss of function. These injuries usually seek medical attention, and appear on the boards as well.

Compartment Syndrome

CASE STUDY

You are presented with a child who was running in on a fast break while playing basketball. He was stopped by an opponent who was completing his 7th year of high school varsity ball, and who stepped on his ankle and lateral leg. You note no deformity, just a bruise and marked swelling. The foot has a strong dorsal pulse, with some diminished sensation to pinprick and light touch. What is the most appropriate next step?

THE DIVERSION

You might be tempted to choose ice, since that is the most appropriate immediate step in an ankle sprain. There is no deformity or evidence of a displaced fracture, and pulses are intact, so getting the swelling down would be top priority. What could be wrong with ice? Probably nothing, except it would be the wrong choice on the boards for this question.

ANSWER REVEALED

The signs and symptoms described are consistent with compartment syndrome, and therefore *obtaining compartment pressures would be the correct choice*. The presence of a pulse and lack of paralysis simply means that it is in the early stages, and does not rule out compartment syndrome.

The signs and symptoms of compartment syndrome can be remembered as the 5 P's

Pain

Paresthesias

Pallor

Paralysis

Pulselessness

The last two are late findings in compartment syndrome and their absence as in the case above does not rule it out.

Ice won't help, and a compression dressing will make it worse. These will, of course, be among the diversionary choices you might be given.

Osteogenic Picture Imperfecta

Osteogenesis Imperfecta

Here are the essentials, along with clues for memorizing them and keeping them osteogenically perfectly straight.

Osteogenesis Imperfecta (OI) Type 1 is the one with the really **blue sclerae. Fractures occur during the preschool years. Rarely are they born with fractures**. Remember, this is autosomal **dominant.** The majority will develop **hearing loss** by the time they are adults.

Hearing loss (both conductive and sensorineural) is considered to be a major feature of OI type 1.

You may be asked to distinguish Type 1A, with good teeth, from Type 1 B, with bad teeth (dentinogenesis imperfecta). Hopefully, they won't get that esoteric, but we included it here just in case.

To remember that Type 1**B** is associated with **b**ad teeth just associate B for Bad and "**b**lue moon" since there is only one moon (type one), which "dominates the sky" (autosomal dominant).

OI Type 2

This is the most severe form of the disease, and is usually lethal. Born with multiple fractures, these infants **rarely live past the postnatal period**. If they describe any "child" that gets past infancy, OI Type 2 cannot be the diagnosis. OI Type 2 is inherited as either a dominant new mutation or "germinal mosaicism".[1]

Children with OI Type 2 are described as having a **"bag of bones"** appearance and are usually **stillborn**. The head is large in proportion to the rest of the body. One would assume this would be included on the pathology boards, but you never know.

OI Type 3

Type 3 is known as the **progressive deforming type**. Children with OI Type 3 are **born with fractures** and the deformities are progressive. They are born with **gray sclerae that lighten over time. Macrocephaly and short stature are other characteristics.**

Picture 3 children (Type 3) in a vertical circle holding hands, like that big wheel in *Pirates of the Caribbean*. They manage to roll down the street, they get gray and dusty from all the dirt (sclerae), and sustain progressive fractures.

OI Type 4

I wouldn't spend a lot of time on this one. Just like with Type 1, the A subcategory has good teeth and *B has bad teeth.*

 Unlike Type 1, the sclerae are white, not blue.

---

[1] Germinal mosaicism is when the defect exists in germinal cells but not in regular somatic cells. Therefore, it can be transmitted as a dominant trait, but appear to be recessive since it is not an expressed phenotype in the parents.

Achondroplasia

CASE STUDY

You are presented with an infant who has the following physical findings: *macrocephaly, frontal bossing, midface hypoplasia, and proximal shortening of the limbs*. You astutely and correctly identify this as a child with achondroplasia. Of course this would be clearly obvious if you have already read through the Genetics chapter in this book, or at least glanced at the section heading two inches or so above. You now must either answer "What is the *inheritance pattern*" and/or "The most likely *cause of sudden death* in this infant…"

THE DIVERSION

The first diversion might be your inability to write the answer with your arm pinned behind you as you pat yourself on the back congratulating yourself for making the correct diagnosis. The inheritance pattern you will simply have to know, and the most likely cause of death can be deduced if you forget. You might be tricked into believing respiratory or cardiac failure, assuming these are associations and therefore most likely to cause sudden death. This would violate the "if-your-shoemaker-could-pick-a-choice-it-is-probably-wrong rule."

ANSWER REVEALED

The most common cause of sudden death in children with achondroplasia is *cervicomedullary junction compression*. The inheritance pattern is *autosomal dominant; however, >80% of cases* occur as a *spontaneous mutation*.

Similar but Different (Crooked Necks)

Congenital Torticollis

BUZZ WORDS

"An infant with head tilted to one side, a **mass in the sternocleidomastoid muscle**, and/or facial asymmetry."

Congenital torticollis requires **daily stretching and physical therapy**. If this therapy is not implemented or is not effective after one year, surgical intervention will be necessary.

Congenital torticollis can be associated with hip dysplasia.

Craning your neck to differentiate the causes of neck tilt

Cause of Neck Tilt	Distinguishing Characteristics
Muscular Torticollis	Muscular torticollis probably results from positioning or trauma; for example, bleeding into the sternocleidomastoid muscle after birth. This is similar to torticollis seen in older children after a minor injury.
Paroxysmal Torticollis	This is a migraine variant that can manifest in infants. Infants will be described with repeated attacks of head tilting, which *only last for minutes at a time*. These require no intervention, and are often accompanied by vomiting, irritability, and pallor.
Posterior fossa tumor	Head tilt secondary to a brain tumor will include physical findings consistent with an upper motor neuron process, including **increased deep tendon reflexes.** This would require an MRI to establish a diagnosis.

Klippel-Feil Syndrome

Klippel-Feil syndrome can also be considered a form of congenital torticollis; however, here you will have **fusion of the cervical vertebrae.** Additional findings include *short neck* and *low occipital hairline* and may include:

· *Scoliosis*

· *Spina bifida*

· *Renal problems (missing one kidney)*

· *Sprengel deformity*

· *Deafness*

"Clipper File" syndrome. Picture a file of hedge clippers instead of a neck - now THAT would be one stiff neck. You can also picture the clippers delivering a bad haircut, resulting in a "low occipital hairline."

Sprengel Deformity

Sprengel deformity results from **poor fetal development and the failure of the scapula to descend to its normal position.**[2] The affected side of the neck will seem broader and shorter.[3] Therefore, it **mimics torticollis.**

Picture a "scapula made of sprinkles on someone's neck."

Developmental Dysplasia of the Hip (DDH)[4]

Here's a disorder that actually occurs more frequently in **females**, and is associated with a strong **family history**. It also occurs **more frequently on the left** than the right side, and is diagnosed by **ultrasound** in young infants. However, after 4 months, plain x-ray would be indicated instead of ultrasound.

The reason for the name change from "congenital dislocation of the hip" is to acknowledge that it is a progressive problem; it can be normal in the first couple of days and present later on.

- **Barlow** is the part of the exam done in adduction with downward pressure.
- **Ortolani** is the attempt at relocating a dislocated femoral head.

They might also show or describe **asymmetric gluteal folds**.

Treatment is with the Pavlik harness, which holds the hips in a position of abduction, flexion, and external rotation. This is more reliable than double or triple diapers.

---

[2] Typically there is an abnormally high and medially rotated position of the scapula.

[3] Of course, there is a scapula sitting there.

[4] Formerly known as CDH (Congenital Dislocation of the Hip) but now known as DDH since joining the witness protection program for diseases that cooperate with the FBI.

Double diapering is an ineffective form of treatment, and is inappropriate. The diapers applied are often loose and fail to provide any degree of abduction.

Risk Factors for DDH

Risk factors for DDH in the newborn include:
- Breech positioning
- Family history of DDH
- Female
- First born

Leg length discrepancy and DDH

Leg length discrepancy can be an important sign of previously undiagnosed DDH. It is also possible that DDH wasn't apparent prior to the patient ambulating, thus the change in terminology from congenital hip dysplasia to DDH.

Watch for the presentation of a child with a "waddling gait" who immigrated here from the developing world. This would be a red flag that DDH is the correct diagnosis.

Infections

Toxic Synovitis (Post-Infectious Arthritis)

Toxic synovitis is a misnomer, since it is not that toxic at all. Look for the following in the history: "**recent URI**," "some **passive ROM**," "**normal ESR,**" "negative gram stain," and "normal or slightly elevated temperature."

Waffling on Waddling Gait

While a waddling gait is a typical description of a child with DDH, there are other causes you should consider, depending on the context they give. For example:

Rickets can be the correct answer if you are presented a waddling gait. However, they would also describe leg bowing and other findings consistent with rickets. **Legg-Calvé-Perthes** disease could be described as a patient with a waddling gait and a limp. This would likely be described in a child around age 7. **Slipped capital femoral epiphysis** could present this way; in addition to a waddling gait, would likely include knee pain in an overweight young adolescent.

B19 Bomber

Although a very benign picture is typically presented, there could be moderate swelling in addition to pain. This is particularly the case following infection with Parvovirus B19, the "B 19" bomber that seems to cause anything and everything. They might describe flushing of the cheeks to suggest Fifth disease and the B19 bomber leaving its mark.

There are other viral etiologies that can cause post-infectious arthritis, including influenza, hepatitis B, rubella, and Mr. Ebstein Barr Virus.

No matter how severe the pain, "toxic" synovitis requires nothing more than reassurance. It is a **diagnosis of exclusion** after other more serious infections are ruled out.

Septic Arthritis

Septic arthritis is much more serious, and requires aggressive intervention. It is usually due to hematogenous spread.

Look for the following in the history: "high fever," "warm to touch," "difficult or impossible to induce any passive range of motion," "positive gram stain," and "increased joint space on x-ray." It typically occurs in a child younger than age 2.

Also important to note is that there will be a "warm," "red," and "swollen" joint. Patients present with "guarding" around the joint and/or "rigidity" and **elevated ESR.**

Ultrasound, MRI, CT and bone scan are **not** helpful in making the initial diagnosis of septic arthritis. They **are**, however, useful to rule out osteomyelitis.

The key steps are **joint aspiration and initiation of antibiotic therapy** to cover *Staph aureus*, which is the most common organism in all age groups. However, in a neonate, group B strep is also possible. Rapid intervention plays an important role in prognosis. IV antibiotics should be started pending culture and sensitivities. Once there is clinical improvement, PO antibiotics can be continued for another 3 weeks.

In general, the septic hip is the most difficult joint to diagnose. If the history suggests a septic hip, then choose antibiotics and treatment. Treatment should begin even before the diagnosis is confirmed.

> **CASE STUDY**
>
> **You are presented with a patient who recently immigrated from a developing country. He presents with a sore ankle that is painful to both passive and active movement, red, and mildly swollen. This was preceded by similar symptoms in the knee yesterday (which is better today). There is also a diffuse macular rash. You are asked for a diagnosis to explain the presentation.**
>
> **THE DIVERSION**
>
> You might be tempted to pick several diversionary choices including meningococcemia, septic arthritis, or even post viral synovitis.
>
> **ANSWER REVEALED**
>
> However, the key here is their noting that the patient is a recent immigrant. This usually means an infectious disease that is either 1) rare due to immunization, or 2) an oldie but a goodie, a disorder that is not seen very often. In this case, a migratory arthritis involving large joints coupled with a rash should lead you to the correct diagnosis of rheumatic fever.

The treatment of choice for empiric antibiotics for septic arthritis depends on the age.

- **Neonates** - You need to cover Group B strep, staph, and gram negative bacilli with cloxacillin/gentamicin.
- **Infants through 3 months** – you need to cover strep, staph, and *H. flu* with cefuroxime or cefotaxime
- **Older children** – *Staph aureus, Strep pneumoniae,* and Group A strep may be covered with cefazolin.
- **Adolescents**- You must also consider the possibility of GC arthritis, and must add azithromycin to ceftriaxone or cefixime

For children with sickle cell disease, you must extend coverage for *Salmonella,* using cefotaxime

If the question hints that MRSA is prevalent, vancomycin should be included in the correct choice.

Ordering Ortho

Involvement of the hip, knee, and shoulder require orthopedic consultation. Joint drainage is often necessary.

Legg Calve Perthes Disease

> Trivia: Young **Forrest Gump** had Legg Calve Perthes in the movie.

Legg Calve Perthes Disease is **avascular necrosis of the femoral head,** usually found in *boys* age 4-8 years. They could show the classic x-ray, **with one femoral head being smaller than the other**.

Remember, **hip pain can frequently be referred to the knee**.

You Say Infection, I say Infarction

Bone scans are useful early, when the exact location of the infection needs to be identified and the infection is too early to be detected on plain film. Bone scan can pick up abnormalities within 3 days of onset. X-ray findings in osteo do not generally appear until 10 to 14 days after infection.

MRI with contrast is much more specific and can distinguish infection from other causes of inflammation. For example, if you are presented with a child who has sickle cell disease, the distinction between infarction and infection would be identified on MRI, not bone scan.

Osteomyelitis

Osteomyelitis is infection of the bone, as opposed to septic arthritis, which is infection of the joint. The most common organism causing osteomyelitis is also *Staph aureus.*

It begins with localized tenderness over the metaphysis, as well as pain on weightbearing.

Some important points to keep in mind regarding osteomyelitis are as follows:

· Know that osteomyelitis <u>begins</u> with an episode of bacteremia, resulting in the seeding of the metaphysis.

· Although it is initially seeded hematogenously, it then <u>spreads</u> by local extension.

· Diagnosis is made by direct aspiration of the metaphysis, which is sent for culture and sensitivity.

Causes of Osteomyelitis through the Ages

Osteomyelitis in the Neonatal Period

The infection usually results from hematogenous spread, typically involving the tibia or femur. In neonates, group B streptococci and *Escherichia coli* are the most common causes.

 Although it is typically contracted via hematogenous spread, a septic joint is present 50% of the time among neonates with osteomyelitis.

Beyond the Neonatal Period

A septic joint is rarely seen with osteomyelitis beyond the neonatal period. The most common cause is *Staph aureus*. Other causes include Group A strep and *H. flu* type b

In children with sickle cell disease, the most common cause of osteomyelitis is *Salmonella*.

PO Meds and Osteomyelitis

PO Meds can be used with osteomyelitis after:

1. There is **a good initial response to IV meds,** and a **specific organism is identified,**
2. **A trial of PO antibiotics and good serum levels are documented while still in the hospital,**
3. You have **compliance assured (parental reliability)**

Treatment should continue for 4-6 weeks as follows:

Etiology of Osteomyelitis.	Treatment of Osteomyelitis
Staph aureus / Group A strep	Oxacillin / Nafcillin 1st / 2nd generation cephalosporin Clindamycin (for patients who are pen allergic)
H. flu	2nd or 3rd generation cephalosporin
Children with sickle cell suspected of having osteomyelitis	Have to assume *Salmonella* is highly likely, and starting with a 3rd generation cephalosporin would be the correct initial course until culture and sensitivity back
Concurrent **puncture wound**	Would need to cover for pseudomonas and/or anaerobic organisms.

Unable to Shake the Pelvis

Pelvic osteomyelitis is prone to abscess formation; read the question carefully to determine if this is what they are alluding to.

BUZZ WORDS Pelvic osteomyelitis is seen more frequently in boys around age 8, and is typically right sided. The cause is *Staph aureus*.

PERIL WARNING The pain is often referred to the hip or thigh. It can present as **abdominal pain**. WBC will be normal, and plain film may be negative. MRI and bone scan would be the studies of choice.

HOT TIP The most common complication of osteomyelitis is recurrence. Surgical intervention might be required with chronic infection, especially when an abscess is suspected.

Osteochondritis Dissecans

DEFINITION Osteochondritis dissecans is the result of **necrosis of the articular surface of a joint** (typically the knee). It is **diagnosed with MRI**.

TREATMENT Treatment is immobilization and surgical removal of fragments "down the road" if there is no improvement.

BUZZ WORDS "**Chronic knee pain that locks and swells**", typically in adolescent boys.

Osgood-Schlatter Disease

DEFINITION Osgood-Schlatter disease *is the result of stress from excessive activity at the insertion of the patellar tendon at the anterior tibial tubercle.* The tibial tuberosity is the location of a specialized growth center called the *apophysis*. This is the site where the quadriceps muscle attaches via the patellar tendon. This is why adolescents are prone to this "overuse injury" during the period of rapid growth.

BUZZ WORDS Osgood-Schlatter disease is typically described in "an athletic adolescent who presents with **pain just below** the knee."

TREATMENT Treatment consists of a couple of weeks' rest with gradual resumption of activity and NSAIDs for pain and inflammation.

Observing the Occult

You could very well be presented with a patient with an occult fracture.

The history will imply or clearly note that there are no systemic symptoms, no recent viral illness, no signs of infectious etiology, and no history that would lead you to suspect a trauma that was missed.

A "toddler's fracture" can occur during the course of a toddler learning to walk. This can also be missed on x-ray. On physical exam there will be point tenderness, and this could be the only clue in the question pointing to this diagnosis.

Since ligaments are stronger than underlying bone in children, a sprained ligament will not likely be the correct answer. Force strong enough to cause a ligament tear in a child would more likely result in a fracture.

Scoliosis

With scoliosis, you will need to know when treatment is needed and when observation alone is okay. A typical case would be 1) a referral from the school triggering parental concern, or 2) the pediatrician discovering possible scoliosis on routine screening. They might describe "*asymmetry of the hips and/or scapula*" on the physical exam, without telling you it is scoliosis. Here are your guidelines:

- ❑ **Curvature of less than 25 degrees requires observation only**.
- ❑ If there is **more than 2 years of growth still expected (child is still growing), bracing** is required for curvature **between 25-40 degrees**.
- ❑ Surgery will be **needed for a lumbar or thoracic curvature greater than 40 degrees**.

There are 3 subtypes of scoliosis as follows:

1) **Congenital scoliosis** - failed segmentation or formation of spinal elements. As noted below, it can also be associated with fused ribs and/or spinal cord anomalies. Natural course/progression is variable.

    Congenital scoliosis may be seen at any age.

2) **Neuromuscular or paralytic scoliosis** is seen in children with either a congenital or an acquired neuromuscular condition. This would include children with muscular dystrophy,

myopathies, spina bifida, or those who have sustained a spinal cord injury. The degree of curvature tends to progress.

3) **Idiopathic scoliosis**- this is isolated scoliosis, with no identified cause. This represents 80% of the cases in practice, but not necessarily 80% of the cases on the boards. These tend to worsen by 1 degree per month during the growth spurt, until skeletal maturity.

Young premenarchal patients with large initial curves are at risk for the highest degree of progression.

If the degree of curvature increases by more than 1 degree per month during the growth spurt, then this may be more than just idiopathic scoliosis, warranting an MRI.

If they describe interventions such as "manipulation" or "electrical stimulation," it will be the wrong answer. (Rolfing, mud therapy, and aerobic psychotherapy have not received FDA approval yet either.)

You will need to distinguish between idiopathic scoliosis and cases associated with other causes. Watch for signs of delayed pubertal development, neurological deficits, or dermatological lesions. Neurofibromatosis is an example of a disorder where scoliosis may be more commonly seen.

School screening for scoliosis is no longer considered to be routine.

Congenital Scoliosis

Although congenital scoliosis is associated with other malformations more than half of the time, most cases are *not* hereditary.

For congenital scoliosis, bracing is not helpful as primary treatment. However, it would be the correct answer for post-op treatment.

Children with congenital scoliosis should be screened with **renal ultrasound** and **cardiac echo**, due to the high association with renal and cardiac disease. Spinal MRI would also be indicated, since there is also a high association with spinal abnormalities.

Chromosome analysis, ophthalmologic evaluation, and head ultrasound are **not** routinely indicated.

Kyphosis

Kyphosis is the convex alignment of the thoracic spine in the sagittal plane (also known as the side view).

The normal range is 20-40 degrees; therefore, don't be intimidated into thinking this is abnormal.

For kyphosis less than 60 degrees, no intervention is needed other than follow-up. Pulmonary function studies would not be indicated in an asymptomatic patient unless kyphosis is well above 60 degrees.

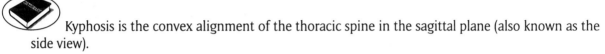

CASE STUDY **You are presented with a teenage patient who "can never stand up straight" and has chronic upper back pain. You note kyphosis on physical examination along with a "distended abdomen." You are asked for the most likely diagnosis.**

THE DIVERSION Among the diversionary choices will be chronic poor posture, scoliosis, spinal tumor and vertebral osteomyelitis.

ANSWER REVEALED The combination of "bad posture, kyphosis and back pain" in a teenager should lead you to a diagnosis of **Scheuermann disease**. Scheuermann disease is a "fixed kyphosis" which presents at puberty. Treatment is primarily with NSAID medication, physical therapy and observation over time.

Caffey Disease

Caffey disease is also known as **infantile cortical hyperostosis,** and it typically occurs during the **first 6 months of life.** Its prominent feature is swelling of the bone shafts, but it **only involves cortical bone**. X-rays show progressive cortical thickening.

Since this is essentially the swelling of bones, consider memorizing Caffey disease as "Café" disease with "bones full of hot café or coffee."

Caffey disease can be confused with abuse, but **in abuse the periosteum will be involved**. This is a classic example where they might imply child abuse by emphasizing progressive cortical thickening but "non-accidental" injury or child abuse won't be the correct diagnosis.

Subluxed Radial Head (Nursemaid's Elbow)

The classic description is of a child that was pulled by the arm, is now not using the involved arm, and was brought in by an hysterical relative. The "best way to manage" the problem will be to reduce it, **but only after checking for other injuries**.

If there is no swelling or discoloration, *x-rays will not be necessary.*

Bone Cysts

Unicameral bone cysts, or **simple bone cysts**, are fluid-filled cysts (usually seen prior to skeletal maturity) that are typically found at the proximal humerus or femur. These are *not* precancerous.

These typically are asymptomatic and are diagnosed as pathological fracture after minor trauma.

Aneurysmal bone cysts are typically seen on the tibia or femur. These present with pain, which can be in the absence of swelling. They can be associated with underlying bone tumors and may require orthopedic referral if this is on the exam.

If present on vertebrae, can have signs of nerve compression.

Viral Myositis

Typical presentation is with weakness and tenderness localized to a muscle. Neurological exam will be unremarkable. Lab findings would include elevated creatinine kinase. They will likely include a history of a recent respiratory illness or influenza. No treatment is necessary.

Metabolic myopathies due to mitochondrial dysfunction might present with a similar picture; however, there will also be rhabdomyolysis noted in the history.

Shouldering Shoulder Diagnosis

Even though this is not the orthopedic or sports medicine boards, you are still expected to shoulder the burden, if you will, of distinguishing between subtle differences in the differential diagnosis of shoulder injuries.

The following table outlines the typical buzz words and the injuries they are typically associated with.

Mechanism of injury / Physical findings	Diagnosis they are looking for
The patient falls back on a posteriorly rotated, abducted arm	Anterior humeral dislocation
Pain over the distal clavicle, with a prominence noted over the area of point tenderness.	Acromioclavicular injury
Direct force to the posterior shoulder. Pain over the sternoclavicular joint, with possible respiratory discomfort.	Posterior sternoclavicular dislocation
Shoulder and upper arm pain in the absence of asymmetry	Proximal humeral fracture
Shoulder pain with elevating and lowering the arm, without any deformity. In addition, this will present as chronic pain, most likely in the absence of acute injury.	Rotator cuff injury

Back Pain

By now, if you have been sitting long enough reading through all of this, your back is probably killing you. However, if you are presented with a patient who has back pain this will not be one of the choices. You must sit at the table listed below to answer these questions correctly.

Main Categories	Subcategories	Associations
Infectious	Diskitis	Usually caused by *Staph aureus*
	Spinal Epidural Abscess	
	Vertebral osteomyelitis	
Developmental	Spondylolysis	
	Spondylolisthesis	Progression of spondylolysis, leading to stress fractures and subluxation of vertebral bodies
	Scheuermann kyphosis	
Traumatic Causes	Herniated disc	
	Vertebral Stress Fracture	
	Overuse syndrome	
Tumors	Osteoid osteoma	Night pain relieved by NSAIDs
	Osteoblastoma	Osteoid osteoma greater than 1.5 cm
	Aneurysmal bone cyst	
	Osteosarcoma	
	Ewing sarcoma	

Club Foot

For those who prefer Latin, Club Foot is called *Talipes Equinovarus*. Simply put, the **foot is internally rotated and the Achilles tendon is contracted**.

Treatment consists of stretching, serial casting, and possible surgical release of the tendon late in the first year of life.[5]

---

[5] Club Foot is also a Mediterranean vacation spot for tired podiatrists, and would be correct if it were one of the choices.

Genu Varus (Bow Legged)

With few exceptions, genu varus is a normal condition, requiring only reassurance.

Intervention would be required with abnormal **findings**, such as **when it is unilateral**, **worsens after age 1, or does not resolve after age 2**. X-ray findings of physeal and epiphyseal distortion would also indicate the need for intervention.

If genu varus is present **after age 2,** then more significant causes, such as **rickets or Blount's disease**, should be considered. When this is the case, there will be something in the history to tip you off.

Blount's Disease

In Blount's disease, there is actual pathology of the proximal tibial physis and epiphysis. There are 2 types:

Infantile Blount's Disease

Infantile Blount's disease is seen in **African Americans** and **shouldn't be confused with rickets**. Note that rickets can also occur more frequently in African Americans due to decreased absorption of UV light. **No treatment is needed** for infantile Blount's disease.

If they are referring to rickets, then other signs of the disorder will need to be presented in addition to genu varus.

Adolescent Blount's Disease

The adolescent is **usually overweight**. As is the case with infantile Blount's disease, adolescent Blount's disease also occurs **more frequently in African Americans**.

Here treatment is some form of intervention, ranging from **bracing to surgery**.

> ### Slippery Wrist/Syndromes with Little or No Radius
>
> **TAR**
> TAR is easy because the name describes it: **T**hrombocytopenia **A**bsent **R**adius.
>
> **Fanconi's Anemia**
> The mnemonic for Fanconi's anemia is a "fan blade" cutting off the thumbs and radius.[6]
>
> **VATER**
> The **R** represents absent "Radius".[7]

---

6 Additional material is in the "Heme/Onc" chapter.

7 The rest is covered in the "Genetics" chapter.

Salter Harris Fracture Classifications

Being familiar with the Salter Harris Fracture classification will surely come in handy on the exam.

Salter Harris Fracture Classifications

There are five types.

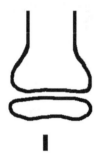

Type 1

This is identified by **separation of the epiphysis and metaphysis**. The fracture is directly through the physis. **X-ray may be negative, with tenderness being the only sign**.

 Casting is needed for 2-3 weeks.

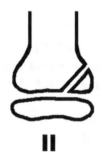

Type 2

With Type 2, **a piece of the metaphysis splits, as well as some physis.**

 It is managed by closed reduction casting for 3-6 weeks.

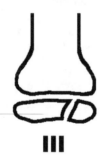

Type 3

The fracture is **through the growth plate, extending through the epiphysis.**

 Open reduction may be necessary.

Everyone has trouble remembering which is Type 2 and which is Type 3. Just remember that **Type 3 is worse because it goes through the epiphysis into the joint space.**

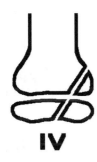

Type 4

There are cracks through everything, all layers.

Type 4 requires reduction in the OR to avoid growth disruption.

IV

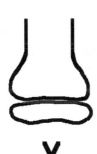

Type 5

This is a crush type injury/compression fracture causing microvascular compromise. It is associated with a high rate of poor growth after the injury.

V

Snuff Box Pain

Pain over the anatomical snuffbox suggests scaphoid bone fracture (wrist), even with a negative x-ray. In fact, a negative x-ray is quite common.

Adding Salt and Pepper

One way to memorize the Salter Harris classification is as follows:

S Type 1   **S**traight through the physis, separated

A Type 2   **A**bove the growth plate

L Type 3   **L**ower-through the lower portion

T Type 4   **T**otally through the metaphysis, growth plate and epiphysis

R Type 5   c**R**ush to remember this is a compression fracture.

The Skinny on Fat Pads

Should they mention the visibility of the **posterior** fat pad on x-ray of the elbow, it suggests fracture and accumulation of fluid. However, an anterior fat pad is a normal finding.

Regarding fat pads, remember **P** = **P**oor (**P**osterior) and **A** = **A**ll right (**A**nterior) fat pad.

SCFE (Slipped Capital Femoral Epiphysis)

"A teenage **male** (usually obese), with knee pain." The knee pain is actually referred hip pain. They may describe the hip as **extended and externally rotated**. SCFE can be diagnosed with x-ray.

SCFE could show up on the board exam as an x-ray. If you look at this once, it will be obvious on the exam. One hip will be normal and the other will look like an ice cream scoop falling off the cone. The ice cream scoop is the acetabular head.

SCFE can occur with various endocrinopathies. Keep this in mind when there are any lab values included in the history, especially those that are endocrine-related. **Keep hip pathology in mind with any description of knee pain on the Boards**. This typically presents as knee pain!

SCFE is treated with immobilization, no weight bearing, and stabilization with pins and/or bone grafts.

Subluxation of the Patella

This is typically due to indirect trauma. Watch for a description of a "pop" after a change in direction off a pivoted knee. On physical exam they will describe pain over the lateral aspect of the patella, with possible deformity over the medial aspect. This may represent patellofemoral instability.

Developing and maintaining quadriceps and hamstring strength, as well as flexibility, is the management take home point for such a case.

Intoeing

There are 3 causes of intoeing

> 1. Metatarsus adductus in infancy
> 2. Tibial torsion in toddlerhood
> 3. Femoral anteversion in early childhood

Tibial torsion is one of the causes of in-toeing, a.k.a. Pigeon Toeing. Tibial torsion and femoral anteversion almost always resolve spontaneously, which is the answer they are seeking on the boards.

The use of bars and other devices has not been shown to correct natural "in-toeing." Most will resolve by school age.[8]

Neither Dennis Browne bars, sleeping on the back, sleeping in bars, Buster Brown® shoes, nor the dog that lives in the Buster Brown® shoes[9] is the answer they are looking for. The good news is that some of the fastest runners in the world have in-toeing.

ALL infants have physiologic femoral anteversion.

Polydactyly

Although polydactyly can be associated with various syndromes, it is usually an isolated autosomal dominant trait. In fact, if you encounter such a patient in real life, you will often note that the parents had an extra digit surgically removed.

You are expected to know the basic management of polydactyly. With simple postaxial polydactyly (which occurs off the 5th finger/toe and amounts to little more than a skin tag), surgical transection/removal is sufficient.

For the simplest form of postaxial polydactyly (type B), tying off or transection of a small skin tag may be sufficient. For more complicated cases involving bone, soft tissues, and tendons, referral to a hand surgeon may be necessary.

---

[8] Our podiatry colleagues vacationing at Club Foot state otherwise, but they aren't writing Pediatric Board questions.

[9] Most of you are too young to remember Buster Brown shoes. Google it.

Chapter 25

Skin Deep: Dermatology

The old summary of the field of Dermatology - "if it's dry, wet it; if it's wet, dry it; and if all else fails, use steroids" - could apply to any field in medicine.

The Dermatology section, more than any other, will require you to follow along with a good atlas. You can also review this in "Pictures Worth 100 Points" by Medhumor Medical Publications, LLC which contains schematics and drawings of many important dermatological findings covered on the exam. We provide the key points and differences on which to focus your attention while reading the atlas.

"Just going through it" won't work. Terms like "vulgaris" don't need translation. However, much of Dermatology is Latin based; for example, ichthyosis means "fish skin." For those who do not have the time to take a quick Podcast™-based course in Latin or have access to somebody who has, we present you with the basics.

There will be many dermatology questions that are not depicted as a picture. In these cases, you will need to recognize the disorder or symptoms of a larger disorder based on the key words in the clinical history. This is the focus of this chapter.

Puffing up: Neonatal Pustular Lesions

Neonatal Herpes

Neonatal herpes could be described as **clustered or grouped vesicles on an erythematous base.**

IV acyclovir would be the treatment if this were suspected. **Wright stain** would contain **multinucleated giant cells and eosinophilic intranuclear inclusions.**

Lesions frequently appear on the buttocks or scalp. Watch for lesions that were not present at birth, or the mention in the question of the use of a scalp pH monitor.

If they tell you the infant's mother has a history of herpes, they are probably trying to trick you. Most cases of neonatal herpes occur without a known history of maternal herpes.

Incontinentia pigmenti would also present as vesicles, but in a **linear pattern without an erythematous base**.

Neonatal Pustular Melanosis

"**Multiple pustules, brown macules, vesicles, and pustules on a non-erythematous base**" is your phrase. Tzanck smear will show sheets of neutrophils. It is usually described in an African American infant. Another possible buzz word would be " leaving a collarette".

No treatment is necessary. Think pustular "Leave-Em-Alone-osis".

Neonatal Pustular Melanosis vs. Staph Infection

Benign Neonatal Pustular Melanosis is a benign eruption that, if present, is **usually present at birth**. This will be described as **pustules** and **hyperpigmented macules** with **peripheral scale**, usually seen in African American infants.

If the rash starts out as pustules, they generally become hyperpigmented macules within a few days. Gram stain or Wright stain will show PMNs *without organisms*.

A **staph infection**, usually involving hair follicles, will reveal both PMNs and gram-positive cocci on gram stain.

Erythema Toxicum Neonatorum

Erythema Toxicum Neonatorum, often known as **E-Tox**, is a very common rash seen in newborns. It is benign, only requiring reassurance.

"Yellow pustules with erythematous base," and "erythematous macules" in the center, along with a description of a *solitary papule* or "*occasional vesicle*" is how erythema toxicum neonatorum will likely be phrased. The rash is frequently **not** present at birth.

Wright stain will reveal eosinophils, which makes sense: **E** Tox and **E**osinophils both begin with the letter "E." Tzanck smear will also show eosinophils and perhaps some neutrophils, but otherwise it will be negative. The rash is benign and will typically fade within 5-7 days.

E. Tox does not appear on the palms or soles. In addition, it is rarely seen in preterm newborns. Remember that it is not present at birth — this is important in differentiating it from other newborn rashes, especially on the boards.

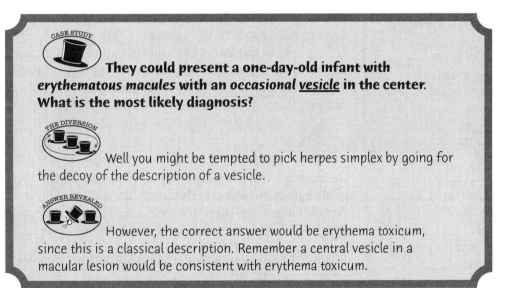

They could present a one-day-old infant with *erythematous macules* with an *occasional <u>vesicle</u>* in the center. What is the most likely diagnosis?

Well you might be tempted to pick herpes simplex by going for the decoy of the description of a vesicle.

However, the correct answer would be erythema toxicum, since this is a classical description. Remember a central vesicle in a macular lesion would be consistent with erythema toxicum.

Cutaneous Candidiasis

Cutaneous candidiasis will present as **diffuse scaling** and **erythematous papules** and **pustules**.

Dry Scaly Skin

Eczema

By definition, eczema is a rash that involves erythema, edema, vesicle formation, exudate, and scaling.

Technically speaking, even though the two are used interchangeably by physicians, atopic dermatitis and eczema are not synonymous. Nummular eczema and contact dermatitis would be considered forms of "non-atopic eczema."

Atopic Dermatitis

Pulling Your Footing

If you are presented with patient who has a rash on the foot, it is very easy to slip up and immediately pick tinea pedis (or "athlete's foot," as it is called in the locker room).

Tinea pedis will be described as a pruritic rash with scaling and peeling. It will involve the plantar aspect and sometimes the lateral aspect of the foot. However, the dorsal aspect will be spared. There will typically be maceration.

Atopic dermatitis *that involves the foot will be scaly, but instead of maceration will be described as being dry, with lichenification. The dorsal aspect of the foot will be involved.*

"Lichenification with scratching" is a key phrase that tells you they are talking about *atopic dermatitis*. They could describe a distribution pattern **behind the knees** and **elbows** with dry and chapped hands. **Itching is an important component of atopic dermatitis.** In toddlers they will likely describe the rash as appearing on the antecubital and popliteal fossas. This is because older children tend to scratch these areas.

Heredity plays a big role. If the family history is emphasized in the question, then they are pointing you to atopic dermatitis. The mention of **allergic rhinitis** and **asthma** are classic co-existing conditions. If both parents have any of these disorders, and if they should happen to mention a **high IgE** level in the cord blood, you have been given a gift. Unwrap it.

Factors that can worsen atopic dermatitis include chemical irritants, heat, physical trauma, and drying elements.

Food and Atopic Dermatitis

Food can be a factor. With a subset of patients, skin testing will identify a specific food allergy. Their eczema will flare up after eating this food. When presented with an infant with eczema, there is up to a 30% chance that food allergy is a factor. Milk, eggs, soy, wheat, and peanuts are likely culprits.

Negative testing helps rule out a food allergy, but a positive result is not as accurate (this type of testing has a lower positive predictive value).

Eliminating these foods is not usually recommended, since food allergy is not a factor in up to 70% of cases of atopic dermatitis. Unnecessary food elimination is not recommended because of the potential negative impact on nutrition.

Breast-feeding for at least 3 months may delay the development of eczema.

Superinfection and Atopic Dermatitis

With eczema that is not improving with emollients and high potency steroids, consider a **superinfection** as the reason. Just remember not to ever use the word "superinfection" when talking to a patient.

Watch for a description of multiple pustules that are oozing and crusting, in the context of eczema that is not responding to usual treatment modalities.

Treatment should be directed to *Staph aureus*.

Eczema Herpeticum

As the name implies, this is invasion of eczematous skin by herpes. If they describe **inflamed eczema which is not responding to antibiotics**, consider this diagnosis if it is among the choices. Of course, if the words **"vesicular lesions"** appear, this is where they are leading. The classic description will include the words **"vesicles"** and **"crusted erosions."** This often occurs on the face, in which case it is usually a primary herpes infection. It is also seen in the occasional young child who sucks his/her thumb or finger. Management includes confirmation with a Tzanck smear and treatment with acyclovir.

Nummular Eczema

This typically presents as coin-shaped plaques on the extensor surfaces of the extremities. It is usually due to dry skin, and responds to topical steroids.

Allergic Contact Derm Trick

Because it requires multiple exposures, they may try to trick you by stating that the child has "worn this necklace for years," etc. It can still be allergic contact dermatitis.

Other Considerations:

Remember to consider **Wiskott–Aldrich Syndrome** if they also note evidence of a possible immunodeficiency. Likewise, **hyperimmunoglobulin E syndrome** can present with eczema. **Scabies** can present with an eczematous picture; however, distribution on the palms and soles and presentation of other family members with a similar rash will be your clues that they are talking about scabies.

Seborrheic Dermatitis

This could be described as **greasy yellow patches** on the **scalp[1]**, **face**, and **skin folds during the first 2 months of life**. There can also be post-auricular lesions.

If you are required to choose a treatment, topical antifungal agents or mild topical steroids would be appropriate.

If they include other features like profuse ear discharge and/or profuse urine output, then consider histiocytosis X.

Contact Dermatitis

As noted above, contact dermatitis, technically speaking, is a form of eczema. It is divided into two types: **allergic** and **primary irritant.**

Allergic contact dermatitis

This is a delayed hypersensitivity reaction that requires multiple exposures. It results in a rash, which is red, vesicular, and sometimes crusting. Jewelry and poison ivy are typical examples.

Primary irritant contact dermatitis

Here there is no delay in reaction. Soaps and detergents are typical agents that can trigger this reaction.

---

[1] Cradle Cap.

Poison Ivy

Poison ivy would typically be described as linear vesicles and papules.

It is a Type 4 reaction. This is easy to remember because **IV** is the Roman numeral for 4. The rash and reaction can spread for several days. However, it is not contagious.

The rash may be prevented or made less severe by washing with soap and water immediately after exposure. In severe cases, oral steroids may be required for up to 21 days.

There are lots of myths around poison ivy that are ripe for diversionary tactics on the exam. Keeping the following facts in mind will be worth at least a point or two:

· Exposure to poison ivy during the winter **can** result in a rash.

· Fluid from the vesicles does not spread the rash.

· Once the chemical sap from the plant is removed from clothes, the rash does not spread.

· Barrier preparations can protect from exposure, but there are no desensitization treatments available.

Psoriasis (the Heartbreak of)

They could describe or show "**silvery**" lesions on the **elbows** or **knees** or scaly lesions on the scalp or even the groin. When these silvery plaques are picked off, or come off, they leave behind "bleeding spots" the size of pins: this is called **Auspitz sign.** Perhaps they will describe some blood where the rash has been scratched and/or picked off. Typical buzzwords could include: "**erythematous plaques surrounded by thick adherent scales**," "**pinpoint areas of hemorrhage**," and/or "**thick scales on the scalp.**"

Psoriasis needs to be differentiated from rashes that can sound quite similar to it when described. If you pay close attention to the buzzwords, you will not be misled. Follow the bouncing Auspitz sign:

· **Non-bullous impetigo** – could be described as *oozing* and *crusting (*unless they are describing your infected fingers from biting your nails to the quick while studying).

· **Nummular eczema** – could be described as *round, oozing, crusting erosions, and dry macules with a fine scaly pattern.*

- **Pityriasis rosea** – could be described as **small oval, thick scaling plaques,** with the **long axis of the lesions parallel to the lines of skin stress.**

- **Tinea corporis** – will present with scaly lesions; however, they will be described as being **thin** rather than thick, with **central clearing.**

Pityriasis Rosea

Look for the catchphrases "**winter and early spring,**" and/or "**scaly patch on the trunk.**" They could show or describe the classic **herald patch.** The rash follows skin folds in a "Christmas tree" pattern.

There is no treatment except for exposure to the sun or other light.

This is easy to remember when you think of "Christmas lights," and link that to the Christmas tree pattern of the rash.

Additional buzzwords would include: "**small oval**" and "**thick scaling plaques,**" with the **long axis of the lesions parallel to the lines of skin stress (you knew that already).**

The palms and soles of the feet are spared in pityriasis rosea.

Pityriasis can be confused with, and must be distinguished from, the following other rashes:

- **Secondary Syphilis** – The rash may appear similar, but patients with secondary syphilis will also present with **fever** and **generalized lymphadenopathy.** Secondary syphilis often involves the palms and soles of the feet.

- **Nummular eczema** and **Tinea Corporis** – The herald patch can be confused with these two other rashes. So keep in mind that tinea corporis will be described as having an *elevated border with central clearing.* Nummular eczema will be described as *crusting erosions,* which will distinguish it from the herald patch of pityriasis rosea.

- **Tinea Versicolor** – may mimic pityriasis because of a similar distribution on the trunk and back. This rash, rather than being described as plaques, will be described as **hyper- or hypo-pigmented scaling macules.**

Ichthyosis Vulgaris (Ugly Fish Skin)

 A typical description of ichthyosis vulgaris would be dry skin with **thin scales that have a pasted-on appearance,** just as you would expect fish skin to be described. It usually presents during the preschool years.

Treatment is with **keratolytic agents,** like **ammonium lactate** creams. In addition, **alpha hydroxy acid** and **urea-containing emollients** would be correct choices.

50% will also have atopic dermatitis, so don't be fooled by that red herring (pun absolutely intended).

Swimming Pool Granuloma

They could describe or show a papular lesion on the sole of the foot in a child walking barefoot. It is caused by **atypical mycobacteria.**

Tinea Corporis

The important point to remember here is to distinguish "ringworm" from "granuloma annulare." Annulare is not scaly and tinea is.

CASE STUDY

You are presented with an 8-year-old girl who has a pruritic rash on the soles of her feet. Symptoms of the rash include minimal scaling, thickening of the skin, and hyper-linearity of the distal soles. The interdigital skin is normal. You have to choose the proper treatment.

THE DIVERSION

It might be quite tempting to assume this is athlete's foot, or tinea pedis, and pick an anti-fungal cream such as clotrimazole or miconazole. But if you did that, you would have picked the wrong answer and the patient would still be picking at her feet.

ANSWER REVEALED

The key to answering this question correctly is noting the minimal scaling and noting that the interdigital skin is not involved. In addition, athlete's foot rarely occurs before puberty. This rules out tinea. The description is of **juvenile plantar dermatosis**, which is a form of contact dermatitis. It is a result of occlusive shoes and synthetic socks. Appropriate treatment is with a steroid cream such as **triamcinolone**.

Granuloma Annulare

EITHER OR CHOICES

The key phrase is **"non-scaling"** – look for this (and write it out in the margin!!) This tells you it isn't ringworm.

Should they want more information, granuloma annulare (GA) is a benign inflammatory condition that manifests as annular lesions *without epidermal involvement.* We really don't know what causes it.

EITHER OR CHOICES

Swimming pool granuloma presents with a break in the skin; with **granuloma annulare** there won't be a break.

Infectious rashes

Impetigo

This can be caused by *Strep* or *Staph.* However, you are expected to know that *Staph aureus* is the most likely cause of both bullous impetigo and crusted impetigo.

PERIL WARNING **Treatment of the *Strep* skin infection does not prevent post-strep GN.**

> The most likely cause of a skin and soft tissue infection following a child stepping on a nail is *Pseudomonas aeruginosa*, not *Staph.*

Staphylococcal Scalded Skin Syndrome (and other Skin Disorders that can "Burn" you)

You will need to know about several skin disorders that are easily confused with each other. Here are the distinguishing points of each.

Staphylococcal Scalded Skin Syndrome (SSSS; AKA Ritter's Disease)

BUZZ WORDS This is typically described in a preschooler. It starts out very tender and red, and spreads to become a "**sheet-like loss of skin,**" with erythema and tenderness. A **toxin** causes all of this, and antibiotics are the treatment of choice.

PERIL WARNING They may throw in earlier treatment with an antibiotic to lead you into thinking it is erythema multiforme.

Erythema Multiforme

DEFINITION Erythema multiforme is a *hypersensitivity reaction* in response to a variety of triggers. There are two forms: erythema multiforme minor and major.

Erythema Multiforme Major

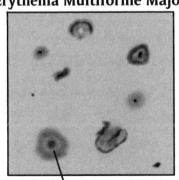

©Medhumor Medical Publications, LLC

Pathognomonic target lesion

Erythema Multiforme Minor

Rarely will a child younger than 3 present with erythema multiforme minor. It is typically triggered by an infection or medication. The most likely trigger will be a primary or recurrent infection with **Herpes Simplex.** The rash appears abruptly; it starts on the extremities and then spreads to the trunk. It will often be described as "edematous macules."

Treatment is geared toward the triggering agent, i.e., stopping the medication or treating the illness (for example, acyclovir would be administered if HSV is the trigger).

> **You could be presented with a child who, after completing an antibiotic regimen, develops a rash on the distal extremities described as "maculo-papular, with some lesions appearing to be *dusky* in the center." There may be 1-2 lesions on the mouth. The child is otherwise well *appearing*. What is the diagnosis?**
>
> Well, with what sound like target lesions, 1-2 lesions appearing on the mouth, and a recent course of antibiotics, you might be tempted to pick erythema multiforme major, or Stevens Johnson syndrome.
>
> However, the description given in this vignette (especially the fact that the child is *well appearing*) makes the correct diagnosis erythema multiforme minor, not major.

Erythema Multiforme Major

Erythema multiforme major is Stevens Johnson Syndrome[2]. On the extreme of the erythema multiforme major spectrum is Toxic Epidermal Necrolysis (TEN).

Stevens Johnson Syndrome

With Stevens Johnson Syndrome, the rash is preceded by fever, muscle aches, and joint aches. Initially the rash is similar to EM minor, but it spreads more quickly, progressing from primarily

---

[2] There is controversy about whether EMM is more related to herpes and distinct from SJS. It all depends on whom you ask or what book you read, so hopefully they will not hold you responsible for such a fine difference. After all, these are the pediatric boards, not the dermatology boards.

cutaneous to **mucous membrane involvement,** including **conjunctiva, oral mucosa, and anogenital mucosa.** The lesions involving the mucosa frequently become encrusted.

Typical medications triggering EM major are sulfa drugs, anticonvulsants, and NSAIDs.

Treatment is geared toward infection and dehydration, and patients are frequently managed in burn units.

The typical **bullous or target lesions** are classic. The lesions are typically discrete and sometimes coalesce. There is no separation of the skin in sheets as there is in scalded skin syndrome.

Toxic Epidermal Necrolysis (TEN)

This is considered by some sources to be the most severe form of erythema multiforme major. Other sources call it a separate entity. Hopefully you would not be called upon to make such a distinction on the exam. Here, too, the sunburn-like erythema and sheet-like separation of skin can be seen. In addition to the lesions described above, one would see **widespread bullae** as well as **denuded necrotic skin.**

If they ask you how to distinguish scalded skin syndrome from TEN, the answer is biopsy. That is because **TEN involves the dermis (as does Stevens Johnson) and SSSS usually does not**. In fact, if they show exfoliating skin that is not red, then the answer will be SSSS; if it IS red, then TEN is the answer.

Erythema Multiforme and TEN have **E's** in them to remind you of the **E**rythema.

You will be expected to differentiate TEN from Staphylococcal Scalded Skin Syndrome (SSSS). The most important point to remember is that SSSS will appear or be described as white, since it only affects the upper epidermis. TEN, on the other hand, involves the full thickness of the epidermis and is therefore red (thus the name).

In addition, SSSS usually affects infants and younger children, whereas TEN involves older children. Mortality is much higher for TEN than for SSSS.

Toxic Dumps

The following are caused by **toxin-producing bacteria**:

Staph Scalded Skin Syndrome	Due to an exotoxin produced by *Staph aureus*
Toxic Shock Syndrome	Caused by toxin production either by *S. aureus* or *Strep*; the mortality of *Strep* TSS is much higher than *Staph* TSS
Scarlet Fever	Also due to a toxin caused by *Strep*[3]

 Toxic epidermal necrolysis (TEN) is **not** due to a toxin despite its name. It is a hypersensitivity reaction.

TEN: Picture somebody whose skin is hypersensitive to dimes.

Pyoderma Gangrenosum

 Key descriptions include **"boggy" and "blue" ulcers with a necrotic base**. It is usually associated with a systemic disease.

Toxic Shock Syndrome presents with fevers, hypotension, and rash. Any kid who comes in with a sepsis-like picture (i.e., fevers and hypotension) and a rash should make you consider TSS. Even though tampons do NOT cause most cases of TSS anymore, they may imply its use in the question (e.g., by noting the Tanner staging in an adolescent girl in septic shock).

Treatment is with antibiotics and aggressive supportive care.

Cellulitis

Cellulitis will be described in a **febrile child** with a tender, **well-demarcated area of erythema** and **induration containing several bullae.** The most common causes are *Strep pyogenes* and *Staph aureus*.

---

[3] It is caused by an erythrogenic exotoxin produced by Group A strep. It occurs most commonly in association with Strep pharyngitis.

Treatment will depend on several factors as follows:

· Mild cases can be treated with topical mupirocin.

· If the cellulitis is more advanced or if they note that MRSA is prevalent in the community, then the following would be indicated: clindamycin, trimethoprim-sulfamethoxazole, or doxycycline (in a child older than 8).

· Cephalexin or amoxicillin-clavulanate may be used empirically if there is low likelihood of MRSA.

Pests of Life (Scabies, Lice and Other Creatures)

Scabies

The key descriptors are "**linear lesions**" that are "**papular**" or "**pustular**," which do not respond to antibiotic treatment. Additional descriptions might include **erythematous papules, some crusted, on the volar aspects of the wrists, axilla,** and **groin.** They may or may not note involvement between the digits.

The absence of symptoms in family members does not rule out scabies.

Diagnosis is usually clinical, but can be confirmed by identifying mites and eggs in skin scrapings. Infestation with the scabies mite causes intense itching (pruritus), and is highly contagious. The S-shaped track (burrow) on the skin is pathognomonic.

Scabies is treated with **permethrin cream (Elimite®).** All household contacts must be treated as well.

Scabies in infants can appear on the palms and soles of the feet.

Lindane (Kwell®) is potentially neurotoxic and not as effective as permethrin. All family members must be treated with **Permethrin 5%** (Elimite®) regardless of their symptoms. This is the treatment of choice for both *adults* and *infants*.

Scabies leaves track marks; they can be **stopped with a "permanent train" (permethrin).**

Head Lice

Head lice will typically be described in 1-2 children in the same family, possibly with excoriation on the nape of the neck and/or behind the ears. They will describe nits on the hair shafts as "white dots that cannot be removed." Don't expect them to mention that classmates were diagnosed; that would be too easy.

The treatment consists of *permethrin cream rinse*, which should be repeated a week after the first application. *Malathion* is another treatment option. The house should be thoroughly cleaned, and close household contacts should be treated as a preventive measure. *Asymptomatic classmates do not need to be treated.*

Lindane is no longer a first line treatment due to potential neurotoxicity.

Even after successful treatment, itching can continue. *This does not constitute treatment failure.* ***It represents an inflammatory reaction, and this can be treated with steroid creams.*** Severe itching may also be helped with diphenhydramine or hydroxyzine.

Head Lice vs. Crabs

While head lice are common in children, pubic crab lice are not. **Pubic lice is strongly suggestive of sexual abuse.**

If they describe **maculae caeruleae (which are blue-gray macules on the abdomen or inner thigh)**, this is a clinical sign consistent with pubic lice.

Believe it or not, you are expected to know about the life cycle of the crab louse and the (plural) crab lice. You are expected to know several exciting facts about these fascinating creatures, including the following:

- **They can last 36 hours without a blood meal**
- **Fresh eggs on hair shafts can hatch 10 days later**
- **Despite their name, pubic lice can also exist in other locations, such as on facial hair[4]**
- **Pubic lice are much slower moving than head lice**
- **Pubic lice impact all races equally, while head lice rarely infest African-Americans.**

---

[4] Insert your own inappropriate or perverse joke here.

Treatments of choice for pubic lice are

· **Permethrin 1%**
· **Pyrethrin with piperonyl butoxide**
· **Permethrin 5%**

Alternatives:

· **Malathion** (flammable, irritating to the groin and expense makes it irritating to the wallet)
· **Lindane** (toxic if swallowed or applied incorrectly, contraindicated in pregnancy and in neonates)

 For crabs in the eyelashes, petroleum jelly applied three times a day for 10 days is often sufficient treatment.

Molluscum Contagiosum

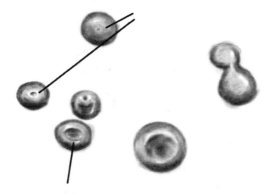 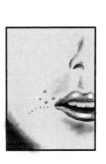

 If they show or describe "pearly papules with central dimpling," think of molluscum contagiosum. It often occurs on the back, but can also appear around the eyes and other parts of the body.

 No therapy is needed; it will clear in months to years.

Remember, a clam is a mollusk, so picture a small clam attaching to a child's back.

Molluscum is differentiated from warts and comedones by the central umbilication. In addition, Wright staining will reveal viral inclusion bodies.

Papular Urticaria

 Here they could describe or show "pink and excoriated" pruritic lesions on the **extensor surfaces** of the arms and legs. They are frequently described as **episodic** and **"erupting at night."** They could also be described as **clustered erythematous papules** with a **central punctum. They could present as recurrent papules lasting up to 10 days.**

 No other family members are affected, differentiating this from scabies.

 Papular urticaria is due to a delayed hypersensitivity reaction to an insect bite.

 Don't expect them to trace it to an individual insect bite or suggest the history of one. They won't. *However, the correct answer for the best management is to identify the "causative" agent* (so the family can then go about the business of eliminating the causative agent).

 There are several rashes that can be easily confused with papular urticaria; however, with close attention to the descriptive buzzwords, you won't be fooled into picking the wrong answer.

- **Non-bullous impetigo** – could be described as **honey colored crusted lesions** that are **not recurrent or episodic.**

- **Molluscum contagiosum** – could be described as **translucent papules** with **central umbilication**. There will not be any period with complete absence of lesions, unlike papular urticaria.

- **Scabies** – appears as **small papules** that *do not appear in clusters.*

They could present you with a toddler who has a 2 month history of a recurrent pruritic rash of clustered erythematous papules. They focus on the recurrent rash and its pruritic quality and throw in that "nobody else in the family is similarly affected."

It will be very tempting to pick the diversionary choice, scabies, chalking up the absence of symptoms in other family members as a deliberate attempt to throw you off track. After all, haven't we all seen cases of scabies where only one family member is affected, at least on initial history? Resist all temptations to scratch that irresistible itch, since this is the boards and no history means <u>no</u> history.

The correct diagnosis is papular urticaria.

Acrodermatitis Enteropathica/Zinc Deficiency

If they show you a child with perioral dermatitis with alopecia, consider *acrodermatitis enteropathica*. It is an inherited condition where zinc is not absorbed well.

A typical presentation is an infant who has an extensive eczematous eruption and is growing poorly. The lesions are typically around the mouth and perhaps in the perianal area.

Picture a RED SINK (ZINC) replacing a mouth (perioral dermatitis). The drain of the sink is clogged with hair, to help you link this to alopecia.

It is autosomal **recessive**.

To distinguish this from eczema, acrodermatitis enteropathica has no lichenification. (Lichenification is a classic word associated with eczema).

Biotin deficiency can present with a similar picture (oral rash and alopecia). However, with biotin deficiency, **ataxia** is also part of the picture.

Acne Vulgaris

This section is full of myths and misconceptions perpetuated not only by the general public but also by physicians.

Acne appears on the chest, back, and face, primarily in teens, although it could appear as early as 8 years of age.

It is important to first gain an understanding of what acne is. Once demystified, it will be easy to answer all questions on acne correctly.

There are 4 primary stages of acne development:

1. Abnormal follicle keratinization and obstruction of hair follicles
2. Excessive production of sebum
3. Bacterial proliferation[5]
4. Inflammation

Let's take a closer look.

Abnormal follicle keratinization and obstruction of hair follicles

Abnormal follicle keratinization and obstruction of hair follicles begins with the plugging of the follicle and thickening of the epithelial lining — thus begins the heartache of the teen years (well, at least one of the heartaches of the teen years). In addition, this results in the **microcomedone.**

Excessive production of sebum

Sebum is produced in response to *androgen* production, which is the case in both males and females. This forms a plug, resulting in the "mature" **comedones** seen in more mature teenagers.

---

[5] For those who are really into genus and species names, it is formally known as *Propionibacterium acnes*.

Bacterial proliferation

This is the perfect environment for proliferation of the archenemy of teenagers everywhere: *Propionibacterium acnes*.

Inflammation

While the *Propionibacterium acnes* bacteria does not trigger many "compliments" regarding the teen's appearance, it does trigger the "complement pathway," resulting in inflammation.

Acne vulgaris[6] is divided into 2 major categories, which have additional subcategories. It is important to note these, since treatment is different and will separate the "haves" (passing grade) from the "have nots" (those taking the exam again). Let's go to the blackboard vulgaris.

Acne is divided into inflammatory and non-inflammatory.

Non-inflammatory

Non-inflammatory consists of **comedones** as follows:

Closed Comedones

Closed comedones ("**whiteheads**") are follicles that are plugged but are covered with epithelium.

Open Comedones

Open comedones are "**blackheads**," which have no epithelial covering.

The black color comes from melanin, not dirt (which is a common misconception). This, like any myth, can come back to haunt you during the exam.

The appearance of comedones prior to age 8 could be a sign of precocious puberty. If this is presented to you on the exam, routine management of acne is not what they are after.

---

[6] I believe this is Latin for nasty.

Endocrine workups are not warranted for acne unless there is evidence of hirsutism or menstrual dysfunction, in which case a workup for polycystic ovary disease would be indicated.

Inflammatory Acne (the good, the bad, and the papule)

These consist of papules, pustules, and nodules (cysts)

Papules

 Papules are small, red, solid lesions.

Adenoma sebaceum can be mistaken for acne. If "acne" is placed in quotes, then you are likely being presented with adenoma sebaceum, which are also known as angiofibromas. These are small papules that are firm and may appear pink, red, or brown (or somewhere in between) in color.

This is especially the case with "acne" that is resistant to treatment, often on the nose and cheeks.

Pustules

 Pustules are superficial and are filled with pus.

Nodules (cysts)

These are much deeper, located in the dermis, and are red and painful. These can lead to permanent scarring.

If they were to get very technical, these cysts are *not true cysts.*

 Neonatal acne requires no treatment. **Systemic steroids** can lead to acne. This appears primarily on the trunk, and they would have to give a history of a disorder where systemic steroids would be used (in order to point you in this direction). **Anticonvulsants** such as phenobarbital and phenytoin (Dilantin®) can lead to acne as well.

Chocolate does not cause or accelerate acne, despite popular belief.

Treatment

 Treatment depends on:

- Type of lesions
- Age of the patient
- Distribution of the lesions

 Acne is not caused by poor hygiene or improper bathing habits. For psychological reasons they expect you to know that teens need to be reassured that this is a normal part of growth and development.

Vigorous scrubbing and squeezing of pimples can lead to permanent scarring.

Topical Treatments

Benzoyl peroxide

Benzoyl peroxide is primarily *bacteriocidal.* It can be irritating to the skin, but this can be reduced if the right formulation is used.

Topical antibiotics

Topical antibiotics, in addition to being *bacteriocidal,* are also *anti-inflammatory.* Topical clindamycin and erythromycin are the most commonly used topical antibiotics. They are used primarily for *inflammatory acne.*

Azelaic acid cream

Azelaic acid cream is used to treat mild acne, color changes secondary to inflammation, and comedones.

Tretinoin

Tretinoin, derived from vitamin A, can play an important role in *preventing acne* by halting the process that plugs hair follicles.

 Topical tretinoin can result in an "initial flare-up" of acne.

Systemic Treatment of Acne

PO Antibiotics

Like topical antibiotics, PO antibiotics have anti-inflammatory qualities. The use of oral antibiotics is reserved for *severe inflammatory acne.* It is particularly effective against acne on the *trunk.* The most commonly used oral antibiotics are *tetracycline, doxycycline, and minocycline.*

Bacterial resistance is a problem, and therefore continued use would not be appropriate. The condition can be controlled, but oral antibiotics do not "cure" acne.

Oral Contraceptives

Because of the anti-androgenergic effects of estrogen, OCP's have been helpful in treating severe acne.

This of course should only be used in female patients. Therefore, check the gender of the patient in the question. Picking OCP's for males would be a careless, costly error indeed.

Isotretinoin (Accutane®)

This powerful agent does it all:

- Antibacterial
- Reduces sebum production
- Anti-inflammatory
- Destroys comedones
- Some have claimed it even cleans windows and washes floors!

Isotretinoin is now used often in combination therapy (often alongside benzoyl peroxide), especially in patients with with multiple inflammatory lesions (since it helps reduce the formation of new lesions).

Check the wording of the question to see if there is a history of steroid use. This can sometimes worsen symptoms when taken at the same time. Remember to "rule out pregnancy" when isotretinoin (Accutane®) is prescribed. Pregnancy should be ruled out before, during, and after treatment.

 Side effects to be aware of include: dry lips, dry skin, dry eyes, nosebleeds, and headaches.[7]

 Androgen is responsible for acne in both males and females.

Alopecia Hairpecia

You need to identify different hair loss patterns. This is Pediatrics, so unless the question is about the funny Canadian on *Whose Line is it Anyway*, "male pattern baldness" will not be one of the correct choices. There are only a limited number of alopecia patterns you need to know.

Tinea Capitis

 "Black dots" or "broken hairs" are common descriptors. Additional descriptions would include kerions, which are tender boggy areas of induration. Fungal culture is the gold standard for diagnosis.

You will either be shown or have described for you some inflammation and bogginess of the surrounding tissue.

Tinea capitis is treated with PO griseofulvin for 6-12 weeks.

Routine labs prior to using griseofulvin are *not* necessary.

Alopecia Areata

This is easy to pick out because there will be no inflammation described or shown. The cause of alopecia areata is unknown.

---

[7] Similar to the side effects of studying for the Boards in dry, poorly aerated rooms.

CASE STUDY You are asked to evaluate a child with areas of "complete hair loss," with no other scalp lesions noted. Other than the alopecia just described and nail pitting, the rest of the physical exam is negative. The hair is tightly braided. What is the most likely diagnosis and treatment?

THE DIVERSION You will be very tempted to pick "hair braid alopecia" (aka traction alopecia) as the diagnosis and "unbraid the hair" as the correct treatment. If you do, you will be pulling your own hair out, because you just blew another easy question.

ANSWER REVEALED The correct answer, especially given the nail pitting, would be alopecia areata, and the management would simply be reassurance. If your reassurance doesn't cure it, the next step would be corticosteroids.

Telogen Effluvium

"Round patches," "well defined," and **complete areas of hair loss** are your buzzwords.

This is the sudden loss of large amounts of hair during routine activities such as washing and brushing the hair. It is often triggered by stressful events like a febrile illness, surgery, or emotional stress.[8]

 This is distinguished from other forms of hair loss in that there is no inflammatory reaction and the "telogen bulbs" can be seen under shedded hairs on microscopic exam.

Trichotillomania (Hair Pulling Mania)

"Irregular patches" of hair loss or **"incomplete"** patches of hair loss may be described. "Hair shafts of different lengths" is an important characteristic they might include, which would differentiate this from other forms of alopecia.

---

[8] Might be the explanation for any hair loss you experience while studying for the Boards.

Alopecia Totalis (Systemic Causes)

This consists of more than bald patches on the scalp. The "totalis" part says that all the rest of the hair will also be affected (think nutritional deficiencies, hypothyroidism, lupus, or other chronic diseases). This will include the absence of eyebrows as well. They will typically provide something in the description to tip you off.

Pigmented Lesions

Urticaria Pigmentosa

They may present this to you as **"pigmented lesions" that turn into hives and develop blisters, particularly *with rubbing*.** It is typically described in an infant during the first 6 months of life.

This is also called Darier Sign (easy to remember if you picture it occurring on the *derriere).*

No treatment is needed. However, if they ask, these infants should **avoid narcotic pain relievers, radiocontrast material, and NSAIDs.**

Tinea Versicolor

The classic description is **hypopigmented patches** that get **worse with exposure to the sun.** A fungus causes it, and KOH prep confirms the diagnosis.

Treatment is with **astringents** (to strip the superficial layers that are primarily involved) or **topical antifungal creams.** It can take a few months of sun deprivation to get rid of it. This is mortifying news for sun worshipping coastal teens.[9]

Oral *ketoconazole, fluconazole,* and *itraconazole* are also considered appropriate in certain situations and could be the correct answer they are looking for. *Topical selenium sulfide* is also acceptable.

---

[9] Support groups probably exist on Facebook for these sad adolescents.

Look at both tinea versicolor and ash leaf spots side by side in your atlas and know the distinguishing characteristics. With ash leaf, they will very likely include the other characteristics of tuberous sclerosis.

Xeroderma Pigmentosum

This is an **autosomal recessive disorder**. UV damaged DNA is not repaired (due to an enzyme deficiency); therefore, **vulnerability to skin cancer as well as metastatic disease is high**. The death rate in childhood is high. **Avoidance of UV light is a key to management**.

"Zero Derma Pigment Ton Sun." Zero skin pigment results in tons of sun getting through and, therefore, skin damage. To remember that it is recessive, picture the patient "receding" into the shade for protection.

Management is frequent evaluations for the appearance of malignancies.

Neurocutaneous Syndromes

Neurocutaneous Stuff

Sturge Weber

They could show what looks like splattered red wine (port wine stain) on the side of the face (in a trigeminal distribution). Additional signs of Sturge Weber syndrome could include **cognitive deficit** and/or **seizures.**

The port wine stain is often associated with a **venous leptomeningeal angiomatosis,** which needs to be identified by **MRI.**

The size of the port wine stain does <u>not</u> correlate with the extent of CNS involvement of the lesion. In fact, **one can have a venous leptomeningeal angiomatosis even when there is no skin lesion.**

The port wine stain itself is merely a cosmetic concern and can be treated by **tunable dye (pulsed dye) laser.**

Klippel Trenaunay Weber syndrome can also present with a port wine stain. However, the associated features are quite different.

Sturge Weber syndrome is associated with **glaucoma.**

Only 8% of those with facial port wine stain lesions have Sturge Weber syndrome. Clearly, this is higher if the port-wine stain is distributed along the branches of the trigeminal nerve.

Neurofibromatosis

Neurofibromatosis is a disorder with skin, CNS, and orthopedic manifestations. There are two types - think of Type 1 as more peripheral and mild, and Type 2 as central.[10]

The neurofibromas typically do not show up until after the onset of puberty. Lisch nodules may not show up until adulthood.

Neurofibromatosis Type 1: Von Recklinghausen Disease

Like a mix and match menu, two (2) of the following seven (7) criteria make the diagnosis of NF1:

- ❏ Café Au Lait Spots (6 or more, which may appear after birth).
  The spots must be >5 mm wide in kids
- ❏ Lisch Nodules (iris hamartomas – can only be seen on slit-lamp exam)
- ❏ Neurofibromas
- ❏ Optic Nerve Glioma
- ❏ Inguinal and Axillary Freckling
- ❏ Bony Defects
- ❏ Family History of NF1 (first-degree relative)

Remember, 2 out of 7 makes the diagnosis. However, for patients with a single clinical finding, there is a genetic test that can be confirmatory. But the mainstay of diagnosis remains clinical.

---

10 In fact, Type 2 is also sometimes known as central neurofibromatosis because of the higher incidence of meningiomas and acoustic neuromas.

Remember this is **Autosomal Dominant** (on chromosome 17), and an affected parent has a 50% chance of transmitting this to any one child. *However, 50% of the cases are due to spontaneous mutation.*

Despite the name, **neurofibromas** have nothing to do with the brain;[11] they are *skin lesions* that appear either on the surface (and are easily seen) or deep in the skin (and can only be found by palpation).

You give me Pheo

Kids with NF1 can get **pheochromocytoma** and **renal artery stenosis,** and need to be monitored often for hypertension. This is a concept that can be tested on the exam.

Change neurofibromatosis to "**Nero Finds a Toaster**" which rhymes with "Neurofibromatosis".[12]

- ❑ Picture Nero in a giant toga. He is playing the fiddle and drinking 6 cups of coffee (**Café Au Lait Spots).**
- ❑ The reason he can do so much at once is that he has bones shaped like giant platters **(Bony Defects).**
- ❑ He keeps playing and he can't see the fire because he has an **Optic Glioma.**
- ❑ Everyone leaves and the fire rages, working its way up so his skin begins to burn (beginning with **axillary freckling).**
- ❑ The freckles get bigger and bigger until they look like "Fish Nodules" – to remind you of "**Lisch Nodules.**" These fish are zoological wonders since their bodies are giant eyeballs (to remind you that **Lisch nodules occur in the eye**).
- ❑ This "Hot" situation is how Nero finds a "toaster." Look this over 5 times, writing it down (some of you might like to draw this to help keep this in long-term memory), and you will have this association locked in.

Neurofibromatosis Type 2

Remember, this is the subtype with the *acoustic neuroma, also known as schwannoma.*

One way to remember this is by imagining the **N** in **N**euroma as the number **2** on its side. It is also associated with chromosome 22.

---

[11] You, of course, knew that already, right?

[12] Nero, the Roman leader who played the fiddle while Rome burned.

Patients usually present with **hearing loss** or **tinnitus** related to their acoustic neuromas. However, **ocular symptoms** may dominate due to *cataracts* or *hamartomas of the retina.* Definitive diagnosis can be made by bilateral cranial nerve VIII masses on **CT or MRI**. Diagnosis can also be made by the presence of **family history** of NF2 along with schwannoma, neurofibroma, meningioma, glioma, or juvenile cataracts.

Picture someone with **2 Giant #2's** replacing their ears to remember that **acoustic neuromas are associated with NF2.**

Tuberous Sclerosis

I like to think of this as the "potato" disease since potatoes are tubers (which is how this was named in the first place). Once again, we use a mix and match menu, which is why there is often confusion with the other neurocutaneous syndromes. Diagnosis is made by the presence of two (2) or more of the following features:

❑ More than 3 **Ash Leaf Spots**

❑ **Periventricular/Cortical Tubers**

❑ **Sebaceous Gland Hyperplasia**

❑ **Shagreen Patch**

❑ **Sub/periungual Fibroma**

❑ **Cardiac Rhabdomyoma** –
  will develop in half the cases – especially seen in infants

❑ **Retinal nodular hamartomas**

❑ **Renal angiomyolipoma**

The adenoma sebaceum can often be mistaken for acne (vulgaris) and they will try to trip you up with that. Therefore, look for tuberous sclerosis hints in the question. Ash leaf macules can be the earliest signs of tuberous sclerosis.

Leather and Leafs

It is important to remember the typical findings, since they will be described or shown on the exam and their more formal terms will not be used.

Ash Leaf Spots – Hypopigmented skin (as in "ash" colored), also known as hypomelanotic macule

Sebaceous Gland Hyperplasia – Really adenomas, and is usually described or shown on the face

Shagreen Patch – Cobblestone appearing skin; shagreen is actually a type of leather that has an orange peel appearance. It would have been infinitely less confusing had they called it an orange peel patch, but confusion, not clarification, seems to be the order of the day

Periventricular/Cortical Tubers – These typically manifest as seizures

Hemangiomas

A hemangioma is a benign neoplasm made up of proliferative and hyperplastic vascular endothelium divided into 3 categories: superficial, deep, and mixed.

Superficial/ Capillary

Capillary hemangiomas, also known by their fruity moniker, **strawberry hemangiomas,** are located in the **upper dermis.**

The **strawberry hemangioma**, which is present at birth, gradually gets larger (as opposed to **Kasabach-Merritt syndrome,** which typically has abrupt onset). Strawberry hemangiomas often resolve completely by age 9 (or younger in many cases).

Treatment is only required when the hemangioma **interferes with vision, breathing, eating, hearing, or other normal functions.** Treatment consists of steroids and laser treatment.

Deep / Cavernous

Deep cavernous hemangiomas are located in the lower dermis, fat, and muscle.

Cavernous hemangiomas will often be **blue.**

Mixed

Mixed, as the name implies, are located in both levels.

Kasabach-Merritt Syndrome

This is a rapidly progressive hemangioma due to the sequestration of platelets into the lesion, resulting in low platelet counts and a vulnerability to bleeding.

Sun, Skin, and Melanoma

Malignant Melanoma

You may be questioned on skin lesions that should be investigated further. These are lesions that are 6 mm or larger, with asymmetric borders and/or irregular colors. Congenital melanocytic nevi are at risk for transformation into melanoma. Giant congenital nevi have the greatest risk for later transformation to melanoma.

The risk for melanoma is cumulative, with more sun exposure over time resulting in higher risk for malignant melanoma and other forms of skin cancer. Other risk factors include family history and fair complexion.

Erythema Confusiosum

I always had a hard time keeping my "erythema" rashes straight. Apparently I am not alone, and this may cause confusion on the exam if all of the "erythemas" are included among the choices.

Whenever I see the word "**erythema**" *fill in the blank* "**–osum,**" my eyes glaze over and everything tends to jumble together. Here is our primer for keeping it straight, so the words or pictures that go with them won't confuse you.

Erythema Multiforme

This is the one associated with Stevens Johnson syndrome. I picture Steve Johnson as someone with a BIG MOUTH who can get oral lesions, thus **Multi ORAL forme** (and that reminds me that other mucous membranes can be involved as well, e.g., anal and genital area). The **foot can also be involved**: with his big mouth, he is always **placing his foot in his mouth**. It starts with fever and other general symptoms.

Erythema Infectiosum

This is "**Fifth Disease:**" slapped cheek. Picture a giant red 5 on the face, which follows an "infection." This will be associated with Parvovirus B19. (Remember, Parvo has a **V** in it, which is the Roman numeral 5, for 5th Disease).

Erythema Chronicum Migrans

Erythema chronicum migrans (ECM) is associated with Lyme disease. Here Lyme disease is seen as a "**CAN**":

Carditis
Arthritis
Neuritis

The CAN "migrates all over the woods," thus chronicum migrans. The classic bullseye rash is present in 70% of cases.

Erythema Nodosum (No Doze em)

Erythema nodosum causes painful bluish lesions on the shin. (Thus, **No Doze,** because you can't sleep with painful shins). This is associated with TB, birth control pills, inflammatory bowel disease, and fungal infections.

Erythema Marginatum

This is associated with **rheumatic fever,** and is one of the major Jones criteria. It is an erythematous macule on the trunk, which clears centrally.

Chapter 26

Rheumatology: Rheum with a View

Driving Arthritis

Typically when you think of arthritis in children, you think JIA[1]. However, there are other conditions that cause arthritis. If you consider how difficult it would be to perform surgery with a thick leather glove, it will be easy to remember the mnemonic **GLOVE.**

Causes of Arthritis in children

GC (Gonorrhea), **G**enetic Syndromes
Lyme disease
Osteomyelitis
Viral (Toxic Synovitis)
Evasive infection (i.e. septic arthritis)

Don't forget that GC can manifest as arthritis. This is easy to forget.

Ankylosing Spondylitis

Ankylosing spondylitis (AS) *mainly* affects the sacroiliac joints, causing eventual *fusion of the spine.* The **HLA-B27 antigen is positive over 90% of the time.** It affects males primarily (3:1), can involve the **eye** (iritis, uveitis), and is also associated with inflammatory bowel disease.

In ankylosing spondylitis, ANA and RF should be **normal,** with a normal or mildly elevated **ESR.**

Look for the "bamboo spine" on plain film in a teenager with **night pain** and **morning stiffness relieved by exercise. Pain of large joints, such as the knee,** could also be a part of the presentation.

Ankylosing spondylitis can also present as a leg and back pain, which is increased when bending over. Systemic symptoms, including a low grade fever and weight loss, can be part of the presentation.

---

[1] JIA stands for juvenile idiopathic arthritis, formerly known as juvenile rheumatoid arthritis (JRA).

Treatment is with NSAIDS, sulfasalazine, and occasionally methotrexate.

Picture a **Giant Eye** replacing the sacroiliac joint to remember to associate AS with uveitis and iritis.

A good way to differentiate the pain of AS from mechanical low back pain is that the pain of AS should improve with activity and get worse with rest – the opposite being true of mechanical low back pain.

Behçet's Syndrome

Behçet's Syndrome is one of those syndromes that they will simply describe and then just come right out and ask you, "What is this?" Knowing the typical presentation will be worth a couple of points on the exam.

Children with Behçet's Syndrome have "**aphthous stomatitis**," "**genital ulcerations**," and "**uveitis**." They can also have other painful **GI ulcers** and **arthritis**.

ANA and Rh factor should be normal.

ESR and **C-reactive protein** will be elevated.

Systemic steroids are the mainstay of treatment.

Picture somebody eating a "long baguette" loaf of bread (=Behçet). They eat it (and get **stomatitis**) and hit themselves in the **eye** with the other end, and then drop it in their lap, causing **genital ulceration**.

Since herpes can also present with oral and genital lesions, in all fairness they should not include **herpes** as one of the choices. However, if they do, they need to include GI symptoms to help distinguish Behçet's from herpes.

Dermatomyositis

They will describe a school-aged kid, **younger than 10 years**. The classic description or picture will include the **"heliotrope" rash on the face,** similar to that found in lupus, as well as tight **shiny or scaly skin** on the **extensor surfaces of the extremities or over the interphalangeal joints** (Gottron's sign). The rash can be very itchy and, if on the scalp, may cause hair loss. They can also present with **periungual lesions**.

Dermatomyositis can frequently affect the esophagus and lungs, so don't miss these important clues.

The heliotrope rash might be described as a **violaceous discoloration of the malar region and/or eyelids.**

The periungual lesions might be described as **nail fold telangiectasias.**

Consider this diagnosis strongly if they present you with a patient who is now having "difficulty getting dressed or climbing steps," is "clumsy," or presents with "voice change" or "difficulty swallowing," along with some of the other signs noted.

Suppose they present you with a patient with the typical findings of dermatomyositis. You read through the entire question written in 0.0001 helvetica font and you are astute enough to make the diagnosis. Your diagnosis is confirmed when you complete the hellish task of reading through to the end of the novel, which they call a "question," when they give away the diagnosis and ask you for the most appropriate <u>initial</u> step in evaluating the patient.

You are down to 3 perfectly logical and seemingly correct choices: EMG, MRI, and creatine kinase levels. Which one is the most appropriate <u>initial</u> step?

EMG is a bit invasive and, therefore, not the correct initial choice. MRI is not an appropriate initial test. The most appropriate initial study, that is relatively non-invasive and readily available, is the creatine kinase level.

Diagnosis is based on clinical findings. However, if you were forced to make a choice on the exam regarding diagnosis, then the correct answer is **creatine kinase concentration.** EMG is also sometimes used, but it would usually not be the first step.

Dermatomyositis and **polyserositis** can have similar presentations. Remember, dermatomyositis has a typical rash and polyserositis does not.

Treating Dermatomyositis (showing door-mat-myositis the door)

Dermatomyositis is treated using high-dose steroids, often with methotrexate (or other immunosuppressives or cytotoxic agents) and IV gamma globulin. Antimalarials may also be used. Patients need to avoid sunlight and use sunscreen.

Ehlers-Danlos Syndrome

Typical presentation is skin that stretches and joints that are hypermobile like Spongebob Squarepants. These kids also have **poor wound healing,** so keep this diagnosis in mind if poor wound healing is included in the question.

Most types of Ehlers-Danlos Syndrome have a **normal life expectancy.**

"**Elbow Dancing** syndrome."

Lowe's syndrome is also associated with hypermobile joints. With Lowe's syndrome, there is also **blindness, intellectual disability,** and **hypotonia.**

Low tone, **Lower** ability, and **Lower level of vision** in Lowe's syndrome than Ehlers-Danlos syndrome.

Because of easy bruisability, Ehlers-Danlos can be mistaken for child abuse. Watch for the presentation of a child with multiple bruising and other manifestations of Ehlers-Danlos syndrome, to avoid being tricked into assuming child abuse.

Henoch Schönlein Purpura (HSP)

There are always several questions on HSP on the exam, so here are some critical points to remember:

HSP is a generalized **vasculitis** of the skin, **GI tract**, **joints**, and **kidneys**. The etiology is unknown, but it often has *an antecedent bacterial or viral infection*. Boys are affected twice as often as girls. The median age is 5 years.

The rash of "palpable purpura" (usually on the lower extremities and buttocks) is present in all cases of HSP. The colicky abdominal pain is also found in most cases, along with heme positive stools. Often intussusception is the cause of the abdominal pain. They may describe a **recent URI** or other viral illness. The **purpuric rash may blanch with pressure**. Additional signs could include "crampy abdominal pain," **hematuria**, and/or **proteinuria**.

In the labs, look for an elevated BUN and creatinine, heme positive stool, and a urinalysis with proteinuria and hematuria.

Intussusception is a potential complication in HSP, and when it occurs in an **ileoileal** location (versus the more typical **ileocolic** location), it makes detection and reduction by barium or air enema less likely.

This is **periarticular** disease - **not articular disease**. *Not knowing this fact can come back to haunt you on the exam.* Typically, the soft tissues around the **knees** and **ankles** are involved. In about a half of cases, there are also signs of kidney dysfunction.

Remember, there is **no thrombocytopenia,** so look for *a normal platelet count.* *This is often misdiagnosed as abuse;* however, HSP would be apparent from the remaining history.

Patients are usually admitted in order to watch for renal complications and to monitor for GI sequelae. There is no specific treatment – care is supportive only.

The rash of HSP can be mistaken for **erythema marginatum (seen in rheumatic fever).** Since they both also have joint pains, distinguishing them can be difficult.

The joint pain seen in rheumatic fever is more severe and a more prominent feature. In all fairness, they will have to present you with other signs consistent with rheumatic fever or HSP to allow you to make the correct choice. However, you need to know what these features are to answer correctly.

A salmon-colored evanescent rash can be seen with JIA; however, you won't typically see abdominal pain, and the rash will not be purpuric.

Juvenile Idiopathic Arthritis (JIA)

Juvenile Rheumatoid Arthritis has now joined the disease witness protection program and is now known as Juvenile Idiopathic Arthritis or JIA. It is basically a diagnosis of exclusion, and other diseases in the differential must be ruled out first. Other diagnoses to consider include:

Monoarticular disease: Can all be remembered as **beginning with L**

Lyme and other infections

Legg-Calve-Perthes disease

Leukemia and bone tumors

Polyarticular disease: Remember the word FIRE CAM

Fabry and **F**arber disease

Infections

Reactive arthritis (post strep, rheumatic fever, or serum sickness)

E lupus = SLE

Connective tissue disease: SLE, sarcoidosis, and vasculitis, as well as inflammatory bowel disease.

And

Malignancy (leukemia)

General Thoughts on JIA (You say Pauci and I say Oligo)

JIA is regarded not as a single disease, but a category of diseases with three principal types of onset:

(1) Oligoarthritis (formerly known as pauciarticular disease)

(2) Polyarthritis

(3) Systemic-onset disease

For all classifications, the age of onset must be less than 16 years of age, and symptoms must be present for at least 6 weeks in at least one joint.

 Large joint involvement is more common than involvement of small joints.

ANA is often positive, while nodules and positive RF are rare.

Girls are affected much more often than boys (except for systemic onset, in which the gender ratios are equal).

 JIA typically presents with "**morning stiffness**," "**gradual loss of motion,**" and a "**rash.**"

 Since there are loads of false positives, RF in and of itself is of no help in diagnosing JIA. They love to present a positive rheumatoid factor in disorders other than JIA.

 Rheumatoid factor is primarily helpful in distinguishing the subtypes of JIA

The following are the characteristics of the specific subtypes of JIA:

1. Polyarthritis

In **Polyarthritis** JIA, **5 or more joints** are affected.

The following guidelines should help you navigate whether you are seeing "face" of JIA Type 1 on the exam:

- Polyarthritis JIA occurs mostly in **females.**
- **Extraarticular involvement** occurs, but is not very common.
- Typically older patients will be RF+.
- With RF + cases, the disease tends to be more serious, with unremitting joint pain, erosions, and nodules.
- **Younger patients** who present with polyarticular disease tend to be **ANA positive** and have milder disease.
- *Systemic disease is uncommon in polyarticular JIA.*

2. Oligoarthritis/Pauciarthritis

In **Oligoarthritis** JIA, 4 or fewer joints are affected.

Remember the following facts regarding **oligoarthritis** JIA:

· Oligoarthritis is an **ANA-positive** disease in **young females**.

· These are the kids that get bad **chronic uveitis**, which is the main morbidity of this otherwise mild subtype.

· **Rheumatoid factor** is usually negative; however, when it is positive the disease is often worse.

· **Boys** with oligoarthritis are usually **HLA-B27 positive**. *Prognosis for these boys is good.*

3. Systemic JIA

Systemic JIA is referred to as *Still's Disease*.

· Systemic-onset JIA affects **males and females equally**.

· **Extraarticular involvement** is common.

· Prognosis is moderately good.

Systemic manifestations may precede joint manifestations by several months. Presenting symptoms include:

· **High fever** with **shaking chills**

· **Leukocytosis** as high as **30-50,000**

· **Rash** – *small, pale red macules with central clearings which coalesce*

· **Hepatosplenomegaly**

· **Lymphadenopathy**

· **Pleuritis/pericarditis**

Uveitis *is rare* **in systemic JIA.** Both **ANA** and **RF** are usually **negative.**[2] Most of the systemic manifestations are **self-limited.**

---

[2] ANA is only positive about 10% of the time.

JIA vs. Leukemia

When leukemia presents with musculoskeletal symptoms in addition to the hematologic findings, it can be difficult to distinguish from JIA. Here is what you should focus on in the question in order to make the distinction:

JIA	Acute Leukemia
Morning stiffness, spiking fevers, and rashes are typical. Symptoms of JIA are periodic and waxing and waning. JIA usually presents insidiously – by definition, symptoms need to be present for more than six weeks.	The musculoskeletal pain is more likely to **awaken the child at night** and will present as **bone pain that does not involve a joint**. Symptoms should be persistent and worsening. Leukemia presents acutely (hence the name – acute leukemia). Hematologic abnormalities tend to be more severe than those found in JIA.

Lymphadenopathy and hepatosplenomegaly are typical of both disorders, so **will be of no help**; therefore, you can cross this out if you are trying to decide between JIA and ALL.

Treating JIA

Hey, have you heard this one before? Treat the pain with NSAIDS and treat refractory pain and systemic symptoms *with steroids* and *immunosuppressants.*[3]

It used to be that aspirin (salicylate) was the main treatment. It also used to be fine to enter airport security with a container of mango strawberry punch. Times have changed.

1st line treatment is now NSAIDs, most commonly **tolmetin sodium, ibuprofen, and naproxen**. Children with JIA on NSAIDs are at risk for all known side effects of NSAIDs, including GI bleeding and elevated LFT's.

TIN = **T**olmetin sodium, **I**buprofen, and **N**aproxen.

2nd line treatment (if NSAIDs don't work) are steroids and immunosuppressive meds.

---

[3] That was a rhetorical question, by the way.

Gold treatments are no longer commonly used.

Steroids are also used when there is **cardiac involvement** (i.e., carditis and myocarditis).

Non-pharmacological interventions are considered to be just as important in treatment as medications. This may include a multidisciplinary team of physical and occupational therapists, as well as social workers and specialized nurses.

Kawasaki Disease (Mucocutaneous Lymph Node Syndrome)

They love this one on the boards. This is a great answer when presented with a fever of unknown origin (FUO).

Watch for a febrile child treated with antibiotics (who is not responding to treatment), along with the following presentation:

Kawasaki Disease typically presents in children **younger than 4 years, most commonly around age 2.** It is more likely to present in the **winter** and **spring**. It is more common in **males** and in patients of **Asian** descent. The diagnosis requires **acute fever of <u>at least</u> five days' duration.** In addition, **there must be at least four of the following**:

- · Cervical lymphadenopathy

- · Dry/fissured lips or swollen tongue

- · Conjunctivitis

- · Polymorphous exanthem concentrated on the trunk

- · Changes in the extremities, including **erythema /induration** leading to **desquamation on the hands and feet**

Additional features that can be seen but are not required for diagnosis include:

- · Sterile pyuria[4]

- · CNS symptoms such as seizures and aseptic meningitis

- · Polyarthritis that is migratory

- · Hydrops of the gallbladder

---

[4] White cells in the urine.

· The diagnosis <u>cannot</u> be made in a child with less than 5 days of fevers. ANA should be negative in Kawasaki disease. If ANA is positive, the diagnosis is unlikely.

Think of a giant (30 ft) 2 year old riding a Kawasaki motorcycle without a face shield. The result is **conjunctivitis** and **fissured lips.** His **hands desquamate** from turning the accelerator grips, and his **feet desquamate** from trying to brake using his feet while **turning sharp corners**. In addition, he is going so fast that he develops a **high fever** and has an **elevated platelet count**.

Lab Findings in Kawasaki

You will be expected to know the important laboratory findings in Kawasaki disease. Keep in mind the following:

Thrombocytosis by the **5ᵗʰ day** of illness.[5] **Leukocytosis** by the **12ᵗʰ day** of illness.

Normocytic anemia consistent with chronic illness is also part of the laboratory findings.

Acute phase reactants such as **C-reactive protein, ESR,** and **alpha-1 antitrypsin** remain high for **4-6 weeks**.

ANA, RF, and **circulating anticoagulant** will **not be elevated in Kawasaki disease.**

Treatment of Kawasaki disease

Kardiac Manifestations of Kawasaki

The primary concern in Kawasaki disease is **coronary artery disease.**

When the diagnosis is suspected, prompt treatment is essential. In addition, at some point a **cardiac echo** must be done to look for coronary artery aneurysms. **KD is now the leading etiology of acquired heart disease in kids younger than 5 years of age (surpassing rheumatic fever).**

Monitoring is primarily via **2 dimensional cardiac echo** done at:

· Time of Diagnosis,

· 2-3 weeks later, and

· 6-8 weeks after the onset of illness

---

[5] Remember to write the word in the margins when presented with a very high platelet count, since you are remembering descriptive terminology which is hard to pick out of a sea of numbers.

In the absence of any findings, no continued followup or followup at 1 year would both be correct (but probably not tested since there is no consensus — but you never know!)

KD is treated with:

· An initial dose of IVIG, 2 g/kg

· **Aspirin** is given ***initially*** *at very high doses* (80 mg/kg/day for 24-48 hours)

· **Aspirin maintenance is** then given at a lower dose (5 mg/kg/day for 2 months)

Patients with Kawasaki disease need to be followed by a cardiologist to monitor for coronary artery disease.

When you are presented with a patient with Kawasaki disease, you will also be given choices in the differential that can easily be confused for Kawasaki disease. However, if you pay attention to the following fine details, you will be well prepared to make the important distinctions:

Drug Reactions – This will be tempting, especially if they present a patient on antibiotics who has not responded to treatment and has developed a macular papular rash. However, in a drug reaction one would not expect high fever or the other clinical criteria associated with Kawasaki disease.

JIA/Systemic Type – This will also present with *fever and rash, as well as* adenopathy. However, the **fever will not be acute**, and the rash will be described as an **evanescent, reticular rash** that appears when the **fever peaks.** They would also have to describe other signs of JIA, including *hepatosplenomegaly, pleural effusions, or cardiomegaly.* ***Cardiomegaly is not a sign of Kawasaki disease.***

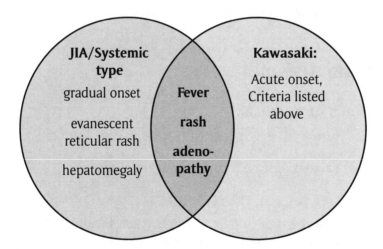

Measles – Seen primarily on the boards and very likely to be one of the choices when presented with a case of Kawasaki disease. Both measles and Kawasaki present with fever and conjunctivitis; however, **measles presents with an _exudative_ conjunctivitis.** The **rash starts at the hairline and progresses downward to the extremities.**

Scarlet Fever – The rash in scarlet fever is seen primarily in flexural areas of the extremities.

Lyme Disease

This is a topic that is full of myths and misconceptions. Here are some important points to remember:

 Lyme disease is caused by infection with the spirochete *Borrelia burgdorferi* and the *body's immunologic response to this infection*. The spirochete is carried to the victim by the Ixodes deer tick, for those interested in entomology!

Hitting the ECM Rash Bullseye

The classic "Bullseye" rash is called "**erythema chronicum migrans**"*(ECM)*.

The rash does not appear in 25% of cases. Therefore, its absence in the clinical history does not rule out Lyme disease. You will most likely be presented a patient with lyme arthritis **without a distinct history of ECM rash or deer tick bite**.

Progression of the Disease

Early Disease First Two Weeks	*Erythema chronicum migrans rash at the site of the tick bite.* *Very vague flu-like symptoms*, with severe arthralgia and extreme fatigue. Even though malaise and fatigue are such common early signs, their non-specificity often leads to a delay in diagnosis.
Several Months	The second stage of Lyme disease is characterized by CNS, cardiac, and arthritic disease. Here you *can* picture the symptoms "migrating" (to remind you that the rash is called "migrans") as a "lime in a **CAN**" where CAN stands for **C**arditis, **A**rthritis (pauciarticular), and **N**eurological Signs (CNS). This also includes Bell's Palsy (a common finding).
Years	Progression of some of the "CAN" symptoms in stage 2, especially arthritis.

Lyme Arthritis

The **Arthritis** is **pauciarticular,** involving **large joints** (especially the knee)**.**

While the knee may be tender and appear swollen, the pain is not unbearable (as it will be with other forms of acute arthritis, such as septic arthritis).

Lyme, Labs, and Difficulties

Lab confirmation is no easy task with Lyme disease. **Remember that detectable levels of serum antibodies don't build up until 4-6 weeks, so false negatives are common,** especially initially. The most commonly seen tests are antibody-based, but these can be confusing. The current recommendations first call for a *Lyme antibody titer and then a Western blot to confirm.*

If treatment is implemented during this time, immunologic response is blunted, and lab results are unreliable. In addition, **false positives with other disorders are common**. This includes autoimmune diseases like **SLE, dermatomyositis,** and other **rickettsial** diseases.

Treatment is with doxycycline for those 8 years and older. For those younger than 8 years of age, amoxicillin is recommended (or cefuroxime in the case of penicillin allergy). Watch for the age of the patient in the presentation. The typical treatment course is 14 to 21 days, with maximum duration of therapy 4 weeks.

Exploding Lymes

If they tell you about a child treated for bona fide Lyme disease who then develops chills and fevers and possibly hypotension with a sepsis-like picture, they are describing the **Jarisch-Herxheimer reaction**, which is the result of lysis of the organism and the release of endotoxin.

Marfan Syndrome

Marfan syndrome is an **autosomal dominant**[6] connective tissue disorder associated with **skeletal, ophthalmologic, and cardiac** disorders**.** There can be **great variation of the morphology among affected family members.**

---

[6] 15% of cases represent a new mutation.

Skeletal abnormalities of Marfan

Skeletal abnormalities associated with Marfan include:

- · Tall stature
- · High arched palate
- · Dental crowding
- · Hyperextensible joints
- · Pectus abnormalities

 Mitral valve prolapse is **not** one of the major criteria.

> ### The Major Criteria for Marfan
>
> You need to be familiar with the major criteria for diagnosing Marfan syndrome
>
> 1. Dilitation and dissection of the ascending aorta/aortic root
> 2. Lubosacral dural ectasia
> 3. Ectopia lentis
> 4. Four skeletal manifestions

Cardiac Abnormalities

Watch for murmurs associated with aortic or mitral valve regurgitation. They could give you a tall teenager presenting with a spontaneous pneumothorax.

Patients with Marfan syndrome are at risk for sudden death associated with aortic rupture. **Close cardiac followup is important.** Referral of other family members for genetic testing would be appropriate. **Marfan syndrome is caused by mutations on chromosome 15 (in the fibrillin gene).**

Ophthalmologic Manifestations of Marfan syndrome

The ophthalmologic manifestation of Marfan syndrome to keep in mind is *ectopia lentis*, or anterior displacement of the *lens of the eye*.

Serial slit lamp evaluation is important.

Post Infectious Arthritis

 Watch for a child who develops mild non-specific arthritis several weeks after an infection, either viral or bacterial. Parvovirus B19 is a common cause of post-infectious arthritis, as well as the cause of almost everything else, or so it seems. Watch for this in a patient with a clinical presentation consistent with **fifth disease or erythema infectiosum**.

Remember, Lyme disease can cause a post infectious arthritis. **Group A beta hemolytic strep** can be associated with arthritis during acute infection or shortly afterward. Other causes of post-infectious arthritis could include *Neisseria gonorrhoeae, Staphylococcus aureus,* influenza A or B, hepatitis B, rubella, or Epstein-Barr.

Patients with fifth disease who develop post infectious arthritis can also present with positive ANA or rheumatoid factor. Don't be fooled into thinking it is anything more exotic than post infectious arthritis.

It is self-limited, requiring only supportive care and analgesics.

CASE STUDY

You are presented with a patient who has vague joint aches but is otherwise doing well. They casually note that the patient received the MMR vaccine several weeks ago, but has otherwise not been ill. You are asked for the most likely explanation for the joint aches.

THE DIVERSION

The most logical choice may seem to be something more serious, since these are the boards and everything is serious. It couldn't possibly be post infectious arthritis, since there was no mention of a recent viral or any other type of illness.

ANSWER REVEALED

Since the MMR is a live vaccine, post infectious arthritis can occur from the rubella component, and this would be the correct answer. This is especially so in a post-pubertal female.

Reactive Arthritis

Like ankylosing spondylitis, reactive arthritis[7] falls under the category of **"seronegative spondyloarthropathy,"** which is just a fancy way of saying that, like anklylosing spondylitis, the ANA and RF factors should be normal.

Just like ankylosing spondylitis, reactive arthritis also can be associated with HLA-B27.

Reactive arthritis presents with **urethritis**, **iritis,** and **arthritis**. The following mnemonic can get you an easy point:

---

[7] Reiter's syndrome is now called reactive arthritis. Panush, RS, Wallace, DJ, Dorff, RE, Engleman, EP. Retraction of the suggestion to use the term "Reiter's syndrome" sixty-five years later: the legacy of Reiter, a war criminal, should not be eponymic honor but rather condemnation. Arthritis Rheum 2007; 56:693.

With reactive arthritis, you hurt at your **knee** (arthritis), where you **see** (uveitis), and where you pee (urethritis). Just remember "can't see, can't pee, and can't climb a tree."

Reactive arthritisoften occurs post-infection with either enteric *(Yersinia, Shigella, or Salmonella)* or venereal *(Chlamydia)* organisms. Obviously, most cases in children will be post enteric, while postvenereal is a consideration for sexually active teenagers.

The urethritis/cervicitis is **nongonococcal and is not due to chlamydia**.

A typical history might consist of **dysuria, injected conjunctiva, and swelling of the foreskin,** with a **benign urinalysis.**

There is no specific diagnostic test – the constellation of a documented bacterial infection followed by the typical symptoms is diagnostic.

Treatment is supportive, with NSAIDS and antibiotics.

You could be presented with a patient with some of the manifestations of reactive arthritis, of course without being told right out that it is reactive arthritis. You would then be asked to pick from among several choices the other signs and symptoms to expect in this patient.

For example, you might be presented with a child with a few swollen tender joints and conjunctivitis and asked to pick other possible manifestations, with the correct choice being urethritis.

Rheumatic Fever

The following are clues for rheumatic fever:

- History of pharyngitis or URI

- **Elevated ESR, ASO titer**, and/or **C reactive protein**

- On physical exam,

    - **Migratory arthritis** of the large joints. *The combination of joint pain, recent URI, and a new heart murmur is a gift*

Splitting Hearts in RF

If they describe **a persistent new murmur** along with **mild congestive heart failure**, this may be **aortic regurgitation**.

Mitral valve regurgitation, which is the **most common murmur etiology in RF**, will be described as a murmur "**heard best at the apex.**"

Further clinical signs:

Emotional lability, coupled with purposeless rapid movements of the extremities and muscle weakness, is either a description of Kanye West at the MTV VMAs, or a patient with **Sydenham's chorea**.

Murmurs related to mitral insufficiency and aortic insufficiency are the most common murmurs in rheumatic fever.

Getting your Jones on

The criteria for the diagnosis of RF were first proposed by original Rolling Stones founder Brian Jones, in the late 60's, two hours before he was found dead in his swimming pool with a copy of Nelson's Pediatrics. That and the constant bickering with Mick Jagger and Keith Richards are his greatest legacies.[8]

You will need to commit the Jones criteria—both **major and minor**—to memory and know them cold. Again, you need a **recent group A strep infection,** as well as:

2 major symptoms

or

1 major <u>and</u> **2 minor** symptoms

 It is easy to forget that a recent group A strep infection is a part of the requirement.

Arth**ritis** is a major criterion, and arth**ralgia** is a minor. They would love to catch you on that one; don't let them.

Major Jones Criteria

J – Joints = Polyarthritis – occurs in 75% of cases

♥ – Carditis (CHF, new murmurs, cardiomegaly)

N – Nodules (subcutaneous) – firm and painless on the extensor surfaces of wrists, elbows, and knees

E – Erythema marginatum

S – Sydenham chorea – rapid, purposeless movements of the face and upper extremities

---

[8] Folks, that is a joke. Please do not send us letters that the Jones Criteria were proposed by T. Duckett Jones; we know that.

Minor Jones Criteria

The minor criteria are much less specific:

- ❑ Fever
- ❑ Arthralgia
- ❑ Elevated acute phase reactants (ESR, C-reactive protein)
- ❑ Prolonged PR interval

 To **help** remember the **minor** criteria, remember the word **help,** since the minor criteria by themselves are not adequate (they need *help*):

H (hot) – as in fever
E (elevated) – as in elevated acute phase reactants
L – to help remember that this minor criterion is arthra–**L**–gia, and not arthritis
P (prolonged) – as in prolonged PR interval

Boning up on the Jones Criteria

Let's take a closer look at the specific aspects of the Jones Criteria.

Arthritis: Remember that arth**ritis** is one of the major criteria and that arthr**algia** one of the minor. The arthritis is "migratory," and usually involves the larger joints (knees, ankles, elbows, and wrists). Each episode lasts from a week up to one month.

The rash is called erythema **marginatum**, but the arthritis is **migratory**. Do not confuse erythema marginatum (RF) and erythema migrans (Lyme).

Treatment: Acute Rheumatic Fever

There are 3 primary treatment goals:

1) Eliminate Group A strep infection
2) Alleviate symptoms
3) Prophylax to prevent recurrence

Elimination of infection is best accomplished with **penicillin** to eradicate Group A beta hemolytic strep – whether confirmed or not! It is an empiric, prudent measure that does not alter the course of the disease. Penicillin is also used for prophylaxis.

Aspirin is used to treat the *migratory arthritis,* and to some degree *fever.*

Steroids would be indicated to treat **carditis (although this is increasingly controversial for mild carditis).**

Haldol may help with *chorea.*

Digoxin is used in *heart failure.*

Strep Mining and Mining for Strep

The following are some of the tests they want you to order when you suspect a diagnosis of rheumatic fever.

If they just hint at a recent strep infection, it isn't enough to make a diagnosis of rheumatic fever. You also need to <u>document</u> the infection.

Rapid Strep/Throat Culture

A positive **throat culture will not distinguish chronic carrier state from recent infection.** A negative **rapid strep** does **not** rule out a recent infection.

ASO Titers and Streptozyme

ASO titers and positive streptozyme correlate very well with a recent strep infection. Definitive documentation of a recent strep infection is usually the answer they are looking for.

Sarcoidosis

Sarcoidosis presents with "history of weight loss and fatigue, with hilar adenopathy." They may describe it in the absence of any respiratory symptoms. It is seen more frequently in **African Americans** than Caucasians.

Watch for an otherwise healthy child who fatigues easily during sports despite being afebrile

Additional findings include **noncaseating granulomas,** as well as **bilateral peribronchial infiltrates on CXR.**

The granulomas actually secrete a form of Vitamin D, which causes **hypercalcemia** and **hypercalcuria.** This results in **renal disease** and **eye disease.**

Sarcoidosis often involves the heart, and the presentation of an EKG with a rhythm disturbance could help distinguish a diagnosis of sarcoidosis from tuberculosis. **A negative PPD will be your clue that you are not dealing with tuberculosis.**

Depression and other problems can also explain fatigue and a child dropping out of a sports program. They will have to give you a sign of sarcoidosis, such as a **chronic cough**, if that is the answer they are looking for.

Scleroderma

Scleroderma results in a thickening and tightening of the skin, often with induration. Literally, this means "hard skin." **Females** are affected much more frequently than males.

There are two main forms of scleroderma.

Localized Linear Scleroderma

The localized form of scleroderma will begin as a *linear hyperpigmented patch* that becomes more and more fibrotic. It only involves skin and adjacent subcutaneous tissue. Initially, patches of skin are "painful and tender." Additional descriptions might include *shiny hypopigmented skin with a brown border.*

Localized scleroderma is more common and has a better outcome than the systemic form. The localized form requires minimal treatment and is self-limited.

Treatment *of the localized form consists of topical lubricants and, occasionally,* photo-chemotherapy. In the presence of widespread progressive disease, other treatment modalities could include **steroids, antimalarials, and immunosuppressives.** This would include **methotrexate** and **penicillamine,** among other agents.

Treatment to prevent the progression to the systemic form would be incorrect.

Systemic Scleroderma

The systemic form is rarely seen in children, but just in case it does pop up on the boards:

 The systemic form may also present with **sclerodactyly,**[9] **pulmonary fibrosis,** and **reflux/dysphagia from lower esophageal sphincter incompetence**.

Most people present with **Raynaud's,** and almost everyone has this at some point in their course. **ANA is almost always positive.**

Septic Arthritis

> ### Serum Sickness
>
> Serum Sickness is a type III hypersensitivity reaction and will be presented as a combination of **fever**, **urticaria**, and **arthralgia** a few weeks after an antigen exposure. Lymphadenopathy could also be a part of the presentation. Treatment is with antihistamines and steroids.

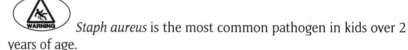 Remember, septic arthritis can easily be confused with **oligoarticular (pauciarticular) JIA**. However, **septic arthritis** will have a much more *acute onset*.

Staph aureus is the most common pathogen in kids over 2 years of age.

If you are presented with a teenager, consider *Neisseria gonorrhea.*

Diagnosis is made by aspirating the joint and examining and culturing the fluid.

Treatment is long-term parenteral antibiotics.

If it cannot be differentiated based on the data they give, then treatment for septic arthritis is the correct choice, since there is no time to wait.

Systemic Lupus Erythematosus

SLE is caused by **the formation of antigen-antibody complexes in a variety of tissues. It is almost always found in** women, though the **gender ratio is more equal in younger children**. It is four times more common in **African Americans** than in Caucasians.

---

[9] Localized scleroderma of the digits.

A diagnosis of SLE is suggested[10] when 4 or more of the following features present over time. *Arthralgias and fatigue are the most common presenting symptoms.*

· Malar rash

· Discoid lesions

· Photosensitivity

· Oral or nasal ulcerations

· Arthritis

· Hematological Complications of Lupus

· The presence of anti-ds-DNA, anti-DNA and anti-SM antibodies.

· Persistent cellular casts in the urine

· Pleuritis or pericarditis (serositis)

· Psychosis or other neurologic problems

In addition to general signs such as fever, rash, and arthritis, lupus also presents with weight loss, fatigue, and malaise. A common presentation of SLE would be fever, arthritis, oral ulcers, and a low WBC. In addition, thrombocytopenia could be a lab finding included in the history. If they present you with an adolescent female with chronic idiopathic thrombocytopenia or ITP, it could be a hint that the patient has SLE.

Screening for Lupus

Antibodies to double-stranded DNA **(anti-ds-DNA)** are very specific for SLE since positive results are rarely seen in other patients, including those with other rheumatological disorders.

Severity of disease flareups can also be tracked via anti-ds-DNA levels, which fluctuate accordingly. The severity of disease can also be traced via C3 and C4 levels, which are inversely proportional to disease severity. C3 and C4 levels go down in more active/acute disease states.

Acute Hemolytic Anemia

Acute hemolytic anemia is another manifestation of lupus. Remember this when presented with hemolytic anemia with unknown (to you) etiology.

---

[10] With 96% accuracy, which is close enough for the exam.

Thromboembolic disease and SLE

Due to the presence of the "lupus anticoagulant," patients with lupus are at increased risk for thromboembolic disease.

Watch for a patient with SLE presenting with signs of thromboembolus in the leg and respiratory distress consistent with a pulmonary embolus. For example, lower leg pain followed by tachypnea, respiratory distress, and chest pain.

The lupus anticoagulant also results in a false positive serology for syphilis.

Raynaud Triad

Raynaud Triad (Raynaud's Phenomenon) can be **a part of Lupus**. The triad consists of the following, which I remember with the **white**, **blue**, and **red** of the French Flag. Raynaud was French, wasn't he?

❏ Ischemia of the Distal Fingers **(white)**

❏ Cyanosis **(blue)**

❏ Cold Fingers **(red)**

Drug Induced Lupus (DILE)

Remember, lupus can be induced by medications, but in these cases the condition is **reversible**. Remember **D-SLE: D**=Drugs for the Heart, **S**=Sulfonamides, **L**=**Li**thium, **E**=Epilepsy (anticonvulsants).

These categories of drugs may all be linked to DILE, but the three most common are procainamide, hydralazine, and quinidine.

ANA is still the most sensitive test, even in drug induced lupus.

Polyserositis

This affects any organ that has a "**pleural covering**", which includes primarily the heart (pericarditis) and lungs (pleurisy).

Renal Disease in Lupus

This is an important component of SLE. Look for signs of nephritis along with other signs of lupus presented in the question.

The following are signs of **active renal disease in SLE:**

- **Increased anti-DNA titers**
- **Decreased** levels of complement: **C3, C4, and CH50.**

Lupus Cerebritis

This is a result of areas of **microischemia and vascular disease**. It results in **seizures**.

Neonatal Lupus

When neonatal lupus does occur, there are *usually no clinical signs*; however, without clinical signs there would be no board exam, just blank pages. The signs on the Boards to look for are rashes on the trunk and, **most importantly, 3rd degree heart block**. A newborn presenting with **bradycardia** should tip you off that they could be alluding to a diagnosis of neonatal lupus-which could also be associated with **hydrops fetalis.** The heart block can lead to failure, and the baby may need a pacemaker.

Heart block would be the most likely explanation for death in an infant born to a mother with SLE.

Dermatological signs include a scaly erythematous rash involving the face but not exclusively. The rash is self-limited and has, at worst, some residual orange atrophic skin.

Hematological signs include **thrombocytopenia;** therefore, petechiae would be a sign that they are describing neonatal lupus.

Most newborns born to women with SLE do NOT develop neonatal lupus. If presented with a neonate with heart block or low heart rate, they will almost certainly not mention a history of lupus in the mom. In fact, in many cases the mom doesn't know she has SLE.

Smoothly rowing your boat to diagnosis

Anti-SSA antibody is closely associated with neonatal lupus. Notably, most infants with congenital heart block have mothers who test positive for anti-SSA or anti-SSB antibodies.

Treating Lupus

Normalization of C3 and C4 levels is the best indication of a good response to treatment.

Like many rheumatologic/immunologic diseases, treatment is with pain management and immunosuppression.

Mild Disease

Mild disease (arthralgia) is treated with **NSAIDs and hydroxychloroquine.** Dapsone may be used for skin manifestations. Low doses of **prednisone** may be used to help maintain disease control.

Ototoxicity is a rare side effect of *hydroxychloroquine*. Much more common are **ophthalmological** side effects, ranging from temporary blurring to permanent retinal damage.

Severe Disease

More severe disease is characterized by unremitting arthralgias, kidney involvement, serositis (pleuritis, carditis), or CNS effects (seizures, cerebritis). These patients need pulses of high dose steroids and possibly immunosuppressants like cyclophosphamide and azathioprine. **Cyclophosphamide** is used particularly for serious organ involvement.

Mycophenolate mofetil may be used for maintenance therapy after a course of cyclophosphamide.

When **steroids are being tapered,** having fevers or worsening joint pains may not be an indication to resume steroids. Some of the medications used to treat mild disease (i.e., NSAIDs) are appropriate treatments in this case.

Lupus patients undergoing treatment with immunosuppressive agents are at risk for serious infections such as varicella.

Patients with lupus on steroids are at risk for the all complications associated with chronic steroid use, including cataracts, glaucoma, osteoporosis, high blood pressure, glucose intolerance, and cushingoid features.

Pick a fact-ANA facts

The ANA is an extremely sensitive screening test (negative rules it out) – it will be positive in almost all SLE, but it is also positive in many other inflammatory disorders.

If the ANA is negative, it is very unlikely to be lupus (because it is a highly *sensitive* test).

On the other hand, the *dsDNA* test is very *specific*. Positive rules it in.

Remember – a sensitive test is how you screen for a disease. A specific test is how you secure the diagnosis.

Benign Stuff

Here, like everywhere else in the book, **consider some of the more benign causes of joint aches and pains**.

Growing Pains: This will be described as being "bilateral," "worse at night," "walking with a limp," and "joint pain without swelling."

Hypermobility: This will be described as "loose joints" (we're not talking about the kind of people with pinky rings at a Saturday night slam) in people who get injured and sustain sprains easily. They need to be counseled to stretch before sports and to be vigilant in the sports they play. No other intervention is needed.

Wegener Granulomatosis

Wegener Granulomatosis is a rare multisystem vasculitis that involves the **sinuses**, **lungs**, and **kidneys**. It is rare in children, and it occurs mostly in Caucasians.

The typical presentation is with upper respiratory symptoms (sinusitis, rhinorrhea), but the severity of disease is related to the extent of kidney involvement. Patients will also have vague constitutional

---

symptoms. Labs will show a̱ntineutrophil c̱ytoplasmic a̱utoantibodies (c-ANCA). If they give you a positive c-ANCA in someone with joint pain, fevers, and sinusitis, think Wegener.[11]

Aggressive treatment with cyclophosphamide is recommended. Steroids are also used. Despite intervention, morbidity and mortality are significant.

To remember the association with c-ANCA, think of it as Wage Earners Giant Matosis. Think of a "wage earner" saying, "Thankya" after getting paid with **giant** *coins shaped like* **kidneys** *and* **lungs**. *He deposits them in a ceramic piggy bank[12] that looks like a sinus.*

Synovial Fluid

They will give you Synovial Fluid to look at, and based on the findings you may have to mix and match. Here are some Guidelines:

Synovial Fluid	*Color*	*Viscosity*
Normal Synovial Fluid	Yellow or clear	Normal or slightly increased viscosity; WBC less than 200
Arthritis secondary to Trauma	Clear or bloody	Increased viscosity; WBC less than 2,000
Lupus	Yellow or clear	Normal viscosity; WBC 5,000 and LE cells
Rheumatic Fever	Yellow-cloudy	Decreased viscosity; WBC 5,000
JIA	Yellow-cloudy	Decreased viscosity; WBC 15,000-20,000
Reactive arthritis	Yellow-opaque	Decreased viscosity; WBC 20,000
Septic Arthritis	Yellow	Variable viscosity; WBC 50,000-300,000 and low glucose and bacteria

---

11 c-ANCA is a fairly common immunologic marker – like ANA. It is fair game.
12 No doubt a gift from a pharmaceutical rep.

Chapter 27

The Eyes Have It

Remember, ophthalmology is spelled with 2 H's and we cover most of it in other sections. Here we pick out some important pieces of information on which they will test you.

The Rhythm of Nystagmus

You could very well be called upon to identify a variety of forms of nystagmus and try to keep them straight until you actually experience pendular nystagmus yourself. What's pendular nystagmus? Follow the bouncing eyeballs and we will explain.

Pendular Nystagmus

Pendular nystagmus is equal velocity movements in both directions (to and fro). It is often a sign of an underlying disorder such as multiple sclerosis or spinocerebellular disease.

Jerk Nystagmus

Jerk nystagmus is characterized by a slow phase back to the central position with a quick gaze laterally.

Jerk nystagmus can be normal when a child gazes far upwardly or laterally.

> ### A Benign Nod
>
> **Spasmus nutans** is a benign, transient disorder without known cause that is characterized by pendular nystagmus, intermittent head tilt, and nodding or head bobbing.
>
> It can be mistaken for muscular torticollis. It is a benign condition that self resolves.

Pseudostrabismus and True Strabismus

Strabismus is deviation of the alignment of one eye in relation to the other.

Pseudostrabismus, also known as "false strabismus," is when the eyes appear to deviate but it is actually due to other factors. These include extra skin that covers the inner corner of the eye, a broad, flat nose, or eyes set unusually close together or far apart.

Distinguishing between **pseudostrabismus** and **true strabismus** is key. They will very likely show this on the exam.

> Esotropia is a subcategory of strabismus and is the most common type of strabismus in infants. Children with esotropia do not use their eyes together. Early surgery is usually needed to align the eyes in order to obtain binocular vision.

They could also describe the "cover test:" the child "fixes" on a distant object while the other eye is covered The process is repeated with the other eye covered. **The eye with strabismus "deviates" instead of fixating on the object**. When a child cannot (or will not) cooperate in this adventure, the corneal light reflex test (Hirschberg test) is used.[1] **Here you shine a penlight on both eyes and expect a *symmetrical light reflex*.**

This is very helpful in ruling out **pseudostrabismus**.

Screening for strabismus is crucial, and they want you to know that. **Untreated strabismus results in amblyopia** (loss of use of the nondominant eye and permanent loss of binocular vision) if not detected by age 6.

Port Wine and the Eye

Remember that infants born with Sturge Weber are at risk for **glaucoma**, so if they describe a child born with a port wine stain, it is the glaucoma that should be addressed first.

Violaceous discoloration is another way of describing a port wine stain.

Strawberry Hemangiomas and the Eye

These, in general, resolve without any intervention unless they are on or near the eyelid *and are interfering with vision,* in which case they may need to be dealt with early on.

Cataracts

If you are presented with an infant with congenital cataracts, **rubella** and **galactosemia** are two important associations to know.

---

[1] It is pretty much a simple test named after the famous doctor and sushi chef.

Styes, Tears and Chalazion

Styes

 Styes are also known as "external hordeolum," and they are the result of inflammation and infection (usually *Staph*) of sebaceous glands in the eyelid.

Warm compresses and, possibly, topical antibiotics are the mainstay of treatment. It is due to inflammation and possible infection of the follicles and/or sebaceous glands. Incision and drainage might be needed if there is no improvement, but PO antibiotics will **not** be the correct answer.

Dacryocystitis

Dacryostenosis

The initial treatment for a dacryostenosis blocked nasolacrimal duct is massaging the duct 2-3 times a day. If there is evidence of infection, then topical antibiotic treatment is indicated.

Oral antibiotics will be the incorrect choice in treating a blocked nasolacrimal duct in an infant.

If blocked duct is not resolved by 12 months of age, then ophthalmological consultation would be in order.

CASE STUDY You are evaluating a 2-month-old with excessive tearing of the left eye and mucoid discharge. When you evaluate the crying infant, you notice that the tears pool on the left eyelid and cheek. The parents note that child has nasal congestion and coughs occasionally. The pregnancy and delivery were unremarkable.

What is the appropriate management?

THE DIVERSION You could be presented with several diversionary choices here, including systemic treatment with antibiotics for a presumed diagnosis of chlamydia. In addition, you will be presented with the option of prescribing topical antibiotic drops for a presumed diagnosis of bacterial conjunctivitis.

ANSWER REVEALED None of these would be correct. Noting the nasal congestion is a diversion. Even the occasional cough is a diversion. For a diagnosis of chlamydia pneumonia, they would have to describe a more persistent staccato cough or chest x-ray findings (neither of which are noted in the vignette). For chlamydi conjunctivitis, they would have to describe bilateral eye discharge.

The correct diagnosis is a blocked nasolacrimal duct, for which the appropriate management would be conservative measures, i.e., massage and warm compresses. Topical antibiotics would only be indicated when erythema and other signs of infection are described.

Chalazion

DEFINITION Chalazion is a lipogranuloma, and is caused by chronic inflammation of one of the small oil-producing glands secondary to retention of secretions. *It is due to chronic inflammation, not bacterial infection,* and is typically *painless.*

Orbiting Cellulitis

You will be expected to distinguish between a patient with orbital and periorbital cellulitis.

Orbital Cellulitis

Since this is an infection involving the tissue immediately surrounding the eye, it is the more serious of the two.

The key buzz words in the description which should tip you off are "compromised vision," "proptosis," and "decreased extraocular movement." This can be caused by spread of skin infections, including insect bites. Watch for retro-orbital pain exacerbated by eye movement. Edema of the eyelid is another sign.

Since *H. influenza* type b can cause this, pay particular attention if they describe a patient who has incomplete immunizations. If they note the patient immigrated from a developing country, this means they are assumed to be unimmunized.

Periorbital Cellulitis

Periorbital cellulitis is the less serious of the orbiting twins. However, periorbital can lead to orbital cellulitis.

In the absence fever or compromised EOM, you are most likely dealing with periorbital cellulitis. If they describe high fever, decreased EOM, and proptosis, they are more likely describing orbital cellulitis.

Corneal Abrasions

The presentation of corneal abrasion on the exam will likely include photophobia, tearing, and intermittent sharp pain. They might also describe an irregular red reflex or a dulled corneal light reflex. Positive fluorescein staining of the cornea would be a slam dunk, but that is unlikely to be included in the description.

Remember to include a corneal abrasion in the differential of an irritable infant.

After confirmation with fluorescein, all that is needed is topical antibiotic treatment.

In the past, a semi pressure patch for 24 hours was considered to be routine, but this is no longer considered to be routine treatment for corneal abrasions.

If you are presented with a patient with symptoms of corneal abrasion following mild trauma, the *first thing to do is fluorescein stain the eye, not prescribe topical antibiotic.*

You are presented with a patient with a 4-month history of a painless nodule on her upper eyelid. What is the appropriate treatment?

If you read this question quickly and didn't note that this is a chronic painless nodule, you might have mistaken it for a stye and quickly picked topical antibiotics and warm compresses. In the blink of an eye you would have chosen the incorrect answer.

When answering a question about a nodule on the eyelid, pay careful attention to the details of the history. If you are dealing with a chronic painless nodule, "referral to ophthalmology for surgical excision" is the correct answer. Once again, ophthalmology is the one specialist referral that is often a correct choice.

Don't Shoot if you see the Red in their Eyes

If you are presented with a patient with "red eye" who is wearing contacts, pause and read the question carefully.

In this case, referral to ophthalmology for definitive care would be the correct answer.

Papilledema, Papillitis and Picking Out the Differences

You are expected to know the descriptive differences between papilledema, papillitis, and other causes of retinal swelling that impact vision. The table below outlines these differences:

	Funduscopic Exam	Clinical Presentation
Papillitis	Optic disc is engorged and inflamed. Difficult to distinguish from papilledema other than the clinical description and presentation	Usually unilateral, preceded by a viral illness; transiently decreased visual acuity
Retrobulbar optic neuropathy	Optic discs appear normal	Loss of visual acuity
Papilledema	Loss of arteriovenous pulsations	The blind spot is enlarged but visual acuity remains normal

Keep Your Eyes on the Retina

It is very likely that you will be presented with at least one funduscopic view of the retina. In this section, we include black and white illustrations of the retina.[2]

Retinitis pigmentosa

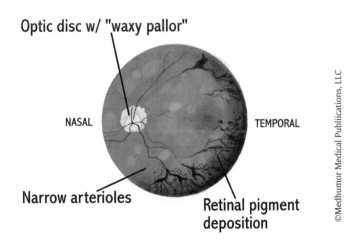

Optic disc w/ "waxy pallor"

NASAL

TEMPORAL

Narrow arterioles

Retinal pigment deposition

©Medhumor Medical Publications, LLC

---

[2] "Pictures Worth 100 Points" contains color drawings of several funduscopic views of retinal diseases.

With **Retinitis pigmentosa**, look for the following:

· Pallor in the center of the optic disc.

· Narrow arterioles coming off the optic disc.

· Retinal pigment deposition on the periphery.

 Retinitis pigmentosa can be seen with Usher Syndrome.

Retinal hemorrhages

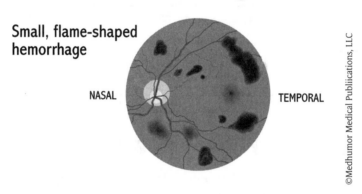

Small, flame-shaped hemorrhage

NASAL

TEMPORAL

©Medhumor Medical Publications, LLC

For **Retinal Hemorrhages**, look for flame-shaped hemorrhage

This is typically seen where child abuse is suspected, or, on the boards, where it is hinted at in the history.

Roping In ROP

Which infants should be screened for ROP?

- Birthweight less than 1500 grams or GA less than 32 weeks
- Birthweight 1500 - 2000 grams with an unstable clinical course, judged to be at risk

When to screen? 31-34 weeks postconception or 4 -6 weeks after birth, whichever is *later*.

 The greatest risk factor for developing ROP is prematurity, with a gestation less than 28 weeks.

Do not go for the bait by choosing oxygen therapy in and of itself as being the greatest risk factor. Oxygen therapy is a contributing factor, but the primary risk factor is <u>prematurity</u> with <u>low birth weight</u>. If presented with an infant greater than 37 weeks gestation on oxygen, the risk for ROP is very low, since retinal vascularization is almost complete at that gestational age.

CASE STUDY **You are presented with an infant who has developed retinopathy of prematurity. You are asked to select from several choices the *most likely risk factor for ROP*.**

THE DIVERSION This is a question where you need to put on the brakes before picking the answer that was previously consistent with conventional wisdom. In this case, when the oxygen fastball is thrown down the middle, you want to be caught looking, looking at the correct answer, that is.

ANSWER REVEALED The correct answer in this case is *very low birth weight or prematurity*. Studies have shown that exposure to oxygen or the maintenance of oxygen saturations above 95% over time does not influence the progression of ROP. The incidence of ROP is inversely proportional to birthweight and gestational age.

Retinopathy of Prematurity

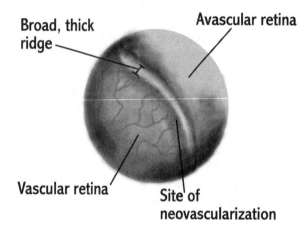

Broad, thick ridge

Avascular retina

Vascular retina

Site of neovascularization

©Medhumor Medical Publiications, LLC

In retinal detachment, look for sparsity of vessels as well as a retinal tear, flap, or corrugated fold.

Looks very similar to an artist rendition of the Mars horizon. The main difference is that the landscape of Mars is much easier to spot on a funduscopic exam with dilated pupils.

Chapter 28

See No Evil, Hear No Evil, Speak No Evil: ENT

Upper respiratory disease is a big part of a general pediatric practice; therefore, ENT is an important section that is highly represented on the exam. Distinguishing the profound from the insignificant will be the key to getting the questions correct on the exam as well.

Ears

Hearing Loss

Hearing loss is broken down into sensorineural and conductive.

Conductive Hearing Loss

This occurs when sound fails to progress to the cochlea. Obstruction can occur anywhere along the way from the external canal to the swinging ossicles.

The most common cause of conductive hearing loss is an effusion, usually due to otitis media. By definition, the effusion is present in the *absence of inflammation.*

Clues of a **mild conductive hearing loss** would include **ignoring commands** and **slight increasing of the television volume.**[1]

Remember, this could be noted in the question. Conductive hearing loss is often correctable with *surgery* or *hearing devices,* as opposed to sensorineural causes. There are only so many causes they can test you on. Here are a few:

> **HOT TIP**
> Hearing loss is associated with CHARGE syndrome and and other syndromes that involve cleft lip and palate.

> **More than Meets the Ear**
> If they present you with a patient with with an external or middle ear malformation, watch for hints that there are also craniofacial, renal, or even associated inner ear malformations.

---

[1] Assuming one does not live in a subway station.

Causes of Conductive Hearing Loss	
Small, Malformed Ears (*Microtia / Aural Atresia* for those who speak Latin)	Very easily corrected.
Perforated Tympanic Membrane	Larger perforations result in significant hearing loss. In addition, post-traumatic hearing loss is usually associated with disruption of the ossicles themselves.
Tympanosclerosis	We have all seen this (basically opacification on the TM), usually after several bouts of OM. They could very well show this to you; remember that this results in **minimal hearing loss**.
OME (OM with Effusion)	This is controversial, but the **hearing loss is minimal and intermittent**.
Cholesteatoma	This is the result of **keratinization of the epithelial cells in the middle ear**.

CASE STUDY

You are presented with a 9 year old boy who has purulent discharge from his right ear over several months despite several courses of antibiotics. On physical exam you note retraction of the tympanic membrane and squamous debris. What do you do next?

THE DIVERSION

You might be tempted to pick higher dose antibiotics or other more conservative measures.

ANSWER REVEALED

This is the description of a cholesteatoma, and, therefore, this is one of those rare times when referral to a specialist will be the correct answer.

BUZZ WORDS

If they describe a **"foul smelling discharge despite treatment of a perforated TM,"** it is a clue to a diagnosis of cholesteatoma.

Sensorineural Hearing Loss

Sensorineural hearing loss can be blamed on malfunction of the *cochlea* and/or auditory *nerve*.

The Loop Diuretics

Furosemide (Lasix®) and ethacrynic acid can cause a temporary hearing loss. When an **aminoglycoside** is also used, the ototoxic effects are amplified.

Picture a Loop earring piercing the cochlea, causing a sensorineural hearing loss.

Aminoglycoside Antibiotics

Remember that aminoglycosides *can result in hearing loss;* **gentamicin** and **tobramycin** are the classics.

Salicylate Ototoxicity

This results in **reversible sensorineural hearing loss**. Hearing can return to normal within a week.

A high-pitched tinnitus is what they will describe.

Viral

Cytomegalovirus (CMV), measles, mumps, and rubella are the most common viral causes of sensorineural hearing loss

Measles, Mumps, Rubella = MMR

Picture an MMR missile and a **C/m**oving **v**ehicle piercing the ear, causing sensorineural hearing loss.

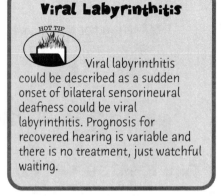

Viral Labyrinthitis

Viral labyrinthitis could be described as a sudden onset of bilateral sensorineural deafness could be viral labyrinthitis. Prognosis for recovered hearing is variable and there is no treatment, just watchful waiting.

Sensorineural Hearing Loss Secondary to Meningitis

Bacterial meningitis is the most common neonatal cause of hearing loss. It tends to occur early in the illness (usually in the first 24 hours). This is an important concept that is often tested on the exam.

PERIL *WARNING* It is not related to the severity of the illness, the age of the patient, or when antibiotics were started.

Sensorineural hearing loss is also associated with *Toxoplasma gondii* infection.

Hearing in Infants

> **Turn Down the Volume**
>
> Repeated exposure to loud sounds, including pounding music through iPod® headphones, can lead to high frequency hearing loss. The same applies to the loud sound produced by power tools.

If you are presented with an infant with any of the following risk factors, they could be indicating that you need to be thinking about potential sensorineural hearing loss.

Risk factors for sensorineural hearing loss include issues associated with prematurity, such as extended assisted ventilation, hyperbilirubinemia, low birth weight, or the use of ototoxic drugs such as gentamicin. Craniofacial abnormalities and syndromes like Waardenburg syndrome are associated with sensorineural hearing loss as well.

Age Appropriate Hearing Tests

Conventional Pure-Tone Audiometry Screen

The conventional Pure-Tone Audiometry Screen is appropriate for **school-age children** who can cooperate with commands. This can **test each ear independently**.

Newborn Hearing Screening

HOT TIP Identification of hearing loss should be done by 3 months of age, and intervention before 6 months is optimal.

There are two screening tests for newborns in the nursery:

1. **Auditory brainstem response (ABR)**
2. **Otoacoustic emissions (OAE)**

HOT TIP It is important for the newborn to be sleeping when the test is done to reduce interference from body movements. **In addition, a normal otoacoustic emission is not an absolute.**

Behavioral Observational Audiometry (BOA)

Behavioral Observational Audiometry (BOA) is used for **infants who are less than 6 months of age**. This is only a screening test, and infants who **fail this must then undergo ABR testing**. Auditory Brainstem Response (ABR) uses electroencephalographic waveforms to determine the child's perceptual threshold. Children older than six months of age may require conscious sedation for an ABR.

Visual Reinforcement Audiometry (VRA)

Visual Reinforcement Audiometry (VRA) is for infants and toddlers.[2] This tests for **bilateral hearing loss** so that intervention to prevent language development impairment can be started.

Hearing amplification devices are available in infants as young as 6 months of age.

If a patient fails a hearing screen or has equivocal results, he/she needs a referral to an audiologist. If you are given a patient that has physical, cognitive, or behavioral concerns that may interfere with administration of the screening, referral to an audiologist would be the correct choice.

Tympanometry

Tympanometry results will invariably be shown or described on the exam. Often, the results are either normal or abnormal due to technique. An example of poor technique in this case includes the probe being wedged against the external canal; this may cause abnormal results.

Tympanometry does not measure hearing sensitivity. You *can* have a normal tympanogram with significant sensorineural hearing loss. On the other hand, a patient can have an abnormal tympanogram and still have normal hearing.

Tympanogram

Flat

A flat line is associated with a "stiff" membrane[3] or with middle ear fluid. If they get fancy, flat will be described as "*low amplitude.*" This is also consistent with an obstructed tympanostomy tube.

---

[2] For those of you without a calculator, this is children between the ages of 6 months and 2 years.
[3] Tympanic, of course.

High

A high line is consistent with a hypermobile TM.

Volume: The Volume of the Graph

Remember high school geometry?[4] Does the volume of the graph measure how large the area under the curve is regardless of the height? Or does it measure your height?

Well, you don't need to remember high school geometry, but you do need to know that the area under the tympanogram curve reflects the area in the external canal. Therefore, high volume is a result of the continuity between middle and outer ear, and correlates with a perforated TM (trauma, myringotomy tubes, or information going in one ear and out the other). It also reflects the absence of pressure and the absence of mobility.

Middle Ear

Otitis Media

Remember, OM is more common in babies fed with propped bottles.

 Erythema of the TM is not enough by itself to hang your diagnostic hat on.

 The most common culprits in acute otitis media are:

· *Streptococcus pneumoniae*
· *H. flu* (non typeable)
· *Moraxella catarrhalis*

The incidence of *H. flu* (non-typeable) has been increasing, and *S. pneumoniae* has been decreasing.

If you are presented with a child with otitis media not responding to first line treatment, then amoxicillin/clavulanate would be the correct answer.

Tympanostomy tubes are now the treatment of choice for recurrent otitis media; this will be the correct answer on the exam. Tympanostomy tubes help prevent cholesteatoma.

---

4 Neither do I.

Mothers want it, advertisers hawk it, and pediatricians often give in to the pressure[5], but antihistamines, decongestants, and other over-the-counter cold remedies as treatment for and/or prevention of acute otitis media have no proven value. So remember: Just Say No To (over-the counter cold remedy) Drugs.

Oral decongestants should not be used in children younger than 6 years of age, at least in those presenting on the boards. Nasal decongestants may be harmful in infants younger than 6 months of age, since rebound nasal congestion may impact respiratory function (infants are nasal breathers).

Confusion over Otitis Media with Effusion

Chronic otitis media with effusion may result in hearing loss and delayed speech and language development.

The appropriate management would be monitoring over time, with periodic checks of TM mobility.

If there is an underlying medical problem such as cleft palate or an immunodeficiency, then prophylactic antibiotics may be indicated (although the risks of potential bacterial resistance must be considered as well in this situation).

You are presented with a 4 year old child with chronic drainage through his perforated left tympanic membrane. The best treatment for this would be:

There are two potential diversions here. One is cholesteatoma and the other is acute otitis media. What is being described here is *chronic suppurative otitis media*. You must first distinguish chronic suppurative otitis media from cholesteatoma. The absence of keratinized epithelial tissue rules the latter out. You now have to pick an antibiotic or recognize the most common cause.

The most common cause is *pseudomonas* and therefore the treatment of choice is *topical ofloxacin*. In addition to *pseudomonas*, chronic suppurative otitis media can be caused by *Staph*.

---

[5] Pardon the pun!

Cholesteatoma and chronic suppurative otitis media can occur together. Therefore read the question carefully to see what they are asking and what the findings are. Keep in mind the following:

· Cholesteatoma can be the result of chronic suppurative otitis media.

· On the other hand, chronic suppurative otitis media can occur without cholesteatoma.

· If chronic suppurative otitis media does not respond to treatment, then they are telling you that a cholesteatoma is the underlying cause.

Prophylaxis with antibiotics is no longer recommended for the prevention and/or treatment of chronic otitis media. Antibiotic prophylaxis is now considered to be a risk factor for colonization with resistant pneumococcus. Tympanostomy tubes are now the treatment of choice for chronic recurrent otitis media; this will be the correct answer on the exam.

Otitis Media and the CNS

If they describe a child who is being treated for OM but not responding and returns with signs of meningitis (classic signs), then it is not a trick question, and workup and treatment for meningitis would be indicated.

Although intracranial suppurative complications of otitis media only occur 1% of the time, the incidence is most likely higher on the boards. Watch for subtle clues in the history, including fever, irritability, and lethargy. More specific signs in a patient with otitis media who is not responding to antibiotics would include headache, double vision, and vomiting.

Recognized Indication for Changing Antibiotics

If after 2-3 days of PO treatment, there is persistent ear pain and/or fever complications, then this may be an indication to switch antibiotics.

The most common intracranial complication of otitis media is meningitis.

Withholding antibiotics

Keep the following in mind when answering questions on basic garden variety otitis media.

- Withholding antibiotic treatment for up to 3 days to see if symptoms persist is considered correct treatment.
- 80% of the time, otitis media will resolve within 2 weeks *without* treatment.
- Treatment would be warranted if they present a patient with rapid onset of symptoms, severe pain, and/or erythema, infants and toddlers under 24 months of age.
- Providing a prescription for antibiotics and advising the parents to wait up to 3 days to see if symptoms persist is okay.

Complications of Myringotomy Tubes

Remember: otorrhea can still occur after the tubes are in place. This is because even though they equalize pressure, they **do not prevent upper respiratory tract infections.**

CASE STUDY

A 5 year old with tympanostomy tubes presents with 3 days of bloody otorrhea as well as nasal congestion. In addition to a copious amount of bloody discharge, the physical exam reveals a large erythematous mass. What is the most likely cause of the bloody otorrhea?

THE DIVERSION

With the mention of a large erythematous mass, you are probably inclined to think this is a tumor that can result in bloody otorrhea including a *rhabdomyosarcoma* or *eosinophilic granuloma* (both typically occurring in the middle ear). You might be inclined to diagnose a good old-fashioned ear infection, or perhaps you will pick the diversionary choice of *cholesteatoma*.

ANSWER REVEALED

However, the correct answer (given the mention of the presence of tympanostomy tubes) would be *tympanostomy tube granuloma*, which is a common complication of tympanostomy tubes.

Otalgia and other Pains in *their* Ear

They could present you with a patient with ear pain that is referred from elsewhere.

Watch for indications that the patient might have TMJ dysfunction, cervical spine abnormality, or a sore throat as the source of the otalgia.

External Ear

Foreign Body

They might give you a hint as to why a child might place a foreign body in his ear, such as developmental delay. In addition, there **is pain on movement of the pinna** (just as there would be with otitis externa, described below). "Otorrhea" might also be described.

Otitis Externa

"Pain when the pinna is manipulated."

They may even describe purulent discharge, which can also be consistent with otitis externa. It occurs most frequently in the summer, which is called "swimmer's ear." *Pseudomonas* is the usual cause.

Treatment is with antibiotic/steroid drops. If there is a question on preventing swimmer's ear, this can be accomplished by acidifying the ear canal with OTC boric acid or acetic acid solutions (before and after swimming), and/or wearing earplugs while swimming.

Hematoma External Ear (Cauliflower Ear)

If you are presented with a patient with swelling and deformity of the external ear following blunt trauma, the correct management would be evacuation of the hematoma immediately by needle aspiration.

Mastoiditis

Mastoiditis is one of the suppurative complications of acute otitis media.

 Treatment of mastoiditis consists of IV antibiotics and surgery.

 "Postauricular swelling and erythema" is the typical description of mastoiditis. Tenderness over the mastoid and outwardly displaced pinna are other important clues to the diagnosis.

The bacteria most commonly causing mastoiditis in children include:

- *Streptococcus pneumoniae*
- *H. flu* (non typeable)
- *S. pyogenes*
- *S. aureus*

Diagnosis is confirmed by **CT** and **tympanocentesis** with **culture.** However, a negative culture would not rule out the diagnosis, especially if they note the patient was already started on antibiotics.

Know Your Nose/Rhinos

They sometimes describe nasal congestion in an adolescent as a clue that cocaine use is a part of the picture.

The "E's" have it. A nasal smear with lots of eosinophils[6] is more likely seasonal allergic rhinitis than anything else.

Rhinitis

Allergic Rhinitis

Nasal steroids are now the treatment of choice for allergic rhinitis. Spread the word.

---

[6] Let's say around 17%.

Chronic Rhinitis

The most common causes are allergy, sinusitis, polyps, cystic fibrosis, and foreign body.

 In pediatric practice, you see lots of runny noses and FACES

Foreign body

Allergies

Cystic Fibrosis

Extra tissue **(Polyps)**

Sinusitis

Pop Goes the Nasal (Polyp)

Nasal Polyps are associated with

- Cystic fibrosis
- Asthma
- Chronic allergic rhinitis
- Chronic sinusitis

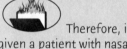 Therefore, if you are given a patient with nasal polyps and are asked which study to order next, the correct answer will be a sweat chloride test.

Choanal Atresia

 "Cyanosis while feeding and resolution with crying."

 CHARGE syndrome is associated with choanal atresia.[7]

Sinusitis

 In pre-adolescents, sinusitis will present as persistent URI, and *not necessarily facial pain* as seen in teens and adults.

 "Nasal congestion," "rhinorrhea," and "cough" will be a typical description of sinusitis.

Timing of Sinuses

You could be tested on when the various sinuses develop.

Here is your program guide:

Maxillary – At birth

Ethmoid – At birth

Sphenoid – start developing age 3 years, fully formed by 7 years

Frontal – Are not fully formed until early teen years

Acute Sinusitis

 This would be described as **"persistent nighttime cough"** and/or "foul breath" after a URI. If they present a patient with a toothache, sore throat, persistent bronchospastic cough, or poorly controlled asthma, the underlying diagnosis could be sinusitis.

---

[7] "C" for coloboma, "H" for heart defects, "A" for atresia choanae, "R" for retardation of growth and development, "G" for genitourinary problems, and "E" for ear abnormalities.

Which Organisms are to Blame?

Most sinus infections are caused by pneumococcus, *H. Flu* (non typeable), or *Moraxella catarrhalis*.[8] *Staph* accounts for a small proportion of sinus infections.

Since these bugs are similar to those that cause OM, the first line of antibiotic should be amoxicillin. However, if they present you with a patient who was recently treated with amoxicillin and/or attends daycare, oral amoxicillin/clavulanate or IM ceftriaxone would be indicated.

Complications: *Orbital cellulitis* is a direct result of *ethmoid sinusitis.* This is easy to remember when you recall that **E**ye and **E**thmoid both start with an **E**. Brain abscess may result from frontal sinusitis (a **frontal assault**). Therefore, any trauma involving a **fracture of the frontal sinus** requires **surgical consult** and repair to **avoid CNS infection**.

Neither nasal swab cultures nor throat cultures correlate well with cultures of sinus aspirates, so ignore that data if they give it to you. PO decongestants and antihistamines do not provide any help for acute sinusitis.

Chronic Sinusitis

Chronic sinusitis, like acute sinusitis, will present as profuse nasal discharge, along with tenderness over the sinuses in a febrile child. An important component will be **nighttime cough**.

> ### Nasal Foreign Body
> This is often described as unilateral, usually blood-tinged, nasal discharge. Foul odor will be your other clue.

The predisposing factors for chronic sinusitis all make sense logically: allergy, immune deficiency, primary ciliary dyskinesis (immotile cilia syndrome), and cystic fibrosis.

Antibiotics (and surgery when necessary) are the treatments of choice.

Imaging studies have no role in managing uncomplicated acute sinusitis. CT would be the study of choice for chronic recurrent sinusitis. MRI would only be indicated if an intracranial complication were suggested in the history.

---

8 Previously known as *Branhamella catarrhalis* and also known as Freddy the dysmorphic acrobat.

Epistaxis

· Epistaxis is usually **due to dry air** and treatment is largely supportive.

· However, read the history carefully and watch for suggestions of a foreign body or vascular anomalies.

· Watch for signs of bleeding disorders in the family history or bleeding/bruising elsewhere.

· Nasopharyngoscopy would be indicated to locate a posterior bleeding source (anterior bleeding sources are often visible on exam).

CASE STUDY

You are presented with a 13 year old boy with recurrent epistaxis. The bleeding is increasing in frequency and severity and takes more time to stop. What is the next step in managing this patient?

THE DIVERSION

You will be tempted by many diversionary choices, such as saline nasal spray or gels, or even more invasive options, such as coagulopathy studies.

ANSWER REVEALED

When presented with a patient with a history of worsening epistaxis on the boards, it is real. It is not the subjective description of a parent. Therefore, the next step would be a *CT scan* to rule out a posterior nasopharyngeal mass such as a *nasopharyngeal angiofibroma*. On the boards they should note the presence of a mass, but even if they do not, consider the CT for worsening epistaxis.

Throat

Infectious Mononucleosis (Mono)

Presenting "Infectious Mono"

 EB virus is usually asymptomatic in preschool children.

For those in school and beyond, the **incubation period** is 2 to 7 weeks. The **prodromal symptoms** are malaise, anorexia, and chills.

Then come the classic symptoms of the "kissing disease:" fever, sore throat, and fatigue, accompanied by **pharyngitis**, **lymphadenopathy**, and headaches.

The high fever can last 1 to 2 weeks.

The **pharyngitis** of infectious mono can include a **thick exudate** and **palatal petechiae**. This can be confused with strep.

Mono can be described as pharyngitis **with exudate**, palpable cervical lymph nodes, and hepatosplenomegaly. They may describe the symptoms in conjunction with treatment with amoxicillin along with subsequent development of a rash. Splenomegaly is common on the Boards, and so is hepatomegaly. In about 30% to 50% of cases, mild hepatic tenderness may be present.

The rash described above is not penicillin allergy, which is awaiting you as the decoy (and, of course, incorrect choice).

In differentiating **strep pharyngitis** from **Epstein Barr (EB) mono**, know that both can have **pharyngitis with exudate, enlarged tonsils, and high fever**. *Hepatosplenomegaly will only be found with mono.*

 Group A Strep can be positive even with EB mono and is, therefore, not a differentiating factor.

Someone can get mono yet be an asymptomatic carrier of strep. **Therefore, serological confirmation is what they are looking for to confirm the diagnosis of mono**. A positive throat culture does not rule out mono.

 The leading cause of pharyngitis in children is viral.

CMV and EBV

The special case of **cytomegalovirus (CMV)** is the illness confused most frequently with EBV-induced infectious mono.

 The children with CMV mono are older. Fever and malaise are the main features.

Mono in Teens

CASE STUDY **You are presented with a child with high fever, swollen lymph nodes, and other signs consistent with mono. They then note that the monospot is negative. What is the next step?**

THE DIVERSION The diversion here is that the monospot screen is frequently negative in children. All of the diversionary choices *including repeating the monospot* and others (i.e., treatment with penicillin), will be incorrect.

ANSWER REVEALED The correct answer will be to obtain EBV IgM/IgG titers to rule out mono.

In adolescents, the classic clinical syndrome consists of the following features:

· Fever
· Lymphadenopathy
· Exudative pharyngitis
· Splenomegaly

Monospot Limitations

❑ The "monospot" is **not as sensitive in children younger than 4**.

❑ Patients who are negative initially **can become positive 2-3 weeks into their illness**.

❑ Antibody titers can be detectable for up to 9 months after the onset of illness, so a positive monospot test does not necessarily mean active/current illness.

 Viral-specific IgM should be done for children younger than 4 who have negative monospot tests but still have symptoms consistent with mono. Lymphocytosis and thrombocytopenia are other lab signs.

IgM antibodies, rather than isolation of the virus, make for a definitive diagnosis.

Treatment Considerations for Mono

Treatment includes restricted activity if the spleen is enlarged, and steroids if the airway is potentially obstructed.

Gee Whiz, GC Pharyngitis

The typical presentation of GC pharyngitis would be a sexually active teenage whom they specifically note has had sexually transmitted diseases in the past. The physical exam will be noteworthy for *erythematous patches*.

You will be expected to test the patient for GC pharyngitis and *other sexually transmitted diseases as well.*

Strep Pharyngitis

Group A beta hemolytic strep is the most common cause of pharyngitis in children who have fever and sore throat in the absence of URI symptoms.

Other causes of pharyngitis include EBV, *Neisseria gonorrhoeae*, and adenovirus. The diagnosis is made by culture and/or rapid strep.

The treatment of choice remains penicillin, and waiting for culture results does not affect treatment outcome. If you are asked, treatment shortens the course *and* prevents the development of complications, including rheumatic fever and abscesses. Ten full days of antibiotics are necessary, even though the patient is feeling better within a few days.

A *negative rapid strep* still requires a throat culture because of the high rate of false negatives. If they present a patient with recurrent symptoms following treatment, the patient should have another culture done. A chronic carrier state is a possibility. The symptoms may also be indicative of a second infection (possibly due to another strain of Group A Strep), or noncompliance is always a possibility as well.

> **GC City**
>
> Don't forget GC with throat pain in an adolescent.

Peritonsillar Abscess

Peritonsillar abscess is typically described as a patient experiencing "dysphagia," with difficulty opening their mouth. Once the mouth is opened (a very common occurrence on the boards), they will have "**unilateral** swelling around the tonsil," and "deviation of the uvula to one side," along with some exudate.

Diagnosis is made by CT. In addition, the WBC will be elevated on CBC

Additional buzzwords include **"trismus"** (whatever that is)[9], **"drooling,"** a muffled **"hot potato"** voice, and **cervical adenopathy**.

Management

Needle aspiration and drainage is critical for diagnostic purposes and to provide symptomatic relief.

---

[9] Actually, trismus is the inability to open one's mouth.

The etiology is usually wide and varied, including group A Strep and anaerobes found in the mouth. The choice of antibiotics should reflect this. The following would be correct antibiotics, if you must choose from among several choices:

- Ampicillin/sulbactam
- Clindamycin
- Amoxicillin/clavulanate (if PO is an option)

Tonsillectomy is indicated **for repeat performances**.[10]

> ### Other Reasons for Tonsillectomy
>
> Additional *indications for tonsillectomy* include the most obvious: malignancy and obstructive sleep apnea.
>
> *Indications for adenoidectomy* would also include chronic sinusitis and/or adenoiditis, as well as obstructive sleep apnea.
>
> Velopharyngeal insufficiency would present with a hypernasal voice, and is a complication of tonsillectomy and/or adenoidectomy.

Retropharyngeal Abscess

If they show or describe the **widening of the retropharyngeal space**, accept the gift and run. Enlarged lymph nodes in a young child may be hinted at. They will describe high fever, difficulty swallowing, and refusal of feedings. On lateral neck film, they will describe widening of the retropharyngeal space. The diagnosis should be confirmed on CT.

The patient's neck may be **hyperextended or held stiffly,** and he/she may demonstrate drooling and/or respiratory difficulties.

This will at least differentiate it from **epiglottitis**, because with epiglottitis, children may drool, but **they lean forward instead of hyperextending their necks or holding their neck stiffly.** Additional findings include decreased PO intake and fever. *Retropharyngeal abscess* will usually be described in a child *younger than four years*. CT scan would be the imaging study of choice to confirm the diagnosis.

Management of Retropharyngeal Abscess

A retropharyngeal abscess is a **surgical emergency**. Needle aspiration under general anesthesia is the best approach. Typical causes include *Strep viridans*, group A *Strep*, and *Staph aureus*, as well as anerobic bacteria. The best choices for antibiotics would include *clindamycin or ampicilllin/sulbactam*. *Throat swab culture is not likely to be helpful.*

---

[10] Repeated peritonsillar abscesses.

You will very likely be called upon to differentiate retropharyngeal from peritonsillar abscess. **Retropharyngeal abscess is more common in patients younger than 4 years of age**. This should be easy to remember since "retro" means to go back to an earlier age in time.

What About the Mouth?

We cover this extensively in the GI chapter, but here are some other bits and pieces to chew on.

Tongue tie (ankyloglossia) requires no intervention, despite the fact that the old timers did it (frenulectomy), and some still tell you it should be done. It will usually be an incorrect choice on the exam.

All Those Oral Lesions

Here's how to keep all those oral lesions straight.

Coxsackievirus Group A

Coxsackievirus Group A gingivostomatitis often presents as "several days of fever, irritability, and decreased appetite," and "4-5 mm ulcers" in the "posterior oral cavity." If they throw in the term **vesiculopapular lesions on the hands and feet**, you've got the answer.

Herpangina

Herpangina will cause lesions on the posterior oral cavity.[11] It is also caused by coxsackievirus group A. Once again, this is the cause of "hand, foot, and mouth disease" where vesicular lesions are noted on the hands, feet, and (you guessed it) mouth.[12]

Note that the **hands and feet can be spared**, so do not let this stop you from identifying coxsackievirus as the etiology.

Herpes Simplex Virus (HSV) (Gingivostomatitis)

Herpes simplex virus infections are cold sores typically described as "vesicles on the **vermilion border**" of the lips, and possibly in the anterior mouth/gums. There is impressive mucosal pain, fever, and adenopathy.

Aphthous Ulcers

Aphthous ulcers are your classic canker sores, the kind you don't want to have when you are drinking lemon juice straight up or on the rocks (or with gin if you prefer).

---

[11] Also known as the posterior mouth, by the way.

[12] Which is not to be confused with the hand, foot and mouth disease seen in cows.

They will be described as having a distinctive grayish-white coagulum surrounded by a thin rim of bright erythema. These resolve on their own over a week or so.

Cold-Induced Panniculitis

Cold-induced panniculitis is a Board classic often described as follows:

An infant "less than a year old," with "**tender red nodules on the cheek,**" afebrile with good PO intake. **Sleeping with a "water-filled pacifier"** or something else very cold is the cause. They are described, or will be shown, as **deep-seated plaques and nodules**.

Remember, no treatment is necessary; the lesion clears within weeks, with no scarring.

"Popsicle panniculitis," as it is also called, helps you remember the appearance and cause.

Delayed Eruption of Teeth

You can remember the common causes of delayed eruption of teeth as the **4 H's plus Rickets**:

> Hypothyroidism
>
> Hypopituitarism
>
> Hypoplasia (ectodermal)
>
> Hypohidrosis (decreased sweating)
>
> **Rickets**
>
> If they describe delayed eruption up by 16 m

Playing Dentist

If they ask you to play dentist, **swelling below the jaw** represents a mandibular dental abscess. **Periorbital swelling** is consistent with a maxillary dental abscess.

Tooth Avulsion

If you are presented with a child with an avulsed *permanent* tooth, know that if it is placed back in its socket within 5 minutes, there is an excellent chance it will survive.

The tooth should reimplanted by any capable adult. If it needs to be reimplanted by a dentist, the tooth should be transported in saliva (preferably the child's, of course) or milk. *Chilled milk* is preferred.

If you are presented with a child with an avulsed *baby/deciduous* tooth, replacing it can cause damage to the incoming permanent tooth, and is therefore contraindicated.

Facial Swelling and Dental Abnormalities

A dental abscess can present with facial swelling that impacts periorbital tissue, which in turn impacts the ability to open the eye. They will, however, have to provide some information hinting at dental disease.

Appropriate treatment would be with penicillin. If the patient were penicillin-allergic, then clindamycin or erythromycin would be appropriate.

Cleft Lip and Palate

The following are some important facts regarding cleft lip and palate that you will be expected to know for the exam.

- Cleft lip (with or without cleft palate) is the most common craniofacial congenital malformation
- Cleft lip/palate is more common than cleft palate alone.
- Cleft lip/palate can occur as a single gene defect, in conjunction with other chromosomal abnormalities, or from teratogenic exposure in utero
- Cleft palate is more likely to be associated with other abnormalities
- Cleft lip/palate occurs more commonly in boys
- Cleft palate occurs more frequently in girls
- Middle ear effusions are almost always present in children with cleft palate

Stridor Cider and Epiglottitis

All that glitters is not croup and epiglottitis. The key again is in the wording, and in the specifics that differentiate similar clinical presentations. They have even been known to take you down the **path of "stridor,"** even showing the **typical steeple sign of croup. Look again at the x-ray and there is a foreign body** sitting there, making "foreign body aspiration" the correct answer. The motto of the story is "know your stridors." Many of the other causes of stridor are covered in the pulmonary chapter as well.

Fortunately, you can answer questions on stridor correctly just by becoming familiar with the buzzwords (in bold in the following sections). On the other hand, you could be the best on-site diagnostician, but get these questions wrong if you do not know these buzzwords cold. This is typical for written Board exams, as clinical skills and test taking skills are different.

Remember that stridor is due to turbulent flow through a narrowed segment of the respiratory tract.

Given how narrow the normal airway is in a newborn, this is a prominent feature of respiratory disease of the newborn. Children older than 2 years of age will have stridor for a variety of other reasons.

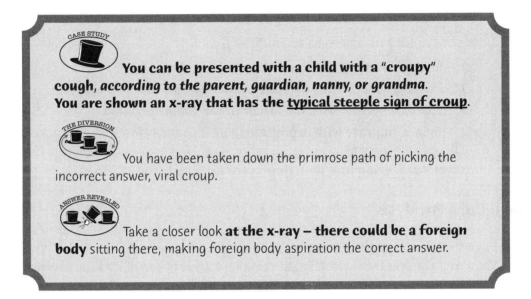

CASE STUDY You can be presented with a child with a "croupy" cough, *according to the parent, guardian, nanny, or grandma.* You are shown an x-ray that has the <u>typical steeple sign of croup</u>.

THE DIVERSION You have been taken down the primrose path of picking the incorrect answer, viral croup.

ANSWER REVEALED Take a closer look **at the x-ray – there could be a foreign body** sitting there, making foreign body aspiration the correct answer.

Inspiratory Stridor

 Inspiratory stridor is caused by *extrathoracic* (above the thoracic outlet) obstruction. All the "structures" above the thoracic outlet are soft and collapse inward with the pressure of inspiration, and that makes for the inspiratory stridor. Extrathoracic includes both supraglottic and glottic and subglottic areas (see below). Inspiratory stridor will always be more prominent, but as you get lower, the chances of also having expiratory stridor increase.

These structures include the tonsils and adenoids, as well as pharyngeal and **hypopharyngeal masses**.

It is easy to remember the causes of inspiratory stridor with the following mnemonic **(INSP)**:

    Immobile Cords (Paralyzed)
    Noid (Adenoid) and tonsil enlargement
    Soft cartilage (laryngomalacia)
    Pharyngeal and hypopharyngeal masses

Laryngomalacia

Laryngomalacia is a condition in which the tissues at the entrance of the larynx collapse into the airway with inspiration.

Laryngomalacia is **the most common cause of congenital stridor.**

Typical descriptions of laryngomalacia include:

- ❏ "Suprasternal and subcostal retractions"
- ❏ In an infants under 1 month of age with stridor, you may see **"worsening with agitation"**
- ❏ Stridor that **worsens with the infant in the supine position**
- ❏ Symptoms **improve with expiration** (pressure from below with expiration "stents" the floppy airway open)
- ❏ Symptoms do **improve with time** as the cartilage becomes firmer

Vocal Cord Paralysis

Vocal cord paralysis is the second most common cause of extra-thoracic airway obstruction and stridor in infancy. It is usually due to **traumatic injury of the recurrent laryngeal** nerve at the time of birth, or to an impairment of the central nervous system.

The cry will be described as weak.

Laryngomalacia also produces inspiratory stridor, but it is "wet" or "variably pitched." **Paralyzed vocal cords** result in a "high-pitched" inspiratory stridor. This is easy to remember because they are fixed like thin guitar strings.

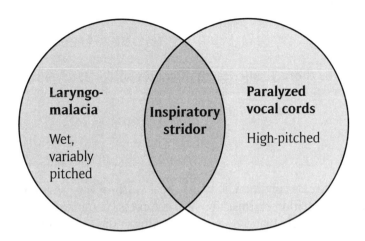

However, **unilateral** vocal cord paralysis would cause **persistent hoarseness**.

Laryngeal webs can also present with a weak cry noted during early infancy. However, **changing position will have no clinical effect on these symptoms.**

Infants with laryngomalacia feed without difficulty and gain weight. If you are presented with an infant who is failing to thrive, laryngomalacia is not the correct answer.

Vocal Cord Nodules

Vocal cord nodules are typically described as being characterized by "progressive hoarseness," which is less severe in the morning, *without stridor or dysphagia*.

Most cases of hoarseness in children are caused by vocal cord nodules. They occur more often in males, and tend to improve with puberty.

Hoarseness may follow endotracheal extubation, so watch for that in the history if you are asked to determine a cause. **Laryngoscopy is often required to diagnose laryngeal and vocal cord disorders.**

You may be presented with a patient who has what seems to be asthma, but is actually vocal cord dysfunction.

No need to lose your voice or sleep over this if you note the following:

As opposed to asthma, a patient with vocal cord dysfunction will have a normal pulse oximeter reading. They will note clear lung fields on physical exam and no response to bronchodilator treatment.

In vocal cord dysfunction, inspiration, rather than expiration, will be problematic.

Expiratory Stridor

Lesions **below the thoracic inlet** cause expiratory stridor. Tracheomalacia and bronchomalacia are classic examples.

Tracheomalacia

Tracheomalacia is a rare condition, in which weak tracheal wall rings **collapse during expiration**. In addition to expiratory **stridor**, extrinsic tracheal compression can also cause fixed wheezing. This can also be the result of chronic ventilation, so watch for this in the presenting history.

With laryngomalacia, symptomatic relief is noted during expiration, which is not the case with tracheomalacia.

A child who has had a TE fistula repair will frequently present later on with tracheomalacia. Consider a diagnosis of tracheomalacia in a patient with a history of TE fistula repair presenting with expiratory stridor.

Another cause of "extrinsic compression" is the **vascular ring** (that wraps around the trachea AND the esophagus). A hint that vascular ring is the problem is "feeding difficulties" in addition to expiratory stridor.

Infants with tracheomalacia can also be described as wheezing.

"Biphasic" (Inspiratory and Expiratory) Stridor

Both congenital and acquired subglottic stenoses (i.e., subglottic hemangiomas) straddle both sides of the anatomical fence (intra-thoracic and extra-thoracic). Stridor is the result; however, the inspiratory component is often louder. Biphasic stridor can also mean a critical obstruction anywhere along the way, so look for clues to this in the question.

With tracheomalacia, if the obstruction is high enough, the stridor may be biphasic. Watch for clues in the question suggesting this disorder

Epiglottitis

Epiglottitis is a supraglottic stenosis, and presents with *"biphasic"* stridor.

Epiglottitis, although now rare thanks to the Hib vaccine, is still fair game on the Boards.

Epiglottitis is typically described in a **4 or 5 year old** with "inspiratory stridor," who is **"leaning forward drooling."**

The phrasing that gives it away is **"drooling, dysphagia, dysphonia, distress and stridor."** The child will be described as being very agitated, refusing to lie down, and insisting on leaning forward.

Lateral neck film will emphasize the **"thumb sign,"** which is the enlarged epiglottis.

Cough will <u>not</u> be included in the description.

5 D's: Instead of the thumb sign, picture the swollen epiglottis as a **Giant Swollen D: D**rooling, **D**ysphagia, **D**ysphonia, **D**istress, and **D**eafening (and frightening) stridor.

They may throw in a parental refusal of all immunizations, or that the child is from another country. The implication here is that the Hib vaccine was not given.

When epiglottitis is suspected, it is a medical emergency that requires rapid attention. Evaluation is done with all equipment for intubation, including having the anesthesiologist (with tacky shower cap and shoe covers) on standby in the room. CBC and blood culture should be obtained, unless the airway is already obstructed or at risk of becoming obstructed momentarily. If in distress, the patient should have minimal stimulation. A third-generation cephalosporin (e.g., ceftriaxone, cefotaxime) directed at *H. flu* should be started empirically.

The vaccine is for ***H. flu* type B. Ear infections are caused by *H. flu* non-typeable**. Therefore, the incidence of *H. flu* ear infections has not gone down since the advent of the vaccine.

How They Are Assessed

Subglottic stenosis	Direct laryngoscopy and bronchoscopy (the latter to assess the patency of the subglottis adequately)
Vocal cord function	Flexible nasolaryngoscopy or direct laryngoscopy, plus CXR and barium swallow
Vascular ring	Barium swallow study

Viral Croup (Laryngotracheobronchitis)

The Scoop on Croup

Etiology: **R**SV, **I**nfluenza, or **P**ara influenza (RIP).

To help remember RIP, think of a dog with a bark-like cough RIPping apart the viruses that cause croup.

They will either describe an **"inspiratory"** stridor or a "biphasic" stridor.

The child they describe, often in the fall or winter, will be younger – **around 18 months** – with a **lower grade fever**. Your clue will be terms like "a hoarse, barking cough." Often laryngotracheitis will be among the listed choices, not viral croup.

More serious signs of respiratory distress would include "tripoding," mouth breathing, and dysphagia. These patients are typically afebrile and non-toxic appearing.

Measles (rubeola) can also cause croup. **Watch out for children who may not have been immunized**, including children of parents who do not like immunizations, and recent immigrants whose immunization status is unknown.

Racemic epinephrine and cool mist are considered short term solutions that are useful. Corticosteroids have now been shown to provide longer-lasting and effective treatment, especially **Decadron®** **(dexamethasone)** and nebulized **budesonide.**

Usually "stridor and barking cough" is the classic description of viral croup. Here are a few facts to help you breathe better:

❏ Viral croup is also known as laryngotracheobronchitis.
❏ The typical age is 2.
❏ URI and mild fever precede stridor.
❏ It is usually caused by parainfluenza, or influenza A and B.

Bacterial Tracheitis

This is also known as "**pseudomembranous croup,**" or "**membranous laryngotracheitis,**" or "Manny the half-witted Money Manager." It is usually caused by *S. aureus*, but can also be caused by *Moraxella catarrhalis*, nontypeable *Haemophilus influenzae*, or oral anaerobes.

Bacterial tracheitis might occur several days into a bout with viral croup. Watch for rapid deterioration of a patient diagnosed with viral croup.

Like viral croup, the words "**inspiratory stridor**" and "**barking cough**" will be described. They may also describe a brassy cough. The patient will typically be described as being toxic-appearing. Bacterial tracheitis presents with thick, purulent secretions which can cause airway obstruction, and, in severe cases, cardiopulmonary arrest. However, this will be followed by fever and severe respiratory symptoms. Patients will be **supine instead of sitting**. They could include a neck film, described as a "**ragged air column**" or "**subglottic narrowing.**"

With epiglottitis, the child will be described as *leaning forward and drooling.* In bacterial tracheitis, they will be more comfortable staying in the supine position.

Since you will likely be presented with a patient who deteriorates rapidly, it is important to know that often intubation is required, as well as clearing of purulent secretions. Broad spectrum antibiotics that provide coverage for *Staph* are also indicated.

Spasmodic Croup

Spasmodic croup is felt to be of allergic etiology and tends to be *recurrent in the absence of a preceding URI.*

Symptomatic treatment, with or without steroids, is the management of choice.

Again, spasmodic croup is probably **allergic in nature**, so they might describe "**nightly recurrences,**" a history of "atopic derm," and "family history of spasmodic croup."

Treatment is essentially the same as for viral croup.

The features are quite similar to viral croup, except there is **no fever** and **no viral respiratory infection**. Therefore, it is essentially **"non-infectious" croup.**

Laryngeal Papillomas

Laryngeal papillomas cause hoarseness, are the most common tumor of the larynx in children, and are usually a result of **human papillomavirus**. It is "managed" by repeated laser excision. They **can** become malignant. In young children, they might have been transmitted at delivery, but child abuse might be what they want you to consider. Read the question carefully.

Thyroglossal Cyst

Unless there are other signs shown to you, any midline lesion on the anterior neck should be assumed to be a thyroglossal cyst; it should have a "Do Not Remove" sign (as in "No Surgical Excisions") hanging over it, since this is often the only functioning thyroid tissue. They will describe the lesion as moving vertically with swallowing or sticking the tongue out. There could be communication with the skin, resulting in draining as well.

Uvula (Bifid) the Punching Bag in the Back of the Throat

If you see this, think submucous cleft palate. They want you to do a tympanometry study to evaluate tympanic membrane mobility.

Craning Your NECK

Neck Masses

Reactive Cervical Adenopathy

Most cases of reactive cervical lymphadenitis in children are **viral or bacterial**. However, other possible causes are also described below. The nodes will likely be described as mobile and tender, but will *not* be described as being erythematous or warm to touch.

Infected Lymphadenitis

If the node itself is infected (rather than reactive), in addition to being tender, it will also be red and warm to touch.

Acute viral cervical lymphadenitis is generally **bilateral. Bacterial lymphadenitis,** on the other hand, is usually **unilateral,** with **more local inflammation.**

HIV Infection

HIV infection should be considered if they present a patient with **chronic cervical lymphadenopathy.**

Adenoviral Lymphadenopathy

The classic presentation of adenovirus infection would be **preauricular adenopathy,** as well as **conjunctivitis.** The key point is the combination of preauricular adenopathy **and** conjunctivitis.

Bacterial Lymphadenopathy

The most common bacterial organisms causing acute cervical adenitis are *Staph aureus* and group A strep.

If they do not provide you with the following labs, then ordering them would be the correct answer: CBC, ESR, blood cultures, PPD, DNA, and DWI.[13]

Treatment

Treatment of choice is antibiotics that can fight the beta lactamase-producers. Amoxicillin/clavulanate and clindamycin are good choices. Erythromycin would be a good choice when penicillin allergy is a factor.

If exposure to cats or kittens is described, then cat scratch disease caused by *Bartonella henselae* may be what they are after.

---

[13] Just kidding on DWI; just making sure you are still with us.

Atypical Mycobacteria

When atypical mycobacteria are the cause of cervical adenopathy, it often requires **surgical excision**.

Needle excision is never the correct answer for atypical mycobacteria lymphadenopathy.

Since atypical mycobacteria will result in a PPD reaction *less than 10 mm*, even a minimal reaction (5 mm) would be consistent with atypical mycobacterial infection.

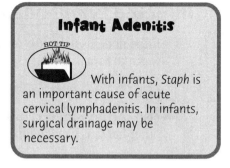

Infant Adenitis

With infants, *Staph* is an important cause of acute cervical lymphadenitis. In infants, surgical drainage may be necessary.

Mycobacterium tuberculosis

Mycobacterium tuberculosis might be what they are after if they present a patient with cervical adenitis who is not responding to antibiotics. They would also likely present other risk factors for tuberculosis.

In an asymptomatic patient with chronic cervical adenopathy, a good first step would be placement of a PPD.

Brucellosis

Brucellosis would present with a picture of **chronic adenopathy and hepatosplenomegaly,** along with a history of exposure to farm animals or ingestion of milk that was not pasteurized.

Other Causes of Enlarged Cervical Lymph Nodes

Neoplasm

If the lymph node is associated with a neoplasm, it will be nontender, firm, and non–mobile/fixed.

Cystic hygroma

A cystic hygroma is dilated lymph vessels. They might be described as being a large soft mass.

Parotitis

You are expected to know the different causes of parotitis and their presentations as outlined in the following table.

Cause of Parotitis	Presentation
Viral Parotitis	Presents in a preschool or school-age child with parotid swelling and vague symptoms, including weakness and fever. There will be **swelling and erythema around the opening of Stensen's duct, but typically no pus can be expressed with parotid massage.** HOT TIP There will be **no erythema of the overlying skin.** If the child is unimmunized, consider a diagnosis of mumps. **HIV infection must be a consideration if the presenting history supports the diagnosis.**
Bacterial parotitis	Occurs before the age of 10. The child will be described as toxic-appearing, with a very high temperature. ***Staph aureus*** is the most common cause of bacterial parotitis.
Salivary gland stone	This will present as recurrent swelling of both parotid glands

CASE STUDY

You are presented with a patient from a developing country who has parotid swelling of a few weeks' duration which is resistant to antibiotic therapy. There is _no information_ on the biological parents. You are told that the patient received multiple vaccines, although it is not well-documented. You are asked for the most appropriate study to help establish the diagnosis.

THE DIVERSION

You would, of course, realize that this is most likely _viral_ parotitis, since this child most likely did not receive an MMR vaccine. Therefore, picking a study such as mumps titers to establish mumps as the correct diagnosis would be automatic.

ANSWER REVEALED

You would have automatically picked the wrong answer. An important part of the history is the _lack of knowledge_ about the biological parents. This, coupled with the information that _some vaccines_ were given, should make you suspicious for _HIV infection_.

Chapter 29

Adolescent Medicine and Gynecology

Adolescent Physiologic Development

The following are some important general patterns and definitions you are expected to know:

- The normal age range for pubertal development is between 9-13 years in both boys and girls (although normal development can take place as early as 8 years of age in girls).

- Traversing from Tanner 2 to Tanner 5 may take as long as five years.

- Adolescent peak height velocity has a lot more to do with Tanner stage than age

---

You say Tanner; I say SMR

What was once called Tanner staging is now known as Sexual Maturity Rating. The names have changed, but the stage is the same.

MALE

	SMR 1 Prepubertal	SMR 2 Beginning of puberty	SMR 3	SMR 4	SMR 5
Pubic Hair	Absent	Fine hair appears	Coarse, curly, and pigmented	Denser and curled, but less abundant than adult	Extends to the inner thigh, adult-like
Phallus Size	Childlike	No change	Increased phallus size	Closer to adult male	Adult size
Testicular Size	Volume < 2.5 mL	Increased size and volume; scrotum more textured	Increased size		Adult size

---

FEMALE

	SMR 1 Prepubertal	SMR 2 Beginning of puberty	SMR 3	SMR 4	SMR 5
Pubic Hair	Absent	Hair along the labia	Coarse, curly, and pigmented	Denser and curled, but less abundant than adult	Extends to the inner thigh, adult-like
Breast	No glandular breast tissue	Small breast buds with glandular tissue	Breast tissue extends beyond the areola	Enlarged areola and papilla form a secondary mound	No longer a separate projection of the areola from the remainder of the breast

Off to the Growth Spurt Races

Pre-puberty Height Velocity – 5-6 cm/ year

Peak Adolescent Height Velocity – 9-10 cm/ year

Delayed Puberty

In a boy, it means no pubertal development by age 14 and in a girl, by age 13.

Growth Spurt

The growth spurt begins with the onset of breast development[1] and ends around menarche. In boys, enlargement of the testes is the first sign of puberty and begins the male growth spurt.

 Elevated alkaline phosphatase values correlate with the adolescent growth spurt, and should be considered normal.

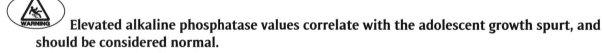 In either case, it is two "bumps" getting bigger.

- Early puberty results in shorter adult height. So the fun of fast maturing males bullying shorter kids with constitutional growth delay is as short lived as their short adult height
- In **constitutional growth delay,** bone age < chronological age (the bones catch up later)
- **Boys** reach **SMR 4** before going through **peak height velocity**
- **Hematocrit increases with the growth spurt**

---

[1] In girls, of course.

Male Pubertal Development

The sequence of male pubertal development is

Testicular growth ➔ Pubarche ➔ Penile growth ➔ Peak height velocity

- Pubertal development occurring prior to age 9 in boys is considered abnormal.
- Constitutional delay is the most common cause for delayed puberty in boys
- The first sign of pubertal development in males is testicular enlargement, with testicular length greater than 2.5 cm indicating the onset of puberty and the end of childhood as the boy once knew it. This typically occurs between age 10 and 11.
- Peak height velocity occurs after SMR Stage 4
- Axillary hair will develop only after pubic hair reaches SMR 5

HOT TIP Pubic hair development and penis enlargement in the absence of testicular enlargement suggests androgen stimulation is coming from outside the gonadal area.

Gynecomastia

If they describe gynecomastia in a male or asymmetric breasts in a female, the choice will usually be "normal; only reassurance is necessary." However, gynecomastia is also associated with Klinefelter syndrome, so watch for other features of Klinefelter in the history.

PERIL WARNING However, if they describe a history of exposure to **ketoconazole** or *bilateral* gynecomastia in males, then it could be considered an abnormal finding. **Galactorrhea** may be due to **marijuana use**. If this does not work as a deterrent for male teens not to smoke pot, I don't know what will.

Female Pubertal Development

Normal Sexual Development

Breast Budding ➔ Pubarche ➔ Peak height velocity ➔ Menarche

- Puberty may begin as young as age 8 in females; prior to age 7 is considered abnormal

Thelarche is the development of breast tissue, and is the first sign of pubertal development in females. It occurs on average around age 10-11. If thelarche does not occur by age 13, a workup is indicated.

Pubarche is the development of pubic hair; in females, it follows breast development by a few years.

Joan of Arche

She was a teenaged French girl and ardent nationalist who fought the British. Even though she preceded him by over 500 years, mysteriously she was an ardent fan of Jerry Lewis (like many of her countrymen and countrywomen today).

Arches occur in Sync

· **Estrogen** is responsible for **breast development**

· **Androgen** is responsible for **hair development**

The two arches, thelarche and pubarche, should occur in parallel. One should not accelerate faster than the other.

· If *thelarche* occurs without *pubarche* (that is, breast tissue without pubic hair), then think androgen insensitivity. In other words, a diagnosis of testicular feminization[2] should be considered.

· *Pubarche* without *thelarche* may occur with an excess of androgens/low estrogen. The absence of breast tissue would also explain this.

Menarche

· The onset of menses will occur, on average, two years after thelarche (at approximately age 12 or 13).

· The first few cycles only last 2-3 days.

· The peak height velocity occurs *before menarche.* One would expect a girl to be at SMR stage 3 or 4 at this point.

---

[2] See endocrinology section for the new nomenclature for "testicular feminization."

Menstruation that persists beyond 10 days is abnormal and requires a workup. However, infrequent menstrual periods during the first 2 years post menarche do <u>not</u> generally require a workup beyond reassurance and followup.

After menarche, girls are within 4cm/ 2inches of adult height.

If you are presented with a girl whose onset of menses was less than two years ago, longer intervals (more than 28 days) can be normal.

Physiologic leukorrhea

Physiologic leukorrhea is a white, odorless, mucoid discharge that precedes menarche by 3-6 months and can continue for several years.

It requires no intervention except followup.

You are presented with an 11 year old girl who is SMR stage 2 and has bloody vaginal discharge. You have to determine the etiology.

One of the diversionary answers could be reassurance, using the logic that this may be the onset of menses, or menarche.

However, if you realized that the onset of menses occurs at SMR state 3 or 4, you would have been spared the indignity of answering this question incorrectly. The correct answer would be another explanation, such as vaginal foreign body, which is a common occurrence in girls this age (i.e., small pieces of toilet paper causing local irritation and mild bleeding).

True Precocious Puberty

True precocious puberty occurs when the sequence of pubertal development follows the normal sequence, but early.

Psychosocial Impact of Delayed or Precocious Puberty

Delayed puberty can have an impact on school performance and self esteem, especially in boys.

Those experiencing **precocious puberty** tend to be shy and withdrawn, preferring to be around those older than them.

Due to their older appearance, expectations (of teachers, etc.) may be higher than expected for their chronological age.

In general, emotional and cognitive development does not always coincide with physical maturation.

Children with precocious puberty may be at higher risk for sexual abuse and/or pregnancy.

The Iso from the Hetero, to the Oh NO

 Isosexual: changes consistent with gender.

 Heterosexual: changes consistent with the opposite gender.

 Non-sexual neurotonogenic: what life become 4-6 weeks prior to the Boards.

Pseudo Precocious Puberty

Pseudo precocious puberty is when things happen out of sequence; for example, the onset of menses without pubic hair development.

Pseudo precocious puberty is usually due to sex steroid production by the adrenals, ovaries, or testes. It can also be due to exposure to exogenous sex hormones.

In males, pseudo precocious puberty would present as the development of secondary sexual characteristics in the absence of testicular enlargement.

Late onset congenital adrenal hyperplasia would be one consideration, and Leydig cell tumors would be another. Anabolic steroids could also be an explanation for this presentation, as well as oral contraceptive pills in females.

Appearance of Axillary Hair

Remember, androgen is responsible for acne <u>and</u> *axillary hair* in boys *and* girls.

In fact, they have presented a picture of a female with acne and asked what hormone is responsible for this; the answer is an androgen.

If a child has signs of premature adrenarche, it is necessary to obtain a bone age and it may be necessary do further lab workup, depending on the results. See the Endocrine chapter for further details.

Search from Top to Bottom

It is always good to think anatomically from top to bottom when working up precocious puberty. This systematic approach can make this potentially complex topic a quick slam-dunk.

Top/Central

Terms like "optic fundus abnormal" and "visual field deficits" tip you off to a CNS lesion, possibly a pituitary mass.

Bottom/Abdominal

For **androgenic**, look for descriptions like "acne", "facial and axillary hair" and "muscle bulk" (in boys). For **estrogenic**, look for a change in vaginal color and more prominent labia minora.

Tools of the Trade

The Friendly Radiologist

Ultrasound will find adrenal (premature appearance of pubic hair) or ovarian masses (premature breast development). **Bone age x-rays** are helpful in drawing a comparison between bone age and chronological age.

Head Imaging

MRI will find many causes of central precocious puberty (true precocious puberty) including:
- Hamartomas
- Hydrocephalus
- Arachnoid or ventricular cysts
- Meningitis
- Encephalitis
- Neoplasms
- CNS trauma

The Friendly Lab

LH, FSH, and adrenal steroids will help differentiate peripheral from central disorders.

Gynecology

Pregnancy

Fertile Facts

· The most likely reason for not using contraception is a desire to become pregnant

· 1/2 of all pregnancies occur within 6 months of the first time experiencing intercourse

· 1/5 occur during the first month

Oral Contraceptives

Not Just for Contraception

· There are other indications and advantages of oral contraceptives besides its descriptive calling card.

· They *decrease the risk* for *ovarian cysts, endometrial cancer,* and even **colorectal cancer**, as well as *osteoporosis.*

· They *reduce* the *risk* for *salpingitis* and *ectopic pregnancy.*

· They provide some protection against **acne** and **iron deficiency anemia** as well.

· Oral contraceptives would be indicated for dysmenorrhea and/or menorrhagia.

IUD New Ideas

The newer IUDs are considered to be safer than in the past, without the increased risk for PID or infertility down the road.

Subcutaneous slow release progesterone options are also available. Other options include contraceptive intravaginal rings.

Since these devices do not require daily compliance, they are considered to be very effective.

Absolute Contraindications

❑ Pregnancy
❑ Liver Disease
❑ Elevated Serum Lipids
❑ Breast Cancer
❑ Coronary Artery Disease
❑ Cerebrovascular Disease

If you need birth control when there are absolute contraindications, you need some serious "**BC HELP**":

Breast Cancer
Coronary Artery Disease (Cerebrovascular Disease)

Hepatic Disease
Elevated
Lipids
Pregnancy

Relative Contraindications

❑ **Hypertension** (I am too tense to have sex anyway)

❑ **Depression** (too depressed)

❑ **Migraines** (not tonight, honey, I have a headache)

❑ **Breast-feeding** (no time for sex)

❑ **Drugs that interfere with absorption**. Anticonvulsants are a classic, so someone with a seizure disorder qualifies as a "relative contraindication." Since absorption may be less than optimal anyway, a backup is needed.

In general, oral contraceptives are not considered to be as effective in adolescents as they are in adults.

You might be asked to pick from among a list of possible absolute contraindications for the use of oral contraceptive pills.

You might be tempted to pick a patient with sickle cell disease because of the increased risk for stroke. Epilepsy might be the diversion that does you in if you remember the relative risk with many anticonvulsants. One of the more benign-appearing choices might be a patient with elevated serum lipids.

If you had picked elevated lipids, you would be correct. Sickle cell disease in the absence of a prior history of stroke is not an absolute contraindication. Epilepsy, even if the patient is taking anticonvulsants, is not an absolute contraindication either.

All contraceptive methods are associated with fewer health risks than pregnancy and delivery.

Indications for a Pap smear

In general, the indications for a pap smear are a bit controversial. The American Cancer Society suggests beginning pap smears 3 years after a female starts having sex, with a recommendation to start screening by age 21 if a woman waits until she is over 18 to have sex.

Sexually Active	Non-sexually active
Any age	By age 21
Every year	Repeated every 3 years[3]

Amenorrhea

During the first 2 years following menarche, infrequent menstrual periods are within the norm and do not warrant a workup.

By definition, primary amenorrhea is the lack of menses by age 16, or 2 years following sexual maturation.

If you are presented with a teenager with primary amenorrhea, keep the following diagnoses in mind:

Polycystic ovary disease

Polycystic ovary disease should be suspected in any female adolescent who, in addition to amenorrhea or dysfunctional uterine bleeding, presents with obesity, hirsutism and acne. Lab findings often include LH:FSH ratio >2.5 and **elevated androgen levels**.

Treatment would include weight loss, oral contraceptive pills, and anti-androgen medications. Spironolactone would be an example of an anti-androgen medication.

While obesity is a common association, it isn't always present, and therefore lack of obesity doesn't rule out polycystic ovary disease.

---

[3] Unless of course they become sexually active before age 21 and then one would assume the category changes to sexually active, and yearly pap smears would be indicated. However, let's hope one would not have to make this distinction on the exam.

Testicular feminization

Testicular feminization[4] will present with normal breast development in the absence of pubic hair.

Turner Syndrome

A typical presentation of Turner syndrome would be an amenorrheic girl with breast development limited to breast budding and no pubic hair development. If they give you with a female with pubertal delay, watch for other features of Turner syndrome in the history. These could include low hairline and low set ears, as well as lymphedema of the hands and/or feet. A karyotype study would be indicated.

Secondary Amenorrhea

Some of the most common causes of secondary amenorrhea are *pregnancy, exercise-induced amenorrhea,* and *PCOS*.

It can also occur in anorexia nervosa, with amenorrhea **preceding** weight loss.

Exercise-induced amenorrhea

The typical presentation is a female teenager who is involved in heavy athletic training whose menstrual cycles gradually become lighter and then stop. Lab values would include low serum estradiol (E2) levels, which increases their risk for low bone density and osteoporosis.

These patients are at increased risk for eating disorders, including anorexia nervosa.

Any patient presenting with secondary amenorrhea needs a pregnancy test to rule this out. Pregnancy is the most common cause of secondary amenorrhea.

---

4 See Endocrinology chapter for revised nomenclature for testicular feminization.

Management would include:

1. Reduction in the intensity of athletic training
2. In the unlikely event they are smoking, they need to stop since this increases the risk for stress fractures
3. Calcium supplements
4. Increase caloric intake

Resumption of menses reduces the risk for bone demineralization

 Hormone replacement would not be the correct treatment

 Delayed puberty is associated with low bone density

Dysmenorrhea

Primary Dysmenorrhea

 Primary dysmenorrhea is crampy lower abdominal pain and pelvic pain that occurs with menses (and is not due to other pelvic pathology). It is due to prostaglandins produced during the ovulatory cycle.

Treatment is prostaglandin inhibitors such as NSAIDs, including ibuprofen or naproxen. Oral contraceptives are only indicated when the NSAID treatment fails.

Primary dysmenorrhea is a significant cause of school absence.

Exercise, healthy diet, acetaminophen, and rest are essentially ineffective in treating bonafide primary dysmenorrhea.

Secondary Dysmenorrhea

Secondary dysmenorrhea is due to underlying pelvic pathology, such as endometriosis. The clue will be pain that occurs during other times besides menstruation.

Dysfunctional Uterine Bleeding

Consider this diagnosis for menstrual bleeding beyond 10 days.

The most common cause of dysfunctional uterine bleeding is anovulation during initial onset of menarche.

If you are presented with a patient with dysfunctional uterine bleeding, consider the following underlying etiologies:

- Tubal Pregnancy/ Threatened abortion
- PID
- Hyperthyroidism
- Bleeding disorder

Treatment is medical with NSAIDs. The possibility of iron deficiency anemia should be addressed.

Heavy bleeding, or menometrorrhagia, may be due to a bleeding disorder, especially if it is cyclical.

Adolescent Behavioral Health

Post Traumatic Stress Disorder

You need to be familiar with the signs and symptoms associated with post traumatic stress disorder, or PTSD, which includes rape-trauma syndrome.

The typical presentation is of a teenage female who, weeks to months after experiencing a sexual assault, presents with *recurrent nightmares, fears of being alone, diminished interest in school,* and/or *decreased appetite.*

Physical symptoms include *lower abdominal pain and vaginal discharge.* These can also be a sign of sexually transmitted diseases and/or pelvic inflammatory disease.

Morbidity and Mortality

The leading causes of death among teenagers:

- · Accidents (mostly MVA)
- · Homicide
- · Suicide

Eating Disorders

Anorexia Nervosa

In order to make the diagnosis of anorexia nervosa the following criteria must be met:

1. Distorted body perception
2. Weight 15% below expected
3. Intense fear of gaining weight
4. Absence of 3 consecutive menstrual cycles[5]

You might be given several signs and symptoms consistent with an eating disorder and will have to pick the one that is *most* important in making the diagnosis.

Many of the choices will seem correct because they do occur with anorexia nervosa, including *excessive exercise, depression, dieting over several months, and/ or taking diuretics.*

These are all diversionary answers since the correct answer is that the patient "thinks" they are fat, despite their weight being normal. This is the most important criteria for making the diagnosis. The other choices are too non-specific.

---

[5] Yes! This criterion applies to females only!

Anorexia nervosa can be distinguished from *Crohn's disease, hypothyroidism, depression, or collagen vascular disease* by the lab findings and information given in the history. In anorexia nervosa, amenorrhea could be the presenting sign prior to weight loss.

Bulimia Nervosa

An important feature of bulimia nervosa is binge eating, which is the consumption of an amount of food larger than most people would eat in one sitting. This is coupled with induced vomiting.

Some of the physiologic and lab findings may be a result of vomiting, including:

- Salivary gland enlargement
- Dental enamel erosion
- Bruises or calluses over the knuckles from forced gagging
- Low potassium
- Low chloride
- Metabolic alkalosis

Indications for hospital admission with bulimia

- Failure of outpatient treatment
- Dehydration
- EKG abnormality
- Mallory Weiss tears
- Suicidal ideation

 Achalasia must be distinguished from bulimia. Key information in the history would include **involuntary** vomiting soon after food is ingested.

There is a risk for developing *hypophosphatemia* during refeeding.

Sexually Transmitted Diseases

With any STD, it is important to note that the partner(s) need to be notified of the diagnosis.

· The most **prevalent** sexually transmitted disease among adolescents is *human papillomavirus*.
· *Chlamydia* is the most common **bacterial** STD.

Anogenital Warts

Anogenital warts are often asymptomatic in males, and this could easily be a question on the exam. Even though human papillomavirus is the most prevalent sexually transmitted disease, genital warts (which are caused by the human papillomavirus) are not the *most common* STD. A small percentage of those with the virus develop warts.

Anogenital warts have a high spontaneous resolution rate. Therefore, it may be a reasonable option to observe for 1-2 years before treatment.

Medical treatment is with podophyllin or podofilox. Surgical excision is another alternative. But most importantly, observation is the initial management.

Physiologic discharge

This is the result of increased estrogen levels during puberty.

It will be described as white mucoid discharge which becomes more copious and watery mid cycle, and stickier and more scant at the end of the cycle.

Bacterial Vaginosis

Bacterial vaginosis is due in part to *Gardnerella vaginalis*. It is associated with the use of anything which disrupts the normal balance of vaginal flora, including antibiotics or IUDs. It is not necessarily an STD. *Gardnerella vaginalis* is a part of normal vaginal flora, but more common in those who are sexually active.

A malodorous fishy = amine odor is diagnostic. Diagnosis can be made by the "Whiff Test," which is testing for the presence of amines after the addition of potassium hydroxide. In addition, clue cells **are diagnostic**.

Trichomonas Vaginalis

Trichomoniasis is one of the most common sexually transmitted diseases.

 Trichomoniasis is often asymptomatic in males, and this could easily be a question on the exam.

Symptoms in women are burning, itching, abnormal vaginal odor, and dyspareunia (pain during intercourse). The key words here are "**flagellated organisms**" on wet mount, "**frothy yellow discharge**," and "**strawberry cervix**" because of friable mucosa.

Well, we will have to revert to something off color here. Because the organism is "**flagellated**," picture an organism that carries a "whip" and **whips the cervix**, which explains the petechia and the "**strawberry cervix.**" In addition, vaginal secretions on a glass slide will show the flagellated organisms.

Treatment

Treatment is **metronidazole** a.k.a. **Flagyl®**, which is easy to remember since it treats **flagellated organisms**. Alternatively, envision a bunch of flagellated organisms riding the metro/subway.

 Partners also need to be treated. The treatment of choice is a 2-gram single dose of metronidazole.

Candida vaginitis

Candida vaginitis may be described as some variation of "milk curd discharge" that is itchy.

Gonorrhea

Gonorrhea is most commonly asymptomatic.

Gon-ARTH-rhea - Gonorrhea may be associated with arthritis. So consider this with any case of arthritis in an adolescent.

GC In Males

Gonorrhea in males presents as dysuria and discharge. Infection can progress to epididymitis, with unilateral pain and swelling of the scrotum.

GC in Females

Females get urethritis and cervicitis, along with dysuria and malodorous discharge. Infection may ascend to any part of the female reproductive tract, and may lead to peritonitis or peri-hepatitis (Fitz-Hugh-Curtis syndrome).

Remember that "Fitz-Hugh-Curtis" is **peri-hepatitis,** not hepatitis. LFT values will therefore be normal, as noted below.

Disseminated gonococcal infection

Disseminated gonococcal infection occurs in about 1%-2% of cases.

Local symptoms are not usually present once dissemination becomes apparent. Rash and joint/tendon involvement are more common. Also possible are meningitis and endocarditis.

Diagnosis is aided by the gram stain showing intracellular gram-negative diplococci. A culture is the gold standard, but empiric treatment is often indicated prior to culture results.

Patients being treated for gonorrhea should also receive treatment for chlamydia.

Genital Herpes

 In females, primary genital herpes infections will manifest as multiple painful ulcers on the labia, along with adenopathy.

 Treatment would consist of oral acyclovir for 7 days.

Topical acyclovir is of no help, and would be the incorrect choice.

Abdominal Pain: Special considerations in Adolescents

Pelvic Inflammatory Disease

CDC on PID

The CDC criteria for diagnosing PID are as follows:

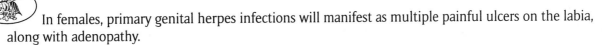

PID Screening

They may present you with an **asymptomatic** sexually active female who has had a 2nd sexual partner since her previous negative pelvic and culture and ask for the most appropriate study. The correct answer will be **urine PCR for chlamydia** or **gonorrhea**. This is only a screen, but it would be an appropriate routine test in a sexually active teenager, since it can pick up asymptomatic cases. The definitive diagnosis is via cervical cultures.

Minimal requirements (when lower abdominal or pelvic pain is present):
- Uterine or adnexal tenderness

    OR

- Cervical motion tenderness

Additional criteria to be sure:
- WBC in vaginal secretions
- Temp > 101°F
- Elevated ESR or C-reactive protein
- Lab evidence of GC or chlamydia at cervix
- Abnormal cervical or vaginal mucopurulent discharge

During a pelvic exam for PID, in addition to obtaining chlamydia and GC cultures, you are also expected to obtain specimens for microscopic examination of vaginal discharge for trichomoniasis and bacterial vaginosis. In addition to GC and chlamydia, PID can be caused by anaerobes and gram-negative rods.

You are also expected to know that you need to obtain a "reactive plasma reagin" for syphilis and HIV testing during that visit. PID is a risk factor for ectopic pregnancy and infertility.

You would be expected to look for evidence of human papilloma virus. In addition, you will be expected to counsel on the HPV vaccine.

Treating PID

Because it is difficult to make a rapid diagnosis and the consequences of missing PID are potentially devastating, the CDC recommends empirical treatment based on minimal criteria, which include:

(1) Lower abdominal tenderness on palpation
(2) Adnexal tenderness
(3) Cervical motion tenderness

Outpatient Treatment

The outpatient treatment of choice is no longer entirely one-stop shopping. Recommended treatment is ceftriaxone 250 mg IM once and doxycycline 100 mg BID for 14 days, with or without metronidazole 500 mg BID for 14 days. See below for additional treatment regimens for PID.

The parenteral therapy may be discontinued 24 h after a patient improves clinically.

PO treatments are indicated for 14 days.

Acceptable Inpatient Treatment of PID
cefoxitin 2 grams IV every 6 hours & doxycycline 100 mg IV or PO every 12 hours, or
cefotetan 2 grams every 12 hours plus doxycycline 100 mg IV or PO every 12 hours, or
clindamycin 900 mg IV every 8 hours plus gentamicin 1.5 mg/kg every 8 hours
Other acceptable outpatient treatment of PID
cefoxitin 2 grams IM with probenecid 1 gram PO x 1, plus doxycycline 100 mg PO BID x 14 days

Inpatient Treatment

If **pain persists** after treatment, **abdominal ultrasound is indicated** to look for tubo-ovarian abscess. Hospitalization is required if follow-up is not assured (as in most teenagers) or symptoms don't improve in 48 hours.

 GC and chlamydia cause **cervicitis**, not vaginitis in adolescents. Do not be fooled by the presentation of vaginal discharge.

Fitz Hugh Curtis

Here is some important additional information (and source of potential diversion) you need to know about regarding Fitz Hugh Curtis syndrome.

 Fitz-Hugh Curtis can be due to chlamydia as well as gonorrhea.

Treatment would be the same as for PID. The right upper quadrant pain due to perihepatitis should resolve within two days after treatment

 In addition to severe right upper quadrant tenderness, as an added diversion they might add in "radiates to the right shoulder," along with nausea. To further throw you off the trail, they might note a negative ultrasound result. If they note that the "only medication" the patient is taking is oral contraceptive pills, they are giving you an important clue to consider an STD as the primary etiology.

 What would be the most appropriate next step in managing this patient?

You will be presented with several choices, including abdominal CT with and without contrast, surgical consult, liver function studies, and serum amylase and lipase. None of these will be correct.

 The correct answer will be a pelvic exam, because the correct diagnosis is Fitz- Hugh Curtis.

Ovarian Cyst

 They will typically present you with a teenager with unilateral abdominal "discomfort," typically mid-cycle. They will probably throw in a positive ultrasound showing a fluid filled cyst on the ovary.

The question will focus on management. Here size is important.

- Cysts smaller than 6.0 cm will only require follow-up ultrasound
- Cysts greater than 6.0 cm or those that are causing significant symptoms beyond discomfort would require laparoscopic cyst aspiration.

Ethical Legal Issues

Even though thankfully this isn't the bar exam, you must know some basic legal issues as they pertain to minors.

Parental Consent

Invariably, a question or two will come up on the exam regarding parental consent, including when parental permission is required and when it is not.

Parental Consent is *not needed*:

- Life threatening emergencies (also sexual assault services)
- Medical care during pregnancy (also family planning)
- Treatment for sexually transmitted diseases (also HIV testing)
- Treatment for substance abuse

Confidentiality must be maintained in these situations if the patient requests it. However, the exception to this rule would be where the patient is a danger to himself or others.[6]

Emancipated minors do not need parental consent to receive treatment.

An emancipated minor is defined as a person under legal age who is no longer under their parent's control and regulation and who is managing their own financial affairs.

In cases where parental consent is not required, informed consent is still required. In such cases the minor is allowed to give informed consent instead of the parent.

Parental consent *is required for*:

Virtually all other medical and surgical procedures require parental informed consent, including blood donation.

---

[6] This is the case for most states in the US, and therefore, would be correct for purpose of the Board exam.

Chapter 30

Sports Injuries

Sports Participation

You will be expected to determine if patients with various conditions are eligible to participate in sports. It is important to note that **children with fevers cannot participate in sports**. Children with **carditi**s and acute **hepatosplenomegaly** (which could include children with mono) cannot participate in sports.

Conditioning Programs

It is important to note that conditioning is encouraged, but know that the following caveats could make their way onto the exam.

 You need to distinguish **weight training** from **power lifting programs**. Weight training involves many reps with low resistance. This is safe for preadolescents. Power lifting is not considered to be safe for preadolescents.

Heat Illness

Heat illness includes both **heat stroke** and **heat exhaustion**, and you need to be able to distinguish them.

Heat Exhaustion

Heat exhaustion is the milder form of heat illness. These patients will present with mild dehydration and a core temperature less than 104 F. They may present a child who has a headache and is thirsty, nauseated, and possibly vomiting.

Patients in heat exhaustion will be sweating; those in heat stroke will not be sweating.

Heat exhaustion should be suspected in anyone who is at risk, is feeling nauseated, and appears to be confused. They should stop exercising and drink fluids.

Heat Stroke

Heat stroke is based on the following:

- Temperature > 105 F
- Flushed, with hot, dry skin (not perspiration)
- CNS depression (confusion, vertigo, syncope, and lethargy)
- Severe dehydration

Heat stroke can lead to **end organ damage** because of the release of **endotoxins** and **cytokines**. Therefore, dehydration is **not** the only cause of problems in heat stroke.

Heat stroke is a medical emergency. The treatment goal of heat stroke is to remove the heat source or cease the activity causing the stress. Then the goal is to decrease the core body temperature. Rehydration is via IV fluids only, with use of vasopressors to maintain BP if needed.

Simple evaporative cooling may be as effective as active cooling via application of ice (and it may be a lot less stressful to the patient and hospital personnel than an ice bath).

Oral rehydration would be inappropriate given the CNS depression seen in heat stroke. Cooling **below 101-102°F** could lead to **hypothermia, and is inappropriate.**

Neurological signs such as delirium, coma, and seizure marks an important distinction between heat exhaustion and heat stroke.

Eye Trauma

In most cases the **"don't refer out to a specialist" rule will not apply here**. The following are the buzzwords indicating referral to an ophthalmologist: **pupil irregularity** and/or **significantly reduced visual acuity**. You also want to watch out for wording that would imply a serious orbital fracture and/or decreased EOM.

Hyphema

 A hyphema is a collection of blood between the cornea and the iris, usually following eye trauma.

 The appropriate **treatment** would either be immediate referral to an ophthalmologist or **admission with bed rest and head at 30-degree angle**. This is to decrease intraocular pressure.

 Patching the eye would not be appropriate; a shield should be used.

Blowout Fracture

A patient with a blowout fracture has a fracture of the orbital wall or floor

The typical history would be a patient who sustains blunt trauma to the eye, has double vision when looking to one side, and/or has a dysconjugate gaze to one side. Pupillary reflexes will usually be intact.

You might be tempted to consider one of the following diagnoses in the differential. We include other possible diagnoses and their clinical presentations.

Diagnoses	Clinical presentations
Corneal abrasion	Severe pain and tearing, with no diplopia or dysconjugate gaze
Hyphema	Presents as blood in the anterior chamber, with possible visual impairment, without *diplopia*
Traumatic iritis	Pain and severe photophobia without diplopia.[1]
Detached retina	Visual deficit in the peripheral field, described as curtain-like. No dysconjugate gaze.

---

[1]Sounds like the beginnings of a nice ophthalmology song parody.

Retinal detachment

Few vessels

Retinal tear, flap, or corrugated folds

Think of an aerial view of Mars
obscured by clouds!

©Medhumor Medical Publications, LLC

CASE STUDY

An 18-year-old girl presents with a red irritated right eye. The symptoms have persisted despite removal of her contact lenses 9 hours ago. On physical examination, there is marked conjunctival irritation, with difficulty keeping her eye open. Her funduscopic exam is normal and her pupils are equal and reactive with no discharge noted. There is diffuse uptake of fluorescein stain, with no focal uptake noted. What is the most appropriate next step in managing this patient?

THE DIVERSION

You will be tempted to take the diversionary path and assume that the diffuse uptake of stain represents a corneal abrasion. You will not be fooled into applying an eye patch with topical antibiotics. However, you could be very easily lulled into choosing to prescribe antibiotic drops rather than refer to an ophthalmologist.

ANSWER REVEALED

Well, you would have been deceived into believing that a corneal abrasion is the correct choice – however, if the correct diagnosis were a simple corneal abrasion, they will describe *a focal uptake of stain*. Diffuse or multifocal uptake in a patient wearing contact lenses could represent a gram-negative infection and/or ulceration of the corneal epithelium. These conditions require urgent followup and management by an ophthalmologist. This is one of the rare occasions where referral to a specialist will be the correct answer on the boards.

Ankle Injuries

Most ankle injuries are inversion injuries involving the lateral ligaments, especially the **anterior talofibular ligament.**

Some important facts to remember include:

· 75% of sports injuries involve the lower extremities

· Contusions and ankle sprains are the most common injury

· 85% of ankle injuries are sprains of the lateral ligaments

Most injuries that occur in the knee and ankle are due to *incomplete healing of a previous injury,* which may not have received appropriate medical attention.

Angling for a Return to Action

Invariably, you will be called upon to answer the question regarding when a child can return to sports after an ankle injury.

The correct answer will be one or all of the following:

· Full range of motion

· Full strength

· No swelling

· No pain

· No joint instability

Anterior Cruciate Ligament Tear

Typically described as an acute knee injury, with the patient describing a *pop.* On physical exam there will be a significant knee *effusion.* Look for a "positive anterior drawer" sign.

The drawer test often results in false positives, so do not rely on the drawer sign alone. Although it can be presumed on clinical findings, definitive diagnosis is done by MRI.

Prepatellar Bursitis

Prepatellar bursitis presents as anterior knee pain over the patella itself, with swelling that is visible.

Treatment consists of NSAIDs and padding during participation in sports that involve recurrent trauma, such as volleyball.

If you are presented with a patient who develops a large area of swelling over his thigh after blunt trauma, do not assume you are being presented with a fracture or an incidental discovery of a lytic lesion. In the absence of other hints, this is likely a soft tissue hematoma, which can be large due to the substantial blood supply to the quadriceps. Other than NSAIDs, ice, and rest, there is no other necessary treatment. If severe, the blood loss may be significant enough to cause a drop in hematocrit, resulting in fatigue and dizziness. In this case, more significant interventions may be necessary.

It's all in the Wrist

If you are presented with a patient who has pain over the "anatomical snuffbox" (which will likely be described as pain over the dorsum of the hand near the base of the thumb), the most likely diagnosis is scaphoid fracture. Scaphoid fractures have a poor prognosis.

You are asked to evaluate a 12-year-old gymnast who has had left wrist pain which has gotten progressively worse over 3 months. However, she does not recall injuring the wrist. On physical exam, there is no swelling, normal range of motion, and no pain noted over the wrist joint itself. Point tenderness is limited to the distal radius.

What is the most likely explanation for the wrist pain? What is the most appropriate management? What would you expect to see on x-ray?

Among the diversionary x-ray findings, you could be presented with scaphoid bone fracture. For diagnosis, you will be tempted to pick wrist fracture or wrist sprain. Regarding management, diversionary choices could include "cease all training," or "continue all physical activity."

Since there is no pain over the wrist joint, scaphoid fracture and/or wrist sprain are not likely. The presentation is consistent with distal radial epiphyseal injury. If the girl were to continue her current training, she is likely to disrupt the growth plate. Therefore, the correct answer would be to rest and splint the wrist until it is healed. **However, this would not mean stopping all training.** She can still engage in training activities that don't involve her wrist, such as running, which would help maintain her stamina.

Pulling over the to Shoulder

The basics of shoulder dislocation are as follows.

The diagnosis is clinical, but x-rays are indicated for confirmation and assessment of other injuries, including fractures. Neurovascular integrity is re-evaluated post-reduction. In addition to immobilization with a sling, you must also fill the space between the arm and body with a pillow or blanket.

Clavicular Fracture

Non-displaced mid-shaft clavicular fractures require no reduction, just a sling and a ticket home.

However, medial clavicular fractures could be more complicated, requiring further evaluation, including a CT scan.

Acromioclavicular separation can present in a similar fashion to a clavicular fracture. However, the pain will be described as distal – superior clavicular pain. In all fairness, they will have to describe a negative clavicular x-ray.

Compartment Syndrome

Compartment syndrome typically will be described as having **4 P's: Pulseless, Pallor, Paresthesias, and Pain.**

You are presented with an athlete with Hemophilia A who sustains an injury to the hand, resulting in numbness. What is the next *most appropriate* step in managing this patient? The most important next step would be to measure *compartment pressures*.

Conclusions on Concussions

Concussion – It is important to know the definition of a concussion, which is an *alteration in the level of consciousness — not necessarily a loss of consciousness*.

Concurring on Concussion

You will be expected to know when a young athlete can return to participating in sports after sustaining a concussion.

Immediately after sustaining an injury and presenting with symptoms consistent with concussion, the patient must be kept out of the game or practice.

The criteria for returning involve a stepwise progress through the following steps, without recurrence of symptoms. If the symptoms recur, the patient must rest for 24 hours before returning to the process, which includes the following:

1. Complete rest, staying at home and relaxing.
2. Walking around / light activity – No weight lifting or activities that involve resistance.
3. Movement consistent with the sport they wish to return to ie, running, skating etc. Minimal resistance training can be introduced.
4. Training drills, but no contact (in cases where that is part of the game, such as football). This is followed by mental status testing.
5. Full-contact training followed by return to full play

The trainer typically serves as a liaison between coaching and medical staff.

Concussion Risky Sports

Participation in the following sports is considered high risk for sustaining a concussion:

· Football
· Boxing
· Ice Hockey
· Basketball
· Rodeo
· Wrestling
· Imitating stunts from MTV's *Jackass* (though not technically a sport – still a popular pastime with unsupervised young people).

Most head injuries occur during football.

Pain in the Neck

Answering questions regarding the management of neck injuries and neck pain, can itself be, uh, a pain in the neck. However, we can help you avoid exam score-threatening injuries with the following important points.

In answering a question regarding an acute injury, you should follow the ABC's of CPR, while keeping the neck in a stable position. In a football player with a neck injury, breathing can be assessed by placing the hand beneath the shoulder pads and jersey to assess chest expansion. If the patient is prone, then the correct step is to log roll them while maintaining neck stability.

Removing shoulder pads and/or helmet is never correct on the field. If airway management is needed, you are supposed to leave the helmet on and remove the face guard only.

The most common sports-related cause of neck injuries is football, not diving. However, diving is an important mechanism for cervical spine injury, and could be presented this way on the exam.

Even if the c-spine film is negative, the patient can only return to sports when there is no pain with motion or palpation of the cervical spine, all neurological tests are negative, and there are no radicular symptoms.

Mouth Guards

Avoiding Contact Sports – Children with hepatomegaly or splenomegaly, as well as those with contagious skin lesions, should avoid contact sports. They can, however, participate in non-contact sports.

Patients with a single kidney should avoid contact sports.

The single organ rule only applies to kidneys. Children with a single ovary or testicle can participate in contact sports. Children can wear protective equipment to safeguard most other single organs. Even protective eyewear is available in the case of a patient with one functioning eye.

CASE STUDY

They could present you with a list of sports and ask which ones require a mouth guard. One of the choices could be "all of the above," or choices can contain a "yes" for some but not all.

THE DIVERSION

Collision sports like football, soccer, basketball, hockey, and wrestling are obvious. However, if you are presented with non-collision sports such as *shot putting* or *discus throwing,* you might be inclined to think to yourself or perhaps even aloud in the exam room, "Discus throwing? Shot putting? There is no contact there! Are these even sports?" You would then pick choices with no mouth guard needed. If you did, you just shot put away a point!

ANSWER REVEALED

Both shot putting and discus throwing require a mouth guard to — believe it or not — protect from dental injuries secondary to teeth clenching. In fact, children with braces are recommended to wear a mouth guard during *any* sport.

Speaking of which, perhaps a mouth guard would be required for NY Mets fans, who have clenched their teeth watching their team supposedly play baseball over the past few years.

The Eyes Have It

Special consideration is given to eye protection. Baseball is the leading cause of sports-related eye injuries, mostly in children younger than 14, often by being hit with a pitched ball.

Therefore, all children younger than 14 should be wearing a face guard when at bat. In addition, children with only one functional eye (corrected vision less than 20/50) need to wear protective goggles when in the field.

HOT TIP

Rather than list each sport's categorization, we will note some of the ones which may not be as obvious. For example: **baseball, squash, and volleyball** are **not** considered to be high contact sports. Team **handball**, on the other hand, *is* a high-impact collision sport.

The following conditions mandate that a child refrain from participating in contact sports:

· Splenomegaly

· Hepatomegaly

· One functioning kidney

· Repeated concussions

> **CASE STUDY** **You are presented with a patient with mono, to imply that the patient has splenomegaly. They could then ask for the best management of this patient and include choices involving medications such as steroids and IV immunoglobulins.**
>
> **THE DIVERSION** The diversion is that you may focus on the medical condition and treatment because you are so proud that you figured out the patient had mono and splenomegaly.
>
> **ANSWER REVEALED** You would be prouder if you realized that the question is really about knowing that splenomegaly precludes participation in contact sports. The correct answer regarding management would be *avoiding contact sports until the splenomegaly is resolved.*

The Juice on Steroid Use

If a teen is suspected of using performance-enhancing substances, a good interview is an important part of making the diagnosis.

The Side effects of Anabolic Steroid Use

The side effects can be *renal, hepatic,* and *psychological.*

Those who use needles are at risk for HIV and hepatitis.

 In **females** you can see:

- · Hirsutism and low voice
- · Early closure of epiphyseal plates

In **males** you can see:

- · Severe acne
- · Gynecomastia
- · High-pitched voice
- · Hypogonadism [2]

---

[2] Yes small testicles and a high pitched voice is an easy image to remember, and one that can probably be used to discourage steroid use among grunting, weight lifting athletes

Trolling for Roids

You will need to know the timing of steroid detection, specifically:

PO Steroids – remain in the urine days – weeks

IM Steroids – remain in the system 6 months or more

Steroids can result in violent behavior. Therefore, if you are presented with a teenager who is experiencing a *sudden change in mood,* withdrawal from steroids could be the cause. **Hypertension** can be seen in both males and females.

Arrhythmias and seizures are *not* signs of steroid use. Cross them out if presented as choices on the exam.

Lab Findings with Steroid Use

Common lab findings they might present you with include:

· Elevated LFTs
· Lower HDL
· Increased LDL
· Oligospermia and azoospermia [3]

Steroid Withdrawal

Hyperactivity is not a characteristic of steroid withdrawal. *Depression,* on the other hand, can be a sign of steroid withdrawal.

Sports, Fluids, and Electrolytes

Significant amounts of sodium are lost in sweat. Therefore, it is essential to consume liquids that also replace electrolytes, e.g., sports drinks.

It is important that young athletes be reminded by staff to keep up with fluid intake; left to their own devices, they will not do so.

Fluid replacement alone is insufficient to protect against heat exhaustion, since it is still possible to produce heat quicker than it can be transmitted to the environment.

---

[3] If the part about the high-pitched voice and small testicles doesn't discourage steroid use, then this certainly should.

The Growth of Growth Hormone

Growth hormone is *not detected in current drug testing,* which accounts for its increasing popularity.

CASE STUDY **You are presented with a teenager who has *nephrotic syndrome in remission*. They will then ask you which restrictions in sports activity are necessary. They may also ask about recommendations for fluid intake.**

THE DIVERSION The diversion is noting that the child had nephrotic syndrome. The key is their mentioning that the child is in *remission*. You might as well cross out any reference to nephrotic syndrome and re-phrase the question. What fluid and sports activity restrictions are required for a normal child??

ANSWER REVEALED If you take this extra step, there will only be one possible correct answer: The patient qualifies for all sports activities and should have full access to fluids during games and practices.

Wrestling with Weight Control in Athletes

It is common for competitive wrestlers to try to lose weight to qualify for a lower weight category, thinking they will be more competitive.

It is important to keep in mind that the weight loss, especially weight loss that occurs in a short period of time, is primarily *water weight loss.* Weight loss in general in these situations results in *lower muscle endurance. Dieting behaviors to alter weight are not limited to females.*

Normal and Abnormal Cardiac Findings in the Athlete

The following findings would warrant **referral to a cardiologist** prior to clearing for participation in sports:

- Syncope, near syncope, or chest pain on exertion
- Palpitations at rest or irregular heart rhythm
- Excessive shortness of breath or fatigue with routine activities
- Family history of Marfan syndrome, cardiomyopathy, long QT syndrome, or clinically significant arrhythmias or premature death
- Weak or delayed femoral pulses
- Any of the following on cardiac exam: fixed split second heart sound, a systolic murmur graded 3/6 or greater, or **any diastolic murmur**
- A patient with Turner syndrome with any chest pain

Any of the following are **contraindications to sports participation:**

- Pulmonary vascular disease with cyanosis and large right-to-left shunt
- Severe pulmonary hypertension
- Severe aortic valve stenosis or regurgitation
- Severe mitral valve stenosis or regurgitation
- Cardiomyopathies
- Vascular form of Ehlers-Danlos syndrome
- Coronary anomalies of wrong sinus origin
- Catecholaminergic polymorphic ventricular tachycardia
- Acute phase of pericarditis
- Acute phase of myocarditis (at least 6 mo)
- Acute phase of Kawasaki disease (at least 8 wk)

Beyond these absolute contraindications, other factors must be considered regarding which sports a specific patient can and cannot participate in. It is very likely that they will test you on this concept.

> **CASE STUDY** They can, and will, present you with a healthy – in fact a very healthy – athletic teenager with findings that would be abnormal in another teenager, but are normal for an athletic teenager. This is an important concept you could be tested on.
>
> **THE DIVERSION** In athletic females, modest **left ventricular hypertrophy** is a normal finding, especially in long distance runners. In athletic males, **left ventricular hypertrophy** can be a normal finding.
>
> **ANSWER REVEALED** No sports restriction will be the correct answer in both of these situations.

The Diabetic Athlete

You may be tested on the concept of exercise in the diabetic patient

While exercise is encouraged, keep in mind the following caveats.

During periods of exercise, increased caloric intake or decreased insulin dose will be needed to avoid hypoglycemia. There could be a delayed response to exercise, hours later resulting in hypoglycemia. Keep this in mind if presented with a question involving this scenario.

During episodes of poor control, especially with ketosis, vigorous exercise should be deferred.

Special consideration for athletes with Down syndrome

Atlantoaxial instability (AAI) is present in an estimated 15% of children with Down syndrome. Although this is under review as of this printing, all children with Down syndrome must have plain neck x-rays (in addition to a thorough neurological exam) before being approved to participate in competitive sports, including Special Olympics.

Chapter 31

Substance Abuse

How are High School Students Getting High?

At least half of high school seniors report having used an illicit drug at least once.

Almost one third report having been drunk within the past month.

Students are now abusing *over-the-counter dextromethorphan*, which is available in cough medicine.

Students are also using prescription drugs, such as *oxycodone*, with increasing frequency.

Where there's smoke, there's more smoke. Use of more than one drug is more common than single drug use in this population.

The earlier a child starts using a drug, the more likely it is that they will develop dependency.

Alcohol is the illicit substance most widely used by high school students. *Alcohol is not an illicit drug* per se, but its use is illegal for this population. *Marijuana* is the most commonly used *illicit drug* in the adolescent population. More ER visits are due to the ill effects of marijuana (and/or drugs that might be mixed in with it) than for alcohol use.

Risk factors for Drug abuse:

Risk factors for drug abuse include the following:
- Low self esteem and poor coping skills
- Alienation from conventional norms
- Homosexuality
- The use of performance-enhancing drugs
- Parental use/abuse of drugs
- Child abuse
- Inconsistent parenting
- Drug use among close friends
- Early academic failure
- Disconnect from family, school, and community

Drug Screening

Associations with Psychiatric Disorders

Psychiatric comorbidity, especially conduct disorder, is more common than the absence of comorbidity in children who use drugs.

The psychiatric disorder often preceded the use of drugs, and often worsens after onset of drug use.

In the case of ADHD, children who are appropriately treated are less likely to abuse drugs than those with ADHD who aren't treated.

Drug abuse can both mimic and/or worsen psychiatric disorders. For example, the use of alcohol or cocaine (or both together) can induce depression (or it can happen the other way around, with depression leading to substance abuse). These substances may also cause psychosis or mimic anxiety disorders.

There is a higher likelihood of physical trauma being reported by children who are abusing drugs.

In general, drug screens reflect substance use within the previous 48 hours. Marijuana (THC), however, can be detected for several weeks. If you are asked how to monitor discontinuation of marijuana use, the correct answer would be serial measurements of *urine THC: creatinine ratio*, which should decrease as marijuana use is discontinued.

Urine specific gravity and the *creatinine concentration* impact the validity of drug tests. Therefore, whenever you obtain a urine tox screen, you should obtain these as well.

Urine tox screens are just that, screens. False positives and false negatives are common. Therefore, *positive results must be confirmed* by gas chromatography and mass spectrometry.

In addition to identifying which drugs are being used by teens, it is important to identify how often and the context within which they are being used.

Pediatricians are not expected to order drug screens on patients solely at the request of the parent. Maintaining confidentiality is expected. However, when a substance abuse problem is identified, a thorough family history for mental illness and drug use/abuse *would be* appropriate. This would, of course, include taking a history from the parents as well.

Obtaining information from the school and/or law enforcement is considered appropriate.

When indicated, urine drug screen specimens should be collected under direct observation.

Confidentiality

The one exception to strict confidentiality would be if the adolescent is at risk of harming him/herself or others.

Know that when an adolescent is placed in a drug treatment program, the pediatrician is expected to track progress.

Random drug screening is not recommended. If the parents request a random test and the teenager objects, obtaining it anyway will be the wrong choice on the exam. The correct answer will be to do a physical exam; obtaining drug testing against their will violates informed consent

Overdose Underquote

Remember: when presented with an overdose victim, the drug they have allegedly taken may not be accurate, especially if the drug is placed in "quotes." It could also be a combination of drugs.

Anticipatory Guidance

You will likely be questioned on appropriate anticipatory guidance. Keep the following in mind when answering questions on this subject.

Parents should be encouraged to discuss and help their teenagers understand the circumstances under which they will be pressured to try drugs. Appropriate actions by the pediatrician would include open ended questions asked in confidence, as well as questioning the adolescent about his /her attitude *in general* regarding drug and alcohol use.

Casual use should not be dismissed. The transition from casual use to dependence may occur much more quickly in adolescents than adults.

On the exam, declining school performance may be a red flag that the problem is substance abuse.

Inhalants

Commonly used inhalants may include paint thinner, fuels, organic solvents, glue, or spray paint.

Immediate effects of Inhalants

Similar to anesthesia: drowsiness, decreased inhibition, and lightheadedness. This leads to ataxia and disorientation.

Extreme Intoxication

Inhalant intoxication may be characterized by generalized muscle weakness, nystagmus, and/or a lack of coordination. Ultimately, they may experience a hangover similar to an alcohol hangover.

Use of inhalants is more common in lower socioeconomic groups, as well as in Hispanic and Native American populations.

Acute Morbidity

The acute effects of inhalants may include

· Asphyxia ➔ death
· Cardiac Arrhythmia ➔ death
· Aspiration ➔ death

 The **most common *fatal complication*** is cardiac arrhythmias.

 The result of both *head CT* and *urine tox screen* will be *negative.*

The presentation can be similar to **alcohol intoxication:** agitation and ataxia. It can also be similar to **PCP** intoxication. However, they will have to give you a clue. First, they might note that the tox screen is negative, and then they will have to note something consistent with the diagnosis, such as **volatile hydrocarbon on their breath**.

Chronic Use

Chronic use of inhalants leads to **encephalopathy**.

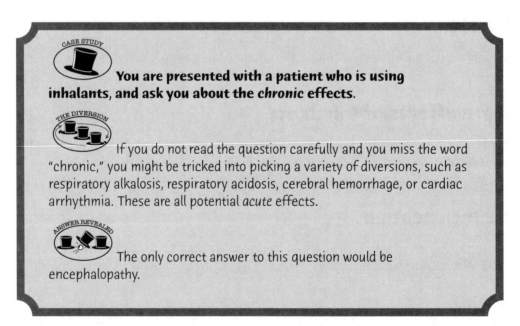

You are presented with a patient who is using inhalants, and ask you about the *chronic* effects.

If you do not read the question carefully and you miss the word "chronic," you might be tricked into picking a variety of diversions, such as respiratory alkalosis, respiratory acidosis, cerebral hemorrhage, or cardiac arrhythmia. These are all potential *acute* effects.

The only correct answer to this question would be encephalopathy.

Organic solvent abuse

The signs of acute solvent abuse include giggling, slurred speech, and ataxia. In addition, urine tox screen will be negative, as will be blood alcohol level.

Death, when it occurs, is due to asphyxia or cardiac arrhythmias.

Combative Behavior

A patient presenting to the ER who is combative could be under the influence of a variety of drugs. Pay close attention to the details for a diagnosis of the specific drug.

 Combating the confusion of the combative patient

Drug	Characteristics	Distinguishing Features
Cocaine	Tachycardia, tremulousness	Hypertension, mydriasis
Alcohol	Combative behavior and agitation	Tremulousness is *not a common feature in a teenager*
Volatile Inhalants	Characterized as a *"quick drunk"* with disinhibition and agitation	Hallucinations, generalized muscle weakness, and nystagmus
Opiates	Can present with agitation	Tremulousness and tachycardia are not part of the profile
Amphetamines	Combative, tachycardia, mydriasis	Nystagmus is *not part of the* profile.
PCP	Combative	Both vertical and horizontal nystagmus

Marijuana

Important points regarding the extent of marijuana use you will be expected to know are:
- Close to half of high school seniors have reported using marijuana at some point.
- 5% have reported using it daily.

Psychologic consequences

Teens using marijuana may experience learning problems, deficits in problem-solving skills, and memory impairment (which may last up to 1 month after they last used marijuana).

Symptoms of mental health problems such as personality disorders, depression, and anxiety can worsen.

School performance is generally worse in children who use marijuana.

Physiologic consequences

Acute Physical Effects of Marijuana

The acute physiologic effects of marijuana include:

· **D**ry mouth
· **D**ilated pupils
· **D**rowsiness
· **D**istortion of time

 All of the acute effects of marijuana begin with a **D**.

Additional physiological consequences may include compromised immune function and decreased sperm count. The latter is reversible, and should serve as motivation to discontinue use.

Impaired coordination can be seen in adolescents using marijuana regularly.

After marijuana use, teens may experience tachycardia (lasting up to 3 hours), along with increased blood pressure.

Chronic effects of Marijuana use

· *Pulmonary* - Just like tobacco smoke, there are carcinogens in marijuana smoke, and significantly more of them.
· *Cardiovascular* - Tachycardia and poor stamina

Withdrawal

Characterized by irritability, insomnia, tremors, and nystagmus. Withdrawal peaks within 4 days and can continue for 2 weeks.

 Gynecomastia is a consequence of chronic marijuana use.

Alcohol Abuse

Alcohol is the most common substance of abuse by young people. 80% of high school seniors report having used alcohol at some point in their lives. There may be a genetic association with alcoholism.

Acute Alcohol Toxicity

They may describe a teenager presenting to the ER with *ataxia, slurred speech, visual disturbance, nausea, and vomiting.* In addition, you need to look for:

- sluggishly reactive pupils, but normal pupil size
- excessive sweating
- flushed skin
- hypoglycemia

With higher doses, look for *irritability, stupor, and even coma.*

Medical consequences of chronic alcohol abuse

The medical effects of alcohol abuse are primarily GI, including *esophagitis, gastritis, and peptic ulcer disease.*

Adolescents have not been using alcohol long enough to have the chronic effects seen in adults such as cirrhosis of the liver. Therefore, do not be tricked into picking any answer that includes the chronic effects of alcohol abuse.

The primary consequences of alcohol use and abuse in teenagers are from **physical trauma** and **overdose.**

The majority of adolescents who binge drink are not at risk for becoming alcoholics as adults. They are at risk, however, for having preexisting depression.

Amphetamine Abuse

Amphetamines primarily have a *sympathomimetic* response in acute overdose, with the following adverse effects:

Short term *physiological signs* of amphetamine toxicity would be adrenergic, including tachycardia, high blood pressure, sweating, agitation, and fever. Hyperthermia can be part of the presentation as well. *Ophthalmological findings* would include dilated pupils with slow reaction to light. The perception that insects are crawling on one's skin may be a sign of amphetamine toxicity. **Nystagmus would not be a finding with amphetamine use**.

If higher doses of amphetamines are ingested, it can lead to fatal arrhythmias.

Treatment of Amphetamine Overdose

Treatment focuses on the specific symptoms, as well as decontamination. If vital signs are unstable, remember to check the ABCs first, including airway protection.

Benzodiazepines are used to treat the high heart rate and high blood pressure, as well as the associated agitation.

Patients with hyperthermia require *aggressive cooling*. Patients should get *activated charcoal*.

Amphetamine Withdrawal

Amphetamine abusers do develop tolerance and may exhibit specific signs following withdrawal. These signs may include drug craving, depression/fatigue, anxiety/aggression, paranoia, and/or difficulty focusing.

PCP intoxication can present in a similar fashion to amphetamine toxicity. However, **PCP** ingestion results in **vertical and horizontal nystagmus**, as well as **muscle rigidity.** In addition, *pupil size will be normal with PCP toxicity.*

Opiates

A teenager who has overdosed on opiates will present with *depressed sensorium, respiratory depression, miosis, indifference to pain, and euphoria.*

Physiologic signs include *decreased blood pressure and low temperature. Constipation* and *urinary retention* are other common findings.

Severe Opiate Overdose

Severe opiate overdose can lead to **pulmonary and other consequences including:**

- **Respiratory arrest**
- **Pulmonary edema**
- **Circulatory collapse**
- **Seizures**

 Cardiac arrhythmias can occur with **propoxyphene** overdose.

They will commonly try to trick you into believing that elevated temperature and hypertension are the result of opiate overdose. The opposite is the case.

As with any acute situation, the ABCs of resuscitation apply. Naloxone is used to reverse respiratory depression.

Since naloxone has a shorter half life than opiates, it may have to be administered repeatedly. The goal is to reverse respiratory depression without triggering withdrawal.

If there is no evidence of withdrawal, a longer acting alternative is nalmefene.

Opiate Withdrawal

Opiate withdrawal may present with a history of *anxiety, poor school performance, rhinorrhea, insomnia, and/or stomach cramps.*

These symptoms can be confused with acute psychosis. Watch for rhinorrhea and stomach cramps as your clue that this is opiate withdrawal and not an acute psychosis.

Barbiturates

Signs and symptoms of barbiturate overdose (including phenobarbital) would include the brady twins (**bradycardia** and **bradypnea**), and the hypo triplets (**hypotension**, **hypothermia**, and **hypoactive bowel sounds**), as well as their hypo cousin (**hyporeactive pupillary reflex**).

Pupil size will be normal. Therefore, if they describe miosis or pinpoint pupils, they are more likely describing opiate overdose rather than barbiturate overdose.

Benzodiazepine Abuse

The physical findings of benzodiazepine abuse include sleepiness and sedation. The pupils are slow to react but normal-sized. Alprazolam would be an example of a benzodiazepine which may commonly be abused.

Physiologic effects of PCP

Sympathomimetic –
Sympathomimetic effects include *tachycardia, hypertension, and increased reflexes*

Cholinergic
Cholinergic effects include *miosis, flushing and diaphoresis*

Cerebellar
Cerebellar effects include *vertical and horizontal nystagmus, ataxia, and lack of coordination*

PCP

PCP is a hallucinogen that leads to *psychiatric disturbances.*

 The following presentations are consistent with PCP use

· Distortion of body image

· Paranoia

· Agitation

· Auditory and visual hallucinations

Therefore, it is important **not to do the following when PCP intoxication is suspected:**

- **Acidify urine** – which will precipitate myoglobin
- **Restraints** – which will worsen rhabdomyolysis

Treatment of PCP intoxication

A cooling blanket will help alleviate the risk for seizures, hypertension, and hyperthermia. In addition, haloperidol, chlorpromazine, or lorazepam would be acceptable treatment.

Rhabdomyolysis

With higher doses, **rhabdomyolysis (symptoms include muscle rigidity) and renal failure** may result.

In addition, "coke fever" can result in rhabdomyolysis. This is a result of hyperpyrexia and muscle rigidity that can be seen in acute cocaine abuse.

Hallucinogens

They will likely present a patient under the influence of hallucinogens as follows. They will present with general signs that could include dizziness, weakness, nausea, and/or visual impairment.

More specific findings could include "smelling colors" or "hearing odors." Time perception will be off.

The major ill effect is damage that can occur as a result of poor decisions due to impaired judgment under the influence of hallucinogens.

Treatment of hallucinogen overdose would be supportive, including a low-stimulation environment and possibly benzodiazepines.

Distinguishing Schizophrenia from Hallucinogen Use

This distinction is difficult to make acutely, because the acute effects of hallucinogen use can be similar to those seen in schizophrenia. The patient should preferably be evaluated after they are off all drugs for 2-4 weeks. The absence of a family history of schizophrenia and the absence of symptoms when the patient is drug-free point away from a diagnosis of schizophrenia.

Visual hallucinations are common with *hallucinogen ingestion.* However, auditory hallucinations and *completely disorganized, delusional thinking* is more consistent with *schizophrenia* than hallucinogen ingestion.

CASE STUDY

What is the most common substance of abuse by young people? What is the most common illicit drug used by young people?

THE DIVERSION

If you do not read the question carefully, you can easily be tricked into getting these easy questions wrong on the exam.

ANSWER REVEALED

The most common substance of abuse by young people is alcohol. The most common illicit drug used by young people is marijuana.

Cocaine Abuse

BUZZ WORDS

Signs of acute cocaine toxicity are general, including tachycardia, hypertension, dilated pupils, and sweating.

More serious complications may include myocardial infarction, stroke, rhabdomyolysis, and possibly renal complications (including renal failure).

With chronic abuse, one can see choreoathetotic movements, due to depletion of dopamine storage.

Acute Cocaine Overdose

At Lower Doses – euphoria and overconfidence

At Higher Doses - aggressive and violent behavior

Death secondary to cocaine ingestion is *not* dose-dependent.

Treatment of Cocaine Toxicity

· Hypertension may be treated with nitroprusside
· Symptoms of psychosis may be treated with haloperidol.

Tobacco Use

Physiologic effects of nicotine

The short term physiologic effects of nicotine include:

· Increased alertness
· Muscle relaxation
· Enhanced memory and alertness
· Decreased appetite
· Decreased irritability

One can see the attraction of nicotine physiologically, and why it can be so addicting.

The **adverse effects of nicotine** include *peptic ulcer disease.* Nausea and vomiting are common *initial* effects that wear off quickly.

The Hazards of Smoking

While most of these hazards seem obvious, you may very well be tested on them. They include:

· Risk for a witch's brew of cancers, from lung to prostate.
· Premature wrinkling of skin.
· Chronic lung disease, including COPD
· Compromised immune function

Second Hand Smoke

Second hand smoke in children leads to *increased incidence of:*
- Otitis media
- URI
- Asthma
- Pneumonia

Smoking Cessation

Smoking cessation is difficult because of the discomfort caused by withdrawal, rather than the absence of pleasurable symptoms. For example, *increased appetite* is one of the more important adverse effects of withdrawal.

Scare tactics about long term ill effects rarely work with adolescents, who view themselves as being immortal.

Chewing Tobacco

Teens are often unaware of the potential immediate risks of chewing tobacco. The nicotine in chewing or smokeless tobacco can cause early fatigue during sports. It can also cause tachycardia and vasoconstriction.

Chapter 32

Psychosocial Issues

Toddler and Preschool

Toilet Training

75% of children will have full bladder and bowel control by age 36 months. Positive reinforcement (praise/rewards) is preferred over punishment-based reinforcement, which rarely works.

Enuresis

Nocturnal Enuresis

The initial workup for new onset enuresis consists of a history, physical exam, and **urinalysis**.

If there is a history of nocturnal enuresis in one parent, there is a 40% chance the child will have it.

If there is a history of nocturnal enuresis in two parents, there is a 70% chance the child will have it.

Short term treatment for enuresis on overnight trips would be **desmopressin acetate** as a nasal spray at bed time. This is only a short term fix to avoid embarrassment, since enuresis *recurs 50% of the time* with desmopressin treatment. Other pharmacological options include oxybutynin or imipramine. These are usually reserved for patients with underlying bladder issues, which should be identified in the question.

Nocturnal enuresis is seen in up to 20% of children at age 5. Therefore, if you are presented with such a scenario on the Boards, a workup may not be necessary.

The most successful method to expedite toilet training is to give positive feedback when the child indicates a need to void.

> ### Overflowing SUDS
>
> The following are some organic causes of enuresis to consider. Look for clues in the question.
>
> **SUDS** = Envision a child with enuresis who is urinating soapsuds instead of urine. This will help you recall organic causes of enuresis.
>
> **S**ickle cell trait
> **U**rinary Tract Infection or Anomaly
> **D**iabetes
> **S**eizure or **S**acral (Lumbar-sacral)

CASE STUDY **If you are presented with a child with a history of nocturnal enuresis who is going on an overnight trip and asked what the appropriate management is, what would be the correct answer?**

THE DIVERSION You may be wise enough to realize that non-pharmacological interventions like bells, whistles, and biofeedback machines will not work in the **short run**. However, you may be faced with two similar medications, including one that would have been the correct answer in years past. If you pick imipramine instead of desmopressin, you may be among the group that experiences post stress enuresis when you learn you got another question wrong.

ANSWER REVEALED Fear not, and put away those plastic sheets. You came to the right source to know that, although imipramine is successful, it is associated with significant risks (especially overdose), and intranasal desmopressin is the correct answer.

- Enuresis alarms are appropriate treatments for **long term** management.
- If a workup for organic causes is indicated, then a simple urinalysis is often the correct answer they are looking for.
- **15% of cases** of enuresis per year will **resolve with no intervention**.
- Non-organic causes of enuresis are related to small bladder, excessive fluid intake before bed, and deep sleeping.

Diurnal Enuresis

If you are presented with a patient with **diurnal enuresis** after a period of daytime continence, **it is most likely due to an organic illness, and thus warrants a workup.**

"Think UTI, DM or DI, or kidney disease."

Remember that 97% of the time the cause is non-organic, even on the Boards. Diurnal enuresis cannot be defined prior to age 3.

If you are presented with a child with new onset diurnal enuresis, the most likely diagnosis is behavioral withholding pattern.

Encopresis

Encopresis is fecal incontinence, also known as "soiling."

The medical aspects of management consist of clearing out the colon and maintaining consistent stool habits. The psychological focus is on education and positive reinforcement rather than punitive, negative reinforcement.

Stool withholding during toilet training

Usually stool is withheld because it is perceived or has been experienced as painful. This results in larger more painful stools, and a vicious cycle ensues.

In older children, laxatives are often used. The premature discontinuation of laxatives often leads to recurrence of encopresis.

In the absence of constipation since infancy, a workup for Hirschsprung's disease is inappropriate. The use of enemas and glycerin suppositories would be incorrect in the absence of encopresis. Mineral oil without the above behavioral interventions would be incorrect as well.

Encopresis tie with UTI

Chronic encopresis may be associated with UTIs because of the pressure on the bladder; and stasis and urinary retention may consequently develop, which may predispose to UTIs.

Family and Environmental Issues

Divorce and Blended Families

A child's response to divorce is developmental stage-dependent. The same holds true for a child's response to an illness in the family.

Somatization and regression of developmental milestones are typical responses to divorce and other stresses.

Divorce and Mediation

As a result of the increase in joint custody arrangements, involvement of divorced fathers in their children's lives has increased.

However, the impact of joint custody can result in increased conflict between parents, which may possibly have a negative effect on the children.

Impact on Adulthood

Children of divorce may have more difficulties with intimate relationships, including marriage, as adults. They may have increased conflict in the workplace as well.

A child's response to divorce will depend on the child's age as outlined in the table below.

Age-based response to divorce:

Age	Typical Response to Divorce
Pre-school (2-5 years)	Regression of the most recently obtained developmental milestone.
Early School Age (6-8)	Overt grieving, fears of rejection, guilt, and fantasies that the parents will get back together.
Late School Age (9-12)	Anger at one or both parents. Open mourning of the loss of the safety and structure of an intact family.
Teenagers	Depression and acting out. Suicidal thoughts and ideation are also possible responses. Teenagers might fake indifference, but **true indifference will never be the correct answer.**

Pregnancy and Postnatal adjustment

Possible Initial Family Grief Reaction to a Child with a Disability

The sequence of reactions is as follows:

> Shock and fear
> Denial and disbelief
> Sadness and anger
> Acceptance

HOT TIP

Initially, a parent may not want to see the child, or may postpone contact after birth by not feeding the child. The correct response is to encourage contact and promote bonding to help work through the fear. Parents may require time to fully comprehend the situation and/or mourn the loss of a "normal" child.

Death in the Family

A child's response to a death in the family will depend on the age of the child, as outlined in the table below. The response is *similar to that of divorce, since both involve a loss.*

Age of Child	Rseponse to Death in the Family
Pre-schoolers	Regression of developmental milestones. *Acting out and tantrums are also possible.*
School-Age	*Somatic complaints* are very common, as well as *sleep disturbance* and *decreased school performance.*
Teenagers	Of course, acting out is a possible reaction. Acting out is always a possibility with teenagers, and can never be the wrong choice on the exam.

PERIL / WARNING Lack of mourning or the appearance of coping well on the surface should never be taken at face value - "no additional intervention" will never be the correct choice for a child mourning a death.

HOT TIP Loss of appetite is common in all age groups; however, overt *failure to thrive is not a common result.* There are also unique factors to consider for each individual situation/relationship with the deceased.

Conversion Disorder

DEFINITION A conversion disorder is a physical symptom that occurs in the context of stress or conflict. It is **un**intentionally produced, but it has no **physiological explanation.**

Conversion disorder occurs equally among boys and girls in childhood. In teenagers, it occurs 3:1 — girls: boys.

Converting to Conversion Disorder

According to the diagnostic criteria, a conversion disorder is defined as follows:

A. One or more symptoms or deficits affecting voluntary motor or sensory function that suggest a neurologic or other general medical condition.

B. Psychological factors are judged to be associated with the symptom or deficit, because the initiation or exacerbation of the symptom or deficit is preceded by conflicts or other stressors.

C. The symptom or deficit is not **intentionally** produced or feigned (as in factitious disorder or malingering).

CASE STUDY A 15 year old female presents with a sudden loss of sensation in her left leg; she reports that she cannot feel anything in the entire leg. There is no history of trauma, and the neurologist has signed off on the case because the neurological exam is normal. Her grandfather recently died of natural causes, and her parents proudly tell you how wonderfully she has coped and accepted his death like an adult. What is the best explanation for the paralysis of her leg?

THE DIVERSION You may be smart enough to not go for the neurological choices such as Guillain Barré syndrome, tethered cord, or metastatic disease involving the spinal cord. So you will then be down to two choices, depression and conversion disorder. Conversion disorder seems a bit farfetched and depression is unlikely since she is coping so well, but a mild depression would be expected. If you went down that path you might be depressed to learn you got the question wrong, and you might have a conversion disorder involving your writing hand.

ANSWER REVEALED Remember: the teen that has "gone through a loss with no problems" does not exist, despite what the parents say. Depression wouldn't explain the physical findings described. The correct answer is conversion disorder. Pick this answer on the exam, and you will be well on your way to converting "board eligible" to "board certified," and, ultimately, "recertified."

Psychosomatic Illness

PERIL WARNING We often hear that asthma, eczema, and a variety of other disorders have "psychological components to them." Psychosomatic illnesses tend to be exacerbated during times of stress. While this is true, **it does not mean that they "cause" the illness**. This is another example of how critical it is to **read the question**. There is a double edged sword to doing an extensive workup in the case of psychosomatic illness, since ordering tests can reinforce the perceived seriousness of the symptoms. You as the physician are expected to overcome your own anxiety and resist the urge to order every test known to man. This will be important if you are presented with a patient who is clearly presenting with a psychosomatic illness or conversion disorder.

Treatment of psychosomatic illness involves recognizing and explaining to the family that the symptoms are real, but there is no organic basis for them.

The key is addressing the stress or anxiety that has led to the symptoms.

Positive feedback is important. It is also important to remove secondary gain, such as missing school.

If weakness is a component of the presentation, limited physical therapy may help.

Somatizations of Stress

"Geez, you know I am really stressed out and I could sure use a nap and some time off." This is not something children will say when they are stressed out. They will complain of, and feel, somatic pain, such as a headache, or even diarrhea and/or abdominal pain.

Organizing the Non-Organic

Conversion disorder – symptoms are incompatible with anatomical and medical logic

Hypochondriasis – preoccupation with illness, frequently in the context of previous illness

Malingering – These patients present with false or exaggerated symptoms, often with a motive

Dysmorphic disorder – despite evidence to the contrary, the patient perceives themselves as being ugly or undesirable

Somatic delusions – belief that something is medically wrong with them, but may take on psychotic dimensions, i.e., their pancreas has wings

Munchausen by proxy – the parent is causing/reporting the presenting non-organic symptoms; the morbidity and mortality can be high. The symptoms disappear when the child is not with the caregiver creating the symptoms.

This may be hinted at or described in the presenting history you are provided with on the exam.

Once again, remember that children may react to stress by somatizing and/or regressing. **Their perceived ability to have some degree of control over the situation is an important component.**[1]

---

[1] Just like adults, I suppose.

Watch for signs of parental anxiety and how they themselves are dealing with stress (the question may clue you in to this).

Recurrent Pain

In the face of recurrent abdominal pain, you are expected to know that a psychosocial history is important. By definition, the seriousness of the problem is related to its interference with everyday life (which, in the case of children, often includes school attendance).

In addition, school may be a factor in causing the recurrent pain.

If the pain persists on weekends, absence from school is unlikely to be a secondary gain factor.

Impact of TV and other Media

Television

The following are the known harmful effects of TV on children:

- · TV often trivializes violence and blurs the distinction between reality and fantasy
- · It may encourage passivity at the expense of activity, unless you consider nimble remote control button pushing to be activity
- · Television definitely **increases aggressive behavior,** and influences the **toys** played with and the **cereals** eaten

Some important facts to know are that, on average:

- · TV watching takes up more time than school
- · Children watch up to 23 hours per week
- · Only the time spent sleeping exceeds the number of leisure hours watching TV

HOT TIP

It is recommended that television watching be limited to 2 hours/day, preferably with the parents watching as well.[2] **Children younger than 2 should not watch TV at all.**

---

[2] Although there is only so much of "Courage the Cowardly Dog®" one can watch in one sitting.

Sleep Disorders

Newborn Sleep Patterns

During a normal sleep cycle, newborns sometimes experience arousal but are not fully awake. Parents may mistake this for the infant being awake, and arouse them from sleep.

 Infants should be able to establish a day/ night schedule by 2 months of age.

By 4 months of age, infants should be capable of sleeping through the night.

A 1 year old should be sleeping 13-14 hours a day. As opposed to the parent of a 1 year old, who sleeps an average of 13-14 hours a week.

In order to avoid an infant being dependent on the presence of a parent to go back to sleep when they arouse during the night, it is best to put the baby to bed sleepy but awake so they learn how to soothe themselves when awake.

In addition, soothing music playing when they go to sleep can also be used to reinforce going back to sleep on their own during the night.

"Sleep training" (where the parents let the baby cry before going back into the bedroom) can begin to take place between 6-8 months of age.

If the infant is not adjusting to a day/night sleep cycle, the correct management is to keep them awake more during the day so they will be more tired at night.

Night Terrors vs. Nightmares

Night Terrors vs. Nightmares

In both cases the child will appear agitated.

Night Terrors

They occur during the **first third of the night and happen rapidly**. There will often be a **family history.** This occurs in **boys** more often than in girls.

They will exhibit **distinctive physical findings**; deep breathing, dilated pupils, and sweating with rapid heart rate and respiratory rate. They can also **become mobile**, which may result in an injury.

If they are woken up, they will be **"disoriented,"** with no recall of the episode.

Most children stop having night terrors by adolescence (when they begin to experience other issues, of course).

The treatment goal is to make sure the environment is safe so they do not injure themselves during the night terror.

Intervening during a night terror may be counterproductive and worsen the child's agitation.

If education and behavioral interventions fail, short-acting benzodiazepines are sometimes used to decrease the amount of slow-wave sleep.

Nightmares

These occur during the **last third of the night**. They can be **woken easily,** and they will **recall the nightmare**, often quite vividly. They are not mobile and, therefore, at no real risk for physical injury.

Chronic Illness and the Family

Impact of Chronic Illness in the Family

The following factors are considered to be protective for siblings of children with chronic disabilities:

- Larger family size
- Female siblings are at higher risk for negative outcomes due to their parentification
- Older siblings are at higher risk for negative outcomes
- Financial resources serve to buffer negative impacts
- Intact families with harmonious relationships help decrease negative effects

Transplant Transitions

Although recipients of liver and kidney transplants in childhood initially go through a growth spurt, they typically do not attain their genetic potential regarding adult height.

Poor compliance is a known problem with adolescents who have received transplants.

There are important psychosocial consequences that go along with receiving an organ transplant. Some of this is due to the side effects of immunosuppressive medications, which may include short stature and/or obesity.

One of the most important interventions that can help the family cope better is to increase home resources.

In general, the scenario of a mother and father responding differently to a child born with a disability is to be expected, and no intervention is necessary unless there is a clear detriment to the child.

Parents who are health care professional and have to use home equipment such as oxygen do not cope better than non-health care professionals

Home monitors are believed to have a role in apnea management in certain patient populations. However, studies show that they tend to increase parental hostility and depression.

Extracurricular Activities and School Performance

Extracurricular activities, such as sports and music, may help improve school performance, with the caveat that over-scheduling can have a detrimental effect.

Enabling Cain and Abel (Sibling Rivalry)

The goal is to have the siblings learn to resolve their conflicts on their own. Parents need to step in when physical or verbal abuse occurs. In those cases, the goal is still to enable them to resolve the conflicts on their own.

Sexual Orientation

You are expected to understand issues around sexual orientation and gender identity as they develop in childhood and adolescence. The following are some important points to consider when answering questions on this subject on the boards:

- Sexual orientation is biologically-based. Influence of adverse life events has not been substantiated.
- Homosexual teens and young adults are at higher risk for substance abuse, suicide, dropping out of school, and being homeless.

Sexual orientation is not a choice.

Sexual activity is a choice.

Same sex experimentation, especially in early adolescence, is not a harbinger of homosexuality.

International Adoption

You are expected to be aware of the physician's role in international adoption.

Before the adoption takes place, the pediatrician should assist the family in reviewing medical records, including information about the biological parents.

 This information may be inaccurate; this should be factored into any question on this subject.

Anticipatory guidance is another role that the pediatrician may play. Included in this should be the advice that the period of transition and attachment may take up to a year.

After the adoption takes place, the pediatrician should do a developmental assessment of the child and recheck every 3-4 months during the first year. Hearing and vision screening should be done at the first visit.

Immunization records should be verified. Screening for TB is mandatory.

Routine blood tests, including CBC, lead level, as well as Hep B, HIV, and syphilis testing are recommended.

If the adopted child is from an area that is endemic for hepatitis C, hepatitis C serology should be measured.

TB testing (via tuberculin skin test) should take place, regardless of whether they received BCG vaccination (they may actually write this out formally as Bacille Calmette-Guérin).

Pediatricians' Role with Children in Foster Care

Here are some of the important points you might be tested on regarding children in foster care and the role of the pediatrician:

- Children in foster care use more mental and general healthcare resources when compared to others in the same socioeconomic strata
- The AAP recommends that children in foster care receive more frequent routine evaluations than their peers
- All children entering foster care require baseline behavioral, mental, and developmental evaluations.
- The pediatrician should communicate directly with the caseworker to facilitate ongoing care, even after the child has been reunited with his/her family.

Chapter 33

Critical Care

Impending System Failure

Vital Signs

Increased Intracranial pressure

When increased intracranial pressure leads to herniation of cerebral contents, it becomes a neurologic emergency.

Hyperventilation is an important vital sign associated with increased intracranial pressure and coma. You must be able to recognize tachypnea that is compensatory for an underlying problem. Look for any underlying problems such as heart failure or toxic ingestion.

The best way to distinguish tachypnea from central hyperventilation is the presence of nonreactive pupils in central hyperventilation

Uncal Herniation

Uncal herniation is characterized by unilateral pupil dilation due to compression of the oculomotor nerve.

Treatment consists of osmotic agents such as mannitol and hypertonic solutions (while waiting for the neurosurgeon to show up).

Malignant hyperthermia

Malignant hyperthermia is a hypermetabolic state that leads to metabolic acidosis, hyperthermia, and **cardiac arrhythmia, as well as a markedly elevated creatine kinase concentration and myoglobinuria**. Additional findings include tachypnea, *muscle rigidity, increased carbon dioxide production, and fever* following the administration of general anesthesia.

Treatment includes hyperventilation, oxygen, and **dantrolene.**

Cushing's Triad

Cushing's triad is an important sign of increased intracranial pressure. It includes:

1. Bradycardia
2. Hypertension
3. Irregular respirations

Hypoxic-ischemic injury can lead to cerebral edema and increased intracranial pressure. Watch for signs of Cushing's triad as a sign of impending cerebral herniation.

Hypertensive Crisis

If you are presented with a patient who has acute onset of hypertension, the correct immediate management is to assess and monitor. The goal is to reduce the blood pressure gradually, by 25% during the first 8 hours and the remainder slowly over the next 48 hours.

Beta blockers can worsen asthma.

Respiratory Failure

Patients with impending respiratory failure will be described as tachypneic, with decreased mentation, poor skeletal muscle tone, and cyanosis.

Agitation is a common sign of hypoxia.

Upper Airway Obstruction

The following description would correlate with a patient experiencing upper airway obstruction: upright posture, which they might describe as tripoding (e.g., with one hand on the exam table). They could describe a patient breathing through an open mouth, having difficulty swallowing secretions, and displaying stridor.

In addition to stridor, a patient with croup could also present with wheezing. *Do not be fooled into ruling out croup based solely on the presentation of a child with wheezing in the absence of stridor.*

Electrolyte Imbalance

Adrenal Insufficiency

The classic presentation is a patient with vague symptoms, including fatigue, vomiting, headache, muscle weakness, weight loss, and *salt wasting.* Electrolyte finding include:

· Hypoglycemia

· *Hyper*kalemia

· Hyponatremia

It is important to know about autoimmune polyendocrinopathy, which can present with **candidiasis** as well as the typical electrolyte imbalances seen with adrenal insufficiency.

In adrenal insufficiency, one can see an elevated ADH level. Do not be fooled into picking a diagnosis of **SIADH.** In this case, the elevated ADH levels may be **appropriate.**

Acute Respiratory Distress Syndrome

Some of you learned this as **"Adult Respiratory Distress Syndrome"**

This starts out as pulmonary edema, which is a result of increased permeability of the alveolar capillary membranes. It is a result of some insult (e.g., in the case of near-drowning, the submersion episode is the insult). The x-ray findings will be described as *"fine reticular infiltrate,"* and 8 hours later things get worse.

The lungs are only the opening act. The headliners include liver, kidney, brain, and bone marrow dysfunction. This multi-organ involvement poses the greatest risk to survival. This is what you want to avoid.

In addition to drowning, ARDS can be secondary to:

· Pneumonia
· Aspiration
· Lung contusion
· Smoke inhalation
· Blood product transfusion
· Sepsis

GCS and ET Tube

Any victim of head trauma with a GCS of 8 or less should be intubated immediately.

Water Intoxication

Consider a diagnosis of water intoxication if you are presented with an *afebrile* patient of typical development with *seizures*, especially if they have no history of trauma or previous seizures.

They might also mention that the child had spent a lot of time swimming, especially in young children. This may be due to swallowing too much water, which can result in euvolemic hyponatremia.

Watch for a previous history of excessive water intake, malnutrition, or feeding with dilute formula. Other associations could include hypotonic IV fluids, glucocorticoid deficiency, or hypothyroidism.

Conditions Requiring Life Support

Near Drowning

Homeward Bound?

If they have been submerged for **less than 1 minute** with no loss of consciousness and required no resuscitation in the field, the patient can usually be observed at home.

Hospital Bound?

Children rescued from near-drowning episodes can look quite **stable** upon **arrival to the emergency department**, and **then go downhill and require advanced life support**.

Duration of asphyxia is the key to prognosis. **The duration of time from submersion to restoration of adequate respiration determines the extent of the damage.**

Any one of the following predicts risk for future deterioration and warrants continued medical supervision:

❑ A history of **apnea and CPR in the field**.

❑ Neurological signs (seizure or disorientation) or respiratory failure from aspiration.

❑ Arterial desaturation and/or tachypnea (specifically, this might be a warning sign of aspiration pneumonia or acute respiratory distress syndrome. See box on previous page.)

Airway and Ventilatory Support

Unfavorable signs that may worsen prognosis include:

- Submersion > 25 minutes
- Apnea or coma at admission
- Initial arterial pH of <7.0

HOT TIP

If the patient requires less than 10 minutes of CPR, there is a good chance they will survive with no neurologic impairment.

Flail Chest/Hemothorax

Flail chest occurs typically after blunt trauma. By definition, there are 2 or more rib fractures in 2 or more locations.

This results in paradoxic chest wall movements, with underlying lung being pulled into the chest cavity during chest expansion and pushed out during chest wall relaxation.

TREATMENT

If you are presented with a history of flail chest with respiratory distress and tachypnea, the most appropriate next step is placement of a chest tube (to decompress the hemothorax and/or pneumothorax).

Pulmonary Edema

If you are presented with a patient with Acute Respiratory Distress Syndrome (ARDS), then PEEP is the key element of ventilatory support.

Splenic Rupture

Splenic rupture will typically be presented in the context of blunt abdominal trauma. A few important caveats are worth reviewing. These may be worth a couple of points on the exam.

- Attention to the ABCs should be the first step in assessing a child with a suspected splenic rupture.
- Peritoneal lavage will be incorrect, since abdominal CT with contrast is a safer and more effective diagnostic tool.
- Baseline CBC, while useful, is not a reliable diagnostic measure.
- Surgery is indicated when there is hemodynamic instability.
- IV fluids and blood products are often indicated, and may be a correct choice on the exam.

Cardiac Failure

Signs of acute heart failure

A typical presentation might be an infant with *poor weight gain, tachycardia, and tachypnea.* CXR will show *cardiomegaly.* Look for an *ejection fraction less than 25 %.* Tricuspid and mitral valve regurgitation may also be described.

An ejection fraction of 55% is normal.

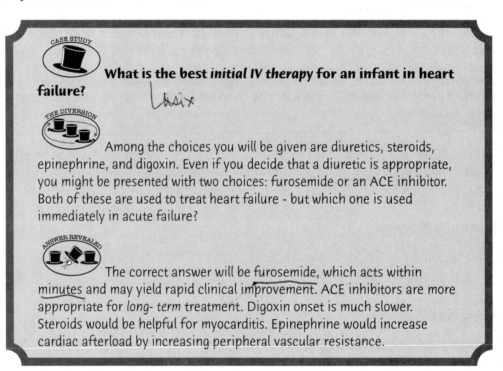

What is the best *initial IV therapy* for an infant in heart failure?

Lasix

Among the choices you will be given are diuretics, steroids, epinephrine, and digoxin. Even if you decide that a diuretic is appropriate, you might be presented with two choices: furosemide or an ACE inhibitor. Both of these are used to treat heart failure - but which one is used immediately in acute failure?

The correct answer will be furosemide, which acts within minutes and may yield rapid clinical improvement. ACE inhibitors are more appropriate for *long- term* treatment. Digoxin onset is much slower. Steroids would be helpful for myocarditis. Epinephrine would increase cardiac afterload by increasing peripheral vascular resistance.

Signs of chronic heart failure

More subtle signs of a more chronic picture will include *failure to thrive* and *poor feeding.*

Cardiogenic Shock/Infants

While cap refill is a good early sign of **shock**, remember that it is not a good predictor of mild dehydration and only a fair predictor of moderate (5-10%) dehydration.

Blood pressure is a very poor indicator of circulatory status in children. Cap refill, urine output, and mental status are better indicators.

They may divert you into over-interpreting diminished cap refill based on environmental factors. If you are presented with a child who had been holding an ice cream bar or had just come in from outdoors, a delayed cap refill will not be reliable. The measurement must be done at room temperature, with no external factors influencing the reading.

Aortic Stenosis

An infant in heart failure with **aortic stenosis** needs to receive prostaglandin E1 to maintain or to reopen the ductus arteriosis, to allow for mixing of oxygenated and deoxygenated blood.

Long QT Syndrome

CASE STUDY

You are presented with a child who collapses or is resuscitated after passing out in a pool. They will then note a history of a close family member who died suddenly and had a history of epilepsy. What is the most likely test to confirm the abnormality in this patient?

THE DIVERSION

Of course, among the choices will be an EEG. If the answer were that simple, anybody with a pulse and an EEG above a flat line could pass the exam. Cardiac echo, angiography, as well as a simple EKG, will be included in the choices.

ANSWER REVEALED

If you did not know anything and simply picked the least invasive of the cardiac answers, you would get it correct. If you knew that congenital long QT syndrome is caused by a variant of ventricular tachycardia, and can result in brief generalized seizures, you would realize that epilepsy may be a misdiagnosis in the close relative. A simple EKG would be the correct answer; it would illustrate a long QT measurement, which is the underlying problem.

Supraventricular Tachycardia

What is the best initial Treatment?

Initial treatment of SVT is with **adenosine.**

Since quick treatment is important, however, the answer may be to place a bag of ice (carefully) on the face while the nurse is getting adenosine. No, it isn't for cooling down the hot situation; it is to increase vagal tone. Valsalva also may work (the patient, not you - it won't help your panic a bit).

If adenosine doesn't work at all, try, try, and try again with an increased dose. If it works but SVT returns right after adenosine is given, then the appropriate treatment is IV **diltiazem.**

Cardiac Tamponade

Cardiac tamponade may present with muffled heart sounds, as well as pulsus paradoxus.

Pulsus paradoxus is decreased systolic blood pressure during inspiration.

Brain Death

Brain death is the irreversible end of brain activity, including the absence of cardiorespiratory function. The absence of vertebral and carotid artery blood flow is consistent with brain death.

In order for a patient to be declared brain dead, there needs to be no other disorders which could obscure neurological functioning (don't forget hypothermia!) If there is any doubt, ancillary imaging studies would be useful in documenting the absence of vertebral and carotid artery blood flow.

The two studies that can be used to document this are a **radionucleotide scan** or **angiography**.

Liver Failure

The most important findings in a child with impending liver failure are an **elevated serum ammonia level** and **change in mental status**.

However, if you are presented with a patient with chronic tremor and anxiety, and lab findings consistent with liver disease, you will want to rule out Wilson's Disease by measuring a serum ceruloplasmin level.

Azotemia

You are expected to distinguish prerenal from renal azotemia. It is much easier to think of it is as "non renal" and "renal intrinsic" azotemia.

Prerenal Azotemia

If they are presenting you with a case of prerenal azotemia, they will likely describe the volume depletion as a history of vomiting, diarrhea, bleeding, or third spacing.

Additional findings may include:

- **Decreased** urine output, with normal urinary sediments,
- **Low** urinary sodium (<10.0 mEq/L)
- **Increased** BUN-to-creatinine ratio.

Renal Azotemia

While renal or intrinsic renal azotemia might also present with dehydration, there will also be a history of direct renal insult. This might include *ingestion of a nephrotoxic agent,* an *ischemic event,* or even *sepsis.*

Watch for a history of *recent treatment for impetigo.* If this is coupled with proteinuria and hematuria, the diagnosis may be post strep glomerulonephritis.

The decreased urine output will be described as oliguria or anuria. Additional urine findings may include red blood cells/casts or granular casts.

Laboratory examination of the urine sediment may demonstrate red blood cell casts, granular casts, and red blood cells, findings seen in glomerulonephritis. When evaluating for possible glomerulonephritis, other appropriate biochemical studies include

Urine the Answer

An important distinction is urine osmolality and urinary fractional excretion of sodium.

Prerenal Azotemia

Increased urine osmolality (>350 mOsm)

Low fractional excretion of sodium (<1% in the older child)

Renal Azotemia

Low urine osmolality (<350 mOsm)

High urinary fractional excretion of sodium (>1% in the older child

streptococcal antibodies, hepatitis B and C panels, and complement studies.

If they also present you with a *low C3*, they are indicating a possible diagnosis of systemic lupus erythematosus, or membranoproliferative or poststreptococcal glomerulonephritis.

In this context, if you are asked to determine additional studies to order, the correct choices would include streptococcal antibodies, including the antistreptolysin O titer, anti-DNAase B titer, and group A antibody to *Streptococcus pyogenes* titer.

In the context of renal azotemia, obtaining hepatitis B and C antigens and antibodies would also be appropriate.

The ABC's of CPR

Remembering a few important points regarding CPR will very likely score you 1-2 points on the exam.

When performing CPR on an infant, the two thumb-encircling hands technique is preferred over the 2 fingers on the sternum technique.

The chest should be compressed 1/3 to 1/2 of the anteroposterior diameter of the chest at a rate of 100 compressions/min.

With 2 rescuers, the correct ratio is 15 compressions to 2 breaths

With 1 rescuer, the correct ratio is 30 compressions to 2 breaths

If an airway has been established, the ventilation rate should be 8-10 per minute *independent of compressions*, which are delivered at the same 100/minute rate without pausing.

Chest compressions can be discontinued if the HR is greater than 60 and perfusion is adequate.

The heart rate greater than 60 beats/min rule is not absolute. If there is still evidence of poor perfusion, e.g., delayed cap refill, weak pulses, or cool extremities, chest compressions should continue.

AEDs (automated external defibrillators) can be used in children **older than 1 year of age**.

Chapter 34

ER

Codes Facts

Remember your ABC's

The first priority for any unresponsive child brought to the ER is to go right to the ABC's (Airway, Breathing, and Circulation). What should you do first? **Establishing an airway** is always the answer they are looking for, regardless of the reason the patient is unresponsive.

CASE STUDY You are presented with a child who has ingested an unknown substance and is unresponsive. What is the first thing you do?

THE DIVERSION Among the diversionary choices, you will be given options to provide inactivated charcoal or intramuscular glucose. What about IM Narcan®?

ANSWER REVEALED Your attempt to pass the boards would be "unresponsive" if you picked these choices. The first thing you should do with any patient who is unresponsive is establish an airway.

ET Tube Size

The child's age plus 16, divided by 4, determines ET tube size. A four year old would be 20/4, which would be a size 5 ET Tube.

Meds that can be given by ET

Consider it a **LANE**:

Lidocaine
Atropine
Narcan®
Epinephrine

Atropine is indicated for bradycardia, not asystole.

 If too low a dose of atropine is given, the bradycardia can worsen.

Calcium could be used with:
- ❏ Hypocalcemia (duh!)
- ❏ Hyperkalemia
- ❏ Calcium Channel Blocker ingestion (hey, it could happen, especially on the Boards)
- ❏ Hypermagnesemia

Convert Numbers to Words

Questions that deal with ER and critical care will be filled with vital signs and lab values. This is another example of where it is critical[1] to write descriptive words in the margins. For example, if you see a temperature of 101.2, write "febrile" in the margin; if HR is 120, write "tachycardia." The picture they are drawing will then become more evident.

 Tidal Volume: 7 mL/kg is the formula used to calculate tidal volume on a vent.

Acute Management of Fever

High Yield Facts regarding High Fever

- A temperature higher than 105.8°F correlates with invasive bacterial infection.
- Consistently using the same method (oral, axillary, tympanic, etc.) to take the temperature is more important than the actual method used. This way it is easier to monitor for body temperature changes.
- Tactile temperature noted by parents is not considered to be reliable.

---

[1] Pun intended.

TREATMENT Fever in **infants younger than 1 month** requires a septic workup and empiric antibiotics, pending culture results.

Infants between 1-2 months require a workup but not necessarily inpatient management and/or empiric antibiotics if initial studies (including WBC, UA, and frequently CSF) are not suspicious for invasive infection.

From **3-36 months**, clinical judgement can play an important role. Watch the history they present. Look for identifiable sources of infection and treat as such. If they present a child that may not have been immunized against pneumococcal disease, for example, workup for occult bacteremia may be indicated. This would include empiric antibiotics pending culture results.

PERIL WARNING Of course, factor in underlying conditions such as sickle cell disease or immunocompromised status if this is part of the history.

Ibuprofen does last longer than acetaminophen.

Fever of Unknown Origin

Non-Infectious causes of FUO:

In addition to the bacterial and viral causes of fever in children, it is important to not lose sight of non-infectious causes of fever.

Remember, FUO can be the presenting sign of JIA.

BUZZ WORDS Typical presentation is a school-aged child with an evanescent rash and **morning stiffness;** the fever will be present for more than one week.

CASE STUDY They may present a variety of 5 year-old children with fever. They will list a few underlying diagnoses and ask which child is in the MOST need of fever-reducing agents (also known as antipyretics).

THE DIVERSION Among the choices will be a child with a history of febrile seizures, as well as a few obviously wrong choices, like a child with an ear infection, and a couple you have to think about, like a child with encephalitis and a child with congestive heart failure. Whenever an answer seems obvious, like, "a history of febrile seizures," you have to assume for at least a moment it cannot be the correct choice. In this case, that would be a wise move.

ANSWER REVEALED The child with a history of febrile seizures that is now 5 years old is just about out of the age of risk, so a febrile seizure is not a high priority. The child with encephalitis needs treatment directed to the encephalitis, and, of course, otitis media is not a priority. However, a child with congestive heart failure would need to have the fever reduced to reduce oxygen demand and subsequent cardiac output demand.

2 Week Old with Fever

We all know that a 2 week old with fever requires an LP, blood culture, and urine culture.

 A chest x-ray is not obligatory in the absence of any respiratory signs.

Anaphylaxis

A patient in anaphylactic shock would be considered unstable. Here, too, it is the ABC's. Airway management is crucial if they ask what is the "first" thing you would do. Fluid maintenance would come afterward.

 Remember it is Epi 1:1000 (not 10,000).

IV Benadryl would also be indicated.

Bites, Fights, and What's Right

Inevitably, kids will bite each other and get close to animals that will bite them. Here is what you need to know:

Cats

Cats bite deeply and make little puncture wounds; therefore, cat bites are worse than dog bites. In addition to anaerobes, consider coverage for *Staph aureus*. *Pasteurella multocida*[2] should also be considered.

Antibiotics/Preventive

The most important first step is wound cleaning via high pressure irrigation – not prophylactic antibiotics.

Antibiotics would be indicated for "dirty cuts," "crush injuries," and "cat bites." Bites that penetrate cartilage, like ears, would also be an indication.

 When you can foresee a problem, give antibiotics. Remember 6 **C**'s:

Clean/Not
Cats and Dogs and Humans (oh my!)
Crush
Cartilage
Cuticles (feet and extremities)
Compromised (Immunocompromised)

The appropriate antibiotic for cat and dog bites would be amoxicillin/clavulanate to help protect against both *Staph aureus* and *Pasteurella multocida*.

> ### Man's Best Friend
>
> Should you have to distinguish this on the picture section, human bites would be half-moon shaped; dog bites are tears; and cats, again, are punctures.

---

[2] An anaerobe; therefore, Augmentin® would be the treatment of choice.

Hymenoptera Stings

Hymenoptera stings are from a variety of insects, including wasps and bees.

These can often cause a triad of systemic reaction:

1. **Hypotension**
2. **Wheezing**
3. **Laryngeal edema**

If a child experiences a localized non-systemic reaction, including angioedema and hives, they are not at increased risk for future systemic reactions and do not require allergy testing or desensitization.

If a child experiences a systemic reaction, they are at increased future risk and need to carry an EpiPen® and obtain an allergy consult.

Spider Bites

There are two primary spider bites to be concerned about creeping up on the boards.[3]

Brown Recluse (Loxosceles reclusa)

Although systemic symptoms can be part of the presentation, typically it is a self-limited local painful lesion that requires no additional treatment.

A target lesion consisting of a red circle surrounding a white ring. This is different than the target lesion associated with Lyme disease, and appears within hours (as opposed to weeks with Lyme disease).

Treatment is largely supportive only.

The Black Widow (Latrodectus mactans)

Often the bite is nothing more than a puncture wound that is barely noticed. However, systemic symptoms can present within 8 hours, including:

· Muscle aches- involving the abdomen, lower back, and chest, as well as the extremities
· Hypertension

---

[3] Pun intended

Treatment consists of narcotic pain killers and antihypertensives, such as nifedipine.

Muscle cramping can be managed with benzodiazepines, narcotic pain killers, and calcium gluconate. Antivenom is only used as a secondary option if these supportive measures do not work.

Wound excision, steroids, hyperbaric chambers, dapsone, and/or watching the movie *The Fly* in rewind mode would not be correct management choices for black widow spider bite on the exam.

Snake Bite / Acute Management

You will need to know if they are describing a snake bite by a venomous or non-venomous snake.

Fortunately you will not be examining a live snake, only a live board question, which can be dangerous and fatal to a passing grade only.

If they describe a snake with a triangular head and fangs, it is likely venomous (insert your favorite lawyer joke here). If they describe a snake with a round head, without fangs or a rattle, it is probably not venomous.

The one exception is a round head with a yellow and red racing stripe. That is a coral snake, which is venomous.

If they describe a snake with such a racing stripe, you know the patient should race to get help. You can also recall, "red and yellow killed a fellow."

Since this is not the herpetology board exam, they will more likely describe the wound itself rather than the snake. If they describe fang marks, assume it is a venomous bite.

Initial signs of venomous bites are local erythema and swelling, followed by enlarged lymph nodes and bulla.

 If the wound appears to be from a non-venomous snake, wound cleaning and tetanus status verification are all that is needed.

If the wound is venemous, the first step in the field is the ABC's of stabilization. Then immobilize the limb and let it hang at the patient's side.

Applying a tourniquet, applying ice, and/or sucking the venom out of the wound are appropriate on episodes of *MacGyver* and even *MacGruber*, but would be incorrect on the boards.

MacGyver might be able to help transport the patient to an appropriate facility, and this would be a correct choice.

Hypothermia

In severe hypothermia, external rewarming alone will cause the following symptoms: peripheral vasodilation, decreased BP, acid base imbalance, and arrhythmias. Therefore, internal rewarming should also be done. This would be best accomplished with warmed IV fluids, as well as gastric lavage with warmed fluids.

Rabies in Cute Pets

Rabies is rare in an immunized cat or dog. In addition, bites from lagomorphs are also **not** an indication for rabies prophylaxis.

What's a lagomorph? Glad you asked! These are rabbits, squirrels, hamsters, rats, mice, and other rodents.

Contrary to popular myth, squirrels are not high risk for carrying rabies.

Carnivores such as raccoons, skunks, foxes, and bats are high risk for rabies.

Rabies

With a suspected bite from a potentially **rabies-infected animal**, the following factors make it riskier:

❑ Bites that are closer to the brain

❑ Unprovoked

❑ An unvaccinated animal that carries rabies

Rabies is **uncommon in small rodents**, including squirrels, chipmunks, rats, and mice. **Rabbits** are also rarely carriers of rabies.

Foxes, bats, raccoons, skunks, and ferrets can transmit rabies. In the US, the animal that most commonly transmits rabies to humans is the bat.

An important source of rabies to consider is **woodchuck**. Add to that **beavers, opossums, coyotes, groundhogs, cats, dogs, and wolves.**

Perhaps it is easier to remember the animals that can carry rabies in pairs, to the tune of **"Frère Jacques"** (repeat the "wolves and coyotes" and "opossums and bats" as best you can).

Foxy ferrets

Cats and dogs

Wolves and coyotes

Groundhogs and woodchucks

Raccoons and skunks

Opossums and bats

Treating Rabies

With a **high index of suspicion, immune globulin is recommended**. Domestic animals can be observed, so Ig can be postponed.

They could very well ask you what to do with a child who was possibly exposed to rabies, so here is the scoop.

- ❑ First, like any wound, **wash and debride** with soap and water.
- ❑ Second, **HRIG** (human rabies immunoglobulin).
- ❑ Third, **5 doses of rabies vaccine** (ouch!)

Any contact with a bat requires treatment, regardless.

Seizures (Acute Management)

IV lorazepam (Ativan®) is the treatment of choice. Lorazepam has a rapid onset and is longer acting than diazepam (Valium®). Once the seizure is under control, a longer acting agent such as phenobarbital should be used.

Phosphenytoin or phenobarbital are the long-acting agents of choice. Phosphenytoin can be given IM if necessary.

If phenytoin is given too rapidly to infants, there is a risk of bradycardia. PR diazepam is an alternative for infants when IV access is problematic.

Status epilepticus

Status epilepticus is treated with phenytoin 20 mg/kg or fosphenytoin 20 mg phenytoin equivalents/kg (loading doses) IV.

Phenobarb is *not* first line treatment for status.

Shock

There are two key points to remember: 1) decreased BP is a late finding, and 2) cap refill is an early sign.

After 3 attempts at IV access or 90 seconds, an intraosseous (IO) line should be used to administer fluids. Most resuscitation meds and blood products can be administered through an IO line.

Warm, Warm a Heart

Warm Shock

An example would be septic shock, as in meningococcemia. The result is poor tissue perfusion, with acidosis and hypotension. Vasopressors such as norepinephrine are helpful. This is because the pipes, not the pump, are the problem.

Cardiogenic Shock (cold shock)

Here the pump is the problem. Therefore, **dobutamine** would be needed to "enhance the pump" (higher doses also have a vasopressor effect). EKG and cardiac echo should be done when cardiogenic shock is suspected.

Cardiogenic shock in an infant will likely be presented as tachypnea and diminished pulses, as well as a gallop rhythm. They might also describe an enlarged liver if there is right-sided heart failure.

> ### Increased ICP
>
> With a Glasgow coma score below 8, intubation would be indicated. Mannitol and Lasix®, along with hyperventilation, are methods to reduce ICP.

Head Trauma

You need to be familiar with the various types of skull fractures and the clues you will see in the question. In addition, you need to know the range of the Glasgow Coma Scale.[4]

---

[4] Not to be confused with the Stupor Index while studying for the Boards.

The clinical impact of increased intracranial pressure can be gradual. In particular, remember that papilledema is often absent initially.

Subdural Hematoma

"Shaken Baby Syndrome" often involves subdural, not epidural, hematomas. In addition, children with Shaken Baby Syndrome may present with retinal hemorrhages and/or bulging fontanelle. The CT picture is also distinctive. They can present later with a headache and drowsiness. The first and second hours are the most critical.

Subdural taps can sometimes remedy subdural hemorrhages without surgery. Severe head injuries, especially those associated with a subdural hematoma, can lead to SIADH. Pay particular attention when they describe a recent head injury and provide you with electrolytes and urine osmolality values.

Epidural Hematoma

This is a Board favorite. They will describe a child sustaining head trauma who then goes through a "lucid period" of improvement, only to deteriorate later. This is the classic presentation for epidural hematoma. The lucid period can be days or hours.

Remember, this can result in a **bloody *atraumatic LP***, so if they describe an "atraumatic" tap with lots of red cells in the question, epidural hematoma is the most likely answer.

Epidural hematomas require surgical intervention.

Retinal Hemorrhages

They have shown retinal hemorrhages in a picture. A vague reference to retinal hemorrhage with no suggestion of abuse in the history might be the only hint you will get. Any child with inexplicable mental status change should be evaluated for retinal hemorrhage. Pay particular attention to this if presented with a child with mental status change and they emphasize no evidence of head trauma on examination. **Retinal hemorrhages can occur even in the absence of external signs of head trauma.**

Glasgow Coma Scale

The higher the number, the better the prognosis. 15 is normal; a score less than 8 is a severe coma (or normal for an HMO coding reviewer). Prognosis is inversely related to the index and **length of time of coma**.

Remember, "Coma 8 ....intubate."

Poor prognostic signs include cerebral bleeding, brain edema, and a coma lasting longer than 6 hours.

Here is another example where you will need to know what is normal and abnormal in the coma index. They might give you a value in the question and "imply" that it is abnormal. Armed with their parameters, you won't be among those who are tricked.

The Glasgow Coma Scale is only useful for head trauma; it is not useful in assessing metabolic coma.

Glasgow for Kids

A common pitfall is that for younger kids, a score less than 5 is normal (i.e., even a healthy 2-year-old won't follow verbal commands). That is why there is a revised Glasgow Coma Scale for infants.

Glasgow Coma Scale			
Response	**Adults and Children**	**Infants**	**Points**
Eye opening	No response To pain To voice Spontaneous	No response To pain To voice Spontaneous	1 2 3 4
Verbal	No response Incomprehensible Inappropriate words Disoriented Conversation	No response Moans to pain Cries to pain Irritable Coos, babbles	1 2 3 4 5
Motor	No response Decerebrate posturing Decorticate posturing Withdraws to pain Localizes pain Obeys commands	No response Decerebrate posturing Decorticate posturing Withdraws to pain Withdraws to touch Normal spontaneous	1 2 3 4 5 6

Hematoma/Nasal Septum

As a general rule, "surgical intervention" is rarely the answer on boards, except when it comes to the eyes. This is another exception to that rule.

If they describe swelling of the nasal septum with any degree of obstruction, immediate ENT consultation is indicated for drainage. If this is not done, there is a risk for significant cartilage damage with saddle nose deformity (the kind you see in hockey players, boxers, and other people who stick their noses where they are not welcomed).

The same is true for hematoma of the pinna, which should be drained and have a pressure dressing applied in order to avoid "cauliflower ear."

Risk Factors for Abuse and Neglect

Child abuse risk factors can be divided into 4 broad categories

1. External factors
2. Parenting skills
3. Vulnerability of the child
4. Psychological factors

Other forms of domestic violence often occur in addition to child abuse.

Also note that abuse may occur in foster care.

External Factors

External factors that increase the risk for abuse include

· Poor housing
· Multiple young children
· Social isolation
· Family discord

Parental Skills

· Unwanted parenthood
· Unexpected parenthood

· Unrealistic expectations

· Parent abused as a child

Vulnerability of the child

Children who are hyperactive are also at increased risk for being abused.

 Children with disabilities and those born prematurely are at higher risk for abuse.

Psychological factors

Alcoholism or **drug abuse,** as well as parental mental illness, all increase risk for child abuse and neglect.

Parents who were abused as children are at high risk for repeating the pattern.

Unrealistic expectations of the child, as well as parental depression, are additional risk factors.

Sibling rivalry and siblings hitting each other is rarely an explanation for serious injury. If this is the explanation given in the history, they are trying to tell you the injury was non-accidental.

In addition, *gender of the child, parental education, and employment status are not important risk factors for child abuse.*

You need to be familiar with the feeding patterns of infants that are beyond normal, which may reflect deeper mother/ infant relationship problems. These include:

· Feeding the child or infant to quiet them down

· Propping the bottle at bedtime

If you are asked a question about the most important intervention, addressing the individual feeding issues are not the most important interventions. Psychosocial intervention is the most important intervention.

Intentional Ingestion

Ingestion that would be unusual for the child's developmental stage may not be accidental. Consider intentional ingestion or abuse if, for example, an infant ingested alcohol. A scenario such as this could represent a parent's attempt to sedate or stop the infant from crying.

Abuse Imitators

This is a Board favorite, and one of the many traps they like to lay down. Like the bizarre characters on Batman, these impostors are likely to make an appearance on the Boards. While the wording of the question will imply abuse, it will usually be the incorrect answer.

Lesions of child abuse are rarely symmetrical.

Fractures

Look for hints that they are talking about osteogenesis imperfecta, such as bluish coloration of the sclerae. Other factors which can result in fractures that are not secondary to abuse are **hypophosphatasia, infantile cortical hyperostosis, and osteoid osteoma.**

· **Infantile cortical hyperostosis (Caffey Disease)** – within 3 months of life; includes fever, swelling of the tissues of the face and jaws, as well as cortical thickening of the long and flat bones

· **Hypophosphatasia** – bowing of the deformities and decreased alkaline phosphatase

Skin Lesions

There are a variety of skin lesions that imitate abuse: "**Mongolian spots**" and **Henoch Schoenlein Purpura** are a couple of examples. What will often distinguish abuse is how it progresses.

If there is variation in color, this usually indicates abuse.

Stevens Johnson Syndrome -Erythema Multiforme (SJS)

This could be misdiagnosed as a burn, but here distribution will be the key, and there will be something in the question to tip you off to SJS. It is the distribution around the mouth that is key. Remember Erythema MultiORALforme.

If they mention that the child is from an Asian culture, in particular Viet Nam or Cambodia, know that cupping and coining of the back are culturally normal and not technically abuse.

Dislocations

Any toddler with a history of being "swung by the arms" will most likely have a subluxation of the radial head (Nursemaid's elbow), rather than a serious fracture.

Periorbital Ecchymoses

Periorbital ecchymoses can be a sign of neuroblastoma, especially on the boards.

Fractures

Skull Fractures

Watch for a toddler who is afebrile and irritable, with bruises to consider a non accidental skull fracture.

In such cases, the correct answer will be to obtain a Head CT and skeletal survey. In fact, a skeletal survey is indicated in a child presenting with a subdural hematoma.

MRI is only useful in determining the age of a subdural hematoma. It is not useful in emergency settings where the quick establishment of an active subdural is important.

The presence or absence of physical signs is never the *sole* deciding factor in deciding whether to obtain a head CT scan following head trauma.

A head CT is indicated for:

- Prolonged LOC
- Protracted vomiting
- Progressing headaches
- Retrograde amnesia
- Lethargy

If you are presented with a toddler who hits his head and is initially described as *stunned for 10 seconds, having an episode of vomiting, sleeping but easily arouses, and with a scalp hematoma, a head CT is NOT indicated.*

When presented with a child in whom a skull fracture or head bleed is suspected, what is the first step you should take?

You might be tempted to choose diagnostic studies such as a head CT, or worse yet, an MRI. However, remember your ABC's with any acute injury.

Your ABC's should lead you to checking airway, breathing, and circulation before doing any diagnostic studies.

Temporal Bone Fracture

A child with a temporal bone fracture will be described with a combination of the following: visible bleeding from the ear or hemotympanum, along with hearing loss and possibly facial paralysis. CSF otorrhea may also be described or hinted at.

Basilar Skull Fracture

They could describe "clear rhinorrhea," which is really CSF. Another important sign is the Battle sign, which is ecchymoses behind the ear. One can also see raccoon eyes, which is periorbital ecchymoses. If basilar skull fracture is suspected clinically, the next step is a CT (not skull x-rays).

This is typically described as a bruise over the mastoid bone and/or "black and blue eyes." It can also involve the "abducens and facial nerve palsy" (6th and 7th cranial nerves) and once again with "discharge from the nose and ears."

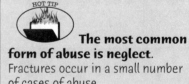

The most common form of abuse is neglect. Fractures occur in a small number of cases of abuse.

The following types of fractures are most likely due to abuse:
- Bucket handle fractures
- Corner fractures (due to pulling an extremity)
- Spiral fractures in infants
- Rib fractures
- Multiple skull fractures
- Spinous process fractures
- Scapula fractures
- Sternum fractures

CASE STUDY

You are asked to choose from a list of fractures to determine which one is most likely secondary to abuse. Included in the list are ones that are easy to eliminate; you are well-prepared and know that *non-displaced linear skull fractures in an infant, clavicular fractures, and supracondylar elbow fractures can all be accidental.*

THE DIVERSION

After eliminating these choices, you might be down to two choices: **bucket handle** fracture and **buckle fracture of the distal radius**. Hmm… you might wonder which one is associated with child abuse — bucket handle or buckle. Well, if you don't know for sure you might have poured another question down the bucket.

ANSWER REVEALED

Buckle fractures are *not* associated with child abuse. Bucket handle fractures are associated with abuse. You can remember this by picturing somebody getting hit by an adult holding a bucket by the handle. It's not a pretty picture – but, then again, neither is failing the Board exam.

Supracondylar Fractures

Pain Management

There is a tendency to undertreat pediatric patients for pain.

You may be tested on this, and it is best to pick choices that manage pain more, rather than less, aggressively.

The risk for respiratory depression with opiates is less than commonly thought, so a correct answer might include a choice of titrating up on the dose to manage pain appropriately.

BUZZ WORDS

Typically occurs in a boy age 5-8 years falling on an outstretched arm which is hyperextended at the elbow.

Fracture Vasculature

Supracondylar fracture of the humerus will impact the vasculature. There may be no external signs in the presence of severe injury/trauma. **Therefore, if trauma to the elbow is mentioned in the question, consider neurovascular compromise**.

BUZZ WORDS

In addition to obvious signs — such as pallor and cyanosis of the distal extremity — watch for **pain on passive extension of the fingers.** A nondisplaced supracondylar fracture might not be obvious on x-ray. Also watch for a **posterior fat pad**.

An anterior fat pad is a normal finding and not suggestive of a fracture.

Similar elbow injuries to watch out for on the exam and their differentiating characteristics are as follows:

Elbow Injury	Distinguishing Characteristics
Dislocation of the elbow	Age 11-15; fall on an outstretched arm which is *supinated* with the elbow *partially extended - not hyperextended.* *However, these too can be associated with neurovascular compromise.*
Epiphyseal Fracture	Older children due to direct impact with the arm laterally rotated on impact. Neurovascular compromise less likely.
Lateral condyle fracture	Forearm is supinated, neurovascular compromise very unlikely.
Nursemaid's Elbow	Nursemaid's elbow will not present with elbow swelling and tenderness.

CASE STUDY You are presented with a patient who has an elbow injury. They note that there is decreased grip strength and decreased radial pulse. You correctly diagnose supracondylar fracture of the distal humerus.

THE DIVERSION The choices you will be presented with won't be very humerus at all. You will need to decide if this is a result of direct vascular injury or a transient neurological deficit.

ANSWER REVEALED The correct answer will be transient neurological deficit. This is because the absent radial pulse is likely due to compression of the radial artery, and not direct trauma to the artery. This will resolve with reduction of the fracture. The neurological deficit, manifested as decreased grip strength, is also transient.

Clavicular Fractures

Once again, this occurs with a fall on an outstretched arm or directly on the shoulder. The child will be holding the arm with the opposite hand.

Greenstick Fracture

A Greenstick typically occurs following a fall on an outstretched hand with a cortical break on one side of the bone and intact periosteum on the opposite side.

The break is not through the bone – one side is broken and the other bent. Like a "Green stick" – get it?

Most clavicular fractures will heal without much intervention other than an arm sling. However, **medial clavicular fracture with anterior or posterior displacement will require an evaluation for possible displacement of the trachea or mediastinal structures.**

Orthopedic consult is rarely indicated immediately. Shoulder immobilization will be the correct answer.

Acromioclavicular separation can be distinguished from a clavicular fracture by the presence of a *palpable step-off of the right anterior shoulder joint in the absence of crepitus.*

AC joint separation will occur in older "skeletally mature" teenagers; in younger children a clavicular fracture is more likely, so note the age of the child presented in the question.

You are asked to evaluate a teenage baseball player who sustained a shoulder injury. He has pain over the distal clavicle, with point tenderness over the superior aspect. He cannot raise his arm above his head. X-ray is negative for clavicular fracture, shoulder fracture, and dislocation. What is the most likely injury?

You will be dazzled with lots of tempting diversionary answers, including a variety of tempting "occult" fractures, such as "occult clavicular fracture" and "occult proximal humerus fracture." Another diversionary choice would be a shoulder separation.

The correct answer in this scenario would be acromioclavicular separation. Children younger than 13 are more prone to sustain a fracture of the distal clavicle. In children older than 13, such as the teenager in this vignette, an acromioclavicular separation is more likely. This patient had point tenderness. The typical pain of a shoulder separation would be more diffuse.

Electric Burns

Most electrical burns affect the skin.

When electric current courses through the body, it is called arc exposure, which results in deep tissue burns and internal organ involvement. This can lead to rhabdomyolysis and renal failure.

Arrhythmias are also possible.

 Most injuries involving exposure to household electrical current involve only skin.

Thermal Burns

You will be expected to distinguish between **accidental** and **non-accidental** burns based on the description in the history. The following are suggestive of **non-accidental** causes of burns. Keeping these in mind will help *you* from being burned on the exam.

- Full thickness burns are rarely an accident, since children will usually withdraw before a full thickness burn sets in
- Distinct margins
- Varying depth

Involvement or sparing of interdigital areas can occur in accidental and non accidental burns.

There will be tips in the question if an "abuse imitator" is the cause. Typically, they might show a picture of a **Collodion baby** or a baby with **Stevens Johnson syndrome,** and they will put "child abuse" as the decoy answer.

 A **splash-like** configuration is suggestive of an **accidental** injury.

The classic "**stocking and glove" distribution** would be a dead giveaway that it is **non-accidental** cause.

Infection Prevention in Burns

Automatic administration of antibiotics is not necessary. The first step in a minor burn treatment is debridement and irrigation.

Minor burns should be cleaned gently with mild soap and water.

Remember to consider tetanus immunization status. Also remember the "Rule of Nines," which is used to calculate involved body surface area in a child older than 9.

[RULE OF 9'S]

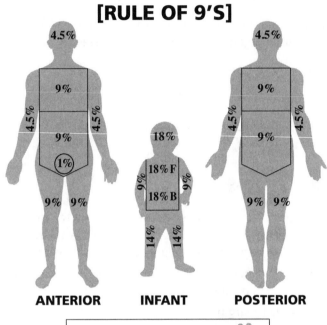

ANTERIOR   **INFANT**   **POSTERIOR**

PALMAR METHOD

By using your own hand you can estimate the extent of a burn.[5]   1%

Rule of Nines

If they ask you to estimate the extent of a burn as a percentage of the total body in a child who is older than 9, here is the rule of 9's.

Arms = 9% each	(9 x 1)
Legs = 18% each	(9 x 2)
Trunk = 36%	(9 X 4)
Head and neck = 10%	(9 X 1)
Perineum = 1%	

Veering from the Vermillion border

Any laceration described as crossing the vermillion border should be referred to a plastic surgeon.

Lacerations

Infection prevention is best accomplished with irrigation and debridement. Irrigate with normal saline under low pressure (but higher pressure may be indicated in very contaminated wounds). Shaving hair is unnecessary.

Nail in my UGG®

BUZZ WORDS

If you are presented with a wound infection due to a puncture wound through a shoe (UGG® or otherwise), the most common causes are *Strep* and *Staph*.

---

5 For a small child you would need to adjust this formula, especially if you have a large hand.

However, you must also consider *Pseudomonas aeruginosa*, especially if they present you with a patient who has a wound infection that is still hanging around 4-5 days after you start treatment.

If the puncture wound presents within 24 hours, irrigation alone might be sufficient treatment. If it presents beyond that point, antibiotics will also be indicated.

If the patient is febrile: IV antibiotics, imaging studies, and ortho referral would be indicated.

Playing Tetanus

Tetanus immunoglobulin (TIG) would be indicated for a patient with a dirty wound who has not completed an initial tetanus series, or if tetanus immunization status is unknown. Pay particular attention to children from developing countries.

This is especially so if they present you with a patient who has a wound contaminated with soil.

In addition to **TIG**, the patient should also be given **Tdap** or **Td (although Tdap is preferred because of concerns of waning pertussis immunity in adolescents).** Whenever TIG is used, one of these vaccines must also be given.

Munchausen Syndrome by Proxy (MSBP)

The tip-off would be a parent in the field of financing rattling off medical terms like a medical dictionary with a blue tooth connection.

They might describe a mother with an MBA from Wharton, whose knowledge and comfort with medical terms rivals the actors on *Grey's Anatomy*, describing her child as "hypovolemic with cap refill greater than 2 seconds" or "a child with repeated ER visits to different ER's on different continents," or "Doctor shopping locally AND on the Internet.[6]"

Sexual Abuse

This will most likely occur by someone close to or known by the family, so look for clues in the question to this effect. They may also describe something that is not abuse, and parental reassurance is the correct answer.

---

[6] If they are doctor shopping at Walmart or Costco, and on the New York City subway system, this is also a significant red flag.

Culture Positive for Sexual Abuse

Neisseria gonorrhea infection on genital, rectal, and pharyngeal secretions cultures should be strongly considered a result of sexual abuse.

Since chlamydia and *Neisseria gonorrhea* are often linked, it is tempting to link them here as well.

 Chlamydia infection in adolescents and adults can be transmitted sexually. Chlamydia can also be vertically transmitted during the birth process and persist in positive cultures for months. However, rectal and vaginal chlamydia infection transmitted at birth should not persist past 18 months of age.

However, sexual abuse should be considered in any prepubertal child beyond infancy who they present with vaginal, urethral, or rectal chlamydia infection.

 The description of a child who acts out by describing explicit adult sexual behavior should be a strong indicator that the child may have observed or experienced inappropriate sexual behaviors.

Condylomata acuminatum is not necessarily sexual abuse.

Hymenal Damage: Since the hymen can be damaged in other ways (like riding a bike), the size of the hymen is not a good way to assess sexual abuse or molestation *in the absence of supporting history and other physical findings.* A common hymen variant lacks tissue above the 3 and 9 o'clock positions. If presented with this information, know that it is too nonspecific in and of itself to confirm sexual abuse.

Labial adhesions and some abrasions can be normal findings in certain injuries, such as bicycle seat injury. Additional findings that are seen as normal variants in girls who have not been abused include gaping hymenal orifice, vaginal discharge, labial adhesions, friability of the posterior fourchette, a linea vestibularis, and vestibule pallor.

An example of when vaginal bleeding in young girls may not represent abuse is urethral prolapse. This often presents in African American girls, ages 3-8 years, as a hyperemic doughnut-shaped mass. Treatment is warm sitz baths and follow-up with an urologist.

"Foreign body," such as toilet paper, might be the answer they are looking for, especially if they describe a foul odor from the vagina.

There will be a clue in the question indicating suspicion of abuse if that is the road they want you to travel down.

Vaginal discharge in a child on antibiotics is usually just a yeast infection when no other information is given.

White discharge can be due to **physiological leukorrhea.** It is due to the desquamation of epithelial cells under the influence of estrogen, typically in a girl around 11 (or just prior to menarche.)

Biological Chemical Weapons

The age of terrorism has reached the Boards, so you must at least be aware of the presentations and treatments you might be presented with, in addition to feeling the terror of preparing for and taking the Boards.

Small Pox

In addition to general signs such as headache, vomiting, and high fever, look for the description of *delirium*, along with a rash which progresses from *papules* ➔ *vesicles* ➔ *pustules* ➔ *scabs*.

It is diagnosed via pharyngeal swab culture or culture of the lesions themselves. Smallpox is spread by direct contact or airborne. Its actual name is *variola*. Treatment is with *cidofovir*, which at the time of publication was experimental. It is still worth noting this.

The lesions associated with varicella and smallpox both start out as flat, red macules, ultimately becoming vesicles.

With varicella, in any area of skin, there will be lesions in different stages of evolution.

With smallpox, in any given area the lesions will all be in the same stage of evolution. Lesions in other parts of the body might be in different stages of evolution, but the lesions in any one area will all be in the same stage of progression.

Don't confuse varicella from variola in the heat of the battle, or viola from violin for that matter.

Chapter 35

Pharmacology

Much of pharmacology is covered within the relevant chapters under treatment. In this chapter we review some specific pharmacological concepts and medications.

Alternative Drugs and Herb interactions

With the increasing popularity of complementary and integrative medicine, you are expected to know the potential side effects and interactions with prescription medications.

Most of these are marketed as "natural remedies." Rest assured that any "natural remedy" that creeps its way onto the Boards is not viewed in a favorable light. Invariably, the question will be about the downside of such remedies. "Naturally," this is what you should be thinking about.

St. John's Wort

This has been used to treat anxiety and depression, presumably as a serotonin reuptake inhibitor. St. John's Wort can also **induce the P-450 pathway, increasing the elimination of other drugs including:**

> · Oral contraceptives
> · Iron preparations
> · Digoxin
> · Anticoagulants
> · Antiretroviral drugs

Therefore, **any female taking oral contraceptives and St. John's wort should also use back-up contraception,** since St. John's wort can increase oral contraceptive metabolism and elimination.

Echinacea

Echinacea is a popular herb marketed to help with the treatment/prevention of upper respiratory tract infections. There are even echinacea lollipops on the market. Echinacea is believed to act by modulating cellular immunity.

Therefore, **echinacea is contraindicated in patients taking immunosuppressive drugs**.

Ginseng

Ginseng is marketed as a "rejuvenating agent" which is something most pediatric patients aren't seeking. However, just in case it should make its way onto the exam, here are the important concepts to keep in mind:

Ginseng can interact with:

- · Anticoagulants
- · Antiplatelet medications
- · Steroids
- · Hypoglycemic medications
- · Diuretics

Valerian Root

 Valerian root can be **sedating** and is often used to treat insomnia. Once again, this is not a common problem among children; however, that won't stop it from appearing on the exam.

 Therefore, valerian root should not be used with alcohol and other sedating drugs.

You Watch What you Eat

You are expected to know which medications should be taken with food, which should not be taken with food, and which foods should be taken with which drugs.

Before you lose your own lunch keeping track of this, we will outline some of the more important associations that might make an appearance on the exam.

Isotretinoin and griseofulvin should be taken with fatty foods because they are lipophilic agents. Their bioavailability is enhanced by these foods.

Dare not take Dairy

Tetracycline, doxycycline, and ciprofloxacin are chelated by dairy products. Therefore, no dairy with these three.

Dairy products are **C**ontraindicated with **T**hese medications: **D**oxycycline, **C**iprofloxacin, and **T**etracycline.

Drug Eat Drug World

You are expected to know which drugs impact the half life of other drugs

The following table will help sort this out

Drugs	Impact
Cephalosporins and fluoroquinolones	Decreased bioavailability of calcium, magnesium, iron, or aluminum compounds
Erythromycin, ciprofloxacin, cimetidine, and omeprazole have inhibitory effects on hepatic enzymatic systems	This reduces theophylline, codeine, beta blockers, antidepressants, corticosteroids, warfarin, and metronidazole metabolism, resulting in increased bioavailability and toxicity
Rifampin, phenobarbital, carbamazepine, and phenytoin are potent enzymatic inducers	Therefore, these medications will decrease the levels of other medications. Therefore, other medications might require their dosing increased accordingly.

Elimination of drugs in infants is unpredictable, which is the reason why levels must be closely monitored. In particular, aminoglycosides are excreted almost exclusively by tubular filtration.

Specifically, quinidine and amiodarone may inhibit renal metabolism of digoxin, resulting in elevated levels.

Medications that are eliminated by the liver will not be impacted in a patient with renal disease. The same rule would apply for a medication that is eliminated by the kidney in a patient with primary liver disease.

A steady state is achieved after 4-5 half-lives.

Antibiotic Reactions

Cefaclor

Cefaclor has a high rate of **serum sickness** reaction; i.e., **fever, swollen lymph nodes, joint aches** and **rash.**

HOT TIP

The chances of a child who had a previous skin reaction to penicillin having a similar reaction to a cephalosporin are less than 10%.

Steroids and Adrenal Insufficiency

CASE STUDY

You are presented with a patient who is treated chronically for adrenal insufficiency with oral mineralocorticoid and hydrocortisone. The patient will either be going for surgery or will have an acute febrile illness, including vomiting.

CASE STUDY

You will be presented with several diversionary choices including oral hydrocortisone, IV/ IM mineralocorticoid, and a variety of oral medication variations, including doubling or tripling the usual oral dose.

ANSWER REVEALED

Since there is no such thing as a parenteral mineralocorticoid, that choice will always be wrong. In the context of a patient who is vomiting or is going in for surgery, they should be given parenteral hydrocortisone, typically hydrocortisone hemisuccinate.

Beta Blockers for Teens

Beta blockers can result in sexual dysfunction. Therefore, if you are presented with a teenager who is not improving clinically after being treated with beta blockers, e.g., for SVT, consider non-compliance as the cause.

Let's face it – the spectrum of sexual dysfunction would hardly be a motivating factor to take beta blocker medication for a member of an age group that usually feels relatively invincible and highly interested in sexual function.

Additional side effects of beta blockers you need to be aware of include:

- · CNS → Difficulty sleeping and subsequent fatigue
- · Smooth muscle → Bronchospasm and cold extremities.
- · Cardiac → Bradycardia and heart block

Remember that beta blockers can therefore exacerbate asthma

Prescription Compliance

In general, if you are presented with a teenager on a given medication, poor compliance is often the most likely explanation for variable effect and/or drug levels.

Diuretics

Acetazolamide

Acetazolamide is a **carbonic anhydrase inhibitor (CAI),** which **blocks the reuptake of bicarbonate,** resulting in **alkaline urine** and **metabolic acidosis**.

"Acid Soul Amide" will help you remember that it results in **metabolic acidosis**. It works on the proximal tubule by preventing the reuptake of bicarbonate, which makes for **alkaline urine.**

Furosemide/Lasix®

"**Loop Diuretics**" **block the absorption of** $Na+$ **and** $Cl-$. They also result in the **wasting of calcium and** K^+ **and** H^+. The bottom line result is **hypokalemic alkalosis.**

 Picture a giant word, "Lasix," and a giant loop of Henle. The loop changes to a **H**oop through which **H hops out**, and Lasix changes to Lasi**K**s (which is how most patients pronounce it), a giant Lasso grabbing the **K** (**K**loride, and **K**alcium), and kicking them out. The result: **hypochloremic hypokalemic alkalosis.**

In addition, you are expected to know that **ototoxicity** and **renal toxicity** are potential dose-related side effects of furosemide.

Hydrochlorothiazide

Sodium and **chloride** are lost at the distal tubule, resulting in hyponatremia and hypochloremia. Since it operates on the distal tubule, water is also lost, resulting in **contraction alkalosis**. In addition, bicarb is retained as a negative anion[1] to replace the lost chloride anion. This results in **metabolic alkalosis**.

Picture a giant "thigh" blocking fluid from re-entering the kidney.

Mannitol

This simply exerts osmotic pressure, **pulling fluid from IC to EC space,** with no **acid base effect**. It also **blocks fluid reabsorption at the kidney level, further decreasing IC fluid levels**.

Spironolactone

Sodium is spiraled out and **potassium is taken in**; therefore, it is **potassium sparing**.

A way to remember that spironolactone is potassium (K) sparing, is to think of it as "spiral-no-lack-K-tone." It is a spiral that **does not lack K**.

---

[1] Yes, we know this is a redundancy (all anions are negative), so no e-mails on that one.

NSAIDs and Aspirin

Aspirin

In addition to Reyes syndrome, you are expected to know that the **most likely adverse effect is GI irritation**. Another adverse reaction is tinnitus, which is dose-related.

How to be Cognizant of Conscious Sedation

You are expected to be well-versed in the changing definitions for conscious sedation and related new terminology, while remaining conscious yourself. Good luck! This is what you are expected to know

Minimal sedation (formerly anxiolysis) – The patient retains the ability to respond normally to verbal commands, and cardiorespiratory functions are unaffected

Moderate sedation (formerly conscious sedation) – The patient retains the ability to respond normally to verbal commands, and cardiorespiratory functions are unaffected.

Deep Sedation – The patient responds to repeated or painful stimuli. With deep sedation, there is further depression of the level of consciousness, with partial or complete loss of protective airway reflexes and need for assistance with airway protection.

General Anesthesia – Unarousable with any stimulation. There is a complete loss of consciousness and airway protective reflexes. Vital signs must be maintained and monitored.

5 Star General Anesthesia – Beyond general anesthesia, this corresponds with the level of boredom you must be experiencing at this point while trying to keep these details straight.

Despite these definitions, sedation varies from patient to patient, and you are expected to know that monitoring is required in case a patient slips into a deeper form of sedation.

Therefore, the following are required for monitoring during conscious sedation:

· One staff member who is PALS certified must be available to monitor, without other duties.

· Patients should be monitored with pulse oximeter and non invasive blood pressure monitor. Vitals should be documented in writing every 5 minutes

· Bag mask respiratory equipment, as well as oxygen, should be immediately available.

· Reversal agents such as naloxone and flumazenil should be available to reverse the effects of opiates and benzodiazepines, respectively.

 In the absence of an underlying cardiac history, EKG monitoring is **not** required.

Chapter 36

Behavior and Mental Health

Much of what you will see in general pediatrics practice is behavior-related. Because of this, behavioral and mental health issues have emphasis on the boards.

Behavioral Concerns

Maternal Infant Bonding

Maternal infant bonding is important immediately after birth.

 If you are asked which is more important to do in the first hour of life and offered choices of

    1) vitamin K administration,

    2) erythromycin eye drops, or

    3) maternal-infant skin-to-skin contact,

The correct answer would be skin-to-skin contact.

Colic

Remember that colic is a diagnosis that is based on history. The physical exam rarely shows anything, and there are no labs that confirm the diagnosis. The good news is that it stops after 3-4 months of age.

Since there are no "proven" methods to treat colic, there are loads of "unproven methods," many of which can be dangerous. Watch out for these "wrong choices."

> ### The Crying Game
>
> Anyone with an infant should know that they are in for the crying game. You must be familiar with the normal crying patterns of infants.
>
> Birth – 6 weeks – up to 2 hours a day can be normal
>
> 6 weeks and beyond – 3 hours a day can be normal

BUZZ WORDS

A typical presentation would be crying episodes in an otherwise healthy infant. The crying usually *starts suddenly.*

TREATMENT

The correct management is to reduce parental frustration by having another caretaker take over. Medications or changing formula are rarely going to be the correct answers on the exam.

HOT TIP

Often, disturbing sleep patterns may just be part of the "temperament" of the infant, with no intervention required.

CASE STUDY

You are presented with a mother who is beside herself because her 2 month old infant "cries continuously." The infant typically cries 2 hours in the early morning around 5 AM, and around 1 hour at night, usually around 1 AM. What should the parents do?

THE DIVERSION

The diversion here is the timing. Anyone can relate to the frustration of an inconsolable infant crying for an entire hour at 1AM and then another 2 hour cycle at 5AM. The timing of the crying is the diversion. Your choices will include thickening formula, Tylenol, antacids, and single malt whiskey nipples (for the parents). If you go for any of these diversionary answers, you might be the one crying for 3 hours a day.

ANSWER REVEALED

When you are presented with a crying infant, add up the *total hours crying.* **If it equals only 3 hours, this is normal and nothing more than "parental reassurance" is needed.**

Temper Tantrums

Most children have temper tantrums at some point in their lives. This is especially common in toddlers. If tantrums are caused by frustration with a task, redirecting them or distracting them before the tantrum can occur is a useful strategy. A consistent daily routine is helpful for most children this age.

Parents should be advised to ignore tantrums if possible, unless the child is in danger of harming himself/herself. The child should be allowed to calm down in a safe place. Physical restraint is not usually a good idea, because it may increase the child's frustration.

Breath-holding Spells

The typical presentation is a toddler who is angry, frustrated or *in pain.* It can occur between the ages of 6 -18 months. The child then cries and then:

- **Simple Breath-holding spell** – the child becomes *pale* or *cyanotic*
- **Complex Breath-holding spell-** the child then continues to cry until he/she is unconscious

> ### Anemia and Breath-Holding Spells
>
> Anemia is not considered to be a cause of breath-holding spells, even though treatment of anemia stops recurrent breath-holding spells. This is a minor difference in the wording, and you need to read the question carefully to see what they are asking.

Occasionally it can progress to a *hypoxic seizure with a postictal period.* However, this is still considered a breath-holding spell, not a seizure disorder.

There is an *association* between anemia and the incidence of breath-holding spells.

The best management is behavioral modification.

Setting Limits with Toddlers

A golden rule of behavior management is to praise a child's desirable behaviors and ignore undesirable behaviors if possible. When a child displays undesirable behaviors, the parent or caregiver should withdraw all attention. This is called extinction. Initially the behavior may worsen (which is called an extinction burst), but if the parent can endure, the behavior should decrease in frequency.

Time out and other forms of Discipline

You could be tested on the appropriate way to manage a behavioral problem with different age groups, including the following:

Time Out - This is time out from negative behavior; sort of a penalty box, for you hockey fans out there. This works best for age 1 and up. Time-out should last one minute per year of the child's age.

Time In -This is positive feedback, where a parent makes nonverbal contact when a child is engaging in appropriate behavior, thus establishing positive reinforcement.

Extinction – Here the parent withdraws attention when a child is misbehaving. Sometimes this can be difficult, and the extinction can be a gradual process.

Token Economy – Where the child receives a "token" for positive behavior. This is most effective and appropriate for ages 3-7 years.

Head Banging

If you are presented with a child between the ages of 8 months - 4 years exhibiting head-banging behavior, especially around bed time, it is considered normal and no intervention is necessary. Therefore, head banging does not necessarily indicate a sensory deficit. It is even normal for grown people to head-bang from time to time – especially at heavy-metal concerts.

If they present you with a toddler with language delay, poor eye contact, and head banging, don't automatically assume a diagnosis of autism. They may describe other signs of neglect such as missed pediatrician appointments, which will clue you into child neglect being the actual diagnosis.

If they present a child older than 4, or signs and symptoms consistent with a chronic neurological condition, such as Lesch-Nyhan Syndrome, then that is your clue that this falls outside the normal range of head-banging behavior.

Thumb Sucking

The best **initial intervention** for thumb sucking in a **toddler** is **positive reinforcement (praise)** when the child is not engaging in thumb sucking. Prolonged thumb sucking beyond age 4 can lead to dental problems, including malocclusion.

Active measures should not be undertaken until the age of 4, since it is likely to be something the child will outgrow. Most thumb sucking is considered to be harmless and no intervention is indicated, especially on the boards.

Biting Behavior

Biting may be considered a normal behavior (as a reaction to frustration) up to age 3.

The correct management is for parents to redirect, remove any positive reinforcement, and/or place the child in time out.

It is not recommended to bite or hit the child back.

Figuring out Fears and Phobias

A **fear** is age-appropriate discomfort over a situation that is realistic within the context. A **phobia** is anxiety that is excessive based on the potential danger posed, after accounting for age and developmental level. By definition, a phobia needs to interfere with daily function for at least 6 months.

Phobias may be managed through desensitization via gradual controlled exposure to the feared situation or object. Alternatively, cognitive behavioral techniques (where the child is shown how to reframe the situations triggering the phobia) may be useful.

Medications will not likely be the correct answer, since effectiveness of medications for phobias has not been well-studied as of the time of publication of this book.

CASE STUDY

You are presented with a preschool or school age child who is masturbating. They will then ask for the most appropriate intervention.

THE DIVERSION

They could throw in misleading information in the history, like the mother travels a lot on business, or the parents are divorced and the child was with the father over the weekend.

ANSWER REVEALED

Masturbation in children is considered normal to a certain extent - they may also include something in the history regarding vulvovaginitis, recurrent UTI, or the use of bubble baths — all of which would increase sexual self-stimulation behavior in children. However, if they were to describe a child imitating sexual activity, this would not be a normal finding.

Adolescent Parents

Most of the information on this subject that you may be tested on is common sense, but it is still worth emphasizing here.

Teen parents typically do not stay together very long. Unrealistic expectations may contribute to misinterpretation of age-appropriate behavior. For example, a 15 month old eating with their hands and making a mess might be misinterpreted as insubordination. Situations such as this may result in inappropriate punishment. In general, involvement of the teen father is beneficial to the child, but it can be very dependent on the nature of his relationship with the mother.

Mental Health Concerns

ADHD

The core symptoms of ADHD

- ❑ Inattentiveness (ADHD- predominantly inattentive subtype)

- ❑ Hyperactivity/Impulsivity (ADHD- predominantly hyperactive/impulsive subtype)

- ❑ Both inattention and hyperactivity/impulsivity (ADHD- combined type)

Facts

The ADHD-predominantly hyperactive subtype affects males more than females. ADHD-inattentive subtype is more common among girls. Recent estimates are that approximately 7% of kids may be affected with ADHD. While it is often diagnosed upon entering school, there is usually retrospective evidence of symptoms during the toddler and preschool years as well (e.g., sleep disturbance, behavioral concerns).

Studies have shown that maternal tobacco and/or alcohol use, as well as lead exposure may lead to an *ADHD-like* presentation. About half of affected individuals will outgrow the symptoms in adulthood. The hyperactivity component may manifest as fidgety behavior in adulthood.

Symptoms can be easily repressed in the office setting, especially at the initial visit. Since the office visit itself constitutes a novel and therefore "stimulating" experience, it may not even represent an *active* repression of symptoms.

In practice, ADHD is quite distinctive, and conditions in the differential rarely cause ADHD symptoms. Once again, this is the Boards' world and we just live there, so **on the Boards, items on the differential often DO cause ADHD symptoms**.

Absence seizure can be similar to ADHD- inattentive subtype. However, history alone can of*ten rule it out, and ordering an EEG may not be the correct answer. The buzzwords for absence seizures are "suddenly stops speaking"* and then *"snaps out of it and comes to."* They may describe odd movements like "twitching of eyelids or lips." Remember, absence seizures can be induced through hyperventilation; ADHD cannot.

Remember, **symptoms of ADHD are typically present before age 7 years.** Depression and anxiety may be in the differential; either may result in "inattention" and/or "acting out behaviors." When there is no past history of inattention or depression, think of substance abuse, especially in teens.

Ruling Out Organic Causes of ADHD

Ruling out organic and medical conditions that can mimic ADHD is critical on the Boards. Often the labs and data in the question already do this, but not always.

Sugar and diet do not cause or contribute to ADHD or hyperactivity. The following must be considered:

- ❏ Visual or hearing deficits
- ❏ Iron deficiency/anemia
- ❏ Lead toxicity
- ❏ Hyperthyroidism
- ❏ Past CNS infection/head trauma
- ❏ Medications on board (They could slip that in)
  Phenobarbital may have cognitive effects, including ADHD-like symptoms. Antihistamines may also do this.
- ❏ Fragile X and fetal alcohol syndrome (FAS) are both associated with ADHD

In most vignettes on the exam, they will not include previous history suggestive of ADHD, even though a history of symptoms present before age 7 is usually required to make the diagnosis.

If they describe classic ADHD, look for clues in the question that they are getting at something else. For example, if they add "lethargy," "abdominal pain," or "poor appetite," they could be hinting at **lead toxicity**.

Families will often seek out alternative treatments for ADHD and other chronic illnesses. Most complementary/alternative strategies to treat ADHD have not been proven in terms of efficacy. The best proven treatment modalities are a combination of pharmacological and behavioral therapy or pharmacotherapy alone (primarily *stimulants)*.

· Stimulant medication will improve attention in children (and adults) who do not have ADHD. Therefore, improved attention span on stimulants is not diagnostic of ADHD.

· Stimulant medication may be indicated in adolescence and beyond.

·Neurodiagnostic imaging is not part of a *routine* workup for ADHD in the absence of other neurological concerns.

Limited studies have shown no known increased risk for fetal congenital anomalies among pregnant mothers taking methylphenidate for ADHD.

The granddaddy of pharmacological treatment of ADHD is stimulants, including methylphenidates and amphetamines. Atomoxetine is an available non-stimulant alternative.

Adverse effects are primarily short term, including irritability, sleep disturbance, and appetite suppression.

Stimulant medications may unmask tic symptoms in children who are predisposed to tic disorders such as Tourette syndrome. However, stimulants do not cause Tourette syndrome.

The isolated appearance of motor tics while on stimulant medications is usually transient; this is not a contraindication to the use of stimulants.

Stimulant medication use after school is often necessary to complete homework. The administration of medication outside of the school setting may provide an opportunity for parents to observe for any adverse effects.

Drug holidays are not necessary, and will be an incorrect choice.

Depression in Children

The most important thing is to **distinguish normal variation from true blue** depression. In addition to the usual signs - somatization, withdrawal, appetite changes, and falling grades - **acting out may be a sign of depression**. However, it is important to keep in mind that adolescents may have mood swings without being depressed. If depressive symptoms are interfering with daily functioning and are beyond the limits of normal, depression is likely.

Parental depression increases the risk for depression in children, both from a genetic and environmental perspective. Children with chronic illnesses are at increased risk for depression, especially those taking glucocorticoids and immunosuppressive agents. Keep in mind that comorbid conditions such as anxiety, ADHD, or substance abuse may be present in pediatric patients with depression.

Fluoxetine is the only FDA-approved medication for the treatment of depression in children and adolescents, although citalopram or sertraline could also be correct answers on the exam as well.

Cognitive behavioral therapy (CBT) is considered to be the most effective psychotherapeutic treatment for depression in children and adolescents.

> ### School Phobia
>
> **School phobia occurs more frequently when there is only one caretaker (for example, a single mother).** The best way to deal with it is to have mom go to the school with the child and wean the amount of time spent.
>
> Separation anxiety can be a normal developmental stage in preschool children.
>
> Pure truancy may be a component of oppositional defiant disorder.

Suicide

One suicide in a community can have a domino effect. The reasons for this are controversial, but the amount of media attention in the community is thought to have a role in increasing the risk of multiple suicides.

Screening for suicidal ideation by asking a depressed teen about suicidal thoughts would likely be a correct choice on the exam. It does not "put the idea in his/her head." Dismissing a suicidal gesture that "seems" to be superficial would also not be a correct choice. However, a gesture undertaken alone (with no rescue available) is one that should be more concerning.

Risk Factors for Suicide:

- Previous suicide attempt
- Family history of suicide
- Native American male teens are at highest risk
- African American females are at lowest risk
- Females engage in self harming behavior more often than males. However, males are more likely to commit suicide.
- Underlying psychiatric diagnosis is a significant risk factor. True suicidal ideation requires hospitalization.

· They can still present you with a patient at risk for suicide who does not have any of these risk factors.

The increased risk for suicide with SSRIs may not be as high as once believed. However, there is still a black box warning. Careful monitoring is recommended when starting or changing medications for depressive disorders.

Normal Rebelliousness vs Conduct Disorder

You will be expected to distinguish adolescent rebellious behavior which is appropriate for their developmental phase from pathological features of a conduct disorder.

In the history of conduct disorder, they would have to describe severe behavioral concerns (such as lying, stealing, setting fires, or cruelty to animals) that are consistent over the course of at least 6 months.

Treating a conduct disorder involves a team approach, including management of comorbid conditions such as ADHD or depression if present. The entire family may be involved in behavior therapy, and structured parent training programs may be beneficial.

Schizophrenia

Schizophrenia is more common in adolescence than in childhood. Children and adolescents with schizophrenia experience auditory or visual hallucinations, delusions, unusual speech and/or behavior, or flat affect. Earlier-onset schizophrenia is associated with a worse prognosis.

Distinguishing a Tic from a Toc

The following will help you distinguish tics from other movements on the exam.

Tics follow a pattern, are repetitive, and *improve or disappear during purposeful movement.* Choreiform movements do not follow a pattern and *increase during purposeful movement.*

Rocking and hand flapping are examples of **stereotypies**, which may be seen in children with autism or Rett syndrome.

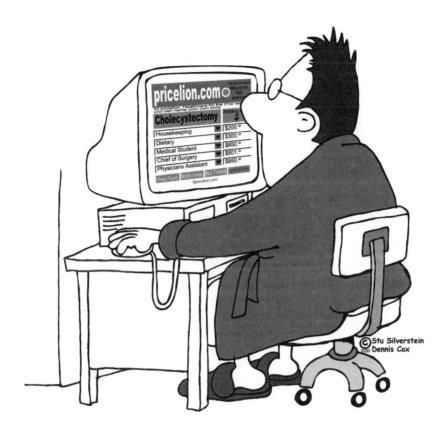

By taking advantage of a cancellation in
Dr. Volpe's schedule, and by bidding on
pricelion.com, Mr. Schlingman was able to get
his cholecystectomy for half of community
standards. And, to promote good will,
Dr. Volpe threw in a bilateral orchiectomy!

Bibliography

1. American Academy of Pediatrics. PREP The Curriculum® Content Specifications. 2010.

2. American Academy of Pediatrics Committee on Bioethics. Ethics and the care of critically ill infants and children. *Pediatrics.* 1996;98(1):149-152.

3. American Academy of Pediatrics Committee on Infectious Diseases. Prevention of varicella: recommendations for use of varicella vaccines in children, including a recommendation for a routine 2-dose varicella immunization schedule. *Pediatrics.* 2007;120(1):221-231.

4. American Academy of Pediatrics Committee on Infectious Diseases. *Red Book: 2009 Report of the Committee on Infectious Diseases.* 28th ed. Elk Grove Village, IL: American Academy of Pediatrics; 2009.

5. American Academy of Pediatrics Newborn Screening Authoring Committee. Newborn screening expands: recommendations for pediatricians and medical homes--implications for the system. *Pediatrics.* 2008;121(1):192-217.

6. American Psychiatric Association. *Diagnostic and Statistical Manual of Mental Disorders.* 4th ed. Washington, DC: American Psychiatric Publishing; 1994.

7. Arnold C, Davis T, Frempong J, et al. Assessment of newborn screening parent education materials. *Pediatrics.* 2006;117(5):S320-5.

8. Bonanni P, Boccalini S, Bechini A. Efficacy, duration of immunity and cross protection after HPV vaccination: a review of the evidence. *Vaccine.* 2009;27 Suppl 1:A46-53.

9. Boppana S, Ross S, Novak Z, et al. Dried blood spot real-time polymerase chain reaction assays to screen newborns for congenital cytomegalovirus infection. *JAMA: Journal of the American Medical Association.* 2010;303(14):1375-1382.

10. Brenner M, Oakley C, Lewis D. The evaluation of children and adolescents with headache. *Curr Pain Headache Rep.* 2008;12(5):361-366.

11. Bukstein O, Bernet W, Arnold V, et al. Practice parameter for the assessment and treatment of children and adolescents with substance use disorders. *Journal of the American Academy of Child Adolesc Psychiatry.* 2005;44(6):609-621.

12. Burton BK. Inborn errors of metabolism in infancy: a guide to diagnosis. *Pediatrics.* 1998;102(6):E69.

13. Centers for Disease Control and Prevention. FDA licensure of bivalent human papillomavirus vaccine (HPV2, Cervarix) for use in females and updated HPV vaccination recommendations from the Advisory Committee on Immunization Practices (ACIP). *MMWR: Morbidity.* 2010;59(20):626-629.

14. Centers for Disease Control and Prevention. FDA licensure of quadrivalent human papillomavirus vaccine (HPV4, Gardasil) for use in males and guidance from the Advisory Committee on Immunization Practices (ACIP). *MMWR: Morbidity.* 2010;59(20):630-632.

15. Centers for Disease Control and Prevention. Knowledge and practices of obstetricians and gynecologists regarding cytomegalovirus infection during pregnancy--United States, 2007. *MMWR: Morbidity.* 2008;57(3):65-68.

16. Centers for Disease Control and Prevention. Updated recommendations for use of tetanus toxoid, reduced diphtheria toxoid and acellular pertussis (Tdap) vaccine from the Advisory Committee on Immunization Practices, 2010. *MMWR: Morbidity.* 2011;60(1):13-15.

17. Cobb K, Bachrach L, Greendale G, et al. Disordered eating, menstrual irregularity, and bone mineral density in female runners. *Med Sci Sports Exerc.* 2003;35(5):711-719.

18. Dietz WH. Critical periods in childhood for the development of obesity. *Am J Clin Nutr.* 1994;59(5):955-959.

19. Friedman DI. Pseudotumor cerebri. *Neurol Clin.* 2004;22(1):99-131, vi.

20. Frush K. Preparation for emergencies in the offices of pediatricians and pediatric primary care providers. *Pediatrics.* 2007;120(1):200-212.

21. Gibbins S, Stevens B. Mechanisms of sucrose and non-nutritive sucking in procedural pain management in infants. *Pain Research.* 2001;6(1):21-28.

22. Greer F, Krebs NF. Optimizing bone health and calcium intakes of infants, children, and adolescents. *Pediatrics.* 2006;117(2):578-585.

23. Johnston LD, O'Maley PM, Bachman JG, Schulenberg JE, eds. Monitoring the Future. National Results on Adolescent Drug Use: Overview of Key Findings, 2005. Bethesda, Md: National Institute on Drug Abuse; 2006.

24. Kozlowski KJ. Ovarian masses. *Adolesc Med.* 1999;10(2):337-50, vii.

25. Lustig D, Saeed R, Abdullah B. Fructose intolerance/malabsorption and recurrent abdominal pain in children [poster]. Presented at: American College of Gastroenterology (ACG) 2010 Annual Meeting and Postgraduate Course; October 15-20, 2010; San Antonio, TX. Abstract P400.

26. Mandelberg A, Amirav I. Hypertonic saline or high volume normal saline for viral bronchiolitis: mechanisms and rationale. *Pediatr Pulmonol.* 2010;45(1):36-40.

27. Neuspiel DR. Marijuana. *Pediatrics in Review.* 2007;28(4):156-7; discussion 157.

28. Ogden C, Carroll M, Curtin L, Lamb M, Flegal K. Prevalence of high body mass index in US children and adolescents, 2007-2008. *JAMA: Journal of the American Medical Association.* 2010;303(3):242-249.

29. Rasquin A, Di Lorenzo C, Forbes D, et al. Childhood functional gastrointestinal disorders: child/adolescent. *Gastroenterology.* 2006;130(5):1527-1537.

30. Wagner C, Greer FR. Prevention of rickets and vitamin D deficiency in infants, children, and adolescents. *Pediatrics.* 2008;122(5):1142-1152.

Index

A

Abdominal Migraines,392
Abdominal Wall Defects,181-182
    Gastroschisis,181
    Omphalocele,181
Acetaminophen Ingestion,132-133
Acetazolamide,190
Achalasia,412
Achievement test,53
Achondroplasia,230, 239, 366, 628
Acidosis and Potassium,205
Acne Vulgaris,668-673
    Azelaic acid cream,671
    Benzoyl peroxide,671
    Neonatal,670
    Oral contraceptives,762
    Topical antibiotics,671
    Tretinoin,672
Acoustic Neuromas,679
Acrodermatitis Enteropathica,667
Acromioclavicular Separation,783
Activated Charcoal,129-130
Acute Lymphocytic Leukemia (ALL),495-496
Acute Mesenteric Lymphadenitis,388
Acute Renal Failure,555
Acute Respiratory Distress Syndrome,461
Acute Transverse Myelitis,607
Acyclovir,109, 169, 311, 312, 314, 578, 584, 649, 653, 660, 773
ADA deficiency,256
Adaptive Immunity,255
Addison Disease,360
Adenovirus,289, 315
    Diarrhea, 395
    Lymphadenopathy,751
    Pharyngitis,738
    UTI,548
Adolescent Sexual Development,755
    Precocious puberty,759
    Pseudo precocious puberty,760
Adrenal Deficiency,360
Adrenal Disorders,360-361
    Congenital adrenal hyperplasia,358
    Primary adrenal deficiency,360
    Secondary adrenal deficiency,361

Adrenal insufficiency,191, 336, 823
Adrenogenital Syndrome,231
Aicardi syndrome,230
    Absence of corpus callosum,230
Airborne Transmission,326
Albendazole,318, 321-322
Alcaptonuria,339
Alcohol Abuse,799
Alkalosis and Potassium,205
Allergic Reactions: Types 1-4,252
Allergic Rhinitis,246-248
Allergies,252-254
    Antibiotics,253
    Milk,253
    Pets,254
    Ragweed,252
Allergy Testing,253
Alopecia,673-675
    Alopecia Areata,673
    Alopecia Totalis,675
    Telogen Effluvium,674
    Trichotillomania,674
Alpers Syndrome,220, 231
Alpha 1- Anti Trypsin Deficiency,231
Alpha fetoprotein,154-155
    Elevated AFP,154
    Low AFP,155
    Trisomy 18,155
    Trisomy 21,155
Alport syndrome,220, 230, 541, 543
Ambiguous Genitalia,355
Amenorrhea,764
    Exercise induced,765
    Polycystic Ovary Disease,764
Aminoglycosides,297
Amphetamine Abuse,800
Anabolic Steroid Use,787-789
Anaphylaxis,248-250, 834
Androgen Insensitivity,228
Anemia,177, 506-523, 556
    Alpha thalassemia,508
    Cooley's anemia,507
    Ferritin,510
    Folate deficiency,512
    G6PD deficiency,514-515

Hereditary spherocytosis,516
Iron deficiency anemia,509-510
Macrocytic anemia,512-513
Newborn,506
Normocytic,514-519
of chronic disease,510-511
Pernicious anemia,513
RDW,509
Sickle cell anemia,517-519
Thalassemia,507-508
Thalassemia major,507
Thalassemia minor,507
Thalassemia trait,507
Vitamin B12 deficiency,512
Angelman Syndrome,227, 599
Anion Gap,191-193
Aniridia,502
Ankle Injuries,781
Ankle Sprains,624
Ankylosing Spondylitis,683
Anogenital Warts,770
Anorexia Nervosa,768-769
Anterior Talofibular Ligament,781
Anthracycline,505
Anthrax,149
Antibiotic Prophylaxis,728
Antistreptolysin-O,592
Anuria,168
Aortic Stenosis,486
Apert Syndrome,180, 219-220, 230
Apgar scores,167
Aphthous Ulcers,740
Apnea,151, 449-450
Central,449
Obstructive,450
Primary apnea,152
Secondary apnea,152
Apparent Life-Threatening Event (ALTE),452
Appendicitis,388
Apt Test,178
Arbovirus,304, 583
California encephalitis,304
Colorado tick fever,304
Dengue fever,304
La Crosse Encephalitis,304
St. Louis encephalitis,304
West Nile encephalitis,304
Western and Eastern equine encephalitis,304
Arthritis,697-698
Post Infectious,697

Ascaris Lumbricoides,318
Ash Leaf Spots,679
Asparaginase,505
Asperger syndrome,49-50
Aspergillosis,324, 326, 457
Aspirin,867
Asthma,246, 435-441
Allergies,439
Asthma in Pre-Schoolers,438
Cough Variant Asthma,438
Prognosis,441
Triggers,435
Asymptomatic Bacteruria,549
Ataxia,231, 255, 448, 495, 589-591, 595-596, 668
Acute ataxia,589
Ataxia Telangiectasia,231, 255, 590
Friedreich ataxia,591
Substance abuse, 795-802
Athlete Normal Findings,790-791
Atopic Dermatitis,652
Atropine,832
Attention Deficit/Hyperactivity Disorder (ADHD),870-872
Atypical Mycobacteria,496, 657, 752
Auditory Brainstem Response,725
Auspitz Sign,655
Autism,49-51
AV Canal Defect,487
Azotemia,829-830

B

Bacterial Endocarditis,479-480
Acute bacterial endocarditis,480
Janeway lesions,479
Osler nodes,479
Subacute bacterial endocarditis,480
Bacteremia,265
Bacterial Lymphadenopathy,751
Bacterial Tracheitis,749
Bacterial Vaginosis,770, 773
Balanitis,574
Barbiturates,802
Bartholin Gland Cysts,569
Bartonella Henselae,279
Basophilic stippling,95
Beckwith Wiedemann Syndrome,181, 227, 336, 502, 571
Behçet's Syndrome,684
Benign Paroxysmal Vertigo,622
Beta Blockers,141, 865
Ingestion,141
Beta Thalassemia,507

Bicarb in DKA,374
Bicycle Safety,124
Bilious vomiting,405
Biological Weapons,855
Biotinidase Deficiency,337
Birth Trauma,161
Black Widow (Latrodectus mactans),836
Bleomycin,505
Botulism,290-292
    Food borne,290
    Infantile,290
    Toxin,291
    Versus myasthenia gravis,292
    Wound,290
Brachial Plexus Injury,161-162
    Erb's Palsy,161
    Horner Syndrome,162
    Klumpke Palsy,162
Brain Abscess,606
BRAT Diet,395
Breast Milk,81-86
    Contraindications,83
    Freezing,82
    Phosphorus,83
    Versus cow's milk,83
Breast-feeding,245
Breath-holding Spells,867
    Complex Breath-holding spell,867
    Simple Breath-holding spell,867
Bronchiectasis,457
Bronchiolitis,316, 441, 455
Bronchogenic cysts,458
Bronchopulmonary Dysplasia,157, 439, 539, 558
Brown Recluse (Loxosceles reclusa),836
Brucellosis,286, 752
Bruton's Disease,257
Bubonic Plague. See Yersinia Pestis
Bulimia Nervosa,769
Bupropion,612

C

Cadmium,129
Café Au Lait Spots,677
Caffey Disease,639-640
Calcium Metabolism,376-378
    Hypercalcemia,377
    Hypocalcemia,377
Campylobacter Diarrhea,399
Campylobacter Fetus,295
Candida vaginitis,771

Candidiasis,322
Car Seats,124
Carbamazepine,863
Carbon Monoxide Exposure,142-143
Carbonic Anhydrase Inhibitor,865
Carboxyhemoglobin,454
Cardiac Arrhythmias ,487-491
    Atrial flutter,487
    Delta Wave,488
    Premature atrial contractions,487
    Prolonged QT Syndrome,488
    Saw-tooth waves,487
    Sinus arrhythmia,488
    Supraventricular tachycardia,490
    Wolff Parkinson White Syndrome,488
Cardiac Failure,826-828
Cardiac Murmurs,483-485
    4th heart sound,485
    Continuous Murmur,485
    Cranial bruits,484
    Diastolic,485
    Hyperdynamic precordium,484
    Systolic,485
    VSD,483
Cardiac Tamponade,828
Cardiogenic Shock,827
Cardiomegaly
    in athletes,791
Cat Bites,835
Cat Scratch Disease,279-280, 751
Cataracts,119-120, 308, 334, 712
Catch-up Immunizations,98
Cauliflower Ear. See Hematoma External Ear
Caustic Substances Ingestion,146-148
    Acidic substances,147
    Alkali Injestion,147
Cefaclor,864
Celiac Disease,417
Cellulitis,662
Cephalohematoma,183
Cephalosporins,298
Cerebral Angiography,621
Cerebral Palsy,619-620
Cerebral Salt Wasting,216
Cerebrovascular Accident,621
Ceruloplasmin,347, 589
Chalazion,714
CHARGE Association,236, 721, 732
Chediak-Higashi Syndrome,523
Chest Pain,491

Chest Wall Trauma,460
Chi Square,36
Child Abuse and Neglect,843-854
    Abuse Imitators,845-846
        Skin Lesions,845
        Stevens Johnson Syndrome,845
    Burns,851
    Fractures,846-850
    Munchausen Syndrome by Proxy (MSBP),853
    Retinal Hemorrhages,841
    Sexual Abuse,853-854
Childhood Functional Abdominal Pain,392
Chlamydia,456, 775
Chlamydia Pneumonia,275
Chloride,205-206
Chlorine Ingestion,144
Choanal Atresia,732
Cholecystitis,429
Cholesteatoma,727
Cholesterol Screening,116-117
Chorea,591
Choreiform Movements,595
Chronic Granulomatous Disease,260, 262, 524
Chronic Hypoxemia,445
Chronic Illness (Impact on the Family),817-818
Chronic Kidney Disease,555-558
Chronic Rhinitis,732
Chronic Suppurative Otitis Media,728
Chvostek Sign,175, 378
Chylothorax,451
Cidofovir,855
Cigarette Cessation in Adolescents,127
Cigarette Smoking,805-806
Cimetidine,863
Ciprofloxacin,863
Clavicular Fracture,161, 783, 850
Cleft Lip/Palate,180, 185, 224, 233, 237, 243, 255, 361, 721, 727, 742, 750
Clindamycin,299
Clostridium Difficile Toxin,399
Club Foot,642
CMV. See Cytomegalovirus
Coagulopathies,532-535
    Hemophilia,533-534
    ITP,530-531
    Thrombocytopenia,529
    Vitamin K–dependent bleeding,533
    Von Willebrand's Disease,534-535
Coarctation of the Aorta,217, 468, 486, 558, 560
Cocaine Abuse,804-805

Coccidioidomycosis,324
Cohort/Prospective Study,39
Cold-Induced Panniculitis,741
Colic,865-866
Colorado,190
Colorectal cancer,762
Colostrum vs. Mature Milk,82
Combative Behavior (Drugs that Cause),797
Common Variable Immunodeficiency,258
Compartment Syndrome,783
Complement Deficiency,261, 262
    CH50,262
Concussions,783-785
Condyloma acuminata (Venereal Warts),576-577, 854
Congenital Lipodystrophy,346
Congenital micropenis,571
Congenital Torticollis,628-629
Congestive Heart Failure,467
Conjunctivitis,694
Constipation,603
Constitutional Growth Delay,756
Contact Dermatitis,654
Contraception,762
    Intravaginal ring,762
    IUD,762
    Oral Contraceptives,762
    Subcutaneous contraceptives,762
Contraction Alkalosis,866
Contraction Stress Test,155
Contrast Media,251
Conversion disorder,812, 814
Cor Pulmonale,243, 448
Cord Compression,503
Corneal Abrasions,715
Court Orders,40
Coxsackievirus,740
CPR,830
Craniosynostosis,236
Cri Du Chat Syndrome,219
Crohn's Disease,420-421
Cross Sectional Study,38
Crouzon syndrome,220
Cryptococcosis,323
Cryptorchidism,238
Cryptosporidium,129
Cushing Syndrome,561
Cutaneous Candidiasis,651
Cyanotic Heart Disease,468-478
    Anemia,469
    Egg shaped heart,477

Increased pulmonary vascularity,477
Oxygen challenge,470
Prostaglandin E1,478
Test Spell,474
Tetralogy of Fallot,473, 487
Transposition of the great arteries,477
Cyclophosphamide,505
Cyclosporin,612
Cystic Fibrosis,417, 446-448
Acute exacerbations,448
Genetics,446
GI manifestations,417
Infancy,447
Sweat test,446
Cystoscopy,540
Cytomegalovirus,302-303, 736

D

Dacryocystitis,713
Dacryostenosis,713
Dantrolene,822
DDAVP,195
Death in the Family,811-812
Dehydration,206-211
CNS,207
Hypernatremic,207
Hyponatremic,206
Treatment,207
Isotonic,206
Oral Replacement Fluid,210
Pseudohyponatremia,200
Delayed Eruption of Teeth,741
Delayed Puberty,756
Demeclocycline,198
Dental abscess,742
Depression,872
Dermatomyositis,603, 685-686
Heliotrope Rash,685
Versus polyserositis,686
Developmental Dysplasia of the Hip (DDH),630-631
Asymmetric gluteal folds,630
Barlow,630
Ortolani,630
Developmental Milestones,53-62
Developmental Screens,62
Dexamethasone,609
Diabetes Mellitus,372
Acanthosis Nigricans,375
DKA,373, 375
Type 1 Diabetes,373

Type 2 Diabetes,375
Diamond-Blackfan Anemia,521-523
Diaphragmatic Hernia,182
Diarrhea,191, 284, 394-403
Acute Infectious Diarrhea,395
Campylobacter,399
Chronic Diarrhea,400-403
Abetalipoproteinemia,403
Cow Milk Intolerance,402
Cryptosporidium,401
Intestinal Lymphangiectasia,403
Malnutrition,402
Toddler's Diarrhea,401
Transient Lactase Deficiency,401
Diarrhea and Feeding,395
E. Coli Diarrhea,396
Enteroinvasive,397
Enteropathogenic,396
Enterotoxigenic,396
Inflammatory Diarrhea,394
Pseudomembranous Colitis,399
Rotavirus,395
Salmonella,284, 397-398
Shigella,398
Watery Diarrhea,394
Yersinia,399
Diazepam,378, 593
Diazoxide,337
DiGeorge syndrome,227, 255-6, 378
Digital clubbing. See hypertrophic pulmonary osteoarthropathy
Dilutional Hyponatremia,199
Diphenhydramine,593
Direct contact transmission,327
Dishwasher Detergent,147
Disseminated Intravascular Coagulopathy,535
Divorce and Blended Families,810
Dog Bites,835
Double Bubble Sign,405
Doxorubicin,505
Doxycycline,863
Drawer Sign,781
Droplet Transmission,326
Drowning,126, 461
Drug Screening,794-795
Duchenne Muscular Dystrophy,220, 228, 604-605
Duodenal Atresia,405
Dysfunctional uterine bleeding,764
Dysmenorrhea,766-767
Dysmorphic disorder,814

Dyspepsia,390
Dystonic Reaction,593, 601
Dysuria,561

E

Eagle Barrett. See Prune Belly Syndrome
Ebstein Barr virus (EBV),302, 735-736, 738
Ecclesiastes,537
Echinacea,861
ECMO,158
Ectodermal Hypoplasia,413
Ectopic urethral opening,562
Eczema,246, 257, 652
Ehlers-Danlos Syndrome,686
EKG Findings,486
Elbow Injury,849
Electric Burns,851
Elfin Facies,241
Emancipated Minors,39, 776
Emotional Lability,370
Empyema,449
Encephalitis,583
    Arboviruses,304, 583
    Cryptococcal,323
    Enteroviruses,583
    Herpes,311, 583
    HIV,314
    MRI for, 622, 671
    Mumps,305, 583
    Varicella,314
Encephalopathy,587
Encopresis,809
Endometrial cancer,762
Entamoeba Histolytica,319
Enterobius vermicularis (pinworms),568
Enterovirus,304
Enuresis,545, 807-809
    Diurnal Enuresis,808-809
    Nocturnal Enuresis,807-808
Eosinophilia,320
Epididymitis,572, 573
Epidural Abscess,606
Epiglottitis,747
Epistaxis ,734
Erythema Chronicum Migrans,682, 695
Erythema Infectiosum,310, 681
Erythema Marginatum,682
Erythema Multiforme,659-661, 681, 845
    Erythema Multiforme Major,660
    Erythema Multiforme Minor,660

Erythema Nodosum,682
Erythema Toxicum Neonatorum,651
Erythrocyte Sedimentation Rate (ESR),363, 683, 699
Esophageal Varices,414
Esophoria,119
ESR. See Erythrocyte Sedimentation Rate
ET Tube Size,831
Ethylene Glycol Ingestion,144
Ewing Sarcoma,493
Exercise Induced Amenorrhea,765
Exercise Induced Asthma,439
Extrinsic Spinal Cord Mass Lesion,607
Eye Trauma,778
    Blowout Fracture,779
    Hyphema,779

F

Failure to thrive,46-47, 555
Familial Nephritis. See Alport Syndrome
Fanconi's Anemia,520-521
Fanconi's syndrome,220
Farber's Disease,346
Fatty Acid Metabolism (Defects),332
Fatty Acids,75
Febrile Seizures,612-613
Female Pubertal Development,757-760
Ferritin,510
Fetal Alcohol Syndrome,233
Fever of Unknown Origin,833
Fifth Disease,310, 681
Firearms,125
Fitz-Hugh-Curtis Syndrome,†770
Flagyl® (metronidazole),319
Flucytosine (5-FC),323
Fluorescent in situ hybridization studies,227
Folate Deficiency,512
Foreign Body Aspiration,442
Foreign Body Ingestion,130-131
Foster Care,820
Fragile X Syndrome,241-242
Friedreich Ataxia,591
Frontal Bossing,239
Furosemide,539, 866

G

G6PD Deficiency,228, 514-516, 518
Galactorrhea,567
Galactosemia,231, 333-334, 336
Ganciclovir,303

Gardner's Syndrome,413, 418
Gardnerella Vaginalis,770-771
Gastric Lavage,130
Gastric outlet obstruction,412
Gastroesophageal (GE) Reflux,407-409
    In Infants,407
    Treatment,409
Gaucher Disease,347-348
    Chronic Juvenile Gaucher Disease,347
    Infantile Gaucher Disease,347
Genu Varus (Bow Legged),643
GI Bleeding,424-426
Ginseng,862
Glasgow Coma Index,842
Glaucoma,244
Glomerulonephritis,552-558
    Berger's Disease (IgA Nephropathy),554
    Focal and Segmental Glomerulosclerosis,553
    Membranoproliferative Glomerulonephritis,553
    Minimal Change Disease,552
    Post Strep Glomerulonephritis,553
Glossoptosis,243
Glue Sniffing. See Volatile Hydrocarbon Abuse
Gonorrhea,772, 775
Granuloma Annulare,658
Griseofulvin,673, 858
Group A beta hemolytic Strep,568
Group A Strep,288
    Necrotizing fasciitis,289
    Strep Cellulitis,289
    Strep Pharyngitis,288
    Toxic Shock Syndrome,289
Group B Coxsackievirus,480
Group B Strep,158, 267, 289
    Early onset,158
    Late onset,159
    Prophylaxis,290
Growth Hormone,789
Growth Spurt,756
Guillain Barré Syndrome,600-601
    Areflexia,600
    Ascending paralysis,600
    Plasmapheresis,601
    Respiratory failure,600
Gynecomastia,567, 757

H

H. (Helicobacter) pylori,301, 390, 415-416
Haemophilus Influenzae,281
Hallermann Streiff Syndrome,242, 413

Hamartomatous Polyps,243
Head Banging,868
Head Lice,664
Head Trauma,840-842
    Basilar Skull Fracture,847
    Epidural hematoma,841
    Hematoma/Nasal Septum,843
    Skull Fractures,846
    Subdural hematoma,841
    Temporal Bone Fracture,847
Headache,584-587
    Increased intracranial pressure,586
    Migraine,585
    Papilledema,586
    Stress/Tension/Emotion,584
Hearing Loss,721-723
    Aminoglycoside,723
    Conductive,721
    Sensorineural,723
Hearing Screen,724-725
    Auditory Brainstem Response (ABR),724
    Behavioral Observational Audiometry,725
    Conventional Pure-Tone Audiometry Screen,724
    Otoacoustic Emissions (OAE),724
    Visual Reinforcement Audiometry (VRA),725
Heat Stroke,778
Heinz Bodies,515
Hemangiomas,680
Hematoma External Ear,730
Hematuria ,537-541, 554
    Hypercalciuria,539
    Low C3 levels,554
    Microscopic,539
Hemihypertrophy,503
Hemolytic Uremic Syndrome,294, 397, 557-558
Hemophilia,533-534
Hemoptysis,462
Hemorrhagic Cystitis,505
Hemorrhagic Disease of the Newborn,178-180
    Early onset,178
    Late onset,178
    Oral vitamin K,178
Hemothorax,825
Henoch Schönlein Purpura (HSP),541, 687-688
Hepatitis,100-101, 431-434
    Hepatitis A,431
    Hepatitis B,100-101, 432
    Hepatitis C,433
    Hepatitis D,434
    Hepatitis E,434

Hepatitis A Vaccine. See Immunizations
Hepatits B Vaccine. See Immunizations
Herald Patch,656
Hereditary Fructose Intolerance,336
Hereditary nephritis,541
Hereditary Spherocytosis,516-517
Herpes Simplex Virus,311, 577, 740
Hib Vaccine,100
Hirschsprung's Disease (Congenital Aganglionic Megacolon),166, 173, 423-424
Histoplasmosis,324
HIV Infection,261, 312-314
    Breast feeding,83
    Encephalitis,314
    Exposure,313
    Lymphadenopathy,751
    Medications,261
    Nevirapine,262, 312
    Nonfunctional antibodies,314
    PCP and,273
    Routine vaccines,103, 106, 108-109, 310, 465, 314
    Testing,774
    Tuberculosis and,121, 274
    Vertical transmission,312
    Zidovudine,261, 312
Hodgkin's Lymphoma. See Lymphoma
Holoprosencephaly,224
Holt Oram Syndrome,225
Home Deliveries,168
Homicide,768
Homocystinuria,339
Human Ehrlichiosis,278
Human Papilloma Virus Vaccine. See Immunizations
Human Thyroid-Stimulating an Immunoglobulin,370
Hunter's Syndrome,240
Huntington's Chorea,231, 592
Hurler Syndrome,231, 240
Hyaline Membrane Disease,156
Hydrocarbon Ingestion,141
Hydrocele,565
Hydrocephaly,45
Hydrochlorothiazide,866
Hydrometrocolpos,568
Hydroxylase Deficiencies (21-hydroxylase),359
Hydroxyprogesterone (17 hydroxyprogesterone),359
Hymenal Damage,854
Hymenoptera Stings,251-252, 836
Hyper IgE,259
Hyper IgM Syndrome,258
Hyperalimentation (HAL),180

Hypercalcemia,70, 241
Hypercapnia,438
Hypercarbia,449
Hyperchromia,517
Hyperimmunoglobulin E Syndrome,654
Hyperinsulinism,336
Hyperkalemia,203-204
Hypernatremia,194-195
Hyperopia,119
Hyperosmolar Diabetic Coma,376
Hyperphosphatemia,70
Hypertension,556, 558-561
Hyperthyroidism
    Dysfunctional Uterine Bleeding,767
    Grave's Disease,370-371
    Hashimoto,369, 371
    Hyperactivity,871
    Tachycardia,491
Hypertrophic pulmonary osteoarthropathy,444
Hyperviscosity Syndrome,177
Hyphema,779
Hypocalcemia,203, 557, 611
Hypochondriasis,814
Hypoglycemia,203, 611
Hypohidrosis,741
Hypokalemia,201
Hypokalemic Alkalosis,866
Hypomagnesemia,203
Hyponatremia,195, 203, 611
Hypoplastic and Aplastic Anemias,519-523
Hypoplastic Distal Phalanges,235
Hypospadias,571
Hypothermia,838
Hypothyroidism
    Alopecia,675
    Addison's disease and,361
    Congenital,368, 424
    Growth deficiency,47, 362, 367-368
    Hashimoto,369
    Hypercholesterolemia,117
    Jaundice,173
    Newborn Screening,330
    Obesity,88
    Secondary,369
    TBG deficiency,550
    Teeth eruption delay,741
    Turner's and,366
Hypoxia,449

I

Ibuprofen Ingestion,134-136
Ichthyosis,657
Idiopathic Thrombocytopenic Purpura,530-531
IgA,541
IgA Deficiency,259
IgM. See Hyper IgM Syndrome
Immunizations,96-114, 310
    DTaP and Td vaccines,96
    Hepatitis A Vaccine,112
    Hepatitis B vaccine,100-101
    Hib vaccine,100
    Human Papilloma Virus Vaccine,103
    Influenza vaccine,107, 112-113
    Meningococcal Vaccine,102
    MMR vaccine,104-108, 310
        after exposure,105
        and PPD administration,106
        and Varicella vaccine,107
        contraindications,106
    Pneumococcal Vaccine,109
    Rotavirus vaccine,110
    Varicella Vaccine,108-109
Immunodeficiencies,254-262
Imperforate Anus,182
Imperforate Hymen,567-568
Impetigo,659
Inborn Errors of Metabolism,193, 350
Increased Intracranial pressure,821
Infantile Botulism,603
    Constipation,603
Infantile Cortical Hyperostosis. See Caffey Disease
Infants of Diabetic Mothers,175, 334
    Hypoplastic left colon,175
Infectious Mononucleosis (Mono). See Ebstein Barr virus
Infectious Rhinitis,247
Infiltrative Ophthalmopathy,370
Inflammatory Bowel Disease,419-421
Influenza, 748
Inguinal Hernia,565
Inhalants,795
Inherited Fructose Intolerance,334
Insect Stings,251-252
Inspiratory Stridor,749
Intellectual Disability,48-49
Intracranial Aneurysms,545
Intussusception,315, 421-422
Iritis,698
Iron deficiency anemia,762
Iron Ingestion,145-146

Irritable Bowel Syndrome,417
Isoniazid,459, 612
Isotretinoin,234, 862
Isovaleric Acidemia,332
Ivermectin,318

J

Jarisch-Herxheimer Reaction,696
Jaundice,171-174
    ABO incompatibility,171
    Acidosis,173
    Albumin,173
    Bronze Baby Syndrome,172
    Exchange transfusion,174
    PDA,173
    Phototherapy,172
    Physiologic jaundice,172
Joan of Arche,758
Job Syndrome,259
Juvenile Idiopathic Arthritis,688-692
    Lymphadenopathy,691
    Oligoarthritis,690
    Polyarthritis,689
    Systemic JRA,690
    Treatment,691
    Versus Leukemia,691

K

Kallmann Syndrome,571
Kartagener Syndrome,231, 457
Kasabach-Merritt Syndrome,531, 680
Kawasaki Disease (Mucocutaneous Lymph Node
    Syndrome),692-695
    Aspirin,694
    Treatment,693
Klinefelter syndrome,221
Klippel-Feil Syndrome,629-630
Knee Injuries,781
Koplik Spots,309
Krabbe Disease,348
Kwashiorkor,89-90
Kyphosis,639

L

Labial Adhesions,567, 854
LAD. See Leukocyte Adhesion Deficiency
Langerhans Cell Histiocytosis,498
Language Deficits,62
Laryngeal Papillomas,750

Laryngomalacia,744
Laryngotracheobronchitis,748
Latex Agglutination,272
Laurence-Moon-Biedl Syndrome,226, 571
Lead Exposure,95-96, 148
Lead Poisoning,512
Learning Disabilities,51-52
Legg Calve Perthes Disease,634
Lesch Nyhan Syndrome,225
Leukocyte Adhesion Deficiency (LAD),260, 525
Lichenification,652
Limb Salvage,494
Linoleic Acid,81
Linolenic Acid,81
Lipogranuloma,714
Lisch Nodules,677, 678
Liver Diseases,426-428
    Biliary Atresia,426
    Cholestatic Jaundice,426
    Gilbert Syndrome,427
    Reye's Syndrome,427
    Wilson's Disease,428
Long QT Syndrome,827
Loop Diuretics,866
Low Set Ears,225
Lowe's Syndrome,686
Lumbar Lordosis,239
Lung Abscess,465
Lyme disease,683, 696
    Erythema chronicum migrans,695
    Jarisch-Herxheimer reaction,696
    Lab results,696
Lymphoma ,496-497
    Hodgkin's Lymphoma,496
    Non-Hodgkin Lymphoma,497
Lysosomal Granules,523

M

Macrocephaly,44
Macrolides,299
Maculae ceruleae,578, 664
Male Pubertal Development ,757
Malignant hyperthermia,822
Malingering,814
Malrotation of the Bowel,406
Mannitol,866
Maple Syrup Urine Disease,335, 338, 350
Marasmus,90
Marfan syndrome,230
Marijuana,797-798

Mastoiditis,731
McCune Albright Syndrome,226
Mean,38
Measles,694
Mebendazole,318, 322
Meconium,165, 166
    Meconium Ileus,166
    Meconium Plug Syndrome,418
Median,38
Menarche,758-759
Meningitis,271
Meningococcal Vaccine. See Immunizations
Menkes Kinky Hair Syndrome,347
Mercury,148
Meta-Analysis,39
Metabolic Acidosis,190-193, 556
    Compensated,189
Metabolic Alkalosis,188
Metabolic Disorders Newborn,174-175
Metabolic Seizure,611
Metabolic Syndrome,376
Methanol,136
Methemoglobin,454
Methemoglobinemia,469
Methotrexate,506, 612
Methylmalonic Acidemia,332
Methylprednisolone,609
Metoclopramide,601
Metronidazole (Flagyl®),301, 771, 863
Microcephaly,46
Micrognathia,243
Micropenis,571
Migraine Headaches,392
    abdominal variant,392
Milk Allergies,253
Mineral Deficiency,72
    Copper,72
    Menkes Kinky Hair Syndrome,72
    Zinc,72
MMR vaccine. See Immunizations
Mode,38
Molluscum Contagiosum,665, 666
MRSA (Methicillin Resistant Staph Aureus),296
Mucopolysaccharidoses,342-343
    Hunter's Syndrome,342
    Hurler's Syndrome,342
    I-cell disease,343
    Leroy I-cell disease,343
    Morquio Syndrome,343
    mucolipidosis II,343

Müllerian Inhibiting Factor,357
Multicystic Dysplastic Kidney Disease (MCKD),544-545
Mumps,305-306, 723
Munchausen by proxy,814
Muscular Dystrophy,604-605
    Becker muscular dystrophy,604
    CPK,604
    Duchenne muscular dystrophy,220, 228, 604-605
    Gower's sign,604
    Hypertrophied calves,604
    Myotonic Muscular Dystrophy,605
Myasthenia Gravis,601-602
    Anti-Smith antibodies,602
    Congenital,602
    Ptosis,601
    Pyridostigmine (Mestinon),602
    Tensilon,601
    Transient,602
Myelomeningocele,608. See Spina Bifida
Myocarditis,480
Myringotomy Tubes,729

N

Nail Patella Syndrome,230
Narcotic Overdose,136
Nasopharyngeal Angiofibroma,734
NBT. See Nitroblue Tetrazolium
Near Drowning,825
NEC,170-171
    Bacterial infection,170
    Hypoxic injury,170
    Thrombocytopenia,170
Necrotizing Enterocolitis (NEC),170-171
Negative Predictive Value,35
Neisseria gonorrhea,569, 854
Neonatal Acne,670
Neonatal Chlamydial Conjunctivitis,168
Neonatal Herpes,649-650
Neonatal Pustular Melanosis,650
Neonatal Sepsis,158-159
Neonatal Vaginal Discharge,567
Nephroblastoma. See Wilms Tumor
Nephrogenic Diabetes Insipidus,195
Nephronophthisis,545
Nephrotic Syndrome,550
Neuroblastoma,498-499
Neurocardiogenic Syncope,489
Neurodiagnostic Testing,622
Neurofibromas,678
Neurofibromatosis,230, 677-679

Acoustic neuromas,679
Lisch Nodules,678
Neurofibromas,678
Neurofibromatosis Type 1 (Von Recklinghausen Disease),677
Neurofibromatosis Type 2,678-679
Optic glioma,678
Pheochromocytoma,678
Neurotoxicity,505
Neutropenia ,525-529
    Chronic benign neutropenia,527
    Cyclic neutropenia,527
    Kostmann agranulocytosis,528
    Shwachman-Diamond Syndrome,528
    Transient neutropenia,526
Newborn Hearing Screening,724
NG Tube,593
Niemann-Pick Disease,349
Night Terrors vs. Nightmares,816-817
Nitroblue Tetrazolium,262
Non Stress Test,155
Non-bullous impetigo,655, 666
Noonan's Syndrome,218
Null Hypothesis,35
Nummular Eczema,653, 655, 656
Nutritional Deficiencies (neonatal),78-79
    Essential fatty acids,78
    Vitamin E,78
    Zinc,79
Nutritional Needs,91
    Malignancies,92
    Renal disease,92
Nystagmus,711
    Jerk Nystagmus,711

O

Obesity,87-89
Occult Bacteremia,265
Occult Spinal Dysraphism,608
Ofloxacin,727
Oligohydramnios,238
Oligohydramnios sequence. See Potter syndrome
Omeprazole,863
Opiate Abuse,800-801
    Opiate Withdrawal,801
Opitz Syndrome,571
Optic Glioma,678
Optic Nerve Glioma,677
Oral Allergy Syndrome,247
Oral Contraceptives ,762-764

Absolute contraindications,762
Relative contraindications,763
Oral Rehydration Fluid,401
Orbital Cellulitis,715
Orchitis,572
Organic Acidemias,330-331
Organophosphate Toxicity,138
Muscarinic effects,139
Nicotinic effects,139
Orthostatic Proteinuria,542
Osgood-Schlatter Disease,636
Osteochondritis Dissecans,636
Osteogenic Sarcoma,493
Osteoid Osteoma,494
Osteomyelitis,634-635, 683
Treatment,635
Osteoporosis,762, 765
Otalgia,730
Otitis Externa,730
Ovarian Cyst,580, 762, 776
Ovarian Torsion,581

P

P Value,36
Pacifiers,453
Pain Management,848
Pancreatitis,428, 505
Acute Pancreatitis,428
Recurrent / Chronic Pancreatitis,429
Panhypopituitarism,357
Papilledema,586, 717
Papillitis,717
Papular Urticaria,666
Parental Consent,776
Parotitis,412
Partial Seizures,616-618
Patterns of Inheritance,228-231
PCBs,129, 149
PCP Abuse,137, 802-804
Pectus abnormalities,697
Pectus Excavatum,219, 340, 466
Pediculosis pubis,578
Pelvic inflammatory disease (PID),762, 767, 773
Penicillin,298
Perchloroethylene,129
Perihepatitis (Fitz Hugh Curtis),772
Pericardial Tamponade,482
Pericardiocentesis,482
Pericarditis,481
Periodic breathing,450

Periorbital Cellulitis,715
Peritoneal dialysis,566
Peritonsillar Abscess,738-739
Permethrin (Elimite),322, 663
Persistent Fetal Circulation,478
Pertussis,282-284
Peutz-Jeghers Syndrome,231, 243, 418
Pfeiffer Syndrome,238
pH Scalp Monitoring,165
Phenobarbital,863
Phenoxybenzamine,561
Phenytoin,863
Pheochromocytoma,561, 678
Alpha adrenergic blockade,561
Beta blockers,561
Phimosis,573
Phosphatidylglycerol,232
Physiologic Growth,43-47
Head Circumference,44
Length,43
Weight,43
Physiologic Leukorrhea,759
Pierre Robin Sequence,243
Pityriasis rosea,656
PKU,341-342
Benign hyperphenylalaninemia,342
Placenta,129
Placental Weight,167
Pneumococcal Vaccine. See Immunizations
Pneumocystis jiroveci (carinii) Pneumonia,273
Pneumonia,463
Mycoplasma,464
Neonatal pneumonia,463
S pneumoniae,464
Viral,464
Pneumothorax,451
Poison Ivy,655
Polycystic Ovary Disease,764
Polycythemia,118-119
Polycythemia (neonatal),177
Polydactyly,224
Polydipsia,545
Polyserositis,706
Polyuria,545
Pompe Disease,344
Port Wine Stain,244, 712
Positive Predictive Value,34
Post Term (Prolonged pregnancy),164
Post Traumatic Stress Disorder,767
Post-Infectious Myelitis,607

Posterior Fat Pad,848
Posterior Fossa (Infratentorial) Tumors,596
Posterior Nasopharyngeal Mass,734
Postpericardiotomy Syndrome,482
Potassium,204-205
Potassium Sparing Diuretics,866
Potter syndrome,237
Prader-Willi Syndrome,226, 571
Precocious puberty,226, 353, 760
 Amenorrhea,764
 Central Precocious Puberty,355
 Premature Adrenarche,354
 Premature Thelarche,355
Prematurity,78, 168-170, 719
 Breast Milk,170
 Calcium,169
 Caloric requirements,170
 Catch up growth,169
 Osteopenia in the premature,78
 Retinopathy,719
Preparing Families for International Adoption,127
Primum non nocere,36
Procarbazine,505
Properdin deficiency,261
Propionic Acidemia,332
Protein/Creatinine Ratio,543
Protein Hydrolysate Formula,78
Proteinuria,542-543, 554
Prune Belly Syndrome,238, 548
Pseudomembranous Colitis,287
Pseudomembranous Croup,749
Pseudomonas,285
 Mechanical ventilators,285
 Osteomyelitis,285
 Otitis externa (swimmer's war),285
Pseudoseizure,609
Pseudostrabismus,711
Psoriasis,655
 Auspitz sign,655
Psychogenic Cough,446
Psychosomatic Illness,813
Ptosis,601
Pulmonary Edema,825
Pulmonary Fibrosis,505
Pulmonary Hypoplasia,238
Pulmonary Interstitial Emphysema (PIE),157
Pulmonary Sequestrations,458
Pulsus Paradoxus,444, 481
Purine and Pyrimidine Disorders,343
Pyoderma Gangrenosum,662

Pyrazinamide,459
Pyridoxine deficiency,611

Q
QT Interval (prolonged),175
Quinolones,300

R
Rabies,838
Ragweed,252
Raynaud's,704
Reactive Arthritis,698
Rebuck Skin Window Test,262
Recurrent or Chronic Abdominal Pain,390-394
 Parasites,393
Recurrent Otitis Media,728
Reed Sternberg. See Lymphoma: Hodgkin's Lymphoma
Regional Enteritis. See Crohn's Disease
Reiter's syndrome. See Reactive Arthritis
Renal Arteriography,561
Renal Dysplasia,544
Renal Salt Wasting,200
Renal stones,541
Renal Tubular Acidosis,191-192
Renal Tubular Acidosis (Type 2),192
 Proximal,192
Renin,561
Respiratory Acidosis,188
Respiratory Alkalosis,188
 Compensated ,190
Respiratory Distress Syndrome,155
Respiratory Failure,443, 822
Retinitis Pigmentosa,545
Retinoblastoma,230, 500
Retinopathy of Prematurity,719
Retrobulbar Optic Neuropathy,717
Retropharyngeal Abscess,739-740
Retrospective Study,38
Rett syndrome,50, 242
Rhabdomyolysis,803
Rhabdomyosarcoma,501-502
Rhett Butler (Clark Gable),242
Rheumatic Fever,682, 699-702
 Arthralgia,701
 Arthritis vs. arthralgia,701
 ASO titer,699
 C reactive protein,699
 Elevated ESR,699
 Emotional lability,700

Major Jones Criteria,700
Migratory arthritis,699
Minor Jones Criteria,701
Mitral valve regurgitation,699
Prolonged PR interval,701
Sydenham's chorea.,700
Rhinitis Medicamentosa,248
Rhizomelic Shortening,239
Rickets,71, 380, 741
Liver disease,71
Rickets of Prematurity,385
Vitamin D toxicity,70
Rickets of Prematurity,385
Rickettsial Diseases,276
Q Fever,278
Rocky Mountain Spotted Fever,276
Rifampin,300, 459, 863
Robin Williams,241
Rocky Mountain Spotted Fever,276
Rose Spots,398
Roseola,307
Rotavirus,110, 317
RSV Infection,316
Rubella,308, 723
Rubeola,309
Rubinstein-Taybi syndrome,238
Russell Silver Syndrome,238, 571

S

Salicylate Ingestion,134
Salpingitis,762
Salter Harris Fracture Classifications,644-645
Sandifer Syndrome,412
Sarcoidosis,702
Scabies,663-664, 666
SCFE (Slipped Capital Femoral Epiphysis) (SCFE),646
Schmidt Syndrome,369
School Phobia,873
Scleroderma,703
Scoliosis,466, 637-638
Seborrheic Dermatitis,654
Second Hand Smoke,806
Secondary Hyperparathyroidism,556
Secondary Syphilis,656
Seizures,179, 612-616, 839
3 per second spike and wave,613
Absence seizures,613-614
ACTH,616
Acute management,839
Benign rolandic seizures,618

Complex partial seizures,613, 616
Hypsarrhythmia,615
Infantile spasms (West Syndrome),615
Myoclonic seizures,615
Neonatal,179
Simple partial seizures,617
Tonic-Clonic seizures,614
Sensitivity,33
Sepsis,193
Septic Arthritis,632, 704
Versus JIA oligoarthritis,704
Septic Newborn,267
Campylobacter Fetus,295
Group B Strep,267
Septic Shock,268
Septicemia,265
Seronegative Spondyloarthropathy,698
Severe Combined Immunodeficiency,256
Sexual Abuse ,853-854
Condylomata acuminatum,854
Hymenal damage,854
Sexual Orientation,818
Sexually Transmitted Diseases,770-773
Shagreen Patch,679
Shock,840
Cardiogenic shock,840
Warm shock,840
Short Stature,362-368, 521
Congenital adrenal hyperplasia,366
Constitutional delay,364
Familial short stature,365
Growth hormone deficiency,362
Hypothyroidism,367
Nutrition deficiency,363
Turner syndrome,366
Shwachman-Diamond Syndrome,528
SIADH,271, 505
Sibling Rivalry,818
Sickle Cell Anemia,517-519, 540
Acute chest syndrome,518
Cerebrovascular accident,518
Functional asplenia,518
Hematuria,540
Sickle Cell and Thalassemia,231
SIDS,452-453
Risk factors,452-453
Silver Nitrate,168
Simple Motor Tic,594
Sinusitis,732-733
Acute,732

Chronic,733
Small Pox,855
    Variola,855
Small Pox vs Varicella,855
Smoking Cessation,806
Snake Bite,837
Somatic delusions,814
Somatization,810, 814
Soto's Syndrome,368
Soy Formula,78
Spasmodic Croup,749-750
Specificity,34
Spider Bites,836-837
    Brown Recluse (Loxosceles reclusa),836
    Black Widow (Latrodectus mactans),836
Spina Bifida,608
Spinal Dysraphism,608
Spinal Trauma,609
Spironolactone,190, 866
Splenic Rupture,825
Sporotrichosis,325
Sprengel Deformity,630
St. John's Wort,861
Staphylococcal Scalded Skin Syndrome,659
Status epilepticus,839
Stippled Epiphyses,235
Stomach Disorders,415-416
    Peptic Ulcer Disease,415
Stomatitis,684
Strabismus,711
Strawberry Cervix,771
Strawberry Hemangioma,680, 712
Strep Pharyngitis,702, 737-738
    ASO titers,702
    Rapid strep,702
    Streptozyme,702
Streptococcus pneumoniae,288
Stridor,742
    Biphasic,746
    Expiratory,746
    Inspiratory,743
Sturge Weber Syndrome,244, 676
Styes,713
Stuttering,62
Subluxed Radial Head (Nursemaid's Elbow),640
Suicide,126, 768
Sunscreen,123
Superior Vena Cava Syndrome,478, 504
Supracondylar Fractures,848-849
Supratentorial Tumors,597-598

Calcification in the sella turcica,597
Craniopharyngioma,597
Pseudotumor Cerebri,598
Supravalvular Aortic Stenosis,241
Supraventricular Tachycardia,828
Surfactant (exogenous),157
Swimming Pool Granuloma,657, 658
Swimming Pools,126
Sydenham Chorea,591, 592
Syncopal episode,609
Syphilis,293
    Congenital,293
    FTA-ABS,293
Syrup of Ipecac,593
Systemic Lupus Erythematosus (SLE),704-708
    3rd degree heart block,707
    Acute hemolytic anemia,705
    Drug induced lupus,706
    Lupus cerebritis,707
    Neonatal lupus,707
    Polyserositis,706
    Thrombocytopenia,707
    Treatment,707
Systemic Treatment of Acne,672-673
    Isotretinoin,672
    Oral antibiotics,672
    Oral contraceptives,672

Talipes Equinovarus. See Club Foot
Tall Stature,367-368
    High caloric intake,368
    Klinefelter syndrome,367
    Marfan Syndrome,368
Thrombocytopenia Absent Radius (TAR),532
Target Lesions,661
Tay Sachs Disease,231, 348-349
Tensilon,601
Teratogens,233-235
    ACE inhibitors,235
    Alcohol,233
    Anticoagulants,235
    Anticonvulsants, 233
    Isotretinoin,70, 234
    Lithium,234
Testicular Cancer,576
Testicular Feminization,228, 356, 765
Testicular Torsion,573
Tetracyclines,300, 863
Tetrahydrobiopterin (BH4),350

Tetralogy of Fallot (TOF),473, 487
The "Schilling" test,513
Theophylline,612, 863
Thermal Burns,851
Third Spacing,200
Thrombocytopenia,178, 529
    Neonatal,178
Thumb Sucking,868
Thyroglossal Cyst,750
Thyroid binding globulin (TBG) Deficiency,372
Thyroid Disorders,368-371. (See also hyperthyroidism and hypothyroidism)
    Congenital hypothyroidism,368
    Graves Disease,370
    Hashimoto thyroiditis,369
    Neonatal Thyrotoxicosis,370
    Thyroid nodules,371
Tibial Torsion,647
Tidal Volume,832
Tinea Capitis,673
Tinea Corpis,656
Tinea Corporis,657
Tinea Versicolor,656, 675
Toilet Training,807-809
Tonsillectomy,739
Tooth Avulsion,741
Total Anomalous Pulmonary Venous Return,471
Total Iron Binding Capacity,510
Tourette Syndrome,595
Toxic Epidermal Necrolysis,661
Toxic Ingestion,132-143
Toxic Synovitis,631-632
Toxocara canis,320
Toxoplasmosis,159-161
Tracheo-Esophageal Fistula,414
Tracheomalacia,746
Tracheoesophageal Fistula,182
Transient Erythroblastopenia of Childhood,521-523
Transient Hematuria,537
Transient Hypogammaglobulinemia of Infancy,259
Transient Proteinuria,542
Transient Tachypnea of the Newborn,152
Transposition of the Great Arteries,477
Transudate,451
Trauma,541
Treacher Collins Syndrome,238
Tremor,595
Tretinoin,672
Trichloroethylene,129
Trichomonas Vaginalis,771

Tricyclic Antidepressants Toxicity,139-141
Trimethoprim with sulfamethoxazole,300
Trisomy 13,224
Trisomy 18,225
Trisomy 21 (Down syndrome),222-224
    Atlantoaxial instability,223
    Brushfield spots,224
    Genetic Variation,222
    Translocation,222
Trousseau Sign,175, 378
True Hermaphroditism,356
Tubal Pregnancy,767
Tuberculosis,274, 458-460, 752
Tuberculosis Screening and Exposure,121-123
Tuberous Sclerosis,230, 239, 679
    Ash leaf spots,679
    Cardiac rhabdomyoma,679
    Renal angiomyolipoma,679
    Retinal nodular hamartomas,679
    Shagreen patch,679
Tularemia,295
Tumor Lysis Syndrome,503
Tunable Dye (Pulsed Dye) Laser,677
Turner Syndrome,217-218, 560, 765
Twins,157
Tympanogram,725
Tympanometry,725-726
Tympanostomy Tubes,728
Type A G6PD Deficiency,516
Type B G6PD Deficiency,516
Type I Error,36
Type II Error,36
Typhoid Fever,285

U

Ulcerative Colitis,419
Umbilical Artery Catheter,163
    Complications,163
Umbilical Cord,162-163
    Oozing,163
    Persistent,162
    Single umbilical artery,163
Uncal Herniation,821
Undescended Testicle,570
    orchiopexy,570
Unstable Bladder,562
Upper Respiratory Tract Infection,248
Urea Cycle Defects,333, 335, 350, 611
Uremia,556
Ureteroceles,546

Ureterostomy,191
Ureteropelvic Junction (UPJ) Obstruction,540, 541
Urethral Strictures,547
Urethritis,574, 698
    Urethral Instrumentation,575
Urticaria,250
    Chronic,250
        Fexofenadine,250
Urticaria Pigmentosa,675
UTI,548
    Enterococcus,548
    Klebsiella,548
Uveitis,684
Uvula (Bifid),750

V

VACTER-L,182, 236
Vaginal Discharge,854
Vaginal Foreign Body,854
Valerian Root,862
Vancomycin,301
Varicella (Newborns),314
Varicella Vaccine. See Immunizations
Varicocele,566
Variola. See Small Pox
VariZIG,109
Vasomotor Rhinitis,247
Venous leptomeningeal angiomatosis,676
Verapamil,490
Vertigo,622
Very Low Birth Weight Infants (VLBW),169
Vesicoureteral Reflux,546
Vinblastine,505
Vincristine,505
Viral Croup,748
Viral Myocarditis,491
Visceral larval migrans,320
Vitamin A (Retinol),67
Vitamin B (B Vitamins),67, 512
    Vitamin B1 (Thiamine),67
        Deficiency,67
        Toxicity,67
    Vitamin B12,512
        Deficiency,512
    Vitamin B2 (Riboflavin),67
        Deficiency,67
Vitamin C (Ascorbic Acid),68
    Deficiency,68
    Toxicity,68
Vitamin D,70-72

1,25 hydroxycalciferol,71
25-hydroxy vitamin D,71
Cholecalciferol,71
Deficiency,71
Ergocalciferol,71
Toxicity,70
Vitamin D Deficient (Nutritional) Rickets,381
Vitamin D Dependent Rickets Type 1,381
Vitamin D Dependent Rickets Type 2,382
Vitamin E (Tocopherol),65, 69
Vitamin K (Phylloquinone),168
    Deficiency,168
Vocal Cord Nodules,745
Vocal Cord Paralysis,744
Volatile Hydrocarbon Abuse,795-797
Volvulus,407
Vomiting,403-412
    Annular pancreas,407
    Antral Web,404
    Cyclic vomiting,410
    DKA,410
    Gastroesophageal reflux,412
    Inborn errors of metabolism,405
    Pyloric Stenosis,404
    Rumination,411
Von Willebrand Disease,231, 534-535
Voriconazole,324
Vulvitis,577
Vulvovaginitis,568-569

W

Waardenburg Syndrome,231
Wegener Granulomatosis,708
Weight Control in Athletes,789
Weight Gain/Full Term Newborn,86
Weight Gain/Preemie,86
Werdnig-Hoffmann Disease,607
Whey/casein ratio,170
Williams Syndrome,241, 560
Wilms Tumor,502
Wilson Disease,231, 347, 588-589, 829
    Ceruloplasmin,589
    Penicillamine,589
Wilson–Mikity Syndrome,158
Wiskott-Aldrich Syndrome,257, 531
Witch's Milk (neonatal galactorrhea),163
Wolman Disease,346
Wound Management,97

X

X- Linked Dominant Disorders. See Patterns of Inheritance
X-Linked Hypophosphatemic Rickets,383
Xeroderma Pigmentosum,676

Y

Yersinia Pestis,295
    Meningeal form,296
    Pneumonic form,296
    Septicemia,296
Your Mother,11

Z

Zellweger Syndrome,333
Zinc Deficiency,667
Zollinger–Ellison Syndrome,416